Methods in Molecular Biology™

Series Editor
John M. Walker
School of Life Sciences
University of Hertfordshire
Hatfield, Hertfordshire, AL10 9AB, UK

For further volumes:
http://www.springer.com/series/7651

Cancer Epigenetics

Methods and Protocols

Edited by

Ramona G. Dumitrescu

Saba University School of Medicine, Saba Island and Georgetown University Medical School, Washington, DC, USA

Mukesh Verma

Division of Cancer Control and Population Sciences, National Cancer Institute, National Institutes of Health, Rockville, MD, USA

Humana Press

Editors
Ramona G. Dumitrescu, Ph.D., M.P.H
Saba University School of Medicine
Saba Island and Georgetown University
Medical School
Washington, DC, USA

Mukesh Verma, Ph.D.
Division of Cancer Control
and Population Sciences
National Cancer Institute
National Institutes of Health
Rockville, MD, USA

ISSN 1064-3745 e-ISSN 1940-6029
ISBN 978-1-4939-6204-4 ISBN 978-1-61779-612-8 (eBook)
DOI 10.1007/978-1-61779-612-8
Springer New York Dordrecht Heidelberg London

Printed on acid-free paper

Humana Press is part of Springer Science+Business Media (www.springer.com)

Preface

The epigenetic regulation plays an important role in normal development and maintenance of tissue-specific genes expression in humans, and the disturbance of these patterns leads to changes involved in tumor formation. Global epigenetic changes and genes' promoter-specific methylation patterns have been observed in many cancer types as playing an essential role in carcinogenesis. More recently, epigenetic changes have been observed in early stages of tumor development and together with the genetic alterations have been defined as abnormalities, necessary for cancer initiation and progression.

Different cancer types not only express distinct methylation patterns but also share common epigenetic changes that are very important in early detection, progression, and prognosis as well as the design of new therapeutic tools against cancer cells.

The technology available to detect these epigenetic changes is evolving rapidly and provides more understanding of these processes in normal and cancerous cells. Several of these technologies are discussed in this book.

Recent studies identified several factors that may play a significant role in the initiation of the epigenetic changes in cancer. Some of the genetic and environmental factors that have been shown to be involved in these processes are also being discussed.

All these epigenetic alterations can be used in clinical practice as biomarkers of early cancerous lesions or markers of progression and prognosis.

Washington, DC, USA — *Ramona G. Dumitrescu, Ph.D., M.P.H.*
Rockville, MD, USA — *Mukesh Verma, Ph.D.*

Contents

Part V Epigenetic Epidemiology

Contributors

RICHARD N. ARMSTRONG • *Queen's University Belfast, Haematology Center for Cancer Research and Cell Biology Belfast, Belfast, Northern Ireland, UK*
KRISHNA K. BANAUDHA • *Department of Biochemistry and Molecular Biology, George Washington University, Washington, DC, USA*
KATJA BIEWUSCH • *Department of Surgery, University Hospital Dresden, Fetscherstraße, Dresden, Germany*
KEVIN BRENNAN • *Division of Surgery and Cancer, Imperial College, London, UK*
KANG MEI CHEN • *Department of Otolaryngology/Head and Neck Surgery, Henry Ford Hospital, Detroit, MI, USA*
HILARY A.A. COLYER • *Haematology, Centre for Cancer Research and Cell Biology Belfast, Queen's University Belfast, Belfast, Northern Ireland, UK*
RINA DAS • *Center to Reduce Cancer Health Disparities, National Cancer Institute, Rockville, MD, USA*
MARGARET DELLETT • *Haematology, Centre for Cancer Research and Cell Biology Belfast, Queen's University Belfast, Belfast, Northern Ireland, UK*
STEFAN DENEBERG • *Center of Hematology, Karolinska University Hospital, Huddinge, Sweden*
ADRIAN M. DUBUC • *Department of Laboratory Medicine and Pathobiology, Division of Neurosurgery, University of Toronto, Toronto, ON, Canada*
RAMONA G. DUMITRESCU • *Saba University School of Medicine, Saba Island and Georgetown University Medical School, Washington, DC, USA*
JAMES M. FLANAGAN • *Division of Surgery and Cancer, Imperial College, London, UK*
ABEL GARCÍA-GARCÍA • *Oral Medicine, Oral Surgery and Implantology Unit, Entrerríos s/n, Santiago de Compostela, Spain*
MARIO PÉREZ-SAYÁNS GARCÍA • *Oral Medicine, Oral Surgery and Implantology Unit, Entrerríos s/n, Santiago de Compostela, Spain*
WOLFGANG GOERING • *Department of Urology, Heinrich Heine University, Duesseldorf, Germany*
ROBERT GRÜTZMANN • *Department of Surgery, University Hospital Dresden, Dresden, Germany*
GLYNIS HARRIS • *Department of Otolaryngology/Head and Neck Surgery, Henry Ford Hospital, Detroit, MI, USA*
SHALETA HAVARD • *Department of Otolaryngology/Head and Neck Surgery, Henry Ford Hospital, Detroit, MI, USA*
MARIE HEYNE • *Department of Surgery, University Hospital Dresden, Dresden, Germany*
SHARAD KHARE • *Hines Veterans Affairs Medical Center, Hines, IL, USA; Department of Medicine, Loyola University Chicago, Maywood, IL, USA*
WUN-JAE KIM • *Department of Urology, College of Medicine, Chungbuk National University, Cheongju, Chungbuk, South Korea*

Yong-June Kim • *Department of Urology, College of Medicine, Chungbuk National University, Cheongju, Chungbuk, South Korea*
Michael Kloth • *Department of Urology, Heinrich Heine University, Duesseldorf, Germany*
Yutaka Kondo • *Division of Molecular Oncology, Aichi Cancer Center Research Institute, Chikusa-ku, Nagoya, Japan*
Unhee Lim • *Cancer Research Center of Hawaii, University of Hawaii, Honolulu, HI, USA*
Qiang Lu • *Department of Obstetrics and Gynecology, Affiliated Hospital of Qingdao University School of Medicine, Qingdao, China*
Dehua Ma • *Department of Obstetrics and Gynecology, Affiliated Hospital of Qingdao University School of Medicine, Qingdao, China*
Stephen Mack • *Department of Laboratory Medicine and Pathobiology, Division of Neurosurgery, University of Toronto, Toronto, ON, Canada*
Ken I. Mills • *Haematology, Centre for Cancer Research and Cell Biology Belfast, Queen's University Belfast, Belfast, Northern Ireland, UK*
Alok Mishra • *Ambedkar Center for Biomedical Research (ACBR), Delhi University, Delhi, India; Dermatology Branch, National Cancer Institute, National Institutes of Health, Bethesda, MD, USA*
Sulma I. Mohammed • *Department of Comparative Pathobiology, Purdue University, West Lafayette, IN, USA*
Paul A. Northcott • *Division of Neurosurgery, The Hospital for Sick Children, Toronto, ON, Canada*
Jong Y. Park • *Division of Cancer Prevention and Controls, H. Lee Moffitt Cancer Center and Research Institute, Tampa, FL, USA*
Christian Pilarsky • *Department of Surgery, University Hospital Dresden, Dresden, Germany*
Gabriela Riscuta • *Division of Cancer Prevention, National Cancer Institute, Rockville, MD, USA*
Wolfgang A. Schulz • *Department of Urology, Heinrich Heine University, Duesseldorf, Germany*
L.M.S. Seeber • *Department of Reproductive Medicine and Gynaecology, Gynaecological Oncology, University Medical Centre Utrecht, Utrecht, The Netherlands*
Daniel J. Sharpe • *Haematology, Centre for Cancer Research and Cell Biology, Queen's University Belfast, Belfast, Northern Ireland, UK*
Keiko Shinjo • *Division of Molecular Oncology, Aichi Cancer Center Research Institute, Chikusa-ku, Nagoya, Japan*
Min-Ae Song • *Cancer Research Center of Hawaii, University of Hawaii, Honolulu, HI, USA*
Sanya Springfield • *Center to Reduce Cancer Health Disparities, National Cancer Institute, Rockville, MD, USA*
Josena K. Stephen • *Department of Otolaryngology/Head and Neck Surgery, Henry Ford Hospital, Detroit, MI, USA*
L. Joseph Su • *Division of Cancer Controls and Population Sciences, National Cancer Institute, Rockville, MD, USA*

Michael D. Taylor • *Department of Laboratory Medicine and Pathobiology, Division of Neurosurgery, University of Toronto, Toronto, ON, Canada*
Alexander Unterberger • *Division of Neurosurgery, The Hospital for Sick Children, Toronto, ON, Canada*
P.J. van Diest • *Department of Pathology, University Medical Centre Utrecht, Utrecht, The Netherlands*
Mukesh Verma • *Division of Cancer Control and Population Sciences, National Cancer Institute, National Institutes of Health, Rockville, MD, USA*
Maria J. Worsham • *Department of Otolaryngology/Head and Neck Surgery, Henry Ford Hospital, Detroit, MI, USA*
Mihi Yang • *Division of Cancer Prevention and Controls, H. Lee Moffitt Cancer Center and Research Institute, Tampa, FL, USA*
Jovanny Zabaleta • *Department of Pediatrics and Stanley S. Scott Cancer Center, Louisiana State University Health Sciences Center, New Orleans, LA, USA*
Shuping Zhao • *Department of Obstetrics and Gynecology, Affiliated Hospital of Qingdao University School of Medicine, Qingdao, China*
Margaret Dellett • *Haematology, Centre for Cancer Research and Cell Biology, Queen's University Belfast, Belfast, Northern Ireland, UK*

Part I

Early Epigenetic Events in Cancer

Chapter 1

Epigenetic Markers of Early Tumor Development

Ramona G. Dumitrescu

Abstract

Cancer patients' outcome and survival depends on the early diagnosis of malignant lesions. Several investigation methods used for the prevention and early detection strategies have specific limitations. More recently, epigenetic changes have been considered one of the most promising tools for the early diagnosis of cancer. Some of these epigenetic alterations including promoter hypermethylation of genes like *P16INK4a*, *BRCA1*, *BRCA2*, *ERα* and *RARβ2*, *APC*, and *RASSF1A* have been associated with early stages of mammary gland tumorigenesis and have been suggested to be included in the models that evaluate individual breast cancer risk. In lung cancer, *P16INK4a* and *MGMT* gene hypermethylation was observed in sputum years before clinical manifestation of the squamous cell carcinoma among smokers. Loss of *GSTP1* function by DNA hypermethylation together with changes in the methylation levels of repetitive elements like LINE-1 and Sat2 was reported in prostatic preneoplastic lesions. Also, DNA hypermethylation for *hMLH1* and *MGMT* DNA repair genes was reported in precursor lesions to colorectal cancer. These epigenetic alterations may be influenced by factors such as xenoestrogens, folate, and multivitamins. Detection of these changes may help determining cancer susceptibility and early diagnosis.

Key words: DNA hypermethylation, Global methylation, Breast cancer, Colorectal cancer, Lung cancer, Prostate cancer, Xenoestrogens, Folate

1. Introduction

It is well recognized that the improvement of the clinical outcomes in cancer patients depends on the early diagnosis of the disease that is translated in a better survival. The rationale of population screening and the surveillance of high-risk patients is that early diagnosis before extensive local proliferation, lymph node spread, and metastasized disease can result in less radical surgical procedure with fewer complications and side effects. The problem is that most of the investigation methods used in cancer prevention programs, like serum tumor markers, radiologic procedures, and endoscopic evaluations, have a limited sensitivity and specificity, can be expensive, and can have issues

Ramona G. Dumitrescu and Mukesh Verma (eds.), *Cancer Epigenetics: Methods and Protocols*, Methods in Molecular Biology, vol. 863, DOI 10.1007/978-1-61779-612-8_1, © Springer Science+Business Media, LLC 2012

with patient compliance. For example, mammographic screening has been shown to reduce breast cancer mortality especially in women over the age of 50 years, and to a lesser extent in younger women, however, the sensitivity of mammography is reduced in some groups of women. Therefore, there is need for a noninvasive, cost-effective procedure that could be used alongside mammography to improve screening sensitivity and specificity. Thus, other molecular markers, like epigenetic markers, need to be evaluated together with several other markers already used. If considered together they will clearly help diagnosis, targeted therapy and evaluate prognosis. DNA methylation events are stable and abundantly present in tumors (1, 2) as well as early stages of carcinogenesis; as a result, DNA methylation is considered one of the most promising tools for the diagnosis of cancer. Here the epigenetic changes reported by several recent studies in premalignant lesions of several cancer types will be discussed.

2. Methylation Changes in Early Tumorigenesis

2.1. Epigenetic Markers of Early Breast Tumor Development

Normal human mammary epithelial cells (HMECs) have been used in numerous studies as a model system for studying epigenetic and genetic changes associated with early breast tumor development (3, 4). It has been found that there are some HMECs in culture that are able to proliferate beyond an in vitro barrier that limits cellular proliferation (5). These variant HMECs in culture present *p16INK4a* promoter hypermethylation. *P16INK4a/ARF* gene has been observed to be hypermethylated in breast cancer specimens at frequencies from 4 to 47%, with the majority reporting a rate of 18–20% (6, 7).

It has been shown that these variant HMECs presenting *p16 INK4a* promoter hypermethylation and consequently lacking *p16INK4a* activity, in addition to this epigenetic change, accumulate abnormalities similar to those that were detected in premalignant and malignant breast lesions (8). These abnormalities include telomeric dysfunction (9), centrosomal dysfunction which generates aneuploidy, increased invasion and stimulation of angiogenesis, decreased apoptosis (10) and activation of a program for targeted DNA hypermethylation (11). In fact, several studies have shown that *p16INK4a* hypermethylation can be observed in histologically normal breast tissue from apparently healthy women without history of breast cancer (5, 12). This finding suggested that this type of cells exists in vivo and they are not the result of cultivation process.

Furthermore, normal HMECs in culture have been shown to overcome a senescence barrier, named stasis that is mediated by the Rb and a stringent barrier that is telomere-length dependent, involving p53. This second barrier is called agonescence or crisis, and once the HMECs overcome this barrier they become immortalized. The immortalized HMECs showed specific gene expression profiles, especially in a set of 30 genes characterized as "cancer proliferation cluster" that included genes expressed during the cell division and after DNA damage. These gene expression changes were similar to those observed in noninvasive breast cancers (13).

Furthermore, the activation of stress pathways, such as COX-2, helps the cells to acquire a mutagenic potential so that they can survive to environmental stresses, can migrate, and can evade apoptosis and immune response. Similarly, markers of premalignant stress activation signaling pathways were found to be overexpressed in breast tissues from DCIS (ductal carcinoma in situ) patients. These epithelial cells are found within the premalignant lesion as well as in morphologically normal tissue that surrounds the lesions. The variant HMECs that exhibit *p16INK4A*-silenced accumulate specific characteristics essential for the malignant transformation (14). Additionally, these normal mammary epithelial cells, which escape senescence in culture, show specific relations between gene silencing, DNA methylation, histone changes, and polycomb association that can be seen in early tumorigenic process (3).

When the frequencies of *p16INK4a/ARF*, *BRCA1*, *BRCA2*, estrogen receptor alpha (*ERα*), and *RARβ2* promoter hypermethylation were examined in the periareolar fine-needle aspiration samples from asymptomatic women at high risk (after the Masood cytology index) for breast cancer development, it was found that the frequency of *p16INK4a* hypermethylation was significantly associated with the combined frequency of promoter hypermethylation of *BRCA1*, *BRCA2*, *ERα*, and *RARβ2*. Thus, the increase in the frequency of *p16INK4a* hypermethylation with the frequency of other genes' hypermethylation suggests that *p16INK4a/ARF* hypermethylation may be a marker of global epigenetic changes at the early stages of tumorigenesis (15).

Furthermore, the hypermethylation of the promoter regions of several other genes was evaluated in ductal lavage fluid from healthy women carriers of *BRCA1* or *BRCA2* mutations, and substantial aberrant methylation was observed, suggesting that methylation analysis of several genes in the ductal lavage fluid can be used to evaluate breast cancer risk in these high-risk women (16). However, we know that only about 5% of breast cancers are the result of *BRCA1/BRCA2* mutations; therefore, the frequency of promoter region hypermethylation of several tumor suppressor genes, namely, *RARB*, *ESR1*, *INK4a/ARF*, *BRCA1*, *PRA*, *PRB*, *RASSF1A*, *HIN-1*, and *CRBP1*, was analyzed in periareolar fine-needle aspiration samples from asymptomatic women at high risk for breast cancer (with family history of breast cancer), and it was found that women without *BRCA1/BRCA2* mutation have a high frequency of hypermethylation (17). This finding brings further evidence that these hypermethylation events occur early during breast cancer development. Also, it has been observed that *RARβ2*, *APC*, and *RASSF1A* promoter methylation occurs frequently in benign breast epithelium, and this epigenetic change is associated with epidemiologic markers that are included in the Gail model that evaluates the increased breast cancer risk (18). More specifically, *RARβ2* methylation is correlated with a personal history of breast cancer, whereas *APC* and *RASSF1A* methylation is associated with the breast cancer risk, calculated by Gail model, particularly in women with prior benign breast lesions. This finding suggests that there are some changes in the benign breast epithelium that may help for individualized breast cancer risk stratification (18).

Furthermore, it has been observed that *RASSF1A* gene methylation was correlated with breast cancer risk as well as with atypical cytology and benign breast disease. In addition, *RASSF1A* methylation showed a linear increase between ages 32 and 55. Another factor that influences breast cancer risk and parity showed an inverse relationship with genes promoter hypermethylation. More specifically, there is less *APC* methylation among women with increased parity. Based on the observation that tumor suppressor gene methylation increases in benign breast tissue and this change is associated with increasing age, it suggests that these epigenetic changes may be included in breast cancer risk models (19).

2.2. Epigenetic Changes in Early Lung Cancer Development

Lung cancer, the leading cause of cancer-related death in the United States, has been associated for a long time with chronic exposure to tobacco carcinogens (20). Similar to other cancer types, the development of lung cancer involves the acquisition of genetic and epigenetic changes throughout the respiratory epithelium (21). Hypermethylation of genes involved in critical cellular functions like cell cycle control, differentiation, adhesion, and death was found to lead to gene silencing in lung tumor tissues (21). Among these genes, *p16INK4a* gene was reported to be silenced by promoter hypermethylation not only in lung cancer tissues but also in early stages of lung cancer development. More specifically, *p16INK4a* hypermethylation was detected in bronchial epithelium of lung cancer cases and in sputum from smokers and former smokers (22) and also in precursor lesions to adenocarcinoma and squamous cell carcinoma (23, 24).

Furthermore, it has been reported that *p16INK4a* and *MGMT* gene hypermethylation was detected even in sputum up to 3 years before the clinical manifestation of the squamous cell carcinoma (25). Then a nested case-control study of incident lung cancer cases found that concomitant hypermethylation of three genes or more is associated with a 6.5-fold increase in the risk of developing lung cancer (26). All these findings suggest that the detection of hypermethylation at the promoter region of several genes in sputum may be a good biomarker for determining lung cancer susceptibility (27). Understanding the factors that can induce these epigenetic changes is important not only for early detection but also for chemoprevention because this may lead to the identification of people that would more likely benefit from the chemopreventive measures.

Moreover, it has been suggested that the impaired DNA repair capacity (DRC) and DNA damage, like single- and double-strand breaks, induced by tobacco-associated carcinogens (28) may play a role in the induction of gene promoter hypermethylation observed in different stages of lung cancer development (21). Further evidence was provided by a study examining the association between DRC, specific genetic variants in DNA repair genes, and the frequency of promoter hypermethylation of several genes in sputum of cancer-free smokers (29). This study found that smokers that present a higher index of methylation (promoter methylation present in at least three genes from a panel of eight analyzed genes) had a reduction in the DRC when compared with smokers that do not show any of these genes methylated in the sputum. In addition, it has been observed that the presence of promoter methylation of several genes is associated with genetic variants in the *MRE11A*, *CHEK2*, *XRCC3*, *DNA-PKc*, and *NBN* DNA repair genes, suggesting that severe DNA damage and reduced DRC could lead to promoter gene hypermethylation.

Additionally, when normal human small airway epithelial cells and immortalized human bronchial epithelial cells were exposed to cigarette smoke condensate (CSC), specific epigenetic changes were detected. CSC exposure was correlated with several histone alterations including a dose- and time-dependent reduction of H4K16Ac and H4K20Me3, an increased of H3K27Me3 levels at the same time with decreased DNA methyltransferase 1 (DNMT1) and increased DNMT3b expression. In addition, hypomethylation of D4Z4, NBL2, and LINE-1 repetitive sequences; upregulation of *H19*, *IGF2*, *MAGE-A1*, and *MAGE-A3*; and hypermethylation of tumor suppressor genes such as *RASSF1A* and *RARβ* were reported in cells exposed to CSC. The finding of progressive genomic hypomethylation and regional hypermethylation in response to CSC, in association with increased clonogenicity, suggests that these epigenetic alterations could be markers of early lung carcinogenesis, especially in smokers (30).

2.3. Epigenetic Changes in Early Prostate Cancer Development

In prostate cancer, it has been found that *GSTP1* gene, encoding the glutathione *S*-transferase (GST), may serve a "caretaker" for prostate cells (31, 32). Normal prostate epithelial cells express GSTP1, while almost all prostate cancer cells fail to express GSTP1, and this lack of expression has been associated with gene promoter DNA methylation (33). Loss of *GSTP1* function also has been found in prostatic intraepithelial neoplasia (PIN) lesions, considered prostate cancer precursors. In addition, the prostate cancer precursor lesions' proliferative inflammatory atrophy (PIA), characterized by proliferating prostatic cells juxtapose to inflammatory cells, has epithelial cells that express increased levels of GSTP1 as a defense mechanism against oxidative damage. However, if *GSTP1* gene expression is altered, the PIA cells are vulnerable to oxidants and electrophiles causing DNA damage that contributes to neoplastic transformation to PIN and prostate cancer malignant progression (31). In fact, *GSTP1* CpG island hypermethylation has been detected in DNA from both PIA and PIN cells (34, 35), suggesting that *GSTP1* hypermethylation could be used for prostate cancer prevention as well as a biomarker for prostate cancer screening, detection, and diagnosis.

Furthermore, the tumor suppressor gene *RASSF1A*, inactivated by hypermethylation in different malignant tumors including prostate cancer (34), has been found to present promoter gene hypermethylation in PIN, in benign prostate tissue, and even in histologically normal prostate epithelial cells, indicating that the quantification of the *RASSF1A* methylation could serve as a biomarker of early prostate cancer development (36). In addition, hypermethylation of *GSTP1* and other genes including *RAR2β* and *APC* has been detected in histopathologically normal prostate tissues from men that subsequently presented positive biopsies for prostate cancer (37).

Moreover, as shown in many tumor types, altered DNA methylation in cancer cells consists of CpG island hypermethylation and genomic hypomethylation and both types of aberrant methylation are frequently found in human prostate adenocarcinoma. When methylation status of several CpG island loci and two repetitive DNA elements, LINE-1 and SAT2, were analyzed in prostate cancer, PIN, and histologically normal tissues, it was observed that the LINE-1 and SAT2 methylation levels decreased with progression of lesion types from normal prostate to PIN to prostate cancer, while promoter regions showed an increase in methylation levels (38). These findings suggested that both methylation alterations are involved in the development of PIN and are early events in prostate cancer tumorigenesis.

2.4. Epigenetic Changes in Early Colon Cancer Development

DNA-methylation-associated silencing of genes expression has been described in colorectal cancers by numerous studies (39). These epigenetic changes play a role in cellular transformation, especially if these changes affect genes involved in maintaining genomic stability.

Aberrant crypt foci (ACF) are surface abnormalities, considered biomarkers of increased colorectal cancer risk, especially if dysplasia is present (40). When ACF were analyzed for promoter hypermethylation for the DNA repair genes *hMLH1* and *MGMT*, increased promoter methylation was observed. Besides, all the lesions with *MGMT* hypermethylation displayed microsatellite instability (MSI)-low phenotype, suggesting that these lesions may be precursors to

MSI-low colorectal cancer (41). In addition, DNA methylation changes, genomic instability, and loss of heterozygosity found in the ACF, similar to cancerous tissues, indicate that these changes could be used as biomarkers of early tumor development (40).

Menigatti et al. (42) analyzed gene promoter methylation status of the DNA repair genes *hMLH1* and *MGMT* in different segments of the colon (cecal, transverse colon, sigmoid, and rectal mucosa) collected from healthy men and women undergoing screening colonoscopy. The investigators found that at least one segment of the colon showed promoter methylation of *hMLH1* and *MGMT* genes in both sexes, and for females in particular, specific age and segment differences were observed. More specifically, promoter methylation increased with age in females, mainly in the right colon, and also hypermethylation of promoters of both genes was observed, more commonly in the right colon. These findings parallel the observations in colorectal cancers that these genes are epigenetically modified and silenced, indicating that these changes may be important aspects of the early carcinogenic process (42).

Furthermore, when DNA methylation of *ERα* and secreted frizzled-related protein 1 (*SFRP1*) was analyzed in normal colorectal mucosa, DNA methylation for both genes was found to be significantly higher in the rectum than in the right colon. Further, an association with age was observed for both genes. More specifically, for each 10 years of age, a 1.7% increase in methylation level was detected for *ERα* and a 2.9% increase for *SFRP1*. Also, race has been shown to play a role in the methylation status of these two genes; thus, African Americans had a decrease methylation of both *ERα* and *SFRP1* when compared with Caucasians and Hispanics (43).

Another epigenetic change that is suggested to be associated with early stages of colorectal cancer is the methylation of microRNA, miR-137. The expression of miR-137 has been observed in normal colon mucosa, and it was inversely correlated with methylation level. It has been suggested that miR-137 acts as a tumor suppressor in the colon, and the silencing in colorectal cancers indicates that methylation of miR-137 could be a marker of early tumorigenesis (44).

3. Factors That Influence the Early Methylation Changes

3.1. Xenoestrogens

It has been shown before that the early exposure to xenoestrogens may increase susceptibility to breast cancer development later in life (45, 46). This increased susceptibility is believed to be the result of increased vulnerability of the breast progenitors to several environmental injuries, including xenoestrogens exposure early in life during development. These breast progenitors are immature cells that divide slowly and are capable of self-renewal and differentiation into different types of breast epithelial cells (45). Furthermore, breast progenitors may transmit the memory of different environment injuries through epigenetic mechanisms to their epithelial progeny that is capable of differentiation.

In previous studies, it has been shown that epithelial progeny exposed to 17β-estradiol and other xenoestrogens, presents hypermethylation in several protein-coding genes (0.5% of them) (46). More recently, hypermethylation in noncoding microRNA genes (9.1% of microRNA), like *miR-9-3*, was also reported. Promoter hypermethylation of *miR-9-3* was found in breast cancer cell lines and primary tumors and also in progenitor-containing mammospheres, an in vitro model to study this epigenetic effect in response to the exposure to xenoestrogens (47). It has been observed that *miR-9-3* plays a role in the p53-mediated apoptotic pathway, and it has been suggested that the epigenetic silencing of this gene can further inhibit the apoptotic process and promotes the proliferation of breast cancer cells. Therefore, it is hypothesized that the hypermethylation of the promoter region of this microRNA gene is an indicator of early breast cancer development (47).

Also, in animal models, it has been found that exposures to estrogens such as bisphenol A during development can impact the prostate epigenome, and these changes may promote prostate tumorigenesis in the adulthood (48).

3.2. Folate Effect on DNA Methylation

Folate, a key component of the one-carbon metabolism pathway, is metabolized to 5-methyltetrahydrofolate, providing the methyl groups for *S*-adenosylmethionine (SAM), a universal donor for the DNA methylation reactions (49). Numerous observations suggest that folate intake modifies cancer risk (50–52). Although the evidence for a relationship between folate availability and cancer risk is quite robust for colorectal cancer, evidence is less extensive and less consistent for the association between dietary folate intake or blood folate concentrations and breast cancer risk (53–57). However, there is consistency for the finding of increased risk of breast cancer intake among women with higher amounts of alcohol consumption and low intake of folate (58). An inverse relationship was observed between folate levels and gene promoter hypermethylation in sporadic colorectal cancers (59).

For lung cancer, several epidemiologic studies suggest that select dietary nutrients and vitamin supplements might have a protective effect against lung cancer development (60). The protective effect of fruits, vegetables, and multivitamins can be explained by the antioxidant activity of these dietary components and vitamins that could reduce DNA damage caused by the tobacco carcinogens. A recent study examined the effect of diet and multivitamins use on the DNA methylation of several genes in cells exfoliated from the aerodigestive tract of current and former smokers (60). The study's hypothesis was that intake of fruits, tomatoes, cruciferous vegetables, leafy vegetables, yellow vegetables, and vitamins is associated with reduced DNA methylation in sputum, whereas animal fat, red and processed meat are associated with increased gene methylation. It was observed that 12 monthly servings of leafy green vegetables and folate intake of 750 μg/day offered a significant protection against methylation. Similarly, the use of multivitamins was found to offer protection against promoter gene methylation (60).

When the association between blood folate levels and promoter gene methylation was analyzed in a multicenter colorectal cancer chemoprevention trial of aspirin and folic acid, it was found that higher RBC folate levels were associated with increased methylation levels for both *ERα* and *SFRP1* methylation (43). These findings raise concerns about the safety of folate supplementary use in healthy individuals, when it is proposed that hypermethylation of several genes in normal tissues may predispose to colorectal cancer development.

4. Conclusions

The identification of these epigenetic alterations in the precancerous lesions may help early diagnosis of different types of cancer and therefore improve the disease outcome and survival. The detection of these epigenetic changes could also help in evaluating the individual risk to cancer development, especially when it is known that different exposures can modulate this risk.

References

1. Chung, W., Kwabi-Addo, B., Ittmann, M., Jelinek, J., Shen, L., Yu, Y., and Issa, J. P. (2008) Identification of novel tumor markers in prostate, colon and breast cancer by unbiased methylation profiling. *PLoS One* 3, e2079.
2. Suzuki, M. and Yoshino, I. (2010) Aberrant methylation in non-small cell lung cancer. *Surg Today* 40, 602–607.
3. Hinshelwood, R. A. and Clark, S. J. (2008) Breast cancer epigenetics: normal human mammary epithelial cells as a model system. *J Mol Med* 86, 1315–1328.
4. Tlsty, T. D., Crawford, Y. G., Holst, C. R., Fordyce, C. A., Zhang, J., McDermott, K., Kozakiewicz, K., and Gauthier, M. L. (2004) Genetic and epigenetic changes in mammary epithelial cells may mimic early events in carcinogenesis. *J Mammary Gland Biol Neoplasia* 9, 263–274.
5. Holst, C. R., Nuovo, G. J., Esteller, M., Chew, K., Baylin, S. B., Herman, J. G., and Tlsty, T. D. (2003) Methylation of p16(INK4a) promoters occurs in vivo in histologically normal human mammary epithelia. *Cancer Res* 63, 1596–1601.
6. Parrella, P., Poeta, M. L., Gallo, A. P., Prencipe, M., Scintu, M., Apicella, A., Rossiello, R., Liguoro, G., Seripa, D., et al. (2004) Nonrandom distribution of aberrant promoter methylation of cancer-related genes in sporadic breast tumors. *Clin Cancer Res* 10, 5349–5354.
7. Silva, J., Silva, J. M., Dominguez, G., Garcia, J. M., Cantos, B., Rodriguez, R., Larrondo, F. J., Provencio, M., Espana, P., and Bonilla, F. (2003) Concomitant expression of p16INK4a and p14ARF in primary breast cancer and analysis of inactivation mechanisms. *J Pathol* 199, 289–297.

8. Tlsty, T. D., Romanov, S. R., Kozakiewicz, B. K., Holst, C. R., Haupt, L. M., and Crawford, Y. G. (2001) Loss of chromosomal integrity in human mammary epithelial cells subsequent to escape from senescence. *J Mammary Gland Biol Neoplasia*6, 235–243.

9. Romanov, S. R., Kozakiewicz, B. K., Holst, C. R., Stampfer, M. R., Haupt, L. M., and Tlsty, T. D. (2001) Normal human mammary epithelial cells spontaneously escape senescence and acquire genomic changes. *Nature* 409, 633–637.

10. Crawford, Y. G., Gauthier, M. L., Joubel, A., Mantei, K., Kozakiewicz, K., Afshari, C. A., and Tlsty, T. D. (2004) Histologically normal human mammary epithelia with silenced p16(INK4a) overexpress COX-2, promoting a premalignant program. *Cancer Cell* 5, 263–273.

11. Reynolds, P. A., Sigaroudinia, M., Zardo, G., Wilson, M. B., Benton, G. M., Miller, C. J., Hong, C., Fridlyand, J., Costello, J. F., and Tlsty, T. D. (2006) Tumor suppressor p16INK4A regulates polycomb-mediated DNA hypermethylation in human mammary epithelial cells. *J Biol Chem* 281, 24790–24802.

12. Dumitrescu, R. G. and Cotarla, I. (2005) Understanding breast cancer risk -- where do we stand in 2005? *J Cell Mol Med* 9, 208–221.

13. Li, Y., Pan, J., Li, J. L., Lee, J. H., Tunkey, C., Saraf, K., Garbe, J. C., Whitley, M. Z., Jelinsky, S. A., et al. (2007) Transcriptional changes associated with breast cancer occur as normal human mammary epithelial cells overcome senescence barriers and become immortalized. *Mol Cancer* 6, 7.

14. Berman, H., Zhang, J., Crawford, Y. G., Gauthier, M. L., Fordyce, C. A., McDermott, K. M., Sigaroudinia, M., Kozakiewicz, K., and Tlsty, T. D. (2005) Genetic and epigenetic changes in mammary epithelial cells identify a subpopulation of cells involved in early carcinogenesis. *Cold Spring Harb Symp Quant Biol* 70, 317–327.

15. Bean, G. R., Bryson, A. D., Pilie, P. G., Goldenberg, V., Baker, J. C., Jr., Ibarra, C., Brander, D. M., Paisie, C., Case, N. R., et al. (2007) Morphologically normal-appearing mammary epithelial cells obtained from high-risk women exhibit methylation silencing of INK4a/ARF. *Clin Cancer Res* 13, 6834–6841.

16. Locke, I., Kote-Jarai, Z., Fackler, M. J., Bancroft, E., Osin, P., Nerurkar, A., Izatt, L., Pichert, G., Gui, G. P., and Eeles, R. A. (2007) Gene promoter hypermethylation in ductal lavage fluid from healthy BRCA gene mutation carriers and mutation-negative controls. *Breast Cancer Res* 9, R20.

17. Vasilatos, S. N., Broadwater, G., Barry, W. T., Baker, J. C., Jr., Lem, S., Dietze, E. C., Bean, G. R., Bryson, A. D., Pilie, P. G., et al. (2009) CpG island tumor suppressor promoter methylation in non-BRCA-associated early mammary carcinogenesis. *Cancer Epidemiol Biomarkers Prev* 18, 901–914.

18. Lewis, C. M., Cler, L. R., Bu, D. W., Zochbauer-Muller, S., Milchgrub, S., Naftalis, E. Z., Leitch, A. M., Minna, J. D., and Euhus, D. M. (2005) Promoter hypermethylation in benign breast epithelium in relation to predicted breast cancer risk. *Clin Cancer Res* 11, 166–172.

19. Euhus, D. M., Bu, D., Milchgrub, S., Xie, X. J., Bian, A., Leitch, A. M., and Lewis, C. M. (2008) DNA methylation in benign breast epithelium in relation to age and breast cancer risk. *Cancer Epidemio. Biomarkers Prev* 17, 1051–1059.

20. Jemal, A., Siegel, R., Ward, E., Murray, T., Xu, J., and Thun, M. J. (2007) Cancer statistics, 2007. *CA Cancer J Clin* 57, 43–66.

21. Belinsky, S. A. (2005) Silencing of genes by promoter hypermethylation: key event in rodent and human lung cancer. *Carcinogenesis* 26, 1481–1487.

22. Belinsky, S. A., Palmisano, W. A., Gilliland, F. D., Crooks, L. A., Divine, K. K., Winters, S. A., Grimes, M. J., Harms, H. J., Tellez, C. S.m et al. (2002) Aberrant promoter methylation in bronchial epithelium and sputum from current and former smokers. *Cancer Research* 62, 2370–2377.

23. Belinsky, S. A., Nikula, K. J., Palmisano, W. A., Michels, R., Saccomanno, G., Gabrielson, E., Baylin, S. B., and Herman, J. G. (1998) Aberrant methylation of p16(INK4a) is an early event in lung cancer and a potential biomarker for early diagnosis. *Proc Natl Acad Sci U S A* 95, 11891–11896.

24. Licchesi, J. D., Westra, W. H., Hooker, C. M., and Herman, J. G. (2008) Promoter hypermethylation of hallmark cancer genes in atypical adenomatous hyperplasia of the lung. *Clin Cancer Res* 14, 2570–2578.

25. Palmisano, W. A., Divine, K. K., Saccomanno, G., Gilliland, F. D., Baylin, S. B., Herman, J. G., and Belinsky, S. A. (2000) Predicting lung cancer by detecting aberrant promoter methylation in sputum. *Cancer Res* 60, 5954–5958.

26. Belinsky, S. A., Liechty, K. C., Gentry, F. D., Wolf, H. J., Rogers, J., Vu, K., Haney, J., Kennedy, T. C., Hirsch, F. R., et al. (2006) Promoter hypermethylation of multiple genes in sputum precedes lung cancer incidence in a high-risk cohort. *Cancer Res* 66, 3338–3344.

27. Belinsky, S. A. (2004) Gene-promoter hypermethylation as a biomarker in lung cancer. *Nat Rev Cancer* 4, 707–717.

28. Shen, H., Spitz, M. R., Qiao, Y., Guo, Z., Wang, L. E., Bosken, C. H., Amos, C. I., and Wei, Q. (2003) Smoking, DNA repair capacity and risk of nonsmall cell lung cancer. *Int J Cancer* 107, 84–88.
29. Leng, S., Stidley, C. A., Willink, R., Bernauer, A., Do, K., Picchi, M. A., Sheng, X., Frasco, M. A., van den, B. D., et al. (2008) Double-strand break damage and associated DNA repair genes predispose smokers to gene methylation. *Cancer Res* 68, 3049–3056.
30. Liu, F., Killian, J. K., Yang, M., Walker, R. L., Hong, J. A., Zhang, M., Davis, S., Zhang, Y., Hussain, M., et al. (2010) Epigenomic alterations and gene expression profiles in respiratory epithelia exposed to cigarette smoke condensate. *Oncogene* 29, 3650–3664.
31. Nelson, W. G., De Marzo, A. M., DeWeese, T. L., Lin, X., Brooks, J. D., Putzi, M. J., Nelson, C. P., Groopman, J. D., and Kensler, T. W. (2001) Preneoplastic prostate lesions: an opportunity for prostate cancer prevention. *Ann N Y Acad Sci* 952, 135–144.
32. Nelson, W. G., De Marzo, A. M., and DeWeese, T. L. (2001) The molecular pathogenesis of prostate cancer: Implications for prostate cancer prevention. *Urology* 57, 39–45.
33. Lin, X., Tascilar, M., Lee, W. H., Vles, W. J., Lee, B. H., Veeraswamy, R., Asgari, K., Freije, D., van, R. B., et al. (2001) GSTP1 CpG island hypermethylation is responsible for the absence of GSTP1 expression in human prostate cancer cells. *Am J Pathol* 159, 1815–1826.
34. Ahmed, H. (2010) Promoter Methylation in Prostate Cancer and its Application for the Early Detection of Prostate Cancer Using Serum and Urine Samples. *Biomark Cancer* 17–33.
35. Nakayama, M., Gonzalgo, M. L., Yegnasub ramanian, S., Lin, X., De Marzo, A. M., and Nelson, W. G. (2004) GSTP1 CpG island hypermethylation as a molecular biomarker for prostate cancer. *J Cell Biochem* 91, 540–552.
36. Aitchison, A., Warren, A., Neal, D., and Rabbitts, P. (2007) RASSF1A promoter methylation is frequently detected in both pre-malignant and non-malignant microdissected prostatic epithelial tissues. *Prostate* 67, 638–644.
37. Troyer, D. A., Lucia, M. S., de Bruine, A. P., Mendez-Meza, R., Baldewijns, M. M., Dunscomb, N., van, E. M., McAskill, T., Bierau, K., et al. (2009) Prostate cancer detected by methylated gene markers in histopathologically cancer-negative tissues from men with subsequent positive biopsies. *Cancer Epidemiol Biomarkers Prev* 18, 2717–2722.
38. Cho, N. Y., Kim, J. H., Moon, K. C., and Kang, G. H. (2009) Genomic hypomethylation and CpG island hypermethylation in prostatic intraepithelial neoplasm. *Virchows Arch* 454, 17–23.
39. Kim, M. S., Lee, J., and Sidransky, D. (2010) DNA methylation markers in colorectal cancer. *Cancer Metastasis Rev* 29, 181–206.
40. Orlando, F. A., Tan, D., Baltodano, J. D., Khoury, T., Gibbs, J. F., Hassid, V. J., Ahmed, B. H., and Alrawi, S. J. (2008) Aberrant crypt foci as precursors in colorectal cancer progression. *J Surg Oncol* 98, 207–213.
41. Greenspan, E. J., Cyr, J. L., Pleau, D. C., Levine, J., Rajan, T. V., Rosenberg, D. W., and Heinen, C. D. (2007) Microsatellite instability in aberrant crypt foci from patients without concurrent colon cancer. *Carcinogenesis* 28, 769–776.
42. Menigatti, M., Truninger, K., Gebbers, J. O., Marbet, U., Marra, G., and Schar, P. (2009) Normal colorectal mucosa exhibits sex- and segment-specific susceptibility to DNA methylation at the hMLH1 and MGMT promoters. *Oncogene* 28, 899–909.
43. Wallace, K., Grau, M. V., Levine, A. J., Shen, L., Hamdan, R., Chen, X., Gui, J., Haile, R. W., Barry, E. L., et al. (2010) Association between folate levels and CpG Island hypermethylation in normal colorectal mucosa. *Cancer Prev Res* (Phila) 3, 1552–1564.
44. Balaguer, F., Link, A., Lozano, J. J., Cuatrecasas, M., Nagasaka, T., Boland, C. R., and Goel, A. (2010) Epigenetic silencing of miR-137 is an early event in colorectal carcinogenesis. *Cancer Res* 70, 6609–6618.
45. Weissman, I. L., Anderson, D. J., and Gage, F. (2001) Stem and progenitor cells: origins, phenotypes, lineage commitments, and transdifferentiations. *Annu Rev Cell Dev Biol* 17, 387–403.
46. Cheng, A. S., Culhane, A. C., Chan, M. W., Venkataramu, C. R., Ehrich, M., Nasir, A., Rodriguez, B. A., Liu, J., Yan, P. S., et al. (2008) Epithelial progeny of estrogen-exposed breast progenitor cells display a cancer-like methylome. *Cancer Res* 68, 1786–1796.
47. Hsu, P. Y., Deatherage, D. E., Rodriguez, B. A., Liyanarachchi, S., Weng, Y. I., Zuo, T., Liu, J., Cheng, A. S., and Huang, T. H. (2009) Xenoestrogen-induced epigenetic repression of microRNA-9-3 in breast epithelial cells. *Cancer Res* 69, 5936–5945.
48. Prins, G. S., Tang, W. Y., Belmonte, J., and Ho, S. M. (2008) Perinatal exposure to oestradiol and bisphenol A alters the prostate epigenome and increases susceptibility to carcinogenesis. *Basic Clin Pharmacol Toxicol* 102, 134–138.
49. Jennings, E. (1995) Folic acid as a cancer-preventing agent. *Med Hypotheses* 45, 297–303.
50. Ciappio, E. and Mason, J.B. (2009) Folate and carcinogenesis: mechanisms. In: *Folate in Health and Disease* (Bailey L & Taylor and Francis LLC eds.).

51. Xu, X. and Chen, J. (2009) One-carbon metabolism and breast cancer: an epidemiological perspective. *J Genet Genomics* 36, 203–214.
52. Miller, J. W., Borowsky, A. D., Marple, T. C., McGoldrick, E. T., llard-Telm, L., Young, L. J., and Green, R. (2008) Folate, DNA methylation, and mouse models of breast tumorigenesis. *Nutr Rev 66 Suppl* 1, S59–S64.
53. Ericson, U., Sonestedt, E., Ivarsson, M. I., Gullberg, B., Carlson, J., Olsson, H.. and Wirfalt, E. (2009) Folate intake, methylenetetrahydrofolate reductase polymorphisms, and breast cancer risk in women from the Malmo Diet and Cancer cohort. *Cancer Epidemiol Biomarkers Prev* 18, 1101–1110.
54. Kim, Y. I. (2006) Does a high folate intake increase the risk of breast cancer? *Nutr Rev* 64, 468–475.
55. Larsson, S. C., Giovannucci, E., and Wolk, A. (2007) Folate and risk of breast cancer: a meta-analysis. *J Natl Cancer Inst* 99, 64–76.
56. Lewis, S. J., Harbord, R. M., Harris, R., and Smith, G. D. (2006) Meta-analyses of observational and genetic association studies of folate intakes or levels and breast cancer risk. *J Natl Cancer Inst* 98, 1607–1622.
57. Ma, E., Iwasaki, M., Junko, I., Hamada, G. S., Nishimoto, I. N., Carvalho, S. M., Motola, J., Jr., Laginha, F. M., and Tsugane, S. (2009) Dietary intake of folate, vitamin B6, and vitamin B12, genetic polymorphism of related enzymes, and risk of breast cancer: a case-control study in Brazilian women. *BMC Cancer* 9, 122.
58. Mahoney, M. C., Bevers, T., Linos, E., and Willett, W. C. (2008) Opportunities and strategies for breast cancer prevention through risk reduction. *CA Cancer J Clin*58, 347–371.
59. van, E. M., Weijenberg, M. P., Roemen, G. M., Brink, M., de Bruine, A. P., Goldbohm, R. A., van den Brandt, P. A., Baylin, S. B., De Goeij, A. F., and Herman, J. G. (2003) Effects of dietary folate and alcohol intake on promoter methylation in sporadic colorectal cancer: the Netherlands cohort study on diet and cancer. *Cancer Res* 63, 3133–3137.
60. Stidley, C. A., Picchi, M. A., Leng, S., Willink, R., Crowell, R. E., Flores, K. G., Kang, H., Byers, T., Gilliland, F. D., and Belinsky, S. A. (2010) Multivitamins, folate, and green vegetables protect against gene promoter methylation in the aerodigestive tract of smokers. *Cancer Res* 70, 568–574.

Chapter 2

Epigenetics of Solid Cancer Stem Cells

Alok Mishra and Mukesh Verma

Abstract

Epigenetics is an emerging science that can help to explain carcinogenesis. The possibility that carcinogenesis may originate in a stem cell process was proposed recently. Stem cells are generated and contribute to tumor formation during the process of tumor development. This chapter focuses on the role of epigenetics and genetics in stem cell formation, different theories about the origin of cancer stem cells (CSCs), and epigenetic mechanisms that occur in solid CSCs. Potential applications of knowledge gained through this field and future prospects for cancer treatment also are discussed.

Key words: Biomarker, Cancer, Differentiation, Genetics, Epigenetic, Histones, Methylation, MicroRNA, Pluripotent, Stem cells, Tumor

Abbreviations

ChIP	Chromatin immunoprecipitation
CSCs	Cancer stem cells
DREAM	Digital restriction enzyme analysis of methylation
HATs	Histone acetyltransferases
HDACs	Histone deacetylases
HDMs	Histone demethylases
HMTs	Histone methyltransferases
iPSC	Induced pluripotent stem cell
LOI	Loss of imprinting
PcG	Polycomb group genes

1. Epigenetics: An Introduction

The term “epigenetics” (Greek: *epi*-over, above genetics) was used first in 1942 by Waddington in explaining embryonic development. Dr. Waddington defined the term as “the causal interactions between genes and their products, which bring the phenotype into being” (1). An epigenetic system should be heritable, self-perpetuating,

Ramona G. Dumitrescu and Mukesh Verma (eds.), *Cancer Epigenetics: Methods and Protocols*, Methods in Molecular Biology, vol. 863, DOI 10.1007/978-1-61779-612-8_2, © Springer Science+Business Media, LLC 2012

and reversible (2). In the current understanding of the biology of chromatin and gene expression, the term "epigenetics" is accepted widely as "the study of heritable changes in gene expression that occur independent of primary DNA sequence." In addition, current knowledge of human biology and medicine recognizes the implications of epigenetics for a variety of biological phenomena that cannot be explained by mere changes in DNA sequences, such as phenotypic variation in clones/monozygotic twins, imprinting and mono-allelic expression, dosage compensation, and origin of divergent cells from common progenitors in development and differentiation. Today's science accepts that cross talk between genetics and epigenetics is involved in molecular mechanisms for gene regulation. The main components that modify chromatin structure and function and ultimately dictate gene expression patterns can be divided into DNA methylation, covalent histone modifications, non-covalent mechanisms (incorporation of histone variants/nucleosome remodeling), and non-coding RNAs, including microRNAs (miRNAs).

2. Normal Cell Epigenetics

2.1. DNA Modifications

The best known and most established epigenetic marker is DNA methylation in the mammalian genome. In mammals, DNA methylation occurs primarily by the covalent modification of cytosine residues in CpG dinucleotides that suppress genes in genomic and non-genomic regions. CpG dinucleotide-rich regions are called "CpG islands" and are present primarily in the 5′ regulatory region of genes and also in repetitive sequences such as the LINE and Alu sequences (3, 4). Aside from the general quenching activity of gene expression, DNA methylation is implicated in X-chromosome inactivation, genomic imprinting, and in preventing chromosomal instability (by shutting off transposons) (5, 6). Many non-CpG regions also are methylated and involved in controlling certain tissue-specific genes, such as Maspin, MAGE, and Oct-4 (7–9). Three major enzymes that are active in the methylation process are *D*NA *m*ethyl*t*ransferases (DNMTs) 3A, 3B, and 1 (10).

2.2. Histone Modifications

Modern, high-throughput, state-of-the-art technologies have interpreted the contextual, spatial, and temporal distribution of histone modification patterns (11, 12). The covalent posttranslational modifications of N-terminal histones in chromatin also are responsible for significant variations in epigenetic control. This results in the compaction of chromatin and recruitment of proteins to execute replication, transcription, and repair (13). More than 50 H2A/H2B sites of modification are known that include acetylation, methylation, citrullination, phosphorylation, SUMOylation, and ADP-ribosylation (14). H3K4me3 is enriched on active 5′ promoters, but H3K9me3 and H3K27me3 are present on repressed promoters (H3 = histone type3, K = lysine residue, me3 = trimethylation). The enzymology of histone modification includes the role of histone acetyltransferases (HATs), histone methyltransferases (HMTs), histone deacetylases (HDACs), and histone demethylases (HDMs) (14, 15). Interestingly, epigenetic codes are decided by the interplay between the DNA methylation and histone modification machineries inside cells, which complicates the scenario (16). The acetylation of histones H3 and H4 is indicative of an open chromatin structure, which can recruit more positive regulatory complexes.

The engagement of non-canonical histone variants in nucleosomal remodeling during epigenetic phenomena is made possible only by non-covalent interactions between DNA-histones/histone-histone. Nucleosomal assembly and disassembly and the presence of 5′/3′ nucleosome-free regions are related to the activation and repression of genes (17, 18). Non-canonical variants of histones, such as H3.3 and H2A.Z, also activate gene transcription (19).

2.3. MicroRNA

Remarkably, microRNA (miRNA) coding genes are regulated by epigenetic machinery. Encoded miRNAs also can epigenetically modulate the downstream expression patterns of DNA methylation and histone medications. A growing number of genes lose activity by miRNA binding at 3′ untranslated regions (UTRs) (20, 21).

2.4. Non-conventional Epigenetics

Looking beyond DNA-associated molecules, prions (infectious proteins) clearly are epigenetic and perpetuate themselves through altered folding states. These states can act as sensors of environmental stress and, through the phenotypic changes they promote, drive evolution (22). In the plant kingdom, migratory small RNA transports from one cell to another are known epigenetic effectors (23).

3. Cancer Cell Epigenetics

3.1. DNA Methylation in Cancer

A distinct aberrant epigenetic landscape has been noted in various cancers. The first molecular epigenetic abnormality in cancer was identified in 1983 by Feinberg and Vogelstein (24). In general, the human cancer epigenome has genome-wide global hypomethylation and site-specific CpG island promoter hypermethylation, as noted by Jones and Baylin (25). Epigenetic genome-wide association studies (EWAS) are planned by the US National Institutes of Health (NIH) under the Roadmap Epigenomics Program, which covers several diseases (http://commonfund.nih.gov/epigenomics/index.asp). Hypomethylation of repeat sequences and retrotransposons induces genomic instability by promoting chromosomal rearrangements (26, 27). Hypomethylation of many genes, such as

GSTP1, *S100*, *Maspin*, and *Ras*, and hypermethylation of promoters of various tumor suppressor genes (*Rb*, *p16*, and *BRCAs*) are being investigated thoroughly in different tumors (28, 29). Silencing of promoters of many transcription factors and DNA repair genes is reported in different cancers (30, 31). Two notable examples of the hypomethylation mechanism are the activation of *PAX2* and the activation of the *let-7a-3* miRNA gene, which has been implicated in endometrial and colon cancer (32). Loss of imprinting (LOI) at the *IGF2* loci is seen in many tumors such as Wilms tumor, and in colorectal and intestinal cancers (33–35).

3.2. Histone Modifications in Cancer

Global loss of acetylated H4-lysine 16 (H4K16ac) and H4-lysine 20 trimethylation (H4K20me3) by overexpressed HDACs has been established in several tumors (36). Because of their ability to reactivate genes, the epigenetic-based HDAC inhibitors currently are one of the most popular anticancer drugs. HMT coding genes such as *EZH* and *NSD3* are extremely active in many solid tumors (19, 37).

3.3. miRNA in Cancer

Misexpression of myriad miRNAs has been seen in a wide spectrum of human cancers. These non-coding RNAs can be classified as growth promoters and tumor suppressors. Some of the most common miRNA-mediated tumor suppression functions in different cancers occur through let-7, miRNA 15, and miRNA 16. Similarly, methylation of gene encoding for miRNA124a is a common epigenetic mechanism in carcinogenesis (37, 38). MicroRNA-based tumor classification has been examined extensively by Lu et al. (38).

4. Cancer Stem Cell Epigenetics

4.1. Cancer Stem Cells: Concept, Biology, and Challenges in the Field

Cancer stem cells (CSCs) are the small number of cells within a tumor that are capable of fueling the tumor's growth. These cells generally represent fewer than 5% of all cells in a tumor. Table 1 shows the CSCs found in different solid tumor types. In contrast to the stochastic (clonal evolution) model, according to the CSC (hierarchical) model of tumors, there is a small subset of cancer cells, called the CSCs/tumor-initiating cells/tumorigenic cells, that can sustain and renew themselves to maintain the whole tumor. This model necessitates revisiting current diagnosis and treatment modalities for all cancers (39). Tumor heterogeneity consists of two types of cells: tumor cells and non-tumor cells (e.g., stromal cells, immune cells). Solid tumors, however, contain cells at various stages of differentiation, which is consistent with the concept of the CSC model. Solid cancers typically contain cells that exhibit divergent nuclear morphologies and differentiation features. The heterogeneity can be explained by the inter- and intra-tumor microenvironment/niche and the prevalent genetic/epigenetic selection pressure. General evidence of the CSC model includes tumor relapse, poor prognosis for less differentiated tumors, and the tritium-labeled molecular studies conducted in the 1960s on acute myeloid leukemia. A 1937 paper by Furth and Kahn validated the CSC model by stating that a single murine cell from culture can initiate a cancer graft (40). This paper can be considered the first experimental proof of the CSC model.

According to the 2006 American Association for Cancer Research (AACR) workshop on CSC, the consensus definition of a CSC is “a cell within a tumor that possesses the capacity to self-renew and to cause the heterogeneous lineages of cancer cells that comprise the tumor” (http://www.aacr.org/home/scientists/publications-of-the-aacr/meeting-reports.aspx) (39). Therefore, a CSC has to self-renew as well as be multipotent to give rise to non-CSCs and to maintain a heterogeneous mass. The only “gold standard” confirmation of CSCs has been an *in vivo* experiment that demonstrated the ability of CSCs to reconstruct the original tumor with the same histology. Solid CSCs are a difficult system to study in comparison to liquid cancers such as leukemias. Known markers exist for each differentiating stage of leukemic cells, but accessing the solid cancer cells and their CSCs is difficult. Solid CSCs and their surface markers may be disturbed mechanically during the process of accessing them, which may alter the actual profile of the surface marker (cluster of differentiation/“CD” markers). In addition, few robust markers have been found that identify many of the solid CSCs, except for some related to brain, breast, prostate, and colon cancers. Thus far, no marker has been identified for all tumor types. It is well known that the frequency of CSCs should be considerably lower in solid tumors, although CSCs may not necessarily be rare, as argued by Strasser and colleagues (41, 42). The frequency of CSCs varies from tumor to tumor and by tumor stage, niche, status of immunity of the host environment, and site of implantation/injection in the case of *in vivo* models. Therefore, to enrich plausible CSCs, investigators should humanize the niche of the injection site, use late-stage tumors with less differentiated cells, and use maximal immune-suppressed mice (NOG) (43). Thus, the convincing population of CSC is strictly a subject of tools and the experimental conditions used. The strength of the evidence supporting the presence of CSCs in tumors has been demonstrated in manuscripts published in high-impact journals as well as from clear proofs of principal obtained from clinical studies (44).

The potential problems of using therapies targeting CSCs are very serious, including depletions of the intrinsic normal stem cell population and a consequent loss of regeneration and healing capacities. Other dangers include the posttreatment evolution of subpopulations of therapy-resistant CSCs and the conversion of non-CSCs to CSCs. These dangers will be resolved only when the mechanisms of CSC origination and variation are better

Table 1
Markers of solid cancer stem cells

Organs	Markers	References[a]
Brain	$CD133^{+}$	(46)
Breast	$CD44^{+}CD24^{-/low}$ Lin-$EPCAM^{+}$	(47)
Colon	$CD133^{+}$	(48)
Head and neck	$CD44^{+}$	(49)
Liver	$CD90^{+}$	(50)
Pancreas	$CD133^{+}$	(51)
Prostate	$CD44^{+}CD24^{-/low}$	(52)
Renal	CD105	(53)
Melanoma	$ABC5^{+}$	(54)

[a] Selected references only

understood. Opponents of the CSC concept have not put forward any concrete explanation of why non-CSCs cannot acquire the CSC phenotype when under Darwinian selective pressure (45).

Markers of solid CSC are mentioned in Table 1.

5. CSC Origin, Evidence, and Relationship to Epigenetics

The hypothesis that cancers arise due to maturation arrest in stem cells was proposed in 1994 for all tissues, based primarily on observations of the origin of teratocarcinomas and hepatocellular carcinomas (55). Brain tumors also arise from normal stem cells (56). In leukemia, it originally was postulated that CSCs arose from normal stem cells (57). Generation of CSCs from progenitor cells also has been reported in blood cancers (58). The same epigenetic patterns in solid precancer and cancers are strong indicatives of the origin of tumors from metastable transient amplifying progenitor cells (59).

An oversimplified depiction of possible CSC generation methods is shown in Fig. 1.

6. Epigenetic Progenitor Model and Solid CSCs

The epigenetic progenitor model suggests that epigenetic modifications, which occur in normal stem or progenitor cells, are the earliest molecular events in the process of cancer initiation. This famous

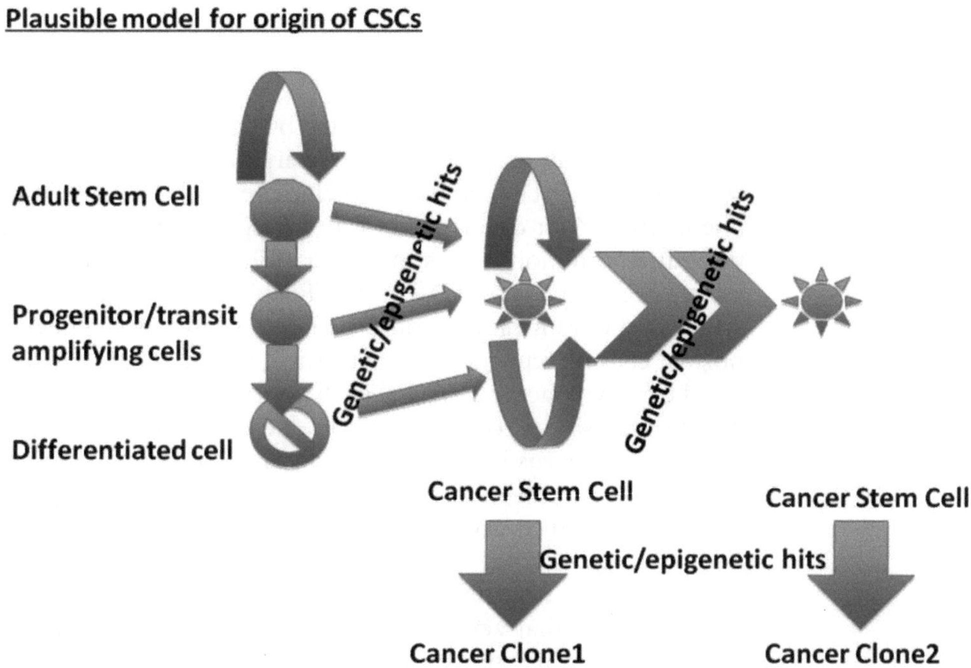

Fig. 1. CSCs can originate from adult stem cells, progenitor cells, differentiated cells, or cancer stem cells (CSCs), per se.

concept originally was proposed by Feinberg *et al.* and today is known widely as the epigenetic progenitor model of the origin of human cancers (60). This concept has been proven clinically, because normal tissues adjacent to tumors have been found to have altered progenitors. At the same time, the idea validates the CSC model of tumor heterogeneity. Ohm *et al.* found a stem-cell-like chromatin pattern that may predispose tumor suppressor genes to DNA hypermethylation and heritable silencing (61).

The similar epigenetic signatures of embryonic stem (ES) cells and cancer cells also strengthen Dr. Feinberg's concept of CSC (28, 62). According to this concept, cancer arises in three steps. The first step is an epigenetic alteration of stem/progenitor cells, mediated by aberrant regulation of tumor-progenitor genes (TPG). This alteration may be due to events in stem cells themselves or to the influence of the surrounding stromal environmental damage. The second step is a gatekeeper mutation (GKM) in tumor suppressor genes in solid tumors. The third and final step involves genetic and epigenetic hits leading to increased tumor evolution with an invasive phenotype (e.g., metastasis).

7. Epigenetic Progenitor Model of CSC: Clues and Views

Several arguments have been presented by CSC proponents regarding CSC origin from progenitors. These are discussed below and presented in Fig. 2. The arguments include reversibility of solid tumor phenotypes (63); occurrence of global epigenetic changes before the initial mutation events in cancer (59, 64); silencing of tumor suppressor genes *p16*, *APC*, and *SFRP* by methylation in the early stages of different cancers; differentiation of melanoma nuclei into normal cells by reprogramming of the genome (65); LOI of insulin-like growth factor 2 (*IGF2*) in the normal colonic epithelium of patients at risk for colorectal cancer (66); and existence of similar epigenetic patterns in human ES cells and cancer cells (human ES cells with cancer cell characteristics, including higher frequency of teratoma-initiating cells; growth factor and niche independence also have been found) (67).

A putative TPG involved in the first step of an epigenetic hit would be one that acts directly on DNA, with both genetic and epigenetic modifications, and mediates epigenetic expansion of progenitor cells, thus increasing their stemness and the potential for self-renewal and pluripotency (POU, Oct-4, Nanog). Polycomb group proteins also can be seen as an important TPG at the first step (68, 69). TPG also might include genes that are silenced, thereby allowing CSCs to escape their niche (60). The second hit will be genetic and tissue specific, such as *APC* in colon cancers. The third and final kind of hit leads to genetic- and epigenetic-induced plasticity and eventually to the generation of metastatic properties.

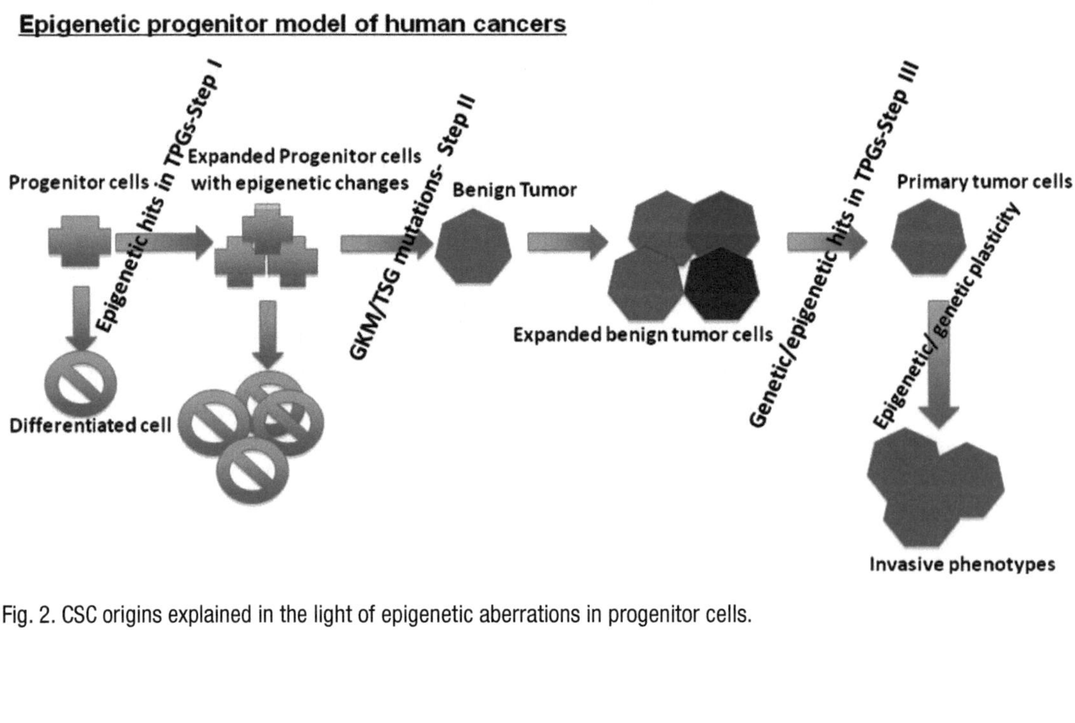

Fig. 2. CSC origins explained in the light of epigenetic aberrations in progenitor cells.

The epigenetic progenitor model of cancer progression is important in understanding the biology of CSCs and tumorigenesis in general. The model can explain tumor heterogeneity, microenvironmental effects, age-onset tumors, cancer risks, and several cancer biology-related questions.

8. Molecular Mechanisms of Epigenetic Changes in CSCs That Lead to Carcinogenesis

The mechanisms of epigenetic changes in CSCs appear to be an unexplored area, at least with regard to solid cancers. As a result, the following discussion is based on observations from different systems such as ES cells, induced pluripotent stem cells (iPSCs), and cancer cells. Laird and colleagues hypothesized that the acquisition of promoter DNA methylation at polycomb group genes (PcG) could lock in stem cell phenotypes and initiate abnormal clonal expansion, thereby predisposing cells to carcinogenic transformation (28). Eric Lander's group demonstrated the existence of a novel chromatin modification pattern, termed a "bivalent domain," consisting of large regions of repressive Lys27 methylation (H3K27) harboring smaller activating regions of Lys4 methylation (H3K4me3) in ES cells (70). It is quite possible that the same mechanism exists in CSCs to maintain their multipotent plastic nature. The mechanism of bivalent histone generation is based on PcG proteins; PcGs also are known to play a role in cancer development (69, 70). Interestingly, Agrelo and Wutz shed light on an aspect of CSC epigenetics through the *Xist* gene silencing pathway linked with X-chromosome inactivation (71). In a very different approach, Bapat described the maintenance and identification of ovarian tumor stem cells based on mitochondrial DNA (72). In addition, Farrar and colleagues extensively reviewed CSC epigenetic modifications in solid tumors in the prostate, liver, kidney, brain, and breast (73).

9. Experimental Methods and Protocols in CSC Epigenetics

9.1. Methods in CSC Biology

Figure 3 presents a laboratory workflow diagram for CSC identification, isolation, and characterization.

9.2. Methods in Epigenetics

Epigenetics employs general experimental methods such as the chromatin immunoprecipitation (ChIP) assay (to study DNA-histone interactions/modifications), DNA methylation assays (to study methylated sequence bisulfite treatment methods), and different arrays (microarray, ChIP-on-Chip, ChIP-Seq).

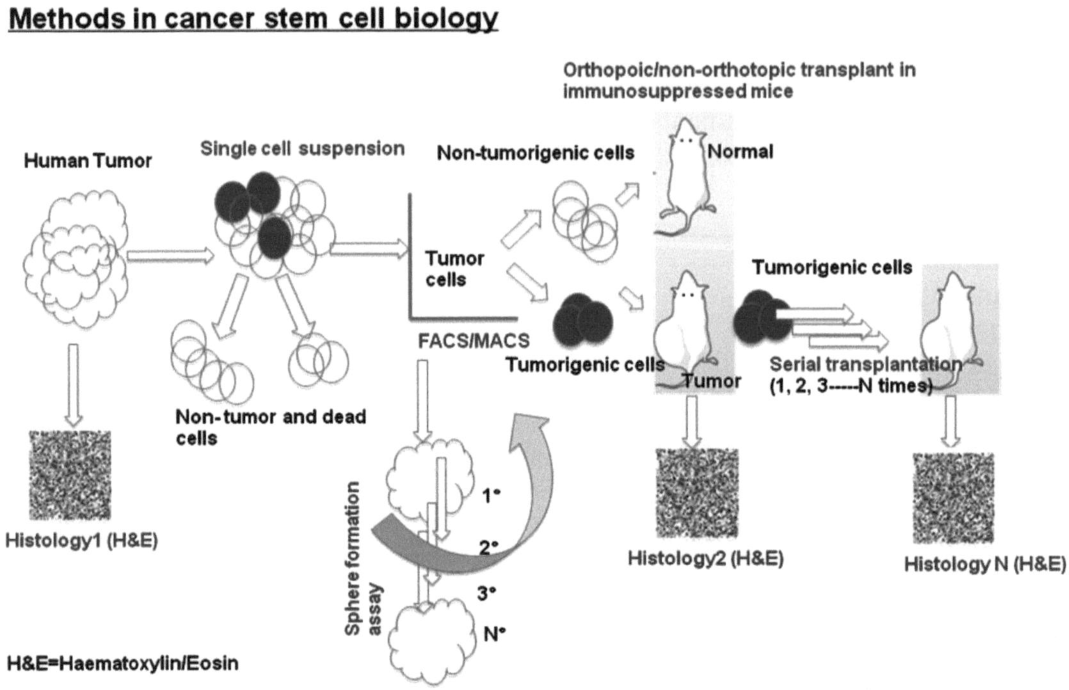

Fig. 3. A general experimental approach to the discovery and validation of CSC research in solid CSCs.

The following Web-based resources can be used for standard laboratory protocols:

- http://www.sigmaaldrich.com/life-science/epigenetics.html (Sigma)
- http://cshprotocols.cshlp.org/cgi/content/abstract/2007/12/pdb.prot4767 (Cold Spring Harbor)
- http://www.qiagen.com/products/byapplication/epigenetics/default.aspx (Qiagen)
- http://www.activemotif.com/catalog/83/epigenetics-chromatin.html (Active Motif)
- http://www.sigmaaldrich.com/life-science/molecular-biology/molecular-biology-products.html?TablePage=103234606 (Sigma)
- http://www.biomol.de/lp/epigenetics.html (Biomol)

Many enzyme-linked immunosorbent assay (ELISA)-based platforms are available commercially to detect DNA methylation. The Imprint™ Methylated DNA Quantification technology kit (MDQ1-48RXN/96RXN) by Sigma, one of the most popular methods, provides a rapid and reliable way to measure global DNA methylation. Up to 200 ng of purified DNA is bound to the wells of the assay strip, and the methylated DNA can be detected within 3 h. The Pacific Biosciences (Benjamin Flusberg) procedure for DNA methylation sequencing saves time by not requiring bisulfite treatment of DNA (74).

State-of-the-art technologies available for epigenome analysis are reduced representation bisulfite sequencing (RRBS), MeDIP-seq, and MethylCap-seq, as well as the array-based Illumina Infinium HumanMethylation27 platform, digital restriction enzyme analysis of methylation (DREAM), 244K CpG island arrays (Agilent), transcriptome-derived deep-sequencing reads (RNA-Seq), and short bisulfite reads (bis-Seq). Streptavidin bisulfite ligand methylation enrichment (SuBLIME) enriches for methylated DNA before bisulfite treatment and deep sequencing by labeling bisulfite-treated DNA with biotin at sites of cytosine non-conversion. A general methodology used in current epigenetic studies is outlined below (75).

9.3. DNA Methylation Method (Bisulfite Modification and Detection of Methylation)

1. Sodium bisulfite modification is performed using a CpGenome DNA modification kit (Intergen).
2. DNA is denatured at 100°C for 10 min, centrifuged briefly, and kept on ice.
3. NaOH is added to a final concentration of 0.3 M in 20-μL volume, and the sample is incubated at 42°C for 20 min.
4. A sodium bisulfite solution is prepared (1.9 g of sodium metabisulfite [Sigma-Aldrich] added to 3.2 mL of 0.44 M NaOH and heated at 50°C to dissolve the bisulfate).
5. After adding hydroquinone (0.5 mL of a 1 M solution), 120 μL of this solution is mixed with each DNA sample.
6. The solution is incubated at 50°C for 16 h in the dark.
7. Sodium bisulfite treatment of DNA converts unmethylated cytosines to uracil, methylated cytosine residues remain unaffected, and the treatment generates methylation-dependent sequence differences in the DNA.
8. The methylation status of different genes is evaluated by combined restriction analysis.
9. Primers are selected to cover the CpG island. Sodium bisulfite-treated genomic DNA is amplified by fluorescence-based, real-time quantitative polymerase chain reaction (PCR).
10. The amplification step is performed with a final reaction mixture of 25 μL consisting of 600 nM of each primer; 200 nM probe; 200 μM each dATP, dCTP, and dGTP; 400 μM dUTP; 3.5 mM $MgCl_2$; 1× TaqMan buffer A and bisulfite DNA. Amplification conditions are 50°C for 2 min, 95°C for 10 min, followed by 42 cycles at 95°C for 15 s and 60°C for 1 min. For controls, one unrelated fully methylated gene, one fully unmethylated gene, and internal reference set to check input DNA also are included.
11. The methylated/unmethylated primers/probes were designed to overlap about five potential CpG dinucleotide sites.

9.4. Histone Modification Method

9.4.1. Immunoprecipitation (IP) Assay

1. ChIP is carried by lysing the cells and precipitating with specific antibodies.
2. Cells are cross-linked in 1% (v/v) formaldehyde for 10 min at 37°C before sonicating to obtain DNA fragments of 200–1,000 bp.
3. The antibodies against protein tags such as Flag are used to precipitate DNA fragments bound by cognate elements.
4. The protein-DNA complex is collected with protein A- or G-Sepharose beads, eluted, and reverse cross-linked.
5. DNA is extracted with phenol-chloroform and precipitated with ethanol. The recovered DNA is resuspended in TE buffer for PCR amplification.

9.4.2. Histone Immunoblotting

1. Cytoplasmic and nuclear extracts are prepared using the NE-PER cytoplasmic extraction reagent (Pierce Chemical).
2. To analyze histone H3 modifications, cells are trypsinized at 37°C for 45–60 s, washed twice with ice-cold phosphate-buffered saline (PBS), and resuspended in 15 μL of chilled lysis buffer per million cells.
3. Samples are incubated on ice for 30 min before centrifugation at 13,000 rpm at 4°C.
4. The supernatant is removed, and pellet resuspended in 4× strength Laemmli's buffer.
5. Samples are stored at −70°C.
6. Sodium dodecyl sulfate-polyacrylamide gel electrophoresis (SDS-PAGE) is run, and resolved proteins are electroblotted.
7. Anti-acetyl K9 antibody, anti-acetyl K14 antibody, anti-acetyl K18 antibody, anti-acetyl K23 antibody, and anti-phospho S10 antibodies are used to detect specific posttranslational modifications on histone H3.
8. Bound antibody is visualized by enhanced chemiluminescence.

10. CSC Epigenetics in Relation to iPSCs

iPSCs are a type of pluripotent stem cell that is derived artificially from a non-pluripotent cell, typically an adult somatic cell, by inducing a "forced" expression of specific genes. In many respects, iPSCs are similar to natural pluripotent stem cells such as ES cells, including in the expression of certain stem cell genes and proteins, chromatin methylation patterns, doubling time, embryoid body formation, teratoma formation, viable chimera formation, and potency and differentiability. The full extent of iPSCs' relation to natural pluripotent stem cells still is being assessed, however.

The interwoven relationships of reprogramming, induced pluripotency, and carcinogenesis provide clear clues to the relationship between iPSCs and natural pluripotent stem cells: (a) four Yamanaka factors that induce iPSC generation have been widely associated with different cancer pathways, (b) the iPSC-generating factor Nanog can be substituted for the *c-myc* oncogene (76), and (c) *p53*-defective iPSCs give rise to tumors in mice (77). Here, loss of cellular identity is due to *p53* inactivation, which in turn is linked to oncogenesis and dedifferentiation pathways. It is also assumed that an inefficient reprogramming phenomenon contributes to many differentiated cells being trapped in the iPS system. In light of these concepts, it is plausible that epigenetic events associated with iPSCs might be active in cancer in general and in CSCs in particular, and possible that pathways and epigenetic events associated with reprogramming into iPSCs might be active in cancers. The CpG island shores with altered DNA methylation in cancer are enriched among the regions that revert their methylation status during reprogramming into iPSCs (78). Because ectopic expression can erase epigenetic memory in differentiated cells while making them iPSCs, it also is plausible that many mutations in somatic cells can generate CSCs. Therefore, aberrant differentiation of progenitor cells as well as of fully differentiated cells can erase their epigenetic memory and cause cells to exhibit the CSC phenotype.

11. Concluding Remarks

Over the last decade, the CSC theory perhaps has generated as much excitement and optimism as any area of cancer research. CSCs are distinct from the other cells that form the bulk of a tumor in that they are self-perpetuating, produce progenitor cells, and consequently recreate the whole heterogeneous tumor as do traditional stem cells. The progenitor cells function to repopulate tumor cells eradicated by treatments such as chemotherapy or radiation.

The existence of CSCs is a subject of debate within biomedical research, because many studies have been unsuccessful in discovering the similarities and differences between normal tissue stem cells and CSCs. Nonetheless, there appear to be potential applications for stem cells in risk assessment, intervention, and treatment of cancer. Understanding the etiology of cancer and the origin of CSCs may help in planning novel strategies in cancer prognosis. Finding the source of cancer cells is necessary for successful cancer treatment. Similarly, if current cancer treatments do not properly destroy enough CSCs, tumor relapse will be likely—as will the possibility that treatments such as chemotherapy, for example, may leave behind only chemotherapy-resistant CSCs, making the resulting tumor most likely resistant to further chemotherapy. If

CSCs are detected early enough, a tumor can be killed off and marginalized with traditional treatment. As tumor size increases, it becomes more difficult to remove the tumor without conferring resistance and leaving enough cells behind for the tumor to reappear. More research is needed in the areas of identifying and enriching CSCs.

References

1. Waddington, C.H. (1942) The epigenotype. *Endeavour* 1, 18–20.
2. Bonasio, R., Tu, S., and Reinberg, D. (2010) Molecular signals of epigenetic states. *Science* 330, 612–616.
3. Bird, A. (2002) DNA methylation patterns and epigenetic memory. *Genes Dev* 16, 6–21.
4. Takai, D., and Jones, P. A. (2002) Comprehensive analysis of CpG islands in human chromosomes 21 and 22. *Proc Natl Acad Sci USA* 99, 3740–3745.
5. Suzuki, M. M., and Bird, A. (2008) DNA methylation landscapes: provocative insights from epigenomics. *Nat Rev Genet* 9, 465–476.
6. Weber, M., Hellmann, I., Stadler, M. B., Ramos, L., Paabo, S., Rebhan, M., and Schubeler, D. (2007) Distribution, silencing potential and evolutionary impact of promoter DNA methylation in the human genome. *Nat Genet* 39, 457–466.
7. Futscher, B. W., Oshiro, M. M., Wozniak, R. J., Holtan, N., Hanigan, C. L., Duan, H., and Domann, F. E. (2002) Role for DNA methylation in the control of cell type specific maspin expression. *Nat Genet* 31, 175–179.
8. Bodey, B. (2002) Cancer-testis antigens: promising targets for antigen directed antineoplastic immunotherapy. *Expert Opin Biol Ther* 2, 577–584.
9. Hattori, N., Nishino, K., Ko, Y. G., Hattori, N., Ohgane, J., Tanaka, S., and Shiota, K. (2004) Epigenetic control of mouse Oct-4 gene expression in embryonic stem cells and trophoblast stem cells. *J Biol Chem* 279, 17063–17069.
10. Kim, G. D., Ni, J., Kelesoglu, N., Roberts, R. J., and Pradhan, S. (2002) Co-operation and communication between the human maintenance and de novo DNA (cytosine-5) methyltransferases. *EMBO J* 21, 4183–4195.
11. Barski, A., Cuddapah, S., Cui, K., Roh, T. Y., Schones, D. E., Wang, Z., Wei, G., Chepelev, I., and Zhao, K. (2007) High-resolution profiling of histone methylations in the human genome. *Cell* 129, 823–837.
12. Wang, Z., Zang, C., Rosenfeld, J. A., Schones, D. E., Barski, A., Cuddapah, S., Cui, K., Roh, T. Y., Peng, W., Zhang, M. Q., and Zhao, K. (2008) Combinatorial patterns of histone acetylations and methylations in the human genome. *Nat Genet* 40, 897–903.
13. Kouzarides, T. (2007) Chromatin modifications and their function. *Cell* 128, 693–705.
14. Jenuwein, T. (2006) The epigenetic magic of histone lysine methylation. *FEBS J* 273, 3121–3135.
15. Hebbes, T. R., Thorne, A. W., and Crane-Robinson, C. (1988) A direct link between core histone acetylation and transcriptionally active chromatin. *EMBO J* 7, 1395–1402.
16. Cedar, H., and Bergman, Y. (2009) Linking DNA methylation and histone modification: patterns and paradigms. *Nat Rev Genet* 10, 295–304.
17. Bai, L., and Morozov, A. V. (2010) Gene regulation by nucleosome positioning. *Trends Genet* 26, 476–483.
18. Schones, D. E., Cui, K., Cuddapah, S., Roh, T. Y., Barski, A., Wang, Z., Wei, G., and Zhao, K. (2008) Dynamic regulation of nucleosome positioning in the human genome. *Cell* 132, 887–898.
19. Jin, C., and Felsenfeld, G. (2007) Nucleosome stability mediated by histone variants H3.3 and H2A.Z. *Genes Dev* 21, 1519–1529.
20. Lewis, B. P., Burge, C. B., and Bartel, D. P. (2005) Conserved seed pairing, often flanked by adenosines, indicates that thousands of human genes are microRNA targets. *Cell* 120, 15–20.
21. He, L., and Hannon, G. J. (2004) MicroRNAs: small RNAs with a big role in gene regulation. *Nat Rev Genet* 5, 522–531.
22. Halfmann, R., and Lindquist, S. (2010) Epigenetics in the extreme: prions and the inheritance of environmentally acquired traits. *Science* 330, 629–632.
23. Mosher, R. A., Lewsey, M. G., and Shivaprasad, P. V. (2010) RNA silencing in plants: Flash report! *Silence* 1, 13.

24. Feinberg, A. P., and Vogelstein, B. (1983) Hypomethylation distinguishes genes of some human cancers from their normal counterparts. *Nature* 301, 89–92.
25. Jones, P. A., and Baylin, S. B. (2002) The fundamental role of epigenetic events in cancer. *Nat Rev Genet* 3, 415–428.
26. Howard, G., Eiges, R., Gaudet, F., Jaenisch, R., and Eden, A. (2008) Activation and transposition of endogenous retroviral elements in hypomethylation induced tumors in mice. *Oncogene* 27, 404–408.
27. Greger, V., Passarge, E., Hopping, W., Messmer, E., and Horsthemke, B. (1989) Epigenetic changes may contribute to the formation and spontaneous regression of retinoblastoma. *Hum Genet* 83, 155–158.
28. Widschwendter, M., Fiegl, H., Egle, D., Mueller-Holzner, E., Spizzo, G., Marth, C., Weisenberger, D. J., Campan, M., Young, J., Jacobs, I., and Laird, P. W. (2007) Epigenetic stem cell signature in cancer. *Nat Genet* 39, 157–158.
29. Long, C., Yin, B., Lu, Q., Zhou, X., Hu, J., Yang, Y., Yu, F., and Yuan, Y. (2007) Promoter hypermethylation of the RUNX3 gene in esophageal squamous cell carcinoma. *Cancer Invest* 25, 685–690.
30. Akiyama, Y., Watkins, N., Suzuki, H., Jair, K. W., van Engeland, M., Esteller, M., Sakai, H., Ren, C. Y., Yuasa, Y., Herman, J. G., and Baylin, S. B. (2003) GATA-4 and GATA-5 transcription factor genes and potential downstream antitumor target genes are epigenetically silenced in colorectal and gastric cancer. *Mol Cell Biol* 23, 8429–8439.
31. Wu, H., Chen, Y., Liang, J., Shi, B., Wu, G., Zhang, Y., Wang, D., Li, R., Yi, X., Zhang, H., Sun, L., and Shang, Y. (2005) Hypomethylation-linked activation of PAX2 mediates tamoxifen-stimulated endometrial carcinogenesis. *Nature* 438, 981–987.
32. Brueckner, B., Stresemann, C., Kuner, R., Mund, C., Musch, T., Meister, M., Sultmann, H., and Lyko, F. (2007) The human let-7a-3 locus contains an epigenetically regulated microRNA gene with oncogenic function. *Cancer Res* 67, 1419–1423.
33. Cui, H., Cruz-Correa, M., Giardiello, F. M., Hutcheon, D. F., Kafonek, D. R., Brandenburg, S., Wu, Y., He, X., Powe, N. R., and Feinberg, A. P. (2003) Loss of IGF2 imprinting: a potential marker of colorectal cancer risk. *Science* 299, 1753–1755.
34. Kaneda, A., and Feinberg, A. P. (2005) Loss of imprinting of IGF2: a common epigenetic modifier of intestinal tumor risk. *Cancer Res* 65, 11236–11240.
35. Fraga, M. F., Ballestar, E., Villar-Garea, A., Boix-Chornet, M., Espada, J., Schotta, G., Bonaldi, T., Haydon, C., Ropero, S., Petrie, K., Iyer, N. G., Perez-Rosado, A., Calvo, E., Lopez, J. A., Cano, A., Calasanz, M. J., Colomer, D., Piris, M. A., Ahn, N., Imhof, A., Caldas, C., Jenuwein, T., and Esteller, M. (2005) Loss of acetylation at Lys16 and trimethylation at Lys20 of histone H4 is a common hallmark of human cancer. *Nat Genet* 37, 391–400.
36. Shi, Y., Lan, F., Matson, C., Mulligan, P., Whetstine, J. R., Cole, P. A., Casero, R. A., and Shi, Y. (2004) Histone demethylation mediated by the nuclear amine oxidase homolog LSD1. *Cell* 119, 941–953.
37. Ventura, A., and Jacks, T. (2009) MicroRNAs and cancer: short RNAs go a long way. *Cell* 136, 586–591.
38. Lu, J., Getz, G., Miska, E. A., Alvarez-Saavedra, E., Lamb, J., Peck, D., Sweet-Cordero, A., Ebert, B. L., Mak, R. H., Ferrando, A. A., Downing, J. R., Jacks, T., Horvitz, H. R., and Golub, T. R. (2005) MicroRNA expression profiles classify human cancers. *Nature* 435, 834–838.
39. Clarke, M. F., Dick, J. E., Dirks, P. B., Eaves, C. J., Jamieson, C. H., Jones, D. L., Visvader, J., Weissman, I. L., and Wahl, G. M. (2006) Cancer stem cells--perspectives on current status and future directions: AACR Workshop on cancer stem cells. *Cancer Res* 66, 9339–9344.
40. Furth, J., and Kahn, M.C. (1937) Transmission of leukemia of mice with a single cell. *Am J Cancer* 31, 276–282.
41. Kelly, P. N., Dakic, A., Adams, J. M., Nutt, S. L., and Strasser, A. (2007) Tumor growth need not be driven by rare cancer stem cells. *Science* 317, 337.
42. Quintana, E., Shackleton, M., Sabel, M. S., Fullen, D. R., Johnson, T. M., and Morrison, S. J. (2008) Efficient tumour formation by single human melanoma cells. *Nature* 456, 593–598.
43. Gupta, P. B., Chaffer, C. L., and Weinberg, R. A. (2009) Cancer stem cells: mirage or reality? *Nat Med* 15, 1010–1012.
44. Park, C.Y., Tseng, D., and Weissman I. L. (2009) Cancer stem cell-directed therapies: recent data from the laboratory and clinic. *Mol Ther* 17, 219–230.
45. Marotta, L. L., and Polyak, K. (2009) Cancer stem cells: a model in the making. *Curr Opin Genet Dev* 19, 44–50.
46. Singh, S. K., Hawkins, C., Clarke, I. D., Squire, J. A., Bayani, J., Hide, T., Henkelman, R. M., Cusimano, M. D., and Dirks, P. B. (2004)

Identification of human brain tumour initiating cells. *Nature* 432, 396–401.

47. Al-Hajj, M., Wicha, M. S., Benito-Hernandez, A., Morrison, S. J., and Clarke, M. F. (2003) Prospective identification of tumorigenic breast cancer cells. *Proc Natl Acad Sci USA* 100, 3983–3988.
48. Dalerba, P., Dylla, S. J., Park, I. K., Liu, R., Wang, X., Cho, R. W., Hoey, T., Gurney, A., Huang, E. H., Simeone, D. M., Shelton, A. A., Parmiani, G., Castelli, C., and Clarke, M. F. (2007) Phenotypic characterization of human colorectal cancer stem cells. *Proc Natl Acad Sci USA* 104, 10158–10163.
49. Prince, M. E., Sivanandan, R., Kaczorowski, A., Wolf, G. T., Kaplan, M. J., Dalerba, P., Weissman, I. L., Clarke, M. F., and Ailles, L. E. (2007) Identification of a subpopulation of cells with cancer stem cell properties in head and neck squamous cell carcinoma. *Proc Natl Acad Sci USA* 104, 973–978.
50. Yang, Z. F., Ho, D. W., Ng, M. N., Lau, C. K., Yu, W. C., Ngai, P., Chu, P. W., Lam, C. T., Poon, R. T., and Fan, S. T. (2008) Significance of CD90+ cancer stem cells in human liver cancer. *Cancer Cell* 13, 153–166.
51. Hermann, P. C., Huber, S. L., Herrler, T., Aicher, A., Ellwart, J. W., Guba, M., Bruns, C. J., and Heeschen, C. (2007) Distinct populations of cancer stem cells determine tumor growth and metastatic activity in human pancreatic cancer. *Cell Stem Cell* 1, 313–323.
52. Collins, A. T., Berry, P. A., Hyde, C., Stower, M. J., and Maitland, N. J. (2005) Prospective identification of tumorigenic prostate cancer stem cells. *Cancer Res* 65, 10946–10951.
53. Bussolati, B., Bruno, S., Grange, C., Ferrando, U., and Camussi, G. (2008) Identification of a tumor-initiating stem cell population in human renal carcinomas. *FASEB J* 22, 3696–3705.
54. Schatton, T., Murphy, G. F., Frank, N. Y., Yamaura, K., Waaga-Gasser, A. M., Gasser, M., Zhan, Q., Jordan, S., Duncan, L. M., Weishaupt, C., Fuhlbrigge, R. C., Kupper, T. S., Sayegh, M. H., and Frank, M. H. (2008) Identification of cells initiating human melanomas. *Nature* 451, 345–349.
55. Sell, S., and Pierce, G.B. (1994) Maturation arrest of stem cell differentiation is a common pathway for the cellular origin of teratocarcinomas and epithelial cancers. *Lab Invest* 70, 6–22.
56. Gil-Perotin, S., Marin-Husstege, M., Li, J., Soriano-Navarro, M., Zindy, F., Roussel, M.F., Garcia-Verdugo J,M., and Casaccia-Bonnefil, P. (2006) Loss of p53 induces changes in the behavior of subventricular zone cells: implication for the genesis of glial tumors. *J Neurosci* 26,1107–1116.
57. Fialkow, P. J. (1990) Stem cell origin of human myeloid blood cell neoplasms. *Verh Dtsch Ges Pathol* 74, 43–47.
58. Cozzio, A., Passegue, E., Ayton, P. M., Karsunky, H., Cleary, M. L., and Weissman, I. L. (2003) Similar MLL-associated leukemias arising from self-renewing stem cells and short-lived myeloid progenitors. *Genes Dev* 17, 3029–3035.
59. Goelz, S. E., Vogelstein, B., Hamilton, S. R., and Feinberg, A. P. (1985) Hypomethylation of DNA from benign and malignant human colon neoplasms. *Science* 228, 187–190.
60. Feinberg, A. P., Ohlsson, R., and Henikoff, S. (2006) The epigenetic progenitor origin of human cancer. *Nat Rev Genet* 7, 21–33.
61. Ohm, J. E., McGarvey, K. M., Yu, X., Cheng, L., Schuebel, K. E., Cope, L., Mohammad, H. P., Chen, W., Daniel, V. C., Yu, W., Berman, D. M., Jenuwein, T., Pruitt, K., Sharkis, S. J., Watkins, D. N., Herman, J. G., and Baylin, S. B. (2007) A stem cell-like chromatin pattern may predispose tumor suppressor genes to DNA hypermethylation and heritable silencing. *Nat Genet* 39, 237–242.
62. Bibikova, M., Chudin, E., Wu, B., Zhou, L., Garcia, E. W., Liu, Y., Shin, S., Plaia, T. W., Auerbach, J. M., Arking, D. E., Gonzalez, R., Crook, J., Davidson, B., Schulz, T. C., Robins, A., Khanna, A., Sartipy, P., Hyllner, J., Vanguri, P., Savant-Bhonsale, S., Smith, A. K., Chakravarti, A., Maitra, A., Rao, M., Barker, D. L., Loring, J. F., and Fan, J. B. (2006) Human embryonic stem cells have a unique epigenetic signature. *Genome Res* 16, 1075–1083.
63. Yuspa, S. H. (1983) Molecular and cellular basis for tumor promotion in mouse skin. *Princess Takamatsu Symp* 14, 315–326.
64. Holst, C. R., Nuovo, G. J., Esteller, M., Chew, K., Baylin, S. B., Herman, J. G., and Tlsty, T. D. (2003) Methylation of p16(INK4a) promoters occurs in vivo in histologically normal human mammary epithelia. *Cancer Res* 63, 1596–1601.
65. Hochedlinger, K., Blelloch, R., Brennan, C., Yamada, Y., Kim, M., Chin, L., and Jaenisch, R. (2004) Reprogramming of a melanoma genome by nuclear transplantation. *Genes Dev* 18, 1875–1885.
66. Sakatani, T., Kaneda, A., Iacobuzio-Donahue, C. A., Carter, M. G., de Boom Witzel, S., Okano, H., Ko, M. S., Ohlsson, R., Longo, D. L., and Feinberg, A. P. (2005) Loss of imprinting of Igf2 alters intestinal maturation

and tumorigenesis in mice. *Science* 307, 1976–1978.

67. Werbowetski-Ogilvie, T. E., Bosse, M., Stewart, M., Schnerch, A., Ramos-Mejia, V., Rouleau, A., Wynder, T., Smith, M. J., Dingwall, S., Carter, T., Williams, C., Harris, C., Dolling, J., Wynder, C., Boreham, D., and Bhatia, M. (2009) Characterization of human embryonic stem cells with features of neoplastic progression. *Nat Biotechnol* 27, 91–97.
68. Bernstein, B. E., Mikkelsen, T. S., Xie, X., Kamal, M., Huebert, D. J., Cuff, J., Fry, B., Meissner, A., Wernig, M., Plath, K., Jaenisch, R., Wagschal, A., Feil, R., Schreiber, S. L., and Lander, E. S. (2006) A bivalent chromatin structure marks key developmental genes in embryonic stem cells. *Cell* 125, 315–326.
69. Valk-Lingbeek, M. E., Bruggeman, S. W., and van Lohuizen, M. (2004) Stem cells and cancer; the polycomb connection. *Cell* 118, 409–418.
70. Muyrers-Chen, I., Hernandez-Munoz, I., Lund, A. H., Valk-Lingbeek, M. E., van der Stoop, P., Boutsma, E., Tolhuis, B., Bruggeman, S. W., Taghavi, P., Verhoeven, E., Hulsman, D., Noback, S., Tanger, E., Theunissen, H., and van Lohuizen, M. (2004) Emerging roles of Polycomb silencing in X-inactivation and stem cell maintenance. *Cold Spring Harb Symp Quant Biol* 69, 319–326.
71. Agrelo, R., and Wutz, A. (2009) Cancer progenitors and epigenetic contexts: an Xisting connection. *Epigenetics* 4, 568–570.
72. Bapat, S. A. (2007) Evolution of cancer stem cells. *Semin Cancer Biol* 17, 204–213.
73. Mathews, L. A., Crea, F., and Farrar, W. L. (2009) Epigenetic gene regulation in stem cells and correlation to cancer. *Differentiation* 78, 1–17.
74. Flusberg, B. A., Webster, D. R., Lee, J. H., Travers, K. J., Olivares, E. C., Clark, T. A., Korlach, J., and Turner, S. W. (2010) Direct detection of DNA methylation during single-molecule, real-time sequencing. *Nat Methods* 7, 461–465.
75. Kumar, D., and Verma M. (2009) Methods in cancer epigenetics and epidemiology. *Methods Mol Biol* 471, 273–288.
76. Nakagawa, M., Koyanagi, M., Tanabe, K., Takahashi, K., Ichisaka,T., Aoi, T., Okita, K., Mochiduki, Y., Takizawa, N., and Yamanaka, S. (2008) Generation of induced pluripotent stem cells without Myc from mouse and human fibroblasts. *Nat Biotechnol* 26, 101–106.
77. Hong, H., Takahashi, K., Ichisaka, T., Aoi, T., Kanagawa, O., Nakagawa, M., Okita, K., and Yamanaka, S. (2009) Suppression of induced pluripotent stem cell generation by the p53-p21 pathway. *Nature* 460, 1132–1135.
78. Doi, A., Park, I. H., Wen, B., Murakami, P., Aryee, M. J., Irizarry, R., Herb, B., Ladd-Acosta, C., Rho, J., Loewer, S., Miller, J., Schlaeger, T., Daley, G. Q., and Feinberg, A. P. (2009) Differential methylation of tissue- and cancer-specific CpG island shores distinguishes human induced pluripotent stem cells, embryonic stem cells and fibroblasts. *Nat Genet* 41, 1350–1353.

Part II

Cancer Specific Type Epigenetic Changes

Chapter 3

DNA Methylation and Histone Modifications in Breast Cancer

Ramona G. Dumitrescu

Abstract

Breast cancer is caused by progressive genetic alterations and epigenetic changes that trigger tumor development. Among the epigenetic alterations descried in breast cancer, DNA promoter methylation has been extensively studied and observed in genes involved in several critical signaling pathways that initiate and promote breast tumorigenesis. In addition to DNA hypermethylation, global methylation levels have been observed to decrease with breast cancer progression. In close connection with DNA methylation changes, histone modifications, especially the acetylation and methylation of histone lysines, play an essential role in the nucleosomes remodeling and gene expression regulation in breast cancer.

Key words: Breast cancer, DNA promoter hypermethylation, Global hypomethylation, Histones acetylation, Histones deacetylases, Histones methylation

1. Introduction

Breast cancer is the second leading cause of death among women in the USA, and it is the most frequently diagnosed tumor (1). Breast cancer is caused by progressive genetic alterations including different mutations in tumor suppressor genes, oncogenes, and other abnormalities but also by epigenetic alterations (2–5). These alterations result in abnormal transcription regulation and change in the expression profiles affecting apoptosis, cellular proliferation, survival, and differentiation. Epigenetic alterations include changes in DNA methylation patterns as well as histone modifications. The DNA methylation changes observed in breast cancer involve the promoter region hypermethylation, associated with silencing of tumor suppressor genes (5, 6), and global hypomethylation, associated with genomic instability and oncogenes' activation (7, 8). In addition to these changes of the DNA methylation patterns, there are several posttranslational modifications of the histones

Ramona G. Dumitrescu and Mukesh Verma (eds.), *Cancer Epigenetics: Methods and Protocols*, Methods in Molecular Biology, vol. 863, DOI 10.1007/978-1-61779-612-8_3, © Springer Science+Business Media, LLC 2012

that have been associated with regulation of the gene expression by modulating chromatin structure. Moreover, both DNA methylation and histone modifications have been found to be influenced by specific regulators that are involved in nucleosomal remodeling (9). Therefore, all these epigenetic changes, DNA methylation changes, and histone modifications interact to each other and lead to nucleosome remodeling involved in gene expression regulation in cancer.

2. DNA Hypermethylation

DNA hypermethylation occurs at the CpG dinucleotides that are usually cluster together to form the CpG-rich regions, called the CpG islands. These CpG islands are located in more than half of genes in the upstream promoter before the exon 1 (10). In the normal cells, these CpG islands of the active genes are usually unmethylated, allowing gene expression. However, in cancer, regional hypermethylation of the CpG islands of several tumor suppressor genes was observed (11, 12), leading to the inactivation of these genes. The first tumor suppressor gene shown to be silenced through DNA hypermethylation was *RB*, the gene associated with retinoblastoma (13). Further, many other tumor suppressor genes have been shown to be silenced in breast cancer through DNA hypermethylation (5).

Based on the Hanahan and Weinberg's detailed overview of the abnormalities that lead to cancer, Jones and coworker described the DNA methylation changes of genes involved in these capacities in breast cancer development (5). These genes are involved in cell cycle regulation (*p16*^{INK4A}, *cyclin D2*, *14-3-3*σ, *p57KIP2*), DNA repair mechanisms (*GSTP1*, *MGMT*, *BRCA1*), hormone regulation pathways (*ER*α, *ER*β, and *PR*), cellular growth–inhibitory signaling (*RAR*β, *TGF*β *SOCS1*, *RASSF1A*, *SYK*, *HIN-1*, *NES1*), programmed cell death (*HOXA5*, *DAPK*, *Twist*, *TMS1*, *GPC3*, *FHIT*), angiogenesis (*maspin* and *THBS1*), and invasion and metastasis (*E-Cadherin*, *CDH13*, *APC*, *prostasin*, *TIMP-3*, *BCSG1* genes) (5, 14).

Furthermore, the impact of aberrant DNA methylation on the clinical outcome of early stage breast cancer patients was analyzed by determining the methylation index (MI) of *MINT17*, *MINT31*, and *RAR*β*2* and it was found that 36% of the tumors had one of these genes hypermethylated and 33% of the tumors had more than one gene hypermethylated. High methylation index was a risk factor for distant recurrence and shorter disease-free survival. Based on this finding, the methylation index was considered an independent prognostic factor for breast tumors, especially for ER-negative tumors (15).

Moreover, when genome-wide analysis was used to characterize the methylation profile of metastatic breast cancers, it has been found that a breast CpG island methylator phenotype (B-CIMP), where a large number of genes are hypermethylated, can provide information about the metastatic potential of the tumors (16). More specifically, the presence of the B-CIMP in tumors showed association with low metastatic risk and survival, while the absence of the B-CIMP was associated with increased risk for metastatic disease and death. These findings suggest that these epigenetic profiles could represent new prognostic biomarkers for breast cancer.

Gene promoter DNA hypermethylation has also been observed in the serum or plasma of breast cancer cases (14), with a good correlation between tumor and blood samples from the same breast cancer patients (17–19). A study by Dulaimi et al. (20) found that DNA promoter methylation was also detectable in the serum of patients with early invasive and preinvasive breast disease, but not in serum samples from normal women, indicating specificity of the markers.

Additionally, a recent study showed that a panel of several genes involved in critical cellular pathways presented concordant hypermethylation in tumor tissue and serum samples and that this panel can be used to develop a blood-based test for breast cancer, which would be able to differentiate between tumor and normal samples, with importance for breast cancer prediction and prognostic (21).

In addition to these protein-encoding genes, several small (20–30 nucleotides) noncoding RNAs, so-called microRNAs (miRNAs) with tumor suppressor function, have been reported to be silenced through DNA methylation (22). MiRNAs are regulatory RNAs, matching the 3′ untranslated regions of target mRNAs that leads to their degradation or inhibition of mRNA translation (18). Several MiRNAs with tumor suppressor role, like the *let-7* family (with at least 11 homologous miRNAs), miR-206, miR-17-5p, miR-125a, miR-125b, miR-200, miR-34, and miR-31, have been shown to be lost in breast tumors (23, 24). Deregulation of the miRNAs has been found to be useful in the classification of mammary carcinomas (25, 26) or for determining the tumors' aggressiveness, for example, in node-negative estrogen receptor-positive tumors (27). In the ERα-positive breast cancer cell lines, it has been found that the increased expression of the miRNA-375 is involved in these cells proliferation. Several events including the loss of H3K9me2 and local global hypomethylation, dissociation of the miR-375 promoter transcriptional repressor, and interactions of ERα with specific regions of miR-375 take place. If miR-375 is inhibited in ERα-positive breast cancer cells, a reduced ERα activation and cell proliferation is observed. Further, RASD1, a target of the miRNA-375, was identified to be involved in the negative regulation of ERα expression (28).

Also, human microRNA-335, which has been shown to be involved in tumor reinitiation in breast cancer, was reported to be inactivated through genetic deletion and epigenetic promoter hypermethylation (29).

3. DNA Hypomethylation

Normal cells have repetitive genomic sequences heavily methylated, and the maintenance of this methylation plays an important role in preventing different chromosomal rearrangements including translocations and gene disruption through the reactivation of transposable elements (7, 30, 31). In cancer cells, global DNA hypomethylation has been suggested to contribute to structural changes in chromosomes, loss of imprinting, microsatellites, and chromosomes instability through abnormal activation of proto-oncogenes and aberrant recombination events and increased mutagenesis (9).

In breast cancer, global DNA hypomethylation has been found to be associated with specific tumor characteristics, including tumor size, stage, and histological grade (32). In addition, promoter hypomethylation of several proto-oncogenes involved in proliferation and metastasis (*synuclein γ* and *urokinase* genes) and drug resistance to endocrine therapy (e.g., *N-cadherin*, *ID4*, *β-catenin*, *annexin A4*, *WNT11* genes) has been reported in breast cancer (9).

Furthermore, extensive cancer-associated hypomethylation of juxtacentromeric satellite DNA and global DNA hypomethylation have been observed in even low-grade breast carcinomas, indicating that the demethylation of the genome is involved in early breast transformation (33).

When genomic methylation of leukocyte DNA was examined by measuring 5-methyldeoxycytosine (5-mdC) in stage I–IIIa breast cancer, it was observed that women with low 5-mdC level in leukocyte DNA have the higher breast cancer risk and that alcohol consumption was inversely associated with the methylation levels (34).

Moreover, when three repetitive elements (LINE1, Sat2, and Alu) were analyzed in invasive breast ductal carcinoma, adjacent normal tissue, and white blood cells (WBC), it was observed that these three repetitive elements show lower DNA methylation in tumor compared to adjacent tissue and WBC DNA. Also, a significant correlation was reported for the methylation of Sat2M1 between tumor and adjacent tissues and WBC DNA and a significant difference in methylation of this element between cases and controls (35). It has been shown before that Sat2 is a good marker of breast and also is associated with global DNA hypomethylation (33).

One of the factors that was associated with global methylation changes is the ionizing radiation (IR). More specifically, the exposure of the rat mammary gland to IR was associated with a loss of genomic cytosine methylation and a reduction in the levels of DNA methyltransferases DNMT1 and DNMT3a and 3b as well as the methyl-binding protein MeCP2. These epigenetic changes took place in the context of activation of DNA repair processes and abnormalities in the cellular signaling pathways and cell cycle control mechanisms (36).

Recently, it has been shown that impaired *BRCA1* function influences the global methylation level by the regulation of the DNMT1 gene, leading to global DNA hypomethylation, loss of genomic imprinting, and an open chromatin configuration and also to increased expression of several proto-oncogenes, including *c-Fos*, *Ha-Ras*, and *c-Myc* (37).

4. Histone Modifications and Nucleosomal Remodeling

DNA hypermethylation promoted gene silencing is closely associated with chromatin modifications with important role in the organization of the DNA in the nucleosome. Understanding the mechanisms that play a role in this interaction could provide insights in the mechanisms involved in these epigenetic changes in cancer. The histones that form the nucleosomes undergo numerous covalent modifications including acetylation, biotinylation, methylation, ubiquitination, phosphorylation, and sumoylation (38–40). Among all these modifications, histone acetylation and methylation have been found to be relatively stable and suggested as potential marks for carrying epigenetic information through cell divisions (41, 42). All these changes influence the chromatin structure, keeping it in the active or repressed state and thus initiating or inhibiting gene expression. More specifically, several modifications are associated with loosening the chromatin structure bringing it to the euchromatic state, when genes are active and the transcription is promoted. These changes that represent marks of active histones include the acetylation of lysine K5, K8, K9, K12, K18 of H3, and K16 of H4 as well as methylation at K4 of H3 (H3K4me) and arginine dimethylation (H4R3me2) (12, 38, 43, 44). Other changes like mono- (me1), di- (me2), or trimethylation (me3) of histone H3 lysine 9 (H3K9), H3K27, and H4K20 are marks of repressive histones, which initiate and maintain the closed chromatin state (heterochromatin), when genes are silenced, thus inactive (9, 12, 45, 46). It has been observed that specific histone modifications, namely, global loss of acetylation of K16 and trimethylation of K20 of histone H4, are hallmarks of human cancers (47). When some of these histone modifications were examined in 880 breast cancer specimens, it has been observed that most breast cancer samples presented low levels of H4K16ac and relatively high levels of H3K18ac and H4K20me3 (48). Also, the level of histones modifications was associated with the tumor size. More specifically, low levels of H4R3me2, H3K9ac, and H4K16ac were associated with large tumor size and vascular invasion (H4K16ac) (48). Reduced levels of histone modifications like lysine acetylation (H3K9ac, H3K18ac, and H4K12ac), lysine methylation (H3K4me2 and H4K20me3), and arginine methylation (H4R3me2) were associated with poor prognostic tumors, for example, basal-like tumors and HER-2-positive tumors. Moreover, when the histological type was analyzed in relationship to these histone marks, it was found that high global histone marks were found in lobular, mucinous, tubular, and mixed tubular breast cancers (48).

All of these covalent alterations represent the histone code that can be "written" by the enzymes involved in these modifications. Histone acetyltransferases (HATs), histone deacetylases (HDACs), histone methyltransferases (HMTs), and histone demethylases (HDMTs) have been found to be part of the nucleosomal remodeling complexes, critical for changing the chromatin structure and controlling gene expression (9, 49).

HATs can be classified into three families based on their highly conserved structural motifs: the GNAT family, the MYST family, and the p300/CBP family (46, 50). Mutations of CBP and p300 have been observed in different cancer types including breast cancers (51). One HAT of the MYST family, Hbo1 that acetylates in particular the lysines 5 and 12 of the H4, has been associated with cancer (52), having an increased expression in hormone-dependent MCF-7 breast cancer cells and in breast carcinomas (53). Also, the *Hbo1* gene is located on chromosome 17 (17q21.3), area prone to amplifications commonly reported in breast cancers. The amplification of this particular region has been associated with poor prognosis and outcome (54). Further, in primary breast cancers, it has been found that the expression of hMOF, a CBP-p300 HAT, is downregulated, and consequently, the acetylation of H4K16 is lost (55).

Eighteen HDACs have been identified in humans, and they were classified in four classes based on their homology to yeast HDACs, enzymatic activities, and cellular localization (9, 50). Class I HDACs includes HDACs 1–3 and HDAC8, class II of the HDACs is divided in two classes: IIa (HDAC4, 5, 7 and HDAC9) and class IIb (HDAC6 and 10), class III includes Sirtuin 1–7, and class IV has a unique member HDAC11. Several studies have found abnormal activity of the HDACs in breast cancer. For example, HDAC1 and 3, but not HDAC8, were observed by Feng et al. to be upregulated in breast cancers (56). In addition, HDAC1 and 3 together with E2F1 and E2F4 were responsible for the downregulation of the *ARH1* gene in breast cancer cells (56). *ARH1* gene was found to be downregulated in more than 70% of breast and ovarian tumors (57). Furthermore, it has been observed that histone H4 acetylation decreases with tumor progression from normal epithelium to ductal carcinoma in situ (DCIS) and to invasive cancer, suggesting that hypoacetylation could be an early event in breast cancer development (58). Zhang et al. found that HDAC6 expression was increased in estrogen receptor positive, low tumor grade tumors and associated with better survival (59). In addition, the inhibition of class II HDACs has been found to have an effect on cell cycle progression, apoptosis, gene expression, and ER signaling in breast tumor cells, being associated with breast cancer progression and estrogen dependence (60).

Furthermore, a recent study found that overexpression of several HDACs, HDAC 1, 6, and 8, is involved in breast cancer invasion and the expression of matrix metalloproteinase-9 (61), suggesting that these changes could be used for the development of targeted therapies for breast cancer metastasis. In addition, in breast carcinogenesis, the abnormal HDMTs and lysine deacetylases activity have been hypothesized to play an important role in the chromatin remodeling and gene expression regulation. It has been observed that histone-lysine-specific demethylase 1 (LSD1) interacts with HDACs in breast cancer cells and that the inhibition of the demethylation and deacetylation of the histones, by using inhibitors of LSD1 and class I and II HDACs, have a synergistic effect on the gene regulation and inhibition of growth, indicating an important target for breast cancer therapy (62).

In addition to these histone changes that promote chromatin remodeling and implicit genes expression, there are other proteins, chromatin-associated proteins, that recognize either the acetylated lysine sites or the methylated lysine sites (49). Among these proteins, EZH2, a component of polycomb repressor complex, can work together with HDACs and methyltransferases to further modify histone tails leading to transcriptional repression. Also, EZH2 has been reported to be involved in maintaining the gene silencing by working with the DNA methyltransferases (63).

5. Interplay Between Histone Modifications and DNA Methylation

There is an interaction between the histone modifications and DNA methylation, involved in nucleosome remodeling and gene expression regulation (12, 64). The polycomb target genes, involved in stem/progenitor differentiation, are generally associated with promoter CpG islands (65) and during epithelial differentiation, EZH2, catalyzes trimethylation of H3K27 on target nucleosomes (63), leading to the recruitment of a second repressor complex, PRC1, resulting in compact chromatin configuration. Following these changes, DNA methyltransferases and methyl-CpG-binding protein are recruited at the promoter inducing CpG islands DNA methylation (66). As a result, epigenetic suppression of several PRC-2 target genes occurs, and this can be heritable through many cell divisions (67).

In the breast progenitor cells, the epigenetic reprogramming can be deregulated by xenoestrogens exposure or inflammatory factors. It has been found that the abnormal signaling involved in the differentiation process may lead to upregulation of EZH2 and other polycomb repressor proteins, like SUZ12, BMI1, G9a, and SUV39H (68–70), resulting in the silencing of tumor suppressor genes and then abnormal proliferation of undifferentiated or semi-differentiated cells. The permanent inactivation of these genes occurs as a result of further accumulation of DNA methylation.

Furthermore, an example of the synergic action of the DNA methylation and HDACs is the finding that the combination therapy of demethylating agents and HDAC inhibitors works together in the reexpression of ER-α in ER-α-negative breast cancer cells, suggesting mechanisms that can be targeted to breast cancer therapy (71).

6. Conclusions

In conclusion, it is very important to understand that there are several epigenetic changes, namely, DNA methylation and histone modifications, that work together in nucleosome remodeling and thus regulation of specific gene expression in breast cancer.

References

1. American Cancer Society. Cancer Facts and Figures 2010. (2010). Atlanta, Georgia, American Cancer Society.
2. Hanahan, D. and Weinberg, R. A. (2000) The hallmarks of cancer. *Cell* 100, 57–70.
3. Polyak, K. (2007) Breast cancer: origins and evolution. *J Clin Invest* 117, 3155–3163.
4. Vogelstein, B. and Kinzler, K. W. (2004) Cancer genes and the pathways they control. *Nat Med* 10, 789–799.
5. Widschwendter, M. and Jones, P. A. (2002) DNA methylation and breast carcinogenesis. *Oncogene* 21, 5462–5482.
6. Baylin, S. B. and Ohm, J. E. (2006) Epigenetic gene silencing in cancer—a mechanism for early oncogenic pathway addiction? *Nat Rev Cancer* 6, 107–116.
7. Eden, A., Gaudet, F., Waghmare, A., and Jaenisch, R. (2003) Chromosomal instability and tumors promoted by DNA hypomethylation. *Science* 300, 455.
8. Feinberg, A. P. and Tycko, B. (2004) The history of cancer epigenetics. *Nat Rev Cancer* 4, 143–153.
9. Lo, P. K. and Sukumar, S. (2008) Epigenomics and breast cancer. *Pharmacogenomics* 9, 1879–1902.
10. Takai, D. and Jones, P. A. (2002) Comprehensive analysis of CpG islands in human chromosomes 21 and 22. *Proc Natl Acad Sci U. S. A* 99, 3740–3745.
11. Esteller, M., Corn, P. G., Baylin, S. B., and Herman, J. G. (2001) A gene hypermethylation profile of human cancer. *Cancer Res* 61, 3225–3229.
12. Esteller, M. (2007) Cancer epigenomics: DNA methylomes and histone-modification maps. *Nat Rev Genet* 8, 286–298.

13. Greger, V., Passarge, E., Hopping, W., Messmer, E., and Horsthemke, B. (1989) Epigenetic changes may contribute to the formation and spontaneous regression of retinoblastoma. *Hum Genet* 83, 155–158.
14. Brooks, J., Cairns, P., and Zeleniuch-Jacquotte, A. (2009) Promoter methylation and the detection of breast cancer. *Cancer Causes Control* 20, 1539–1550.
15. van Hoesel, A. Q., Van, d., V, Kuppen, P. J., Putter, H., de Kruijf, E. M., van Nes, J. G., Giuliano, A. E., and Hoon, D. S. (2011) Primary tumor classification according to methylation pattern is prognostic in patients with early stage ER-negative breast cancer. *Breast Cancer Res Treat*
16. Fang, F., Turcan, S., Rimner, A., Kaufman, A., Giri, D., Morris, L. G., Shen, R., Seshan, V., Mo, Q., et al. (2011) Breast cancer methylomes establish an epigenomic foundation for metastasis. *Sci Transl Med* 3, 75ra25.
17. Hu, X. C., Wong, I. H., and Chow, L. W. (2003) Tumor-derived aberrant methylation in plasma of invasive ductal breast cancer patients: clinical implications. *Oncol Rep* 10, 1811–1815.
18. Mirza, S., Sharma, G., Prasad, C. P., Parshad, R., Srivastava, A., Gupta, S. D., and Ralhan, R. (2007) Promoter hypermethylation of TMS1, BRCA1, ERalpha and PRB in serum and tumor DNA of invasive ductal breast carcinoma patients. *Life Sci* 81, 280–287.
19. Sharma, G., Mirza, S., Prasad, C. P., Srivastava, A., Gupta, S. D., and Ralhan, R. (2007) Promoter hypermethylation of p16INK4A, p14ARF, CyclinD2 and Slit2 in serum and tumor DNA from breast cancer patients. *Life Sci* 80, 1873–1881.
20. Dulaimi, E., Hillinck, J., Ibanez, d. C., I, Al-Saleem, T., and Cairns, P. (2004) Tumor suppressor gene promoter hypermethylation in serum of breast cancer patients. *Clin Cancer Res* 10, 6189–6193.
21. Radpour, R., Barekati, Z., Kohler, C., Lv, Q., Burki, N., Diesch, C., Bitzer, J., Zheng, H., Schmid, S., and Zhong, X. Y. (2011) Hypermethylation of tumor suppressor genes involved in critical regulatory pathways for developing a blood-based test in breast cancer. *PLoS One* 6, e16080.
22. Lujambio, A., Ropero, S., Ballestar, E., Fraga, M. F., Cerrato, C., Setien, F., Casado, S., Suarez-Gauthier, A., Sanchez-Cespedes, M., et al. (2007) Genetic unmasking of an epigenetically silenced microRNA in human cancer cells. *Cancer Res* 67, 1424–1429.
23. O'Day, E. and Lal, A. (2010) MicroRNAs and their target gene networks in breast cancer. *Breast Cancer Res* 12, 201.
24. Veeck, J. and Esteller, M. (2010) Breast cancer epigenetics: from DNA methylation to microRNAs. *J Mammary Gland Biol Neoplasia* 15, 5–17.
25. Blenkiron, C., Goldstein, L. D., Thorne, N. P., Spiteri, I., Chin, S. F., Dunning, M. J., Barbosa-Morais, N. L., Teschendorff, A. E., Green, A. R., et al. (2007) MicroRNA expression profiling of human breast cancer identifies new markers of tumor subtype. *Genome Biol* 8, R214.
26. Liu, J., Getz, G., Miska, E. Alvarez-Saavedra, E., Lamb, J., Peck, D., Sweet-Cordero, A., Ebert, B. L., Mak, R. H., et al. (2005) MicroRNA expression profiles classify human cancers. *Nature* 435, 834–838.
27. Foekens, J. A., Sieuwerts, A. M., Smid, M., Look, M. P., de, W., V, Boersma, A. W., Klijn, J. G., Wiemer, E. A. and Martens, J. W. (2008) Four miRNAs associated with aggressiveness of lymph node-negative, estrogen receptor-positive human breast cancer. *Proc Natl Acad Sci U. S. A* 105, 13021–13026.
28. de Souza Rocha, S. P., Breiling, A., Gupta, N., Malekpour, M., Youns, M., Omranipour, R., Malekpour, F., Volinia, S., Croce, C. M., et al. (2010) Epigenetically deregulated microRNA-375 is involved in a positive feedback loop with estrogen receptor alpha in breast cancer cells. *Cancer Res* 70, 9175–9184.
29. Png, K. J., Yoshida, M., Zhang, X. H., Shu, W., Lee, H., Rimner, A., Chan, T. A., Comen, E., Andrade, V. P., et al. (2011) MicroRNA-335 inhibits tumor reinitiation and is silenced through genetic and epigenetic mechanisms in human breast cancer. *Genes Dev* 25, 226–231.
30. Ehrlich, M. (2002) DNA hypomethylation, cancer, the immunodeficiency, centromeric region instability, facial anomalies syndrome and chromosomal rearrangements. *J Nutr* 132, 2424 S–2429 S.
31. Jones, P. A. and Baylin, S. B. (2002) The fundamental role of epigenetic events in cancer. *Nat Rev Genet* 3, 415–428.
32. Soares, J., Pinto, A. E., Cunha, C. V., Andre, S., Barao, I., Sousa, J. M., and Cravo, M. (1999) Global DNA hypomethylation in breast carcinoma: correlation with prognostic factors and tumor progression. *Cancer* 85, 112–118.
33. Jackson, K., Yu, M. C., Arakawa, K., Fiala, E., Youn, B., Fiegl, H., Muller-Holzner, E., Widschwendter, M., and Ehrlich, M. (2004) DNA hypomethylation is prevalent even in low-grade breast cancers. *Cancer Biol Ther* 3, 1225–1231.
34. Choi, J. Y., James, S. R., Link, P. A., McCann, S. E., Hong, C. C., Davis, W., Nesline, M. K., Ambrosone, C. B., and Karpf, A. R. (2009) Association between global DNA hypomethy-

lation in leukocytes and risk of breast cancer. *Carcinogenesis* 30, 1889–1897.

35. Cho, Y. H., Yazici, H., Wu, H. C., Terry, M. B., Gonzalez, K., Qu, M., Dalay, N., and Santella, R. M. (2010) Aberrant promoter hypermethylation and genomic hypomethylation in tumor, adjacent normal tissues and blood from breast cancer patients. *Anticancer Res* 30, 2489–2496.
36. Loree, J., Koturbash, I., Kutanzi, K., Baker, M., Pogribny, I., and Kovalchuk, O. (2006) Radiation-induced molecular changes in rat mammary tissue: possible implications for radiation-induced carcinogenesis. *Int J Radiat Biol* 82, 805–815.
37. Shukla, V., Coumoul, X., Lahusen, T., Wang, R. H., Xu, X., Vassilopoulos, A., Xiao, C., Lee, M. H., Man, Y. G., et al. (2010) BRCA1 affects global DNA methylation through regulation of DNMT1. *Cell Res* 20, 1201–1215.
38. Schubeler, D., MacAlpine, D. M., Scalzo, D., Wirbelauer, C., Kooperberg, C., van, L. F., Gottschling, D. E., O'Neill, L. P., Turner, B. M., et al. (2004) The histone modification pattern of active genes revealed through genome-wide chromatin analysis of a higher eukaryote. *Genes Dev* 18, 1263–1271.
39. Shiio, Y. and Eisenman, R. N. (2003) Histone sumoylation is associated with transcriptional repression. *Proc Natl Acad Sci U. S. A* 100, 13225–13230.
40. Shilatifard, A. (2006) Chromatin modifications by methylation and ubiquitination: implications in the regulation of gene expression. *Annu Rev Biochem* 75, 243–269.
41. Barski, A., Cuddapah, S., Cui, K., Roh, T. Y., Schones, D. E., Wang, Z., Wei, G., Chepelev, I., and Zhao, K. (2007) High-resolution profiling of histone methylations in the human genome. *Cell* 129, 823–837.
42. Wang, Z., Zang, C., Rosenfeld, J. A., Schones, D. E., Barski, A., Cuddapah, S., Cui, K., Roh, T. Y., Peng, W., et al. (2008) Combinatorial patterns of histone acetylations and methylations in the human genome. *Nat Genet* 40, 897–903.
43. Bernstein, B. E., Kamal, M., Lindblad-Toh, K., Bekiranov, S., Bailey, D. K., Huebert, D. J., McMahon, S., Karlsson, E. K., Kulbokas, E. J., III et al. (2005) Genomic maps and comparative analysis of histone modifications in human and mouse. *Cell* 120, 169–181.
44. Schneider, R., Bannister, A. J., Myers, F. A., Thorne, A. W., Crane-Robinson, C., and Kouzarides, T. (2004) Histone H3 lysine 4 methylation patterns in higher eukaryotic genes. *Nat Cell Biol* 6, 73–77.
45. Jenuwein, T. and Allis, C. D. (2001) Translating the histone code. *Science* 293, 1074–1080.
46. Kouzarides, T. (2007) Chromatin modifications and their function. *Cell* 128, 693–705.
47. Fraga, M. F., Ballestar, E., Villar-Garea, A., Boix-Chornet, M., Espada, J., Schotta, G., Bonaldi, T., Haydon, C., Ropero, S., et al. (2005) Loss of acetylation at Lys16 and trimethylation at Lys20 of histone H4 is a common hallmark of human cancer. *Nat Genet* 37, 391–400.
48. Elsheikh, S. E., Green, A. R., Rakha, E. A., Powe, D. G., Ahmed, R. A., Collins, H. M., Soria, D., Garibaldi, J. M., Paish, C. E., et al. (2009) Global histone modifications in breast cancer correlate with tumor phenotypes, prognostic factors, and patient outcome. *Cancer Res* 69, 3802–3809.
49. Wang, Z., Zang, C., Cui, K., Schones, D. E., Barski, A., Peng, W., and Zhao, K. (2009) Genome-wide mapping of HATs and HDACs reveals distinct functions in active and inactive genes. *Cell* 138, 1019–1031.
50. Dalvai, M. and Bystricky, K. (2010) The role of histone modifications and variants in regulating gene expression in breast cancer. *J Mammary Gland Biol Neoplasia* 15, 19–33.
51. Iyer, N. G., Ozdag, H., and Caldas, C. (2004) p300/CBP and cancer. *Oncogene* 23, 4225–4231.
52. Avvakumov, N. and Cote, J. (2007) The MYST family of histone acetyltransferases and their intimate links to cancer. *Oncogene* 26, 5395–5407.
53. Iizuka, M., Takahashi, Y., Mizzen, C. A., Cook, R. G., Fujita, M., Allis, C. D., Frierson, H. F., Jr., Fukusato, T., and Smith, M. M. (2009) Histone acetyltransferase Hbo1: catalytic activity, cellular abundance, and links to primary cancers. *Gene* 436, 108–114.
54. Hyman, E., Kauraniemi, P., Hautaniemi, S., Wolf, M., Mousses, S., Rozenblum, E., Ringner, M., Sauter, G., Monni, O., et al. (2002) Impact of DNA amplification on gene expression patterns in breast cancer. *Cancer Res* 62, 6240–6245.
55. Pfister, S., Rea, S., Taipale, M., Mendrzyk, F., Straub, B., Ittrich, C., Thuerigen, O., Sinn, H. P., Akhtar, A., and Lichter, P. (2008) The histone acetyltransferase hMOF is frequently downregulated in primary breast carcinoma and medulloblastoma and constitutes a biomarker for clinical outcome in medulloblastoma. *Int J Cancer* 122, 1207–1213.
56. Feng, W., Lu, Z., Luo, R. Z., Zhang, X., Seto, E., Liao, W. S., and Yu, Y. (2007) Multiple histone deacetylases repress tumor suppressor gene ARHI in breast cancer. *Int J Cancer* 120, 1664–1668.
57. Yu, Y., Xu, F., Peng, H., Fang, X., Zhao, S., Li, Y., Cuevas, B., Kuo, W. L., Gray, J. W., et al. (1999) NOEY2 (ARHI), an imprinted putative tumor

suppressor gene in ovarian and breast carcinomas. *Proc Natl Acad Sci U. S. A* 96, 214–219.

58. Suzuki, J., Chen, Y. Y., Scott, G. K., DeVries, S., Chin, K., Benz, C. C., Waldman, F. M., and Hwang, E. S. (2009) Protein acetylation and histone deacetylase expression associated with malignant breast cancer progression. *Clin Cancer Res* 15, 3163–3171.
59. Zhang, Z., Yamashita, H., Toyama, T., Sugiura, H., Omoto, Y., Ando, Y., Mita, K., Hamaguchi, M., Hayashi, S., and Iwase, H. (2004) HDAC6 expression is correlated with better survival in breast cancer. *Clin Cancer Res* 10, 6962–6968.
60. Duong, V., Bret, C., Altucci, L., Mai, A., Duraffourd, C., Loubersac, J., Harmand, P. O., Bonnet, S., Valente, S., et al. (2008) Specific activity of class II histone deacetylases in human breast cancer cells. *Mol Cancer Res* 6, 1908–1919.
61. Park, S. Y., Jun, J. A., Jeong, K. J., Heo, H. J., Sohn, J. S., Lee, H. Y., Park, C. G., and Kang, J. (2011) Histone deacetylases 1, 6 and 8 are critical for invasion in breast cancer. *Oncol Rep* 25, 1677–1681.
62. Huang, Y., Vasilatos, S. N., Boric, L., Shaw, P. G., and Davidson, N. E. (2011) Inhibitors of histone demethylation and histone deacetylation cooperate in regulating gene expression and inhibiting growth in human breast cancer cells. *Breast Cancer Res Treat.*
63. Sparmann, A. and van, L. M. (2006) Polycomb silencers control cell fate, development and cancer. *Nat Rev Cancer* 6, 846–856.
64. Ballestar, E. and Esteller, M. (2005) The epigenetic breakdown of cancer cells: from DNA methylation to histone modifications. *Prog Mol Subcell Biol* 38, 169–181.
65. Meissner, A., Mikkelsen, T. S., Gu, H., Wernig, M., Hanna, J., Sivachenko, A., Zhang, X., Bernstein, B. E., Nusbaum, C., et al. (2008) Genome-scale DNA methylation maps of pluripotent and differentiated cells. *Nature* 454, 766–770.
66. Hinshelwood, R. A., Melki, J. R., Huschtscha, L. I., Paul, C., Song, J. Z., Stirzaker, C., Reddel, R. R., and Clark, S. J. (2009) Aberrant de novo methylation of the p16INK4A CpG island is initiated post gene silencing in association with chromatin remodelling and mimics nucleosome positioning. *Hum Mol Genet* 18, 3098–3109.
67. Cheng, A. S., Culhane, A. C., Chan, M. W., Venkataramu, C. R., Ehrich, M., Nasir, A., Rodriguez, B. A., Liu, J., Yan, P. S., et al. (2008) Epithelial progeny of estrogen-exposed breast progenitor cells display a cancer-like methylome. *Cancer Res* 68, 1786–1796.
68. Dimri, G. P., Martinez, J. L., Jacobs, J. J., Keblusek, P., Itahana, K., van, L. M., Campisi, J., Wazer, D. E., and Band, V. (2002) The Bmi-1 oncogene induces telomerase activity and immortalizes human mammary epithelial cells. *Cancer Res* 62, 4736–4745.
69. Kleer, C. G., Cao, Q., Varambally, S., Shen, R., Ota, I., Tomlins, S. A., Ghosh, D., Sewalt, R. G., Otte, A. P., et al. (2003) EZH2 is a marker of aggressive breast cancer and promotes neoplastic transformation of breast epithelial cells. *Proc Natl Acad Sci U. S. A* 100, 11606–11611.
70. Lehnertz, B., Ueda, Y., Derijck, A. A., Braunschweig, U., Perez-Burgos, L., Kubicek, S., Chen, T., Li, E., Jenuwein, T., and Peters, A. H. (2003) Suv39h-mediated histone H3 lysine 9 methylation directs DNA methylation to major satellite repeats at pericentric heterochromatin. *Curr Biol* 13, 1192–1200.
71. Giacinti, L., Claudio, P. P., Lopez, M., and Giordano, A. (2006) Epigenetic information and estrogen receptor alpha expression in breast cancer. *Oncologist* 11, 1-8.

Chapter 4

DNA Methylation Changes in Prostate Cancer

Wolfgang Goering, Michael Kloth, and Wolfgang A. Schulz

Abstract

Epigenetic alterations contribute significantly to the development and progression of prostate cancer, the most prevalent malignant tumor in males of Western industrialized countries. Here, we review recent research on DNA methylation alterations in this cancer type. Hypermethylation of several genes including *GSTP1* is well known to occur in a consistent and apparently coordinate fashion during the transition from intraepithelial neoplasia to frank carcinoma. These hypermethylation events have shown promise as biomarkers for detection of prostate carcinoma. Many other individual genes have been shown to undergo hypermethylation, which is typically associated with diminished expression. These investigations indicate additional candidates for biomarkers; in particular, hypermethylation events associated with progression can be employed to identify more aggressive cases. In addition, some of genes silenced by aberrant methylation in prostate have been shown to exhibit properties of tumor suppressors, revealing insights into mechanisms of carcinogenesis. Whereas most studies in the past have used candidate gene approaches, new techniques allowing genome-wide screening for altered methylation are increasingly employed in prostate cancer research and have already yielded encouraging results.

Key words: Biomarker, DNA hypermethylation, DNA hypomethylation, Prostate adenocarcinoma, Cancer epigenetics

1. Introduction

Prostate carcinoma is a major health problem of older men in Western industrialized countries. In the United States, more than 217,000 men are diagnosed with this cancer annually at a median manifestation age of 69 years, of which around 32,000 will die from the disease (1). These are typical figures for Western industrialized countries, whereas the incidence of the disease is lower in other regions, especially Asia. Still, recently, a 2,700 years old skeleton of a Scythian king was diagnosed with prostate cancer using modern microscopic and biochemical techniques (2). While prostate cancer is thus not a new disease, its prevalence appears to have

Ramona G. Dumitrescu and Mukesh Verma (eds.), *Cancer Epigenetics: Methods and Protocols*, Methods in Molecular Biology, vol. 863, DOI 10.1007/978-1-61779-612-8_4, © Springer Science+Business Media, LLC 2012

increased, not only because of population aging. In particular, the availability of highly sensitive tests for the prostate-specific antigen (PSA) has led to earlier diagnoses of prostate cancer during the last decades, creating the novel dilemma of how to distinguish indolent cancers, which are better treated by active surveillance or watchful waiting than radical treatment.

Thus, current treatment of prostate cancer faces major clinical challenges. First, due to widespread PSA testing, an increasing number of patients are diagnosed with carcinomas that progress very slowly. These cases can, to some extent, be circumscribed by low grading, i.e., Gleason grades = 3 in biopsies, low PSA, and confinement to the organ according to imaging techniques. However, distinguishing indolent from aggressive forms is far from perfectly achieved by current histopathological and clinical techniques (3, 4). Second, cancers persisting despite surgery and radiotherapy can be restrained over some time by antiandrogenic treatments. However, once they become resistant to this treatment, castration-resistant prostate cancers (CRPC, formerly called HRPC) develop which are essentially incurable and often highly aggressive. The mortality of prostate cancer, nowadays, is mostly due to CPRC. Although many of the mechanisms involved in the progression towards castration resistance are better understood today, it is still difficult to find appropriate treatments, especially because of their diversity. In particular, advanced prostate cancers metastasize preferably to bone, which has a great impact on patient morbidity and contributes to mortality (3). Therefore, uncovering the molecular mechanisms leading to castration resistance and underlying bone tropism are a major focus of clinically oriented prostate cancer research. Moreover, molecular biomarkers that enable differentiating between indolent and aggressive prostate cancers at the time of detection will greatly improve prostate cancer treatment by allowing individualized treatment. DNA methylation changes hold major promise for achieving that latter goal, as will be discussed later in this chapter.

2. Genetic Changes in Prostate Cancer

Many genetic alterations occurring during development and progression of prostate cancer have been identified over the last 2 decades (3). Briefly, recurrent common chromosomal aberrations are losses and gains of chromosome 8p and 8q, respectively, losses at 5q, 6q, 10q, 13q, 16q, 18 and gains at 1q, 3q, 7 and Xq12, respectively (5, 6). Of note, it is not likely that there is a single linear sequence of genetic alterations during prostate cancer progression. Rather, these alterations occur as preferred combinations and to different degrees in cancers with different clinical course.

However, either alone or in combination, they do not allow a sufficiently precise subtyping for clinical practice (7). Although most of the above chromosomal losses or gains have been defined for quite some time, it is still debated which specific genes on each chromosome are associated with prostate cancer. Allelic loss or mutations of "classical" tumor suppressors, *PTEN*, *RB1*, and *TP53*, are predominantly found in advanced stage prostate cancers, and mutations in common proto-oncogenes, such as the *RAS* family, are overall rare.

Intriguingly, more than 50% of all prostate cancers harbor chromosomal rearrangements leading to deregulated expression of members of the *ETS* transcription factor family (8). *ETS* gene arrangements in prostate cancer depend on androgen-stimulated corecruitment of the androgen receptor (AR) and the TOP2B topoisomerase, where the AR mediates chromosomal proximity of the involved chromosomal regions (9, 10) and TOP2B contributes to DNA double-strand breaks (11). Additionally, hypomorphic genetic variants in DNA repair genes like *ESCO1* and *POLI* were linked to oncogenic *ETS* gene arrangements (12). The predominant *ETS* gene arrangement is a translocation on chromosome 21q giving rise to a fusion gene, in which the androgen-responsive *TMPRSS2* promoter drives the expression of a N-terminally truncated, presumably overactive ERG transcription factor. As the two original genes are located around 3 Mb apart, the fusion can occur as an interchromosomal translocation or as an interstitional deletion (13–15).

While it is quite well established that the appearance of *TMPRSS2-ERG* fusions marks the transition from prostatic intraepithelial neoplasia (PIN) to prostate carcinoma (16), the functional consequences of this fusion and novel analogous rearrangements (17) are not fully understood. Most likely, the *ETS* fusion oncogenes cooperate with other alterations. In vivo experiments using transgenic mice expressing truncated human ERG result in a weak PIN phenotype (3), whereas mice with *TMPRSS2-ERG* fusion and loss of *Pten* develop high-grade PIN and adenocarcinoma (18, 19). Additionally, overexpression of truncated *ETS* genes promotes cell migration and invasion in several cell culture models, and conversely, knockdown of different ETS factors in prostate cancer cell lines decreases their invasiveness (3, 16). Recently, whole-genome chromatin immunoprecipitation analyses revealed involvement of ERG in androgen receptor (AR) signaling. ERG binds to AR downstream targets inducing epigenetic silencing of prostate epithelial differentiation pathways (20). Taken together, *ETS* gene rearrangements are strongly AR dependent and likely promote prostate cancer progression by disrupting differentiation pathways and increasing invasiveness.

While the oncogenic nature of the *ETS* fusion genes is now generally accepted, their prognostic value is still under investigation. Three independent studies including watchful waiting (21) and radical prostatectomy (13, 22) as treatments have suggested a poorer outcome for patients with *TMPRSS2-ERG* fusions, especially with 21q interstitional deletions. Several studies report *ETS* fusions to be associated with either higher Gleason grade, increased stage, or decreased PSA recurrence-free survival, whereas other studies indicate no connection to aggressive prostate carcinoma features or, remarkably, correlate *ETS* fusions with a more favorable outcome (16). Additionally, a favorable prognosis of prostate cancer was associated with expression of a fusion transcript from an alternative *TMPRSS2* starting exon (23).

3. The Significance of Epigenetic Changes in Prostate Cancer

Epigenetic alterations, sometimes termed "epimutations," contribute to the development and progression of most human cancers. They cause stable changes in gene expression affecting many aspects of the transformed cell phenotype. For instance, genes silenced by hypermethylation in prostate cancer are involved in DNA repair, apoptosis, cell cycle control, steroid hormone response, and metastasis (24). More fundamentally, epigenetic changes taking place at the initiation stage could contribute to the establishment of a tumor stem cell population, fixing the phenotype of these precursor cells and that of their aberrantly differentiated descendents (25). In its most radical form, the "epigenetic precursor cell" hypothesis posits that epigenetic changes on their own suffice to establish tumor stem cells. As argued elsewhere (26), it is more likely that in prostate cancer, genetic and epigenetic alterations conspire to establish an aberrant precursor cell population and differentiation lineage. The pertinent genetic changes may comprise *ETS* gene fusions, as discussed above, and particular chromosomal changes such as chromosome 8p or 6q loss that characterize subgroups of prostate cancer (27). The most relevant epigenetic alterations in this respect might be a series of DNA hypermethylation events that have been closely linked with the initiation phase of prostate cancer (28–30) and have been interpreted as an "epigenetic catastrophe" (31) in an evocative, but appropriate term. These changes in DNA hypermethylation are evidently related to changes in the expression and activity of chromatin regulator proteins, especially the polycomb complex PRC2. As in other cancer types (32, 33), polycomb target genes are preferentially hypermethylated in prostate cancer (34), and the number of hypermethylation events correlates with the degree of overexpression of the PRC2 catalytic component EZH2 (35). The details of the mechanisms by which polycomb complexes and other chromatin regulators interact with DNA methyltransferases to bring about hypermethylation are still under intense investigation and have been reviewed by others (36, 37). Therefore, the present contribution will largely focus on DNA hypermethylation.

Importantly, aberrant epigenetic regulation is involved not only in the initiation process of prostate cancer but also in the progression phase of the disease. With respect to DNA hypermethylation, this implies that a number of genes, as detailed below, become hypermethylated during the initiation phase of prostate cancer in a very consistent fashion. This means that these events are well suited for detection of the disease, but that they provide little information for prognostic purposes. Other genes are hypermethylated in a fraction of the cases or become hypermethylated only during progression to a metastatic or hormone-refractory stage. A priori, these seem to be better suited for prognostic and predictive purposes.

Other epigenetic changes are likewise associated with progression rather than initiation. These include certain chromatin modifications (38, 39), an increase in polycomb factor expression (35, 40), and the so-called global DNA hypomethylation.

Global hypomethylation evident by the decrease of total 5-methylcytosine (5meC) contents has been found in most cancer types and affects especially retroelements, like LINE-1, ALUs, and HERVs, which are densely methylated in normal cells. Hypomethylation sets in at different cancer stages in different cancer types and can be either associated with cancer initiation or cancer progression (26, 41). For example, in bladder cancer, hypomethylation of LINE-1 or HERV-K retroelements was found in very early cancer stages or even adjacent benign tissue, suggesting that it is associated with the initiation of the disease (42), as in colorectal cancer (43). In prostate cancer, hypomethylation is generally associated with tumor progression, and the depletion of 5meC, as well as comprehensive hypomethylation of retroelements, is regularly found in advanced cancer stages (26, 44). Likewise, hypomethylation-related overexpression of cancer-testis antigen genes is largely restricted to advanced stages (44, 45). In contrast, loss of imprinting (LOI) due to hypomethylation at the differential methylated region (DMR) of the *IGF2* gene was observed in aging benign prostates before carcinomas occur (46, 47). The mechanisms underlying this overall decrease in 5meC and the loss of DNA methylation at repeat sequences in human cancers are still unknown. Several explanations have been proposed (26, 41, 48), including loss of a major regulator of DNA methylation, uncoupling of DNA methyltransferase activity from DNA replication, guanosine base modification due to oxidative stress, and insufficient concentrations of the methyl group donor *S*-adenosylmethionine (SAM).

4. DNA Hypermethylation in Prostate Cancer

The extent and consistency of DNA hypermethylation in prostate cancer is remarkable. By 2007, more than 50 genes had been reported to be hypermethylated in prostate cancer (49, 50). Of these, roughly a dozen genes including *GSTP1*, *RASSF1A*, and

APC are consistently affected in the vast majority of prostate cancer cases and attempts to use DNA hypermethylation for cancer detection focus on those genes.

The best characterized gene encodes glutathione *S*-transferase P1 (GSTP1) and was found to be hypermethylated by Lee et al. (51), a finding confirmed by several independent groups in other populations (52, 53). The high incidence of *GSTP1* promoter hypermethylation implicates this as an early event during cancer development. Indeed, changes in *GSTP1* methylation can be already observed in high-grade PIN precursor lesions (28, 50). Likewise, RASSF1A, a negative regulator of Ras signaling, is downregulated by promoter hypermethylation commonly in 49–99% of carcinomas (24). DNA methylation of *RASSF1A* was also found in benign areas of cancer-carrying prostates, but in a less dense pattern (29, 54). In addition, *RARB2*, *NKX2-5*, and *ESR1* showed age-related changes in CpG-island methylation (55). Such findings suggest that hypermethylation of certain genes in the aging prostate occurs as a "field effect," predisposing to or accompanying the development of carcinomas. Of note, methylation levels of *AR*, *RARB2*, *NKX2-5*, *SPARC*, and *TIMP3* were significantly higher in prostate samples of healthy African-American males compared to prostate samples of Caucasian males, which may contribute to the higher risk for prostate cancer in the former population (56).

For daily clinical practice and for the patients' benefit, prostate cancer diagnostic based on minimal invasive methods would represent a powerful tool for diagnosis and prognosis, supplementing the combination of digital rectal examination and PSA testing in present use. The PSA screening method for early detection of prostate cancer is unfortunately not optimal due to the high proportion of false-positive and false-negative results (sensitivity 90%; specificity 10–31%) (57, 58). As reviewed in ref. (50), *GSTP1* hypermethylation has been explored for detection of prostate cancer by examining CpG-island methylation in clinical samples such as plasma and serum, prostate secretions, voided urine, and prostate biopsy specimens. The most convincing results were obtained by using urine samples after prostatic massage detecting prostate cancer with 98% specificity and 73% overall sensitivity. The ratio of DNA methylation at *GSTP1* and *MYOD1* in tissue samples was likewise proposed as a useful method for prostate cancer detection (59, 60), delivering higher sensitivity than histological analysis alone. Generally, combining DNA methylation analyses of *GSTP1* with other genes revealed better detection rates with improved sensitivity and specificity (Table 1) compared to *GSTP1* DNA methylation alone. Combining DNA methylation analyses of *RASSF1*, *RARB2*, *MDR1*, and *APC* with *GSTP1* uncovered prostate cancer reliably regardless of whether tissue, urine, or blood serum samples were used (29, 61–65). Using a high-throughput

Table 1
Development of DNA-methylation-related biomarkers in prostate cancers

Genes	Analyzed samples	Parameter	References
MLL2, MLL3, NSD1, DNMT3A, MBD4, SRCAP	Prostate tissues	Expression	(39)
RASSF1A, RARB2, APC, GSTP1	Prostate tissues; urine	Methylation	(29, 62, 63)
GSTP1, APC, MDR1	Prostate tissues	Methylation	(65)
GSTP1/MYOD1	Prostate tissues	Methylation ratio	(59)
RARB2, GSTP1	Prostate tissues	Methylation	(61)
FLNC, EFS, ECRG4, PITX2, PDLIM4, KCNMA1	Prostate tissues	Methylation	(61)
APC, HOXD3, TGFB2	Prostate tissues	Methylation	(69)
RASSF1A, RARB2, GSTP1	Serum	Methylation	(64)

MassCLEAVE/MassARRAY method (66) to quantify the methylation status of eight genes including *RARB2*, *GSTP1*, *FLNC*, *EFS*, *ECRG4*, *PITX2*, *PDLIM4*, and *KCNMA1* (61), a combination of *RARB2* and *GSTP1* was revealed as the most useful marker for detecting prostate cancer. Combinations of the remaining six genes improved prediction of biochemical, local, and systemic recurrence of prostate cancer.

As discussed elsewhere (26), in addition to DNA methylation itself, several genes involved in epigenetical silencing were shown to be upregulated in prostate cancer. They include the polycomb-associated protein SIRT1, a NAD^+-dependent histone deacetylase (35, 67), and EZH2, which is elevated particularly in metastatic cases (40). Therefore, expression analysis of genes involved in epigenetic silencing may likewise provide useful tools for prostate cancer detection and prognosis. Very recently, one interesting approach based on expression microarrays revealed a combination of the expression levels of six additional genes involved in epigenetical regulation (*MLL2*, *MLL3*, *NSD1*, *DNMT3A*, *MBD4*, *SRCAP*) as a useful marker set to distinguish nonmalignant from cancerous tissue (39).

Ongoing scientific work will unravel new genes suitable as markers for the detection or prognosis of prostate cancer and identify new putative targets for the treatment of prostate cancer. For instance, the methylation level of *APC* was related to biochemical recurrence and cancer-specific mortality in some, but not all studies (68–70). Of note, the DNA methylation pattern at silenced genes is often not homogeneous, and the results of methylation analyses depend on the chosen method and, more strongly, on the CpG sites examined (71).

Many further single genes have been analyzed for their methylation, their function, and their applicability as biomarkers for prostate cancer detection and prognosis. The studies compiled in Table 2 are often based on investigations of prostate cell lines and small sets of prostate cancer tissues. Typically, they investigate DNA methylation changes in prostate cancers and assess the correlation between promoter DNA methylation and expression of the gene in question. In a typical study of this sort, mRNA and protein expression of HRK, a member of the Bcl-2 family regulating apoptosis, was described as markedly reduced in tissue samples (72). *HRK* DNA methylation was assessed by methylation-specific PCR (MS-PCR), revealing a good correlation between *HRK* DNA methylation and expression. The *SLC5A8* gene coding for a potential tumor suppressor protein showed lower expression in 7 out of 10 prostate cancer samples compared to matched benign samples correlating with dense methylation of its promoter (73). *BTG-3*, a further candidate tumor suppressor gene, was downregulated in prostate cancer cell lines and in a small set of tumors ($n=8$) compared to matched benign cells and samples, respectively (74). Interestingly, the authors reported a decrease of DNMTs activities and an increase of histone acetyl transferase (HAT) activity after treatment of LNCaP and PC-3 cells with the demethylating agent 5-aza-2′-deoxycytidine (5-azadC) and the tyrosine kinase and DNA topoisomerase II inhibitor genistein. Likewise, Sprouty1, a regulator of FGF signaling, exhibits decreased expression in prostate cancer cell lines correlating with promoter methylation. Detailed promoter analysis using luciferase reporter gene approaches revealed a direct link between expression and promoter methylation (75) confirming preliminary results by our group (76). Of note, in all studies mentioned, silenced gene expression was restored in prostate cancer cell lines by treatment with 5-azadC. In summary, such exploratory studies provide candidate genes for prostate cancer detection, prognosis, or treatment, often allowing insights into pathomechanisms.

Several studies listed in Table 2 used larger sets of prostate tissue specimens for additional evaluation of relation to clinicopathologic parameters. For instance, suppressor of cytokine signaling 3 (*SOCS3*) is hypermethylated in about 40% (20/51) of prostate cancer tissues, strongly correlating with higher Gleason scores and a worse prognosis (77). Tissue samples exhibiting *SOCS3* DNA hypermethylation display weaker mRNA and protein expression. Likewise, *TNFRSF10C* and *TNFRSF10D* (commonly referred to as *DcR1* and *DcR2*), encoding two TRAIL decoy receptors, were described as hypermethylated in 50% of prostate cancer cases using conventional MS-PCR (78). Further investigations revealed significant downregulation of *DcR1* and *DcR2* expression due to

Table 2
Hypermethylated genes in prostate cancer: an update

Gene	DNA methylation analysis	Expression analysis	Functional analysis	References
BTG3	BS-Seq	mRNA (qRT-PCR)	–	(74)
CADM2	MS-PCR BS-Seq	mRNA (RT-PCR) Protein (WB, IHC)	+	(95)
Clusterin	BS-Seq	mRNA (qRT-PCR, microarray)	–	(108)
EN1	DNA methylation headloop PCR	mRNA (qRT-PCR)	–	(109)
EPB41L3	MS-PCR	mRNA (qRT-PCR) Protein (IHC)	–	(30)
EPHA7	MS-PCR BS-Seq	mRNA (RT-PCR) Protein (WB, IHC)	+	(110)
FYN	BS-Seq	mRNA (qRT-PCR) Protein (WB, IHC)	–	(98)
ID4	MS-PCR	mRNA (RT-PCR) Protein (WB)	+	(96)
INHBB	DNA methylation headloop PCR	mRNA (qRT-PCR)	–	(109)
HRK	MS-PCR	mRNA (RT-PCR) Protein (IHC)	–	(72)
LPL	BS-Seq	mRNA (qRT-PCR)	–	(111)
MCAM	MS-PCR BS-Seq	Protein (IHC, TMA)	+	(93)
PITX2	QM real-time PCR	–	–	(84)
SCTR	DNA methylation headloop PCR	mRNA (qRT-PCR)	–	(109)
SLC18A2	BS-Seq	Protein (WB, IHC, TMA)	–	(99)
SLC5A8	BS-Seq QM real-time PCR	mRNA (RT-PCR)	–	(73)
SOCS3	MS-PCR BS-Seq	mRNA (qRT-PCR) Protein (IHC)	–	(77)
SOX7	MS-PCR BS-Seq	mRNA (qRT-PCR) Protein (IHC)	+	(94)
Sprouty1	Pyrosequencing	mRNA (qRT-PCR)	–	(75)
TFPI2	BS-Seq	mRNA (qRT-PCR)	–	(112)

(continued)

Table 2 (continued)

Gene	DNA methylation analysis	Expression analysis	Functional analysis	References
TNFRSF10C/DcR1	MS-PCR BS-Seq	mRNA (qRT-PCR)	–	(78, 79)
TNFRSF10D/DcR2	MS-PCR BS-Seq	mRNA (qRT-PCR)	–	(78, 79)

BS-Seq bisulfite sequencing, *IHC* immunohistochemistry, *MS-PCR* methylation-specific PCR, *QM real-time PCR* quantitative methylation real-time PCR, *qRT-PCR* quantitative reverse transcription PCR, *TMA* tissue microarray, *WB* western blot

DNA hypermethylation and detailed methylation analysis using bisulfite sequencing uncovered a patchy methylation pattern (79). Lower expression of *DcR1,* but not *DcR2,* correlates strongly with a poorer clinical outcome (79), and hypermethylation of the *DcR1* promoter was found related to clinicopathologic parameters, like high clinical stage, high Gleason sum, and high serum PSA (80).

Aberrant DNA methylation of the paired-like homeodomain transcription factor 2 (*PITX2*) gene, whose mutation causes Rieger syndrome by physical or functional haploinsufficiency (81–83), was found in several cancers, including AML, breast, and prostate cancer (84–86). This methylation event provides good prognostic values (87), even if examined in blood and bone marrow (88). In prostate cancer, *PITX2* promoter hypermethylation was strongly and independently associated with biochemical recurrence after radical prostatectomy in several studies (61, 84, 89, 90). Strangely, studies assessing the *PITX2* expression in correlation to DNA hypermethylation are rare. In a large set of breast cancer cell lines, DNA methylation correlated inversely with mRNA expression levels (91). In prostate cancer, our group detected dramatically reduced *PITX2* expression in prostate cancer samples and cell lines that correlated highly significantly with *PITX2* DNA methylation (92).

Notably, the correlation between expression and DNA methylation is not universal. For instance, Liu et al. (93) investigated DNA methylation of the melanoma cell adhesion molecule (*MCAM*) in prostate cancer specimens using quantitative MS-PCR. Although 80% (70/88) of the analyzed tumor samples exhibited DNA methylation, no correlation to protein expression assessed by tissue microarray was evident. In addition, treatment with 5azadC showed no effect on *MCAM* expression, revealing regulation independent of DNA methylation. Nevertheless, *MCAM* DNA methylation was associated with higher tumor stage and Gleason score.

In the course of prostate cancer development and progression, DNA methylation may contribute to silencing of tumor suppressor genes. Reconstituting the expression of the respective genes may reduce the tumorigenicity of tumor cells. In fact, ectopic expression of SOX7 suppresses proliferation and inhibits the transcription activated by an endogenous mutant β-catenin in prostate and colorectal cancer cell lines (94). *SOX7* downregulation occurred in 47% of the prostate cancer specimens, and DNA methylation using MS-PCR was found in 48% (10/21) of these samples. Treatment of LNCaP prostate carcinoma cells with 5azadC restored *SOX7* mRNA levels. Likewise, 5azadC treatment reconstituted expression of the cell adhesion molecule *CADM2*, a candidate tumor suppressor gene, in the prostate cancer cell lines DU145 and LNCaP (95). Ectopic CADM2 expression reduced colony-forming ability in soft agar and decreased proliferation in DU145 cells. Similarly, ectopic expression of inhibitor of differentiation 4 (ID4) in DU145, in which it is silenced, decreased proliferation via S-phase arrest and induced morphological changes towards a more epithelial phenotype (96). Of note, the authors selected ID4 as a putative candidate gene from the Oncomine™ (Compendia Bioscience) database (97) by searching for genes downregulated in different independent larger scale expression studies. Such meta-analyses will become more and more attractive for *in silico* preselection of candidate genes. Sorensen et al. (98) found the *FYN* tyrosine kinase gene downregulated in six independent Oncomine studies. They further assessed expression and promoter methylation in a small set of carcinoma and benign samples and found downregulation of *FYN* expression and an aberrant DNA methylation pattern in prostate carcinoma specimens compared to benign samples. The same group reported later the vesicular monoamine transporter 2 (SLC18A2), selected by reanalysis of microarray and SNP array studies, to be downregulated in 90% of a large set of prostate cancer tissues ($n = 506$) compared to benign samples according to a tissue microarray (99). In several prostate cancer, cell lines expression of *SLC18A2* was linked to DNA hypermethylation, which was found to be heterogeneous using bisulfite sequencing. Lowered cytoplasmic expression of SLC18A2 correlated significantly with poorer clinical outcome.

Over the last years, studies using high-throughput analyses in combination with extensive *in silico* methods have become ever more relevant in profiling cancer DNA methylation (100, 101). This development has led to an increasing number of publications reporting hypermethylation of multiple genes in prostate cancer (Table 3). Using automated denaturing high-performance liquid chromatography (DHPLC) in combination with *in silico* based preselection, Murphy et al. (102) detected seven genes (*BIK*, *BNIP3*, *cFLIP*, *TMS1*, *DcR1*, *DcR2*, *CDKN2A*) to be fully or partially methylated in several prostate cancer cells, delivering new

Table 3
Recent genome-wide screening studies for prostate-cancer-related DNA hypermethylation

Genes	Method	References
HOXD3, BMP7, various	Differential CpG-island array	(104)
KRT7, TACSTD2, SLC15A3, GADD45d, IFI30, ANXA2, AQP3	Microarray following 5-aza-2-deoxycytidine treatment	(107)
BIK, BNIP3, cFLIP, TMS1, DcR1, DcR2, CDKN2A	*In silico* preselection; DHPLC	(102)
TNF-α pathway genes	Genome-wide methylation assay	(103)

promising marker for prostate cancer detection or prognosis. Very recently, a large-scale methylation detection approach based on a genome-wide methylation assay (Infinium Methylation Assay; Illumina) detected roughly 1,000 significantly hypermethylated genes in prostate tumor tissues (103). Pathway analysis of the genes with altered methylation patterns identified the involvement of a network of genes regulated by TNF-α. In another high-throughput genome-wide methylation analysis, more than 200 genes were uncovered as differentially methylated between low- and high-grade prostate cancers by genomic CpG-island microarrays (104). In further investigations, methylation of *HOXD3*, which may be involved in TGFβ pathway regulation (105), was described as a good prognostic marker for biochemical recurrence by the same group (69, 106).

Screening for DNA hypermethylation can also be performed by expression microarrays following 5azadC treatment, assuming that demethylation by the drug leads to reactivation of genes repressed by hypermethylation (107). This approach disclosed nearly 3,000 genes upregulated by 5azadC treatment, leading to the detection of at least seven genes (*KRT7*, *TACSTD2*, *SLC15A3*, *GADD45d*, *IFI30*, *ANXA2*, *AQP3*) hypermethylated in prostate cancer.

5. Conclusion

Given the current rapid development of large-scale genome screening and sequencing techniques, it is likely that the coming years will see a comprehensive elucidation of DNA methylation alterations in prostate cancer. This will provide further candidates for biomarker development and further insights into prostate cancer pathogenesis. Already, it is evident that DNA methylation alterations in prostate cancer are highly prevalent and constitute a crucial factor in the development and progression of the disease. The hypermethylation events associated with prostate cancer initiation that were identified in the 1990s and at the beginning of the last decade are already explored as biomarkers for improved detection of prostate cancer delivering promising results, and certain methylation changes are clearly associated with worse outcome. One major open question is whether specific subtypes of the disease might be identified by combinations of hypermethylation (and perhaps hypomethylation) events. This is one of the topics that might be answered by more comprehensive studies. Further open questions are which mechanisms are responsible for the catastrophic change in methylation patterns at the initiation of prostate cancer and which mechanisms underlie the further changes during progression, especially global hypomethylation. The association between deregulation of chromatin regulator proteins such as EZH2 and other polycombs with altered DNA methylation is a first step in this direction, but much further work will be needed. The answer to these questions will also reveal deep insights into prostate cancer pathogenesis. A final question is which of the methylation changes in prostate cancer are functionally important as opposed to those that may occur only as a byproduct or consequence of overall epigenetic dysregulation. Again, upcoming comprehensive analyses of DNA methylation and, in particular, studies integrating genetic, epigenetic, and expression changes will provide a clearer picture of prostate cancer initiation and progression. Nevertheless, we expect that elucidating the functional consequences of DNA methylation changes will present major challenges for research for quite some time yet. As predicted in this chapter, during the preparation of the book, several further large scale studies on DNA methylation changes in prostate cancer have been published (113–117).

References

1. American Cancer Society 2010. *Cancer facts & figures 2010*, American Cancer Society, Atlanta, GA.
2. Schultz, M., Parzinger, H., Posdnjakov, D.V., Chikisheva, T.A. and Schmidt-Schultz, T.H. (2007) Oldest known case of metastasizing prostate carcinoma diagnosed in the skeleton of a 2,700-year-old Scythian king from Arzhan (Siberia, Russia). *Int J Cancer* 121, 2591–2595.
3. Shen, M.M. and Abate-Shen, C. (2010) Molecular genetics of prostate cancer: new prospects for old challenges. *Genes Dev* 24, 1967–2000.
4. Sartor, A.O., Hricak, H., Wheeler, T.M., Coleman, J., Penson, D.F., Carroll, P.R., Rubin, M.A. and Scardino, P.T. (2008) Evaluating localized prostate cancer and identifying candidates for focal therapy. *Urology* 72, S12–24.
5. Ribeiro, F.R., Henrique, R., Hektoen, M., Berg, M., Jeronimo, C., Teixeira, M.R. and Lothe, R.A. (2006) Comparison of chromosomal and array-based comparative genomic hybridization for the detection of genomic imbalances in primary prostate carcinomas. *Mol Cancer* 5, 33.
6. Sun, J., Liu, W., Adams, T.S., Li, X., Turner, A.R., Chang, B., Kim, J.W., Zheng, S.L., Isaacs, W.B. and Xu, J. (2007) DNA copy number alterations in prostate cancers: a combined analysis of published CGH studies. *Prostate* 67, 692–700.
7. Taylor, B.S., Schultz, N., Hieronymus, H., Gopalan, A., Xiao, Y., Carver, B.S., Arora, V.K., Kaushik, P., Cerami, E., Reva, B.,

Antipin, Y., Mitsiades, N., Landers, T., Dolgalev, I., Major, J.E., Wilson, M., Socci, N.D., Lash, A.E., Heguy, A., Eastham, J.A., Scher, H.I., Reuter, V.E., Scardino, P.T., Sander, C., Sawyers, C.L. and Gerald, W.L. (2010) Integrative genomic profiling of human prostate cancer. *Cancer Cell* 18, 11–22.

8. Kumar-Sinha, C., Tomlins, S.A. and Chinnaiyan, A.M. (2008) Recurrent gene fusions in prostate cancer. *Nat Rev Cancer* 8, 497–511.
9. Lin, C., Yang, L., Tanasa, B., Hutt, K., Ju, B.G., Ohgi, K., Zhang, J., Rose, D.W., Fu, X.D., Glass, C.K. and Rosenfeld, M.G. (2009) Nuclear receptor-induced chromosomal proximity and DNA breaks underlie specific translocations in cancer. *Cell* 139, 1069–1083.
10. Mani, R.S., Tomlins, S.A., Callahan, K., Ghosh, A., Nyati, M.K., Varambally, S., Palanisamy, N. and Chinnaiyan, A.M. (2009) Induced chromosomal proximity and gene fusions in prostate cancer. *Science* 326, 1230.
11. Haffner, M.C., Aryee, M.J., Toubaji, A., Esopi, D.M., Albadine, R., Gurel, B., Isaacs, W.B., Bova, G.S., Liu, W., Xu, J., Meeker, A.K., Netto, G., De Marzo, A.M., Nelson, W.G. and Yegnasubramanian, S. (2010) Androgen-induced TOP2B-mediated double-strand breaks and prostate cancer gene rearrangements. *Nat Genet* 42, 668–675.
12. Luedeke, M., Linnert, C.M., Hofer, M.D., Surowy, H.M., Rinckleb, A.E., Hoegel, J., Kuefer, R., Rubin, M.A., Vogel, W. and Maier, C. (2009) Predisposition for TMPRSS2-ERG fusion in prostate cancer by variants in DNA repair genes. *Cancer Epidemiol Biomarkers Prev* 18, 3030–3035.
13. Perner, S., Demichelis, F., Beroukhim, R., Schmidt, F.H., Mosquera, J.M., Setlur, S., Tchinda, J., Tomlins, S.A., Hofer, M.D., Pienta, K.G., Kuefer, R., Vessella, R., Sun, X.W., Meyerson, M., Lee, C., Sellers, W.R., Chinnaiyan, A.M. and Rubin, M.A. (2006) TMPRSS2:ERG fusion-associated deletions provide insight into the heterogeneity of prostate cancer. *Cancer Res* 66, 8337–8341.
14. Iljin, K., Wolf, M., Edgren, H., Gupta, S., Kilpinen, S., Skotheim, R.I., Peltola, M., Smit, F., Verhaegh, G., Schalken, J., Nees, M. and Kallioniemi, O. (2006) TMPRSS2 fusions with oncogenic ETS factors in prostate cancer involve unbalanced genomic rearrangements and are associated with HDAC1 and epigenetic reprogramming. *Cancer Res* 66, 10242–10246.
15. Teixeira, M.R. (2008) Chromosome mechanisms giving rise to the TMPRSS2-ERG fusion oncogene in prostate cancer and HGPIN lesions. *Am J Surg Pathol* 32, 642–644; author reply 4.
16. Tomlins, S.A., Bjartell, A., Chinnaiyan, A.M., Jenster, G., Nam, R.K., Rubin, M.A. and Schalken, J.A. (2009) ETS gene fusions in prostate cancer: from discovery to daily clinical practice. *Eur Urol* 56, 275–286.
17. Berger, M.F., Lawrence, M.S., Demichelis, F., Drier, Y., Cibulskis, K., Sivachenko, A.Y., Sboner, A., Esgueva, R., Pflueger, D., Sougnez, C., Onofrio, R., Carter, S.L., Park, K., Habegger, L., Ambrogio, L., Fennell, T., Parkin, M., Saksena, G., Voet, D., Ramos, A.H., Pugh, T.J., Wilkinson, J., Fisher, S., Winckler, W., Mahan, S., Ardlie, K., Baldwin, J., Simons, J.W., Kitabayashi, N., MacDonald, T.Y., Kantoff, P.W., Chin, L., Gabriel, S.B., Gerstein, M.B., Golub, T.R., Meyerson, M., Tewari, A., Lander, E.S., Getz, G., Rubin, M.A. and Garraway, L.A. (2011) The genomic complexity of primary human prostate cancer. *Nature* 470, 214–220.
18. King, J.C., Xu, J., Wongvipat, J., Hieronymus, H., Carver, B.S., Leung, D.H., Taylor, B.S., Sander, C., Cardiff, R.D., Couto, S.S., Gerald, W.L. and Sawyers, C.L. (2009) Cooperativity of TMPRSS2-ERG with PI3-kinase pathway activation in prostate oncogenesis. *Nat Genet* 41, 524–526.
19. Carver, B.S., Tran, J., Gopalan, A., Chen, Z., Shaikh, S., Carracedo, A., Alimonti, A., Nardella, C., Varmeh, S., Scardino, P.T., Cordon-Cardo, C., Gerald, W. and Pandolfi, P.P. (2009) Aberrant ERG expression cooperates with loss of PTEN to promote cancer progression in the prostate. *Nat Genet* 41, 619–624.
20. Yu, J., Mani, R.S., Cao, Q., Brenner, C.J., Cao, X., Wang, X., Wu, L., Li, J., Hu, M., Gong, Y., Cheng, H., Laxman, B., Vellaichamy, A., Shankar, S., Li, Y., Dhanasekaran, S.M., Morey, R., Barrette, T., Lonigro, R.J., Tomlins, S.A., Varambally, S., Qin, Z.S. and Chinnaiyan, A.M. (2010) An integrated network of androgen receptor, polycomb, and TMPRSS2-ERG gene fusions in prostate cancer progression. *Cancer Cell* 17, 443–454.
21. Attard, G., Clark, J., Ambroisine, L., Fisher, G., Kovacs, G., Flohr, P., Berney, D., Foster, C.S., Fletcher, A., Gerald, W.L., Moller, H., Reuter, V., De Bono, J.S., Scardino, P., Cuzick, J. and Cooper, C.S. (2008) Duplication of the fusion of TMPRSS2 to ERG sequences identifies fatal human prostate cancer. *Oncogene* 27, 253–263.
22. Yoshimoto, M., Joshua, A.M., Cunha, I.W., Coudry, R.A., Fonseca, F.P., Ludkovski, O.,

Zielenska, M., Soares, F.A. and Squire, J.A. (2008) Absence of TMPRSS2:ERG fusions and PTEN losses in prostate cancer is associated with a favorable outcome. *Mod Pathol* 21, 1451–1460.

23. Hermans, K.G., Boormans, J.L., Gasi, D., van Leenders, G.J., Jenster, G., Verhagen, P.C. and Trapman, J. (2009) Overexpression of prostate-specific TMPRSS2(exon 0)-ERG fusion transcripts corresponds with favorable prognosis of prostate cancer. *Clin Cancer Res* 15, 6398–6403.
24. Park, J.Y. (2010) Promoter hypermethylation in prostate cancer. *Cancer Control* 17, 245–255.
25. Feinberg, A.P., Ohlsson, R. and Henikoff, S. (2006) The epigenetic progenitor origin of human cancer. *Nat Rev Genet* 7, 21–33.
26. Schulz, W.A. and Hoffmann, M.J. (2009) Epigenetic mechanisms in the biology of prostate cancer. *Semin Cancer Biol* 19, 172–180.
27. Lapointe, J., Li, C., Giacomini, C.P., Salari, K., Huang, S., Wang, P., Ferrari, M., Hernandez-Boussard, T., Brooks, J.D. and Pollack, J.R. (2007) Genomic profiling reveals alternative genetic pathways of prostate tumorigenesis. *Cancer Res* 67, 8504–8510.
28. Brooks, J.D., Weinstein, M., Lin, X., Sun, Y., Pin, S.S., Bova, G.S., Epstein, J.I., Isaacs, W.B. and Nelson, W.G. (1998) CG island methylation changes near the GSTP1 gene in prostatic intraepithelial neoplasia. *Cancer Epidemiol Biomarkers Prev* 7, 531–536.
29. Florl, A.R., Steinhoff, C., Muller, M., Seifert, H.H., Hader, C., Engers, R., Ackermann, R. and Schulz, W.A. (2004) Coordinate hypermethylation at specific genes in prostate carcinoma precedes LINE-1 hypomethylation. *Br J Cancer* 91, 985–994.
30. Schulz, W.A., Ingenwerth, M., Djuidje, C.E., Hader, C., Rahnenfuhrer, J. and Engers, R. (2010) Changes in cortical cytoskeletal and extracellular matrix gene expression in prostate cancer are related to oncogenic ERG deregulation. *BMC Cancer* 10, 505.
31. Yegnasubramanian, S., Kowalski, J., Gonzalgo, M.L., Zahurak, M., Piantadosi, S., Walsh, P.C., Bova, G.S., De Marzo, A.M., Isaacs, W.B. and Nelson, W.G. (2004) Hypermethylation of CpG islands in primary and metastatic human prostate cancer. *Cancer Res* 64, 1975–1986.
32. Schlesinger, Y., Straussman, R., Keshet, I., Farkash, S., Hecht, M., Zimmerman, J., Eden, E., Yakhini, Z., Ben-Shushan, E., Reubinoff, B.E., Bergman, Y., Simon, I. and Cedar, H. (2007) Polycomb-mediated methylation on Lys27 of histone H3 pre-marks genes for de novo methylation in cancer. *Nat Genet* 39, 232–236.
33. Widschwendter, M., Fiegl, H., Egle, D., Mueller-Holzner, E., Spizzo, G., Marth, C., Weisenberger, D.J., Campan, M., Young, J., Jacobs, I. and Laird, P.W. (2007) Epigenetic stem cell signature in cancer. *Nat Genet* 39, 157–158.
34. Gal-Yam, E.N., Egger, G., Iniguez, L., Holster, H., Einarsson, S., Zhang, X., Lin, J.C., Liang, G., Jones, P.A. and Tanay, A. (2008) Frequent switching of Polycomb repressive marks and DNA hypermethylation in the PC3 prostate cancer cell line. *Proc Natl Acad Sci U S A* 105, 12979–12984.
35. Hoffmann, M.J., Engers, R., Florl, A.R., Otte, A.P., Muller, M. and Schulz, W.A. (2007) Expression changes in EZH2, but not in BMI-1, SIRT1, DNMT1 or DNMT3B are associated with DNA methylation changes in prostate cancer. *Cancer Biol Ther* 6, 1403–1412.
36. Morey, L. and Helin, K. (2010) Polycomb group protein-mediated repression of transcription. *Trends Biochem Sci* 35, 323–332.
37. McCabe, M.T., Brandes, J.C. and Vertino, P.M. (2009) Cancer DNA methylation: molecular mechanisms and clinical implications. *Clin Cancer Res* 15, 3927–3937.
38. Seligson, D.B., Horvath, S., McBrian, M.A., Mah, V., Yu, H., Tze, S., Wang, Q., Chia, D., Goodglick, L. and Kurdistani, S.K. (2009) Global levels of histone modifications predict prognosis in different cancers. *Am J Pathol* 174, 1619–1628.
39. Bianco-Miotto, T., Chiam, K., Buchanan, G., Jindal, S., Day, T.K., Thomas, M., Pickering, M.A., O'Loughlin, M.A., Ryan, N.K., Raymond, W.A., Horvath, L.G., Kench, J.G., Stricker, P.D., Marshall, V.R., Sutherland, R.L., Henshall, S.M., Gerald, W.L., Scher, H.I., Risbridger, G.P., Clements, J.A., Butler, L.M., Tilley, W.D., Horsfall, D.J. and Ricciardelli, C. (2010) Global levels of specific histone modifications and an epigenetic gene signature predict prostate cancer progression and development. *Cancer Epidemiol Biomarkers Prev* 19, 2611–2622.
40. Varambally, S., Dhanasekaran, S.M., Zhou, M., Barrette, T.R., Kumar-Sinha, C., Sanda, M.G., Ghosh, D., Pienta, K.J., Sewalt, R.G., Otte, A.P., Rubin, M.A. and Chinnaiyan, A.M. (2002) The polycomb group protein EZH2 is involved in progression of prostate cancer. *Nature* 419, 624–629.
41. Wilson, A.S., Power, B.E. and Molloy, P.L. (2007) DNA hypomethylation and human diseases. *Biochim Biophys Acta* 1775, 138–162.

42. Florl, A.R., Lower, R., Schmitz-Drager, B.J. and Schulz, W.A. (1999) DNA methylation and expression of LINE-1 and HERV-K provirus sequences in urothelial and renal cell carcinomas. *Br J Cancer* 80, 1312–1321.
43. Suter, C.M., Martin, D.I. and Ward, R.L. (2004) Hypomethylation of L1 retrotransposons in colorectal cancer and adjacent normal tissue. *Int J Colorectal Dis* 19, 95–101.
44. Yegnasubramanian, S., Haffner, M.C., Zhang, Y., Gurel, B., Cornish, T.C., Wu, Z., Irizarry, R.A., Morgan, J., Hicks, J., DeWeese, T.L., Isaacs, W.B., Bova, G.S., De Marzo, A.M. and Nelson, W.G. (2008) DNA hypomethylation arises later in prostate cancer progression than CpG island hypermethylation and contributes to metastatic tumor heterogeneity. *Cancer Res* 68, 8954–8967.
45. Hoffmann, M.J., Muller, M., Engers, R. and Schulz, W.A. (2006) Epigenetic control of CTCFL/BORIS and OCT4 expression in urogenital malignancies. *Biochem Pharmacol* 72, 1577–1588.
46. Fu, V.X., Dobosy, J.R., Desotelle, J.A., Almassi, N., Ewald, J.A., Srinivasan, R., Berres, M., Svaren, J., Weindruch, R. and Jarrard, D.F. (2008) Aging and cancer-related loss of insulin-like growth factor 2 imprinting in the mouse and human prostate. *Cancer Res* 68, 6797–6802.
47. Bhusari, S., Yang, B., Huang, W. and Jarrard, D.F. (2011) Insulin-like Growth Factor-2(IGF2) Loss of Imprinting Marks a Field Defect Within Human Prostates Containing Cancer. *The Prostate*, in press.
48. Franco, R., Schoneveld, O., Georgakilas, A.G. and Panayiotidis, M.I. (2008) Oxidative stress, DNA methylation and carcinogenesis. *Cancer Lett* 266, 6–11.
49. Nelson, W.G., Yegnasubramanian, S., Agoston, A.T., Bastian, P.J., Lee, B.H., Nakayama, M. and De Marzo, A.M. (2007) Abnormal DNA methylation, epigenetics, and prostate cancer. *Front Biosci* 12, 4254–4266.
50. Li, L.C. (2007) Epigenetics of prostate cancer. *Front Biosci* 12, 3377–3397.
51. Lee, W.H., Morton, R.A., Epstein, J.I., Brooks, J.D., Campbell, P.A., Bova, G.S., Hsieh, W.S., Isaacs, W.B. and Nelson, W.G. (1994) Cytidine methylation of regulatory sequences near the pi-class glutathione S-transferase gene accompanies human prostatic carcinogenesis. *Proc Natl Acad Sci U S A* 91, 11733–11737.
52. Jeronimo, C., Henrique, R., Hoque, M.O., Mambo, E., Ribeiro, F.R., Varzim, G., Oliveira, J., Teixeira, M.R., Lopes, C. and Sidransky, D. (2004) A quantitative promoter methylation profile of prostate cancer. *Clin Cancer Res* 10, 8472–8478.
53. Santourlidis, S., Florl, A., Ackermann, R., Wirtz, H.C. and Schulz, W.A. (1999) High frequency of alterations in DNA methylation in adenocarcinoma of the prostate. *Prostate* 39, 166–174.
54. Aitchison, A., Warren, A., Neal, D. and Rabbitts, P. (2007) RASSF1A promoter methylation is frequently detected in both pre-malignant and non-malignant microdissected prostatic epithelial tissues. *Prostate* 67, 638–644.
55. Kwabi-Addo, B., Chung, W., Shen, L., Ittmann, M., Wheeler, T., Jelinek, J. and Issa, J.P. (2007) Age-related DNA methylation changes in normal human prostate tissues. *Clin Cancer Res* 13, 3796–3802.
56. Kwabi-Addo, B., Wang, S., Chung, W., Jelinek, J., Patierno, S.R., Wang, B.D., Andrawis, R., Lee, N.H., Apprey, V., Issa, J.P. and Ittmann, M. (2010) Identification of differentially methylated genes in normal prostate tissues from African American and Caucasian men. *Clin Cancer Res* 16, 3539–3547.
57. Ahmed, H. (2010) Promoter Methylation in Prostate Cancer and its Application for the Early Detection of Prostate Cancer Using Serum and Urine Samples. *Biomark Cancer* 2010, 17–33.
58. Hessels, D., Verhaegh, G.W., Schalken, J.A. and Witjes, J.A. (2004) Applicability of biomarkers in the early diagnosis of prostate cancer. *Expert Rev Mol Diagn* 4, 513–526.
59. Jeronimo, C., Usadel, H., Henrique, R., Oliveira, J., Lopes, C., Nelson, W.G. and Sidransky, D. (2001) Quantitation of GSTP1 methylation in non-neoplastic prostatic tissue and organ-confined prostate adenocarcinoma. *J Natl Cancer Inst* 93, 1747–1752.
60. Harden, S.V., Sanderson, H., Goodman, S.N., Partin, A.A., Walsh, P.C., Epstein, J.I. and Sidransky, D. (2003) Quantitative GSTP1 methylation and the detection of prostate adenocarcinoma in sextant biopsies. *J Natl Cancer Inst* 95, 1634–1637.
61. Vanaja, D.K., Ehrich, M., Van den Boom, D., Cheville, J.C., Karnes, R.J., Tindall, D.J., Cantor, C.R. and Young, C.Y. (2009) Hypermethylation of genes for diagnosis and risk stratification of prostate cancer. *Cancer Invest* 27, 549–560.
62. Hoque, M.O., Topaloglu, O., Begum, S., Henrique, R., Rosenbaum, E., Van Criekinge, W., Westra, W.H. and Sidransky, D. (2005) Quantitative methylation-specific polymerase chain reaction gene patterns in urine sediment

distinguish prostate cancer patients from control subjects. *J Clin Oncol* 23, 6569–6575.

63. Roupret, M., Hupertan, V., Yates, D.R., Catto, J.W., Rehman, I., Meuth, M., Ricci, S., Lacave, R., Cancel-Tassin, G., de la Taille, A., Rozet, F., Cathelineau, X., Vallancien, G., Hamdy, F.C. and Cussenot, O. (2007) Molecular detection of localized prostate cancer using quantitative methylation-specific PCR on urinary cells obtained following prostate massage. *Clin Cancer Res* 13, 1720–1725.
64. Sunami, E., Shinozaki, M., Higano, C.S., Wollman, R., Dorff, T.B., Tucker, S.J., Martinez, S.R., Mizuno, R., Singer, F.R. and Hoon, D.S. (2009) Multimarker circulating DNA assay for assessing blood of prostate cancer patients. *Clin Chem* 55, 559–567.
65. Enokida, H., Shiina, H., Urakami, S., Igawa, M., Ogishima, T., Li, L.C., Kawahara, M., Nakagawa, M., Kane, C.J., Carroll, P.R. and Dahiya, R. (2005) Multigene methylation analysis for detection and staging of prostate cancer. *Clin Cancer Res* 11, 6582–6588.
66. Ehrich, M., Field, J.K., Liloglou, T., Xinarianos, G., Oeth, P., Nelson, M.R., Cantor, C.R. and van den Boom, D. (2006) Cytosine methylation profiles as a molecular marker in non-small cell lung cancer. *Cancer Res* 66, 10911–10918.
67. Huffman, D.M., Grizzle, W.E., Bamman, M.M., Kim, J.S., Eltoum, I.A., Elgavish, A. and Nagy, T.R. (2007) SIRT1 is significantly elevated in mouse and human prostate cancer. *Cancer Res* 67, 6612–6618.
68. Richiardi, L., Fiano, V., Vizzini, L., De Marco, L., Delsedime, L., Akre, O., Tos, A.G. and Merletti, F. (2009) Promoter methylation in APC, RUNX3, and GSTP1 and mortality in prostate cancer patients. *J Clin Oncol* 27, 3161–3168.
69. Liu, L., Kron, K.J., Pethe, V.V., Demetrashvili, N., Nesbitt, M.E., Trachtenberg, J., Ozcelik, H., Fleshner, N.E., Briollais, L., van der Kwast, T.H. and Bapat, B. (2011) Association of tissue promoter methylation levels of APC, TGFbeta2, HOXD3, and RASSF1A with prostate cancer progression. *Int J Cancer*
70. Henrique, R., Ribeiro, F.R., Fonseca, D., Hoque, M.O., Carvalho, A.L., Costa, V.L., Pinto, M., Oliveira, J., Teixeira, M.R., Sidransky, D. and Jeronimo, C. (2007) High promoter methylation levels of APC predict poor prognosis in sextant biopsies from prostate cancer patients. *Clin Cancer Res* 13, 6122–6129.
71. Mikeska, T., Candiloro, I.L.M. and Dobrovic, A. (2010) The implications of heterogeneous DNA methylation for the accurate quantification of methylation. *Epigenomics* 2, 561–573.
72. Higuchi, T., Nakamura, M., Shimada, K., Ishida, E., Hirao, K. and Konishi, N. (2008) HRK inactivation associated with promoter methylation and LOH in prostate cancer. *Prostate* 68, 105–113.
73. Park, J.Y., Zheng, W., Kim, D., Cheng, J.Q., Kumar, N., Ahmad, N. and Pow-Sang, J. (2007) Candidate tumor suppressor gene SLC5A8 is frequently down-regulated by promoter hypermethylation in prostate tumor. *Cancer Detect Prev* 31, 359–365.
74. Majid, S., Dar, A.A., Shahryari, V., Hirata, H., Ahmad, A., Saini, S., Tanaka, Y., Dahiya, A.V. and Dahiya, R. (2010) Genistein reverses hypermethylation and induces active histone modifications in tumor suppressor gene B-Cell translocation gene 3 in prostate cancer. *Cancer* 116, 66–76.
75. Kwabi-Addo, B., Ren, C. and Ittmann, M. (2009) DNA methylation and aberrant expression of Sprouty1 in human prostate cancer. *Epigenetics* 4, 54–61.
76. Fritzsche, S., Kenzelmann, M., Hoffmann, M.J., Muller, M., Engers, R., Grone, H.J. and Schulz, W.A. (2006) Concomitant down-regulation of SPRY1 and SPRY2 in prostate carcinoma. *Endocr Relat Cancer* 13, 839–849.
77. Pierconti, F., Martini, M., Pinto, F., Cenci, T., Capodimonti, S., Calarco, A., Bassi, P.F. and Larocca, L.M. (2011) Epigenetic silencing of SOCS3 identifies a subset of prostate cancer with an aggressive behavior. *Prostate* 71, 318–325.
78. Shivapurkar, N., Toyooka, S., Toyooka, K.O., Reddy, J., Miyajima, K., Suzuki, M., Shigematsu, H., Takahashi, T., Parikh, G., Pass, H.I., Chaudhary, P.M. and Gazdar, A.F. (2004) Aberrant methylation of trail decoy receptor genes is frequent in multiple tumor types. *Int J Cancer* 109, 786–792.
79. Hornstein, M., Hoffmann, M.J., Alexa, A., Yamanaka, M., Muller, M., Jung, V., Rahnenfuhrer, J. and Schulz, W.A. (2008) Protein phosphatase and TRAIL receptor genes as new candidate tumor genes on chromosome 8p in prostate cancer. *Cancer Genomics Proteomics* 5, 123–136.
80. Cho, N.Y., Kim, B.H., Choi, M., Yoo, E.J., Moon, K.C., Cho, Y.M., Kim, D. and Kang, G.H. (2007) Hypermethylation of CpG island loci and hypomethylation of LINE-1 and Alu repeats in prostate adenocarcinoma and their relationship to clinicopathological features. *J Pathol* 211, 269–277.
81. Semina, E.V., Reiter, R., Leysens, N.J., Alward, W.L., Small, K.W., Datson, N.A.,

Siegel-Bartelt, J., Bierke-Nelson, D., Bitoun, P., Zabel, B.U., Carey, J.C. and Murray, J.C. (1996) Cloning and characterization of a novel bicoid-related homeobox transcription factor gene, RIEG, involved in Rieger syndrome. *Nat Genet* 14, 392–399.

82. Flomen, R.H., Vatcheva, R., Gorman, P.A., Baptista, P.R., Groet, J., Barisic, I., Ligutic, I. and Nizetic, D. (1998) Construction and analysis of a sequence-ready map in 4q25: Rieger syndrome can be caused by haploinsufficiency of RIEG, but also by chromosome breaks approximately 90kb upstream of this gene. *Genomics* 47, 409–413.

83. Lines, M.A., Kozlowski, K., Kulak, S.C., Allingham, R.R., Heon, E., Ritch, R., Levin, A.V., Shields, M.B., Damji, K.F., Newlin, A. and Walter, M.A. (2004) Characterization and prevalence of PITX2 microdeletions and mutations in Axenfeld-Rieger malformations. *Invest Ophthalmol Vis Sci* 45, 828–833.

84. Weiss, G., Cottrell, S., Distler, J., Schatz, P., Kristiansen, G., Ittmann, M., Haefliger, C., Lesche, R., Hartmann, A., Corman, J. and Wheeler, T. (2009) DNA methylation of the PITX2 gene promoter region is a strong independent prognostic marker of biochemical recurrence in patients with prostate cancer after radical prostatectomy. *J Urol* 181, 1678–1685.

85. Toyota, M., Kopecky, K.J., Toyota, M.O., Jair, K.W., Willman, C.L. and Issa, J.P. (2001) Methylation profiling in acute myeloid leukemia. *Blood* 97, 2823–2829.

86. Maier, S., Nimmrich, I., Koenig, T., Eppenberger-Castori, S., Bohlmann, I., Paradiso, A., Spyratos, F., Thomssen, C., Mueller, V., Nahrig, J., Schittulli, F., Kates, R., Lesche, R., Schwope, I., Kluth, A., Marx, A., Martens, J.W., Foekens, J.A., Schmitt, M. and Harbeck, N. (2007) DNA-methylation of the homeodomain transcription factor PITX2 reliably predicts risk of distant disease recurrence in tamoxifen-treated, node-negative breast cancer patients--Technical and clinical validation in a multi-centre setting in collaboration with the European Organisation for Research and Treatment of Cancer (EORTC) PathoBiology group. *European Journal of Cancer* 43, 1679–1686.

87. Duffy, M.J., Napieralski, R., Martens, J.W.M., Span, P.N., Spyratos, F., Sweep, F.C.G.J., Brunner, N., Foekens, J.A., Schmitt, M. and Grp, E.P. (2009) Methylated genes as new cancer biomarkers. *European Journal of Cancer* 45, 335–346.

88. Gobel, G., Auer, D., Gaugg, I., Schneitter, A., Lesche, R., Muller-Holzner, E., Marth, C. and Daxenbichler, G. (2011) Prognostic significance of methylated RASSF1A and PITX2 genes in blood- and bone marrow plasma of breast cancer patients. *Breast Cancer Res Treat*

89. Banez, L.L., Sun, L., van Leenders, G.J., Wheeler, T.M., Bangma, C.H., Freedland, S.J., Ittmann, M.M., Lark, A.L., Madden, J.F., Hartman, A., Weiss, G. and Castanos-Velez, E. (2010) Multicenter clinical validation of PITX2 methylation as a prostate specific antigen recurrence predictor in patients with post-radical prostatectomy prostate cancer. *J Urol* 184, 149–156.

90. Schatz, P., Dietrich, D., Koenig, T., Burger, M., Lukas, A., Fuhrmann, I., Kristiansen, G., Stoehr, R., Schuster, M., Lesche, R., Weiss, G., Corman, J. and Hartmann, A. (2010) Development of a diagnostic microarray assay to assess the risk of recurrence of prostate cancer based on PITX2 DNA methylation. *J Mol Diagn* 12, 345–353.

91. Nimmrich, I., Sieuwerts, A.M., Meijer-van Gelder, M.E., Schwope, I., Bolt-de Vries, J., Harbeck, N., Koenig, T., Hartmann, O., Kluth, A., Dietrich, D., Magdolen, V., Portengen, H., Look, M.P., Klijn, J.G., Lesche, R., Schmitt, M., Maier, S., Foekens, J.A. and Martens, J.W. (2008) DNA hypermethylation of PITX2 is a marker of poor prognosis in untreated lymph node-negative hormone receptor-positive breast cancer patients. *Breast Cancer Res Treat* 111, 429–437.

92. Vinarskaja, A., Schulz, W.A., Ingenwerth, M., Hader, C. and Arsov, C. (2011) Association of PITX2 mRNA downregulation in prostate cancer with promoter hypermethylation and poor prognosis. Urol Oncol 30, in press.

93. Liu, J.W., Nagpal, J.K., Jeronimo, C., Lee, J.E., Henrique, R., Kim, M.S., Ostrow, K.L., Yamashita, K., van Criekinge, V., Wu, G., Moon, C.S., Trink, B. and Sidransky, D. (2008) Hypermethylation of MCAM gene is associated with advanced tumor stage in prostate cancer. *Prostate* 68, 418–426.

94. Guo, L., Zhong, D., Lau, S., Liu, X., Dong, X.Y., Sun, X., Yang, V.W., Vertino, P.M., Moreno, C.S., Varma, V., Dong, J.T. and Zhou, W. (2008) Sox7 Is an independent checkpoint for beta-catenin function in prostate and colon epithelial cells. *Mol Cancer Res* 6, 1421–1430.

95. Chang, G., Xu, S., Dhir, R., Chandran, U., O'Keefe, D.S., Greenberg, N.M. and Gingrich, J.R. (2010) Hypoexpression and epigenetic regulation of candidate tumor suppressor gene CADM-2 in human prostate cancer. *Clin Cancer Res* 16, 5390–5401.

96. Carey, J.P., Asirvatham, A.J., Galm, O., Ghogomu, T.A. and Chaudhary, J. (2009) Inhibitor of differentiation 4 (Id4) is a potential tumor suppressor in prostate cancer. *BMC Cancer* 9, 173.
97. Rhodes, D.R., Yu, J., Shanker, K., Deshpande, N., Varambally, R., Ghosh, D., Barrette, T., Pandey, A. and Chinnaiyan, A.M. (2004) ONCOMINE: a cancer microarray database and integrated data-mining platform. *Neoplasia* 6, 1–6.
98. Sorensen, K.D., Borre, M., Orntoft, T.F., Dyrskjot, L. and Torring, N. (2008) Chromosomal deletion, promoter hypermethylation and downregulation of FYN in prostate cancer. *Int J Cancer* 122, 509–519.
99. Sorensen, K.D., Wild, P.J., Mortezavi, A., Adolf, K., Torring, N., Heeboll, S., Ulhoi, B.P., Ottosen, P., Sulser, T., Hermanns, T., Moch, H., Borre, M., Orntoft, T.F. and Dyrskjot, L. (2009) Genetic and epigenetic SLC18A2 silencing in prostate cancer is an independent adverse predictor of biochemical recurrence after radical prostatectomy. *Clin Cancer Res* 15, 1400–1410.
100. Schulz, W. and Goering, W. (2011) Eagles report: Developing cancer biomarkers from genomewide DNA methylation analyses. *World J Clin Oncol* 2, 1–7.
101. Kondo, Y. and Issa, J.P. (2010) DNA methylation profiling in cancer. *Expert Rev Mol Med* 12, e23.
102. Murphy, T.M., Sullivan, L., Lane, C., O'Connor, L., Barrett, C., Hollywood, D., Lynch, T., Lawler, M. and Perry, A.S. (2011) In silico analysis and DHPLC screening strategy identifies novel apoptotic gene targets of aberrant promoter hypermethylation in prostate cancer. *Prostate* 71, 1–17.
103. Kim, S.J., Kelly, W.K., Fu, A., Haines, K., Hoffman, A., Zheng, T. and Zhu, Y. (2011) Genome-wide methylation analysis identifies involvement of TNF-alpha mediated cancer pathways in prostate cancer. *Cancer Lett*
104. Kron, K., Pethe, V., Briollais, L., Sadikovic, B., Ozcelik, H., Sunderji, A., Venkateswaran, V., Pinthus, J., Fleshner, N., van der Kwast, T. and Bapat, B. (2009) Discovery of novel hypermethylated genes in prostate cancer using genomic CpG island microarrays. *PLoS One* 4, e4830.
105. Miyazaki, Y.J., Hamada, J., Tada, M., Furuuchi, K., Takahashi, Y., Kondo, S., Katoh, H. and Moriuchi, T. (2002) HOXD3 enhances motility and invasiveness through the TGF-beta-dependent and -independent pathways in A549 cells. *Oncogene* 21, 798–808.
106. Kron, K.J., Liu, L., Pethe, V.V., Demetrashvili, N., Nesbitt, M.E., Trachtenberg, J., Ozcelik, H., Fleshner, N.E., Briollais, L., van der Kwast, T.H. and Bapat, B. (2010) DNA methylation of HOXD3 as a marker of prostate cancer progression. *Lab Invest* 90, 1060–1067.
107. Ibragimova, I., de Caceres, I.I., Hoffman, A.M., Potapova, A., Dulaimi, E., Al-Saleem, T., Hudes, G.R., Ochs, M.F. and Cairns, P. (2010) Global Reactivation of Epigenetically Silenced Genes in Prostate Cancer. *Cancer Prevention Research* 3, 1084–1092.
108. Rauhala, H.E., Porkka, K.P., Saramaki, O.R., Tammela, T.L. and Visakorpi, T. (2008) Clusterin is epigenetically regulated in prostate cancer. *Int J Cancer* 123, 1601–1609.
109. Devaney, J., Stirzaker, C., Qu, W., Song, J.Z., Statham, A.L., Patterson, K.I., Horvath, L.G., Tabor, B., Coolen, M.W., Hulf, T., Kench, J.G., Henshall, S.M., Pe Benito, R., Haynes, A.M., Mayor, R., Peinado, M.A., Sutherland, R.L. and Clark, S.J. (2011) Epigenetic deregulation across chromosome 2q14.2 differentiates normal from prostate cancer and provides a regional panel of novel DNA methylation cancer biomarkers. *Cancer Epidemiol Biomarkers Prev* 20, 148–159.
110. Guan, M., Xu, C., Zhang, F. and Ye, C. (2009) Aberrant methylation of EphA7 in human prostate cancer and its relation to clinicopathologic features. *Int J Cancer* 124, 88–94.
111. Kim, J.W., Cheng, Y., Liu, W., Li, T., Yegnasubramanian, S., Zheng, S.L., Xu, J., Isaacs, W.B. and Chang, B.L. (2009) Genetic and epigenetic inactivation of LPL gene in human prostate cancer. *Int J Cancer* 124, 734–738.
112. Ribarska, T., Ingenwerth, M., Goering, W., Engers, R. and Schulz, W.A. (2010) Epigenetic inactivation of the placentally imprinted tumor suppressor gene TFPI2 in prostate carcinoma. *Cancer Genomics Proteomics* 7, 51–60.
113. Kim, J.H., Dhanasekaran, S.M., Prensner, J.R., Cao, X., Robinson, D., Kalyana-Sundaram, S., Huang, C., Shankar, S., Jing, X., Iyer, M., Hu, M., Sam, L., Grasso, C., Maher, C.A., Palanisamy, N., Mehra, R., Kominsky, H.D., Siddiqui, J., Yu, J., Qin, Z.S. and Chinnaiyan, A.M. (2011) Deep sequencing reveals distinct patterns of DNA methylation in prostate cancer. *Genome Res* 21, 1028–1041.
114. Kim, S.J., Kelly, W.K., Fu, A., Haines, K., Hoffman, A. Zheng, T. and Zhu, Y. (2011) Genome-wide methylation analysis identifies involvement of TNF-alpha mediated cancer

pathways in prostate cancer. *Cancer Lett* 302, 47–53.

115. Kim, Y.J., Yoon, H.Y., Kim, S.K., Kim, Y.W., Kim, E.J., Kim, I.Y. and Kim, W.J. (2011) EFEMP1 as a novel DNA methylation marker for prostate cancer: array-based DNA methylation and expression profiling. *Clin Cancer Res* 17, 4523–4530.

116. Kobayashi, Y., Absher, D.M., Gulzar, Z.G., Young, S.R., McKenney, J.K., Peehl, D.M., Brooks, J.D., Myers, R.M., Sherlock, G. (2011) DNA methylation profiling reveals novel biomarkers and important roles for DNA methyltransferases in prostate cancer. *Genome Res* 21, 1017–1027.

117. Schwartzman, J., Mongoue-Tchokote, S., Gibbs, A., Gao, L., Corless, C.L., Jin, J., Zarour, L., Higano, C., True, L.D., Vessella, R.L., Wilmot, B., Bottomly, D., McWeeney, S.K., Bova, G.S., Partin, A.W., Mori, M. and Alumkal J. (2011) A DNA methylation microarray-based study identifies ERG as a gene commonly methylated in prostate cancer. *Epigenetics* 6, 1248–1256.

Chapter 5

DNA Methylation in Promoter Region as Biomarkers in Prostate Cancer

Mihi Yang and Jong Y. Park

Abstract

The prostate gland is the most common site of cancer and the second leading cause of cancer death in American men. Recent emerging molecular biological technologies help us to know that epigenetic alterations such as DNA methylation within the regulatory (promoter) regions of genes are associated with transcriptional silencing in cancer. Promoter hypermethylation of critical pathway genes could be potential biomarkers and therapeutic targets for prostate cancer. In this chapter, we updated current information on methylated genes associated with the development and progression of prostate cancer. Over 40 genes have been investigated for methylation in promoter region in prostate cancer. These methylated genes are involved in critical pathways, such as DNA repair, metabolism, and invasion/metastasis. The role of hypermethylated genes in regulation of critical pathways in prostate cancer is discussed. These findings may provide new information of the pathogenesis, the exciting potential to be predictive and to provide personalized treatment of prostate cancer. Indeed, some epigenetic alterations in prostate tumors are being translated into clinical practice for therapeutic use.

Key words: Prostate cancer, DNA methylation, Epigenetic variation, Biomarker

1. Introduction

Prostate cancer is the most common type of cancer and the second leading cause of cancer mortality in the American men. One man in six will develop prostate cancer during his lifetime, and one man in 34 will die of the disease (1). In 2010, it is estimated that 217,730 new cases will be diagnosed in the United States, and 32,050 men will die from the disease (2). The low mortality rate and gradual decrease of incidence rates, from 2000 to 2006, suggest that public awareness of early detection and advanced treatments of prostate cancer has begun to affect prostate cancer

Ramona G. Dumitrescu and Mukesh Verma (eds.), *Cancer Epigenetics: Methods and Protocols*, Methods in Molecular Biology, vol. 863, DOI 10.1007/978-1-61779-612-8_5, © Springer Science+Business Media, LLC 2012

outcomes. However, the probability of developing prostate cancer sharply increases with age, e.g., ~30-fold increase among men over 40 years of age, compared to men under 40 years old. The aging of the current population means that the disease will become an even greater public health problem in the future.

There are substantial individual differences in the risk or progression of prostate cancer. In some patients with prostate cancer, the disease progresses relatively slow. In these cases, patients often die with prostate cancer rather than from prostate cancer. However, some cases grow aggressively and metastasize through the bloodstream and lymphatic system to other parts of the body. Currently, there are two important clinical challenges. The first challenge is the early detection of prostate cancer. Digital rectal examination (DRE) and serum prostate-specific antigen (PSA) are two main diagnostic tools. There is a considerable overlap in PSA levels between patients with prostate cancer and patients with benign prostatic hyperplasia (BPH). Approximately 25% of patients with prostate cancer show no elevation of serum PSA and must be diagnosed by other methods (3). Therefore, the identification of biomarkers that can facilitate the diagnosis of prostate cancer at the early stages could improve the current standard of treatments. The second challenge is to determine which of prostate cancer's clinical forms a patient is presenting with, i.e., aggressive vs. indolent. This is critically important information given the significant morbidity associated with treatment interventions and could eventually help distinguish men who need intensive treatment from those who may be better served by watchful waiting. Currently, the level of PSA, clinical stage, and the grade of tumor (Gleason score) are used to estimate prognosis and determine treatment modalities. To overcome limitations of PSA and DRE, new biomarkers are demanded to improve the outcome of prostate cancer.

2. Role of DNA Methylation in the Promoter Regions in Prostate Cancer

Development and progression of prostate cancer are results of the accumulation of genetic and epigenetic alterations. Although genetic changes are involved in the inactivation of genes with important anticancer functions (e.g., tumor suppressor and DNA repair genes), DNA methylation in a promoter region is an important epigenetic mechanism for the downregulation (silencing) of expression of these genes. DNA methylation in the promoter region of tumor suppressor genes appears to occur at early stages of carcinogenesis and occurs with various frequencies. Therefore, epigenetic changes have the potential to be a new generation of biomarkers. Several types of epigenetic changes have been reported for prostate cancer including DNA hypermethylation, loss of imprinting, and altered histone modification patterns.

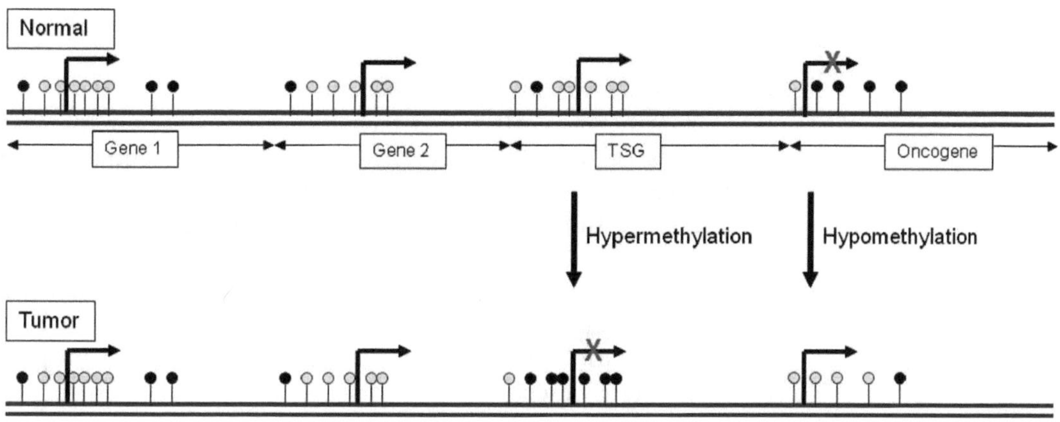

Fig. 1. Role of DNA methylation in cancer: unmethylated and methylated CpG sites are indicated by *white* and *black circles*, respectively. This figure shows a representative region of genomic DNA in normal and tumor cell. The promoter regions in gene1, gene2, and tumor suppressor gene are rarely methylated in normal cells and, therefore, expressed. Cytosines 5′ to guanosines (CpG) islands in promoter region of tumor suppressor gene are methylated, and it results in gene silencing. Conversely, hypomethylation in the promoter region of oncogene in tumor reactivates transcription.

CpG islands are CpG-rich areas of 200 bp to several kilobases in length, usually located near the promoters of highly expressed genes, and are the sites of common methylation in human tumors (4), including the prostate. A common molecular feature associated with tumorigenesis is hypermethylation of cytosines 5′ to guanosines (CpG) within the regulatory (promoter) region of suppressor gene genomic DNA (5–8). 5-methyl cytosine is unstable and mutates to thymine and methylated CpG sites degrade to TpG/CpA. In tumors, many CpG islands exhibit aberrant hypermethylation, resulting in gene silencing (Fig. 1). Many tumor suppressor genes have been found to be silenced by promoter hypermethylation in tumors.

It is firmly established that an increase of methylation across the promoter region affects transcription of genes. However, how methylated genes are downregulated is not completely known. Furthermore, the extent of methylation in the CpG islands required for gene silencing is not clear except for a short list of genes (9–18). Yet, regardless of mechanism, the observation of methylated promoter regions in silenced tumor suppressor genes in prostate tumor tissues suggests that DNA methylation may indicate a significant association with carcinogenesis and progression of prostate cancer.

3. Hypermethylated Genes in Prostate Tumor

The majority of previous publications in epigenetic research in prostate cancer focused on DNA hypermethylation. Indeed, a gene silencing by DNA hypermethylation in the promoter region is a more common event than a gene silencing by DNA mutations in carcinogenesis. Numerous studies on various hypermethylated genes in different cancers suggest that this is a key part of the carcinogenesis and progression of cancer.

Currently, over 40 genes have been investigated for their frequencies of hypermethylation and for their potential role in prostate cancer (Table 1). Most data in Table 1 were obtained from prostate tumor tissues. The functions of tumor suppressor genes in prostate cancer fall into four major categories: tumor suppressor genes, tumor cell invasion/metastasis, metabolism, and DNA repair. Defected function of these genes by promoter hypermethylation can contribute to carcinogenesis and progression of prostate cancer.

3.1. Tumor Suppressors Genes

3.1.1. Caveolin-1 (CAV1)

Caveolin-1 (*CAV1*) is known as a tumor suppressor gene and involved in the vesicular transport, cholesterol balance, transformation, and tumorigenesis. Recent studies reported the dual function of *CAV1* both as a tumor suppressor gene and metastasis-promoting gene (19, 20).

Cui et al. found that 91% (20/22) of cases showed differential hypermethylation in the prostate tumor tissues when compared with adjacent normal tissues (20). Increased DNA methylation of *CAV1* was correlated with biochemical recurrence. Therefore, *CAV1* plays a role as a tumor suppressor gene which is silenced by hypermethylation in carcinogenesis in prostate. A recent study supports that *CAV1* is downregulated in prostate tumor due to hypermethylation in the promoter region of *CAV1* (21). However, Woodson et al. did not observe *CAV1* methylation in prostate tumor tissues (22). Karam et al. reported overexpression of *CAV1* as an established feature of prostate cancer and aggressive PSA recurrence (23). Moreover, *CAV1* is reported to upregulate fatty acid synthase (FASN), a tumor promoter, in the progression of prostate cancer (24). These data suggest that the methylation status of *CAV1* may not be a reliable biomarker for prostate cancer.

3.1.2. Cyclin-Dependent Kinase Inhibitors

The tumor suppressor gene *CDKN2* (*p16*) is one of the cyclin-dependent kinase inhibitors (CDKIs). *CDKN2A* ($p16^{INK4a}$) is a key protein in the signaling pathway, which can be damaged by a variety of genetic and epigenetic changes including hypermethylation in prostate tumors. Aberrant CDKI expression is observed in many tumor tissues including prostate (25–28). The reported frequencies of *CDKN2A* promoter methylation are inconsistent in prostate tumors, ranging from 0 to 77% (25–27, 29–36). Perhaps these inconsistent results are due to different detection methods and/or different targets of methylated loci. For example, Gu et al. identified DNA methylation at the *SmaI* site for 21 of 30 samples and found only one sample had an altered methylation pattern at the *SmaI* site downstream of exon 1 of the *CDKN2A* (32). Since Herman et al. first reported inactivation of *CDKN/p16* by DNA methylation in

Table 1
Frequencies of methylated genes in prostate tumor and biosamples

Gene	Common name	Function	Frequency	References
ALDH1a2	Aldehyde dehydrogenase 1 family, member A2	Tumor suppressor (synthesis of RA)	100% (7/7)[a]	(208)
ALDH1a3	Aldehyde dehydrogenase 1 family, member A3	Tumor suppressor (synthesis of RA)	21% (5/24)	(48)
APC	Adenomatous polyposis coli	Tumor suppressor	12% (2/17)[b]	(194)
			90% (66/73)	(30)
			14% (11/76)[c]	(89)
			92% (36/39)[c]	(165)
			57% (21/37)	(92)
			27% (27/101)	(29)
			100% (118/118)	(25)
			41% (182/447)	(216)
			79% (48/61)	(203)
			65% (117/179)	(121)
			3.0[d]	(51)
			83% (44/53)[c]	(85)
			73% (131/179)	(121)
			27% (21/79)	(50)
			82% (59/72)	(203)
			64% (109/170)	(191)
			83% (65/78)	(88)
			51% (48/95)[b]	(36)
			51% (58/113)[b]	(183)
			51% (18/35)	(120)
			48% (25/52)[b]	(31)
			78% (88/113)	(35)

(continued)

Table 1 (continued)

Gene	Common name	Function	Frequency	References
AR	Androgen receptor	Steroid hormonal response	29% (2/7)[a]	(148)
			13% (2/15)	(145)
			8% (3/38)	(146)
			25% (6/24)	(147)
			15% (16/109)	(56)
			39% (30/76)[c]	(132)
CAV1	Caveolin-1	Tumor suppressor	91% (20/22)	(20)
			100% (4/4)	(21)
			0% (0/8)	(22)
CCNA1	Cyclin A1	Tumor suppressor	79% (19/24)	(48)
CCND2	Cyclin D2	Tumor suppressor	25% (21/83)	(50)
			32% (32/101)	(45)
			99% (117/118)	(49)
			1.78[d]	(51)
CD44	CD44 molecule	Tumor invasion/metastasis (lipid-raft-associated)	78% (31/40)	(219)
			33% (30/90)	(22)
			3% (1/30)[c, e]	(28)
			68% (27/40)	(218)
			32% (36/111)	(177)
			72% (58/81)	(94)
			0% (0/18)[c]	(86)
			20% (2/8)	(256)
			22% (39/179)	(121)

CDH1	E-cadherin	Tumor invasion/metastasis (lipid-raft-associated)	31% (29/95)[b]	(36)
			0% (0/30)[c, e]	(28)
			54% (19/35)	(221)
			70% (14/20)[a]	(222)
			27% (27/101)	(29)
			0% (0/111)	(177)
			0% (0/73)	(30)
			4% (5/114)	(35)
			61% (49/81)	(94)
			30% (6/20)	(159)
			77% (40/52)[b]	(31)
			24% (22/90)	(22)
			69% (70/101)	(45)
			21% (38/179)	(121)
CDH13	H-cadherin	Tumor invasion/metastasis (lipid-raft-associated)	45% (68/151)	(225)
			31% (31/101)	(29)
			54% (96/179)	(121)
CDKN2A (*p16*^{INK4a})	Cyclin-dependent kinase inhibitor 2A	Tumor suppressor	73% (8/11)	(27)
			3% (3/101)	(29)
			6% (4/73)	(30)
			77% (91/118)	(25)
			66% (21/32)	(26)
			13% (3/24)	(34)
			70% (21/30)	(32)
			4% (5/113)	(35)
			37% (19/52)[b]	(31)
			15% (8/53)	(37)
			12% (11/95)[b]	(36)
			10% (3/30)[c]	(28)
			60% (3/5)[a]	(33)

(continued)

Table 1 (continued)

Gene	Common name	Function	Frequency	References
CRBP1	Cellular retinol-binding protein 1	Steroid hormonal response (control of retinoids)	81% (96/118)	(25)
			47% (17/36)	(188)
			34% (34/101)	(189)
P14^ARF	Cyclin-dependent kinase inhibitor 2A	Tumor suppressor	4% (2/53)	(37)
			6% (6/95)[b]	(36)
			37% (19/52)[b]	(31)
			4% (5/118)	(25)
			0% (0/73)	(30)
			3% (1/32)	(42)
			6% (1/16)	(26)
			22% (2/9)	(27)
DAPK	Death-associated protein kinase	Tumor suppressor	36% (39/109)	(56)
			1% (1/101)	(29)
			0% (0/73)	(30)
			28% (27/95)[b]	(36)
			10.9–18.7[f]	(57)
EDNRB	Endothelin receptor type B	Steroid hormonal response (cell adhesion)	49% (36/73)	(30)
			72% (58/81)	(94)
			70% (23/35)	(193)
			100% (80/80)	(87)
			50% (9/18)[b]	(86)
			83% (40/48)	(195)
			66% (8/12)[b]	(194)

EPHA7	EPH receptor A7	Steroid hormonal response (cell differentiation, apoptosis)	42% (20/48)	(197)
Esr1	Estrogen receptor alpha	Steroid hormonal response	90% (28/31) 19% (14/73) 95% (36/38) 41% (64/156)	(157) (30) (146) (156)
Esr2	Estrogen receptor beta	Steroid hormonal response	83% (19/23) 65% (13/20) 79% (30/38)	(160) (159) (146)
FHIT	Fragile histidine triad gene	Tumor suppressor	15% (15/101) 65% (15/23) $>10^6$	(29) (67) (57)
FYN	SRC family tyrosine kinase	Tumor invasion/metastasis (cell differentiation)	67% (12/18)	(242)

(continued)

Table 1 (continued)

Gene	Common name	Function	Frequency	References
GSTP1	Glutathione S transferase P1	Steroid hormonal response (metabolism)	58% (7/12)	(175)
			81% (68/84)[c]	(179)
			39% (31/80)[b]	(179)
			26% (20/76)	(89)
			86% (37/43)	(164)
			85% (89/105)	(176)
			36% (36/101)	(29)
			88% (96/109)	(56)
			84% (99/118)	(177)
			100% (18/18)	(178)
			95% (69/73)	(30)
			87% (32/37)	(92)
			79% (22/28)[b]	(170)
			71% (43/61)	(169)
			95% (112/118)	(25)
			75% (24/32)	(42)
			72% (58/81)	(94)
			79% (89/113)	(35)
			48% (25/52)[b]	(31)
			83% (79/95)[b]	(36)
			42% (71/168)[c]	(87)
			28% (5/18)[c]	(86)
			93% (74/80)	(87)
			100% (20/20)	(168)
			91% (52/57)	(171)
			75% (24/32)	(172)
			44% (4/9)[g]	(180)
			90% (18/20)	(181)
			94% (16/17)	(173)
			42% (71/168)[c]	(182)
			91% (63/69)	(174)

HIC1	Hypermethylated in cancer 1	Tumor suppressor	99% (108/109) 67% (52/78) 100% (73/73)	(56) (75) (30)
LPL	Lipoprotein lipase	Tumor suppressor (metabolism of lipids)	38% (21/56)	(67)
MDR1/ABCB1	Multidrug resistance 1, ATP-binding cassette, subfamily B (MDR/TAP), member 1	Steroid hormonal response	48% (36/76) 83% (15/18)[c] 55% (97/177) 88% (64/73) 100% (35/35) 51% (91/179)	(89) (86) (190) (30) (120) (121)
MGMT	O^6-methylguanine DNA methyltransferase	DNA repair	26% (14/53) 34% (21/62) 2% (2/109) 19% (22/118) 25% (8/32) 76% (28/37) 0% (0/101) 1% (1/73) 19% (10/52)[b] 15% (14/95)[b]	(37) (251) (56) (25) (42) (92) (29) (30) (31) (36)
NEP	Neuroepithelial tyrosine kinase	Tumor cell invasion/metastasis	17% (3/18)[c] 14% (3/21) 73% (16/22)	(86) (243) (245)
NKX3.1		Tumor suppress (defense for oxidative damage)	83% (33/40)	(128)
NKX2.5		Tumor suppress (defense for oxidative damage)	30% (6/20)	(130)
PITX2	Paired-like homeodomain 2	Tumor suppress	3.4[d] 2.99[d] 100% (17/17)	(81) (82) (83)

(continued)

Table 1 (continued)

Gene	Common name	Function	Frequency	References
PTGS2	Prostaglandin-endoperoxide synthase 2	Tumor suppressor	88% (64/73)	(30)
			11% (8/76)	(89)
			71% (38/53)	(85)
			68% (54/80)	(87)
			65% (51/78)	(88)
			0% (0/18)[c]	(86)
RARβ	Retinoic acid receptor beta	Steroid hormonal response	79% (11/14)	(162)
			71% (25/35)	(120)
			91% (39/43)	(164)
			79% (33/42)[c]	(165)
			53% (54/101)	(29)
			78% (85/109)	(56)
			84% (42/50)	(163)
			70% (79/113)	(35)
			35% (18/52)[b]	(31)
			40% (32/81)	(94)
			39% (7/18)[c]	(86)
			62% (59/95)[b]	(36)
RASSF1A	Ras association domain family 1	Tumor suppressor	21% (16/76)	(89)
			71% (37/52)	(91)
			99% (117/118)	(25)
			53% (54/101)	(29)
			96% (70/73)	(30)
			84% (31/37)	(92)
			74% (97/131)	(93)
			73% (38/52)[b]	(31)
			49% (40/81)	(94)
			78% (88/113)	(35)
			78% (74/95)[b]	(36)
			17% (3/18)[c]	(86)
			50% (7/14)	(95)

S100A2	S100 calcium-binding protein A2	Tumor cell invasion/metastasis	94% (32/34) 99% (117/118)	(229) (25)
S100A6	S100 calcium-binding protein A6		52% (14/27)	(229)
SFN	14-3-3σ	Tumor suppressor	87% (45/52)[c] 99% (121/122)	(132) (134)
SLC5A8	Solute carrier family 5, member 8	Tumor suppressor	70% (7/10)	(110)
SLC18A2	Vesicular monoamine transporter 2	Tumor suppressor	88% (15/17)	(114)
TIG1	Tazarotene-induced gene 1	Steroid hormonal response (chloroplast trigger factor)	53% (26/50) 55% (17/31) 70% (43/61) 10% (16/168)[c] 96% (77/80) 42% (75/179)	(163) (204) (203) (182) (87) (121)
TIMP-2	Tissue inhibitor of metalloproteinase-2	Tumor cell invasion/metastasis	60% (25/42)	(234)
TIMP-3	Tissue inhibitor of metalloproteinase-3	Tumor cell invasion/metastasis	41% (37/91)[b] 37% (19/52)[b] 6% (7/109) 97% (114/118) 0% (0/73)	(36) (31) (56) (25) (30)
TNFRSF10C/DcR1	TNF receptor superfamily, member 10c	Tumor suppressor	65% (117/180) 50% (25/50) 78% (46/59) 0% (0/35)	(121) (117) (116) (120)
TNFRSF10D/DcR2	TNF receptor superfamily, member 10D	Tumor suppressor	38% (5/8)	(119)

[a] Cell culture
[b] Urine samples
[c] Serum DNA
[d] Hazard ratio
[e] Bone marrow
[f] Methylation fold compared to normal cells
[g] Ejaculates

prostate tumors (33), other researchers have investigated the role of hypermethylated *CDKN2A* in carcinogenesis and progression of prostate cancer (25–27, 29–35). Nguyen et al. observed methylation of *p16*^{INK4a} only in exon 2. Although methylation at exon 2 may not be functional, this exon 2 methylation may be a potential biomarker for prostate tumor because of a high prevalence of methylation in tumor tissues (27). These results were confirmed by other groups, who reported that methylation occurred in the promoter region in 9%, 15% of tumors in exon 1 (26, 37), and 66% in exon 2 (26). Jeronimo et al. found that the *p16*^{INK4a} gene was frequently methylated in tumor tissues (77%). However, the high frequency of methylation was also found in BPH (25). These data suggested that *p16*^{INK4a} methylation may be a potential biomarker for an early detection of prostate cancer.

Another *CDKI*, the *CDKN2A/p14*^{ARF}, generated from an alternative splicing process that replaces the first exon of *p16*^{INK4a}, has been known as a growth suppressor. Therefore, epigenetic alterations of *p14*^{ARF} may affect *p16*^{INK4a}*/RB1* pathways in the tumorigenesis and progression of prostate cancer. The *p14*^{ARF} promoter has been methylated in various cancers, glioma (38), bladder (39), leukemia (40), head and neck (41), and prostate cancers (25–27, 30, 31, 36, 37, 42). Based upon eight independent studies, frequencies of *p14*^{ARF} methylation in prostate cancer range from 0 to 37% (25–27, 30, 31, 36, 37, 42). With the exception of two studies (27, 31), most studies reported low methylation frequencies that ranged from 0 to 6%. The *p16*^{INK4a} and *p14*^{ARF} are frequently comethylated, which may deregulate the *RB1* or p53 pathway (42). However, promoter methylation in *p14*^{ARF} is rare in prostate tumors. Therefore, methylation in *p16*^{INK4a} rather than *p14*^{ARF} may be the predominant event in the *INK4a/ARF* loci in tumor tissues.

3.1.3. Cyclin A1 (CCNA1) and Cyclin D2 (CCND2)

The cell cycle is controlled by a family of cyclin-dependent kinases (CDKs). Cyclin A1 (CCNA1) activates two different CDKs and functions in both S phase and G2 (43, 44), while cyclin D2 (CCND2) is involved in the regulation of transition from G1 to S (45). Abnormal expression of *CCND2* may disrupt the normal cell cycle, and therefore, it is considered as both an oncogene and tumor suppressor gene. Aaltomaa et al. reported that expressions of *CCNA1* and *CCND2* were interrelated in prostate cancer tissues (46, 47).

Shames et al. observed a higher frequency of hypermethylation of *CCNA1* in both prostate tumors and benign tissues (48). However, Wegiel et al. reported that levels of CCNA1 protein and mRNA expression were significantly higher in prostate tumors than in adjacent benign tissues (47).

Aberrant expression of *CCND2* by DNA methylation has been noted in prostate cancer (45, 49). The frequencies of methylation in *CCND2* were significantly higher in prostate tumors (32%) than in normal tissues (6%) (45). Studies observed a positive correlation between the methylation in *CCND2* and clinicopathological features such as Gleason score and preoperative serum PSA (45, 50). Moreover, methylation status of *CCND2* was significantly associated with the risk for recurrence among prostate cancer patients who underwent a prostatectomy treatment (51). Henrique et al. further reported that *CCND2* methylation levels were significantly higher in prostate tumors compared to tissues of high-grade prostatic intraepithelial neoplasia (HGPIN), BPH, or normal prostate, whereas mRNA expression levels followed the opposite trend (49). They found that high *CCND2* methylation levels correlate with clinicopathological parameters of tumor aggressiveness. Altogether, *CCND2* promoter methylation, but not cyclin A1 gene, may be a useful prostate cancer biomarker for the identification of the aggressive prostate cancer that may benefit from different therapeutic modalities.

3.1.4. Death-Associated Protein Kinase

Death-associated protein kinase (DAPK) is a serine/threonine kinase involved in apoptosis pathway (52). Overexpression of *DAPK* induces apoptosis, whereas loss of its function leads to protection against apoptosis (53). Therefore, *DAPK* may function as a suppressor of metastasis. A repressed expression of *DAPK* by hypermethylation in the promoter region has been shown for various human cancers (52, 54, 55). The methylation frequencies in prostate cancer range from 0% to 36% in four independent studies (29, 30, 36, 56). In addition, Mishra et al. observed that methylation level of DAPK in a prostate cancer cell line (LNCaP) is significantly higher than one in a normal cell line (RWPE1) through global methylation analysis (57). However, *DAPK* overexpression and repressed function in prostate tumors (58) suggest that *DAPK* activity may be damaged at a posttranslational level in cancer cells (59). Based on its unclear function and a persistently low frequency of methylation in both tumors and normal tissues, *DAPK* needs to be further tested for a potential biomarker for prostate cancer.

3.1.5. Fragile Histidine Triad

Fragile histidine triad (*FHIT*) is known as a tumor suppressor gene and frequently methylated in various cancers such as lung (60), leukemia (61), ovarian (62), skin (63), cervical (64), gastric (65), renal (66), and prostate cancers (29, 67). Previous studies indicate that FHIT is a proapoptotic factor (68). Guo et al. (69) reported that downregulation of FHIT protein in more than half of the prostate tumors is determined by immunohistochemistry. However, these results were not confirmed by another study (70). Although there are indications for a potential role of *FHIT* methylation in prostate cancer, previous studies show its limited value due to a persistently low frequency of methylation in tumors and normal tissues (29, 57, 67).

3.1.6. Hypermethylated in Cancer 1

The tumor suppressor hypermethylated in cancer 1 (*HIC1*) is a transcriptional repressor, which is epigenetically silenced in solid tumors (71–73). Loss of heterozygosity (LOH) of the short arm of chromosome 17 (17p) is a frequent genetic alteration in human cancers. Moreover, frequent LOH or DNA methylation changes occur in a more telomeric region at 17p13.3. In the animal study, heterozygous $HIC1^{+/-}$ mice developed spontaneous malignant tumors of different types (74, 75). These results suggest that *HIC1* may be involved in tumorigenesis. Three studies investigated methylation in the promoter region of *HIC1* in prostate tumors. Results of three studies indicated that CpG island at the *HIC1* was methylated in 89–100% of prostate tumors (30, 56, 76). However, the methylation status of *HIC1* in prostate tumors parallels the respective normal tissue, although a high proportion of tumors are methylated. Therefore, DNA methylation sites in *HIC1* gene are not good candidates as prognostic markers for progression or early detection of prostate cancer (30, 76).

3.1.7. Lipoprotein Lipase

Lipoprotein lipase gene (*LPL*) is common locus of the somatic deletions in prostate tumors. Gallucci et al. reported *LPL* deletion in 76% of prostate tumor determined by fluorescence in situ hybridization (FISH) (77). *LPL* deletion was associated with higher stages, biochemical/clinical progression, and Gleason grade. Only one published study evaluated methylation status in *LPL* using 56 prostate tumors and matching normal tissue pairs. Kim et al. found that 21 samples out of 56 primary cancers (38%) were methylated in the *LPL* promoter region, while methylation was not detected in any normal tissues. In addition, the methylation status in *LPL* was positively associated with the preoperative PSA levels (67). These data suggest that biallelic inactivation of *LPL* by gene deletion and hypermethylation may affect progression of prostate cancer.

3.1.8. Paired-Like Homeodomain Transcription Factor 2 (PITX2)

Paired-like homeodomain transcription factor 2 gene (*PITX2*) encodes a member of the RIEG/PITX homeobox family, which is in the bicoid class of homeodomain proteins. The protein acts as a transcription factor, and it is involved in the development of several major organs. *PITX2* expression is induced by the Wnt pathway, and the protein mediates cell-type-specific proliferation by inducing growth-regulating genes (78). Methylation in *PITX2* was reported as one of the best validated methylated genes for predicting distant recurrence outcome of breast cancer by Maier et al. (79). These results were validated by an independent cohort and confirmed by two additional studies. Harbeck et al. reported that *PITX2* methylation can predict outcome in node-negative, tamoxifen-treated breast cancer (80). *PITX2* promoter methylation is also a biomarker for disease recurrence, early distant metastasis, and poor overall survival in breast cancer patients (81).

Recently, two cohort studies ($N=605$ (82); $N=476$ (83)) showed prostate cancer patients with high *PITX2* methylation had threefold higher chance of biochemical recurrence than patients with low *PITX2* methylation. They also showed the prognostic capability of *PITX2* methylation status in patient strata defined by the Gleason score. These results were supported by Vanaja et al. (84). Methylation profile of six genes including *PITX2* was significantly associated with prediction of biochemical, local, and systemic recurrence of prostate cancer. Together, the data show the ability of *PITX2* methylation status to provide prognostic information beyond the traditional Gleason score. Therefore, the prognostic potential of the *PITX2* methylation may help to determine a personalized treatment.

3.1.9. Prostaglandin-Endoperoxide Synthase 2

Prostaglandin-endoperoxide synthase 2 (*PTGS2*) is a key regulator of inflammation and may play a role in prostate carcinogenesis. The two PTGS isoforms, *PTGS1* and *PTGS2*, differ in their expression patterns. While *PTGS1* is constitutively expressed in most tissues, *PTGS2* is usually not expressed and is induced by inflammation, hypoxia, and *Wnt* signaling (85). An elevated expression of *PTGS2* is frequently reported in different human cancer sites including prostate. *PTGS2* overexpression and enzymatic activation can enhance the level of antiapoptotic protein B-cell CLL/lymphoma 2 (*BCL2*) and matrix metalloproteinase (*MMP*) family. Antiapoptotic and proproliferative and inflammatory functions of *PTGS2* support its role in tumorigenesis. However, other studies show that *PTGS2* may not be expressed or downregulated in prostate tumor. Bastian et al. observed *PTGS2* gene is silenced in prostate cancer by hypermethylation (86, 87). Range of methylation in *PTGS2* promoter was 0–88% of prostate tumor (30, 86, 88–90).

Methylation at the *PTGS2* gene was significantly different in prostate tumor and in BPH. These data indicated that methylation in *PTGS2* could be a reliable biomarker which can distinguish tumor from nontumor tissues (88). Moreover, the CpG island hypermethylation at *PTGS2* correlated with seminal vesicle infiltration, capsular penetration, pathologic T-stage, and recurrence (89). However, there was no PTSG2 methylation in hormone-refractory metastatic prostate cancer (87).

3.1.10. RAS Association Domain Family Protein 1 Isoform A

The RAS family of proto-oncogenes plays a key role in signal transduction pathways involved in cellular proliferation and survival, interacting with other regulatory circuits of cell growth and death. Overexpression of RAS may cause reduction of growth factor dependency, resistance to apoptosis, or other features of the tumor phenotype. However, RAS association domain family protein 1 isoform A (*RASSF1A*), a tumor suppressor gene, was known to be associated with the DNA repair proteins and with the apoptotic effect (91). Inactivation by methylation of *RASSF1A* may deregulate the DNA repair pathway and cell-cycle control in the tumor. Methylation in *RASSF1A* promoter gene was found in a large fraction of various tumors including prostate (92). In prostate tumors, *RASSF1A* promoter methylation is a common event, occurring in 21–99% of tumor tissues (25, 29–31, 35, 36, 90–96). *RASSF1A* promoter methylation is also positively associated with aggressiveness of prostate cancer (29, 92, 93). In addition, Aitchison et al. reported that there was over 50% of methylation in normal epithelial cells and benign prostatic tissues as well as prostatic intraepithelial neoplasms (96). These findings indicate that *RASSF1A* promoter methylation may be associated with early event of carcinogenesis and progression.

3.1.11. Solute Carrier Family 5A8 (SLC5A8)

Solute carrier family 5 (iodide transporter) (*SLC5*) is a solute-linked carrier gene family that contains 12 sodium-coupled transporters for several chemicals (97). *SLC5A8* is downregulated by methylation, obesity, or chronic hypoxia, while it is up regulated by lactate, butylate, TNF (tumor necrosis factor)-α, or nitric oxide (NO) (98). The potential function of *SLC5A8* protein in normal prostate tissues is likely to mediate concentrative uptake of butyrate and propionate, all of which are inhibitors of histone deacetylases (HDACs). SLC5A8 can also transport a variety of pharmacologically relevant monocarboxylates, e.g., various nonsteroidal anti-inflammatory drugs such as ibuprofen and ketoprofen (99) especially transport pyruvate into epithelial cells, and may explain a potential tumor suppressive role (100). *SLC5A8* was identified as a differentially methylated gene by restriction landmark genome scanning which provides a global analysis of methylation events in colon cancer cell lines and lung tumor (101, 102). Since then, increasing evidence suggests that gene silencing of *SLC5A8* may contribute to the carcinogenesis and progression of tumors. *SLC5A8* promoter methylation and gene silencing were detected in lung, brain, thyroid, gastric, pancreatic, breast, and prostate tumors (100, 102–112).

We previously reported hypermethylation of *SLC5A8* in prostate (111) and pancreatic tumors (110), and its expression was restored by treatment with either 5-azacytidine or TSA in cancer cell lines (111). Although these results hint a potential role of HDACs on *SLC5A8* expression, aberrant methylation represents the principal mechanism for inactivating *SLC5A8* in prostate tumor.

3.1.12. Solute Carrier Family 18 (Vesicular Monoamine) Transporter 2

Solute carrier family 18 (vesicular monoamine) transporter 2 (*SLC18A2*) transports monoamines, such as dopamine, serotonin, and histamine, from the cytosol into vesicles for storage and/or exocytotic release during neurotransmission or autocrine/paracrine factor release (113). Although *SLC18A2* is expressed in prostate tumors, biological function in normal and tumor prostate tissues is unknown. However, several of the monoamines that are substrates for SLC18A2-mediated transport have been shown to influence growth, proliferation, migration, or apoptosis of prostate cancer cells in vitro and in vivo. Kristiansen et al. reported that 50% of tumor tissues had silenced *SLC18A2* expression, by performing microarray analyses (114). A recent study confirmed that *SLC18A2* is frequently downregulated in tumor tissues by methylation, as compared with nonmalignant prostate tissue samples. Level of expression of *SLC18A2* is also negatively associated with risk for biochemical recurrence after radical prostatectomy (115).

3.1.13. Tumor Necrosis Factor Receptor Superfamily, Member 10C and 10D (TNFRSF10C and 10D)

The TNF receptor superfamily member 10C is one of several TNF-related apoptosis-inducing ligand (TRAIL)-like decoy receptors. *TNFRSF10C* is located on 8p21.3, which is a common prostate cancer susceptibility region (116, 117). *TNFRSF10C* encodes for DCRl and is involved in the inhibition of the apoptosis pathway. TNFRSF10C lacks the intracellular death domain and appears unable to induce apoptosis. The extracellular domains of TNFRSF10C compete with those of DR4 or DR5 for TRAIL binding. Thus, TNFRSF10C inhibits apoptosis induction through DR4 and DR5 (118). Previous studies reported that frequent loss of expression of *TNFRSF10C* by aberrant methylation of promoter regions in human tumor tissues (118, 119) and low expression of *TNFRSF10C* was associated with tumor recurrence (120). Hypermethylation of *TNFRSF10C* promoter region had been reported in prostate tumor tissues, with a range from 0 to 78% (117, 118, 121, 122). A recent German study reported that *TNFRSF10D*, which codes for DCR2, was also downregulated by methylation in tumors (120).

3.1.14. NK3 Homeobox 1 (NKX3.1) and NK2 Transcription Factor Related, Locus 5 (NKX2.5)

The *NKX3.1* is located on 8p21, which is a common prostate cancer susceptibility region (123). This gene is an NK family homeodomain protein and a tumor suppressor gene that is downregulated in the early phases of prostate cancer. Like its cardiac homolog, NKX2.5, *NKX3.1* acts synergistically with serum response factor (SRF) (124).

Loss of function of the *NKX3.1* homeobox gene in the mouse prostate leads to deregulated expression of oxidative damage response genes and increased levels of 8-oxy-dG, correlated with the onset of PIN (125, 126). Downregulation of *NKX3.1* was observed throughout prostate cancer progression (125, 127, 128). In addition, downregulation of *NKX3.1* is frequently observed with overexpression of *MYC*, an oncogene, at the early stage of prostate cancer (125). Asatiani et al. found hypermethylation at CpG sites –921, –903, and –47 of *NKX3.1* in tumors, as compared with adjacent normal cells (129). However, these data were not supported by another study. Lind et al. reported that downregulation of *NKX3.1* expression might not be caused by DNA methylation, but other epigenetic mechanisms (130). Chung et al. reported that

NKX2.5 promoter was significantly highly methylated in prostate tumor, as compared to normal tissues (131). These results were confirmed by another group (132). We expect that further methylation information at their promoters will be available.

3.1.15. Stratifin (SFN/14-3-3σ)

The p53-regulated gene *14-3-3σ* is a putative tumor suppressor gene involved in cell-cycle regulation and apoptosis following DNA damage. In response to DNA damage, *14-3-3σ* enforces a G2/M arrest by inhibiting the cyclin B1–cdc2 complex from entering the nucleus. This allows DNA repair before cell-cycle progression (133). *14-3-3σ* undergoes frequent epigenetic silencing in several types of cancer, including prostate cancer, suggesting that the loss of 14-3-3σ expression may be causally involved in tumor progression (134). However, there were similar high frequency of *14-3-3σ* methylation in both of prostate cancer and BPH (133, 135). Thus, promoter methylation at *14-3-3σ* may not be a specific biomarker for prostate cancer.

3.2. Genes Involved in Metabolism

The specific causes of prostate cancer are not known, but multiple etiological factors, including genetics, hormones, diet, infection, and environmental exposures, are thought to play significant roles. Although the precise role of androgens and their receptors in carcinogenesis and progression of prostate cancer has not been fully studied, previous studies suggest that these processes are important (136, 137). The production of estrogens from androgens is mediated by the aromatase enzyme, the aberrant expression of which plays a critical role in the development of malignancy in a number of tissues (138). Differences in the activities of these enzymes are determined to a large extent by genetic and epigenetic changes in the genes encoding them.

3.2.1. Androgen Receptor

It had been known that androgens stimulate the growth of prostate cells through the androgen receptor (*AR*) (139). There are two well-known AR target genes, *PSA* and *TMPRSS2–ETS* fusion genes. The exact roles of *PSA* and *TMPRSS2–ETS* in prostate cancer are not fully defined yet. While silencing of *AR* expression leads to decrease growth and induce apoptosis in vitro (140–142), overexpression of *AR* also induces growth inhibition and apoptosis (143). In addition to prostatectomy and radiation therapy, androgen deprivation is one of the most effective treatments for prostate cancer. However, many advanced prostate cancers turn into a castrate-resistant cases. Prostate tumor cells in this stage grow aggressively without stimulation of androgens. Androgen receptor is one of the most frequently overexpressed proteins in the castrate-resistant cases (144). Jarrard et al. (145) reported a significant association between *AR* promoter methylation and its expression in vitro using prostate cancer cell lines.

Several groups found *AR* promoter methylation in 8–39% of the prostate tumor tissues (56, 133, 146–149). Frequencies of *AR* promoter methylation are higher in castrate-resistant cases than ones in primary prostate tumor tissues (146, 148). Until now, the biological significance of *AR* silencing by promoter methylation in castrate-resistant prostate cancer is not clear. Recently, Wang et al. reported that *AR* selectively upregulates M-phase cell-cycle genes in castrate-resistant cells, including ubiquitin-conjugating enzyme E2C (*UBE2C*), a gene that inactivates the M-phase checkpoint. They also found that epigenetic marks at the *UBE2C* enhancer are present in castrate-resistant cells and direct *AR*-enhancer binding and *UBE2C* activation (139). On the other hand, Schayek et al. found that progression to metastatic stage in a cellular model of prostate cancer is associated with methylation of *AR*, and *AR* suppresses the insulin-like growth factor-I receptor (*IGF*), therefore suggesting roles of *IGF* for stimulating *AR* signal in castrate-resistant prostate cancer (149).

3.2.2. Estrogen Receptors

Estrogens are effective against androgen-dependent prostate cancer, but paradoxically, estrogens might also be involved in the causation of this malignancy (150). The biological actions of estrogens are meditated by the estrogen receptor (*ER*) (151). There are two ERs which are highly homologous DNA-binding domains but different N-terminus and ligand-binding domains. Stimulation of *ERα* (*Esr1*) leads to aberrant proliferation, inflammation, and premalignant pathology, whereas activation of *ERβ* (*Esr2*) appears to have beneficial effects regarding cellular proliferation and a putative protective role against carcinogenesis (138).

Both *ERs*, *Esr1* and *Esr2*, are downregulated in prostate tumor tissues (152, 153). Promoter methylation is the primary mechanism responsible for low expression of *ERs* (147, 154, 155). *Esr1* expression is associated with a poor prognosis for hormonal therapy (156), and its hypermethylation is correlated with cancer progression (157). The range of *Esr1* methylation in prostate cancer is diverse from 19 to 95% (31, 147, 157, 158). *Esr2* may serve as a tumor suppressor gene because it protects against uncontrolled cell proliferation in normal prostate cells (155). However, high expression of *Esr2* in prostate tumors is associated with increased risk for recurrence and distant metastasis (153, 159). Therefore, *Esr2* may have multiple roles in carcinogenesis and progression. The frequency of *Esr2* promoter methylation ranges from 65 to 83% in prostate tumors (147, 160, 161). The extent of ERs promoter methylation is significantly higher in prostate tumors than in the BPH samples (158, 161). In addition, the percentage of methylated CpG sites in *Esr2* promoter increased progressively from 0.29% (normal) to 35% (grade 4/5 prostate cancer) (154).

3.2.3. Retinoic Acid Receptor β (RARβ)

Retinoic acid receptor β (*RARβ*) is known as a tumor suppressor gene by interacting with retinoic acid. Expression of retinoic acid receptor B (*RARβ*) is reported to be absent or downregulated in tumor tissues (162). The *RARβ2* promoter is aberrantly methylated in many cancers, including prostate cancer (163). Several groups reported that frequencies of methylation of the *RARβ2* promoter range from 40% to 84% of primary prostate cancers but rarely in normal prostate tissues or BPH samples (29, 35, 56, 95, 121, 163–166). Moderate or high frequencies of *RARβ* promoter methylation were also observed in urine or blood samples, respectively (31, 36, 87). Therefore, *RARβ2* gene methylation may be an ideal biomarker candidate for early detection of prostate cancer (56, 163).

3.2.4. Glutathione S Transferase P1

Glutathione S transferase P1 (GSTP1) is involved in the detoxifying process and elimination of potentially genotoxic foreign compounds by conjugating glutathione into toxic chemicals. These processes protect prostate cells from DNA adducts and carcinogenesis (167). Thus, defective *GSTP1* activity may increase DNA mutations and, therefore, may increase the prostate cancer risk (168). Because of its consistently frequent hypermethylation in the promoter region in prostate cancer, *GSTP1* is perhaps one of the most studied genes in prostate cancer.

Lee et al. first reported a high frequency of *GSTP1* hypermethylation in prostate tumor tissues (169). Since then, numerous studies confirmed similar results consistently. Methylation of the *GSTP1* promoter region occurs in 26–100% of tumor tissues (25, 29–31, 35, 42, 56, 88, 90, 93, 95, 169–180). However, this methylation is rarely detected in normal prostate or BPH tissues. *GSTP1* methylation was also detected consistently with high frequency in urine, blood, and ejaculates of prostate cancer patients, while either low or no methylation was detected in the samples from healthy controls (31, 36, 87, 181–183). Different frequencies of *GSTP1* promoter hypermethylation between tumor and normal prostate tissues make an ideal biomarker for prostate cancer. To increase the accuracy of detection, some investigators used multiple gene panel approaches, had commonly chosen *GSTP1*, and studied its promoter hypermethylation as a biomarker for prostate cancer incidence, progress, and recurrence or survival (31, 36, 165, 184).

3.2.5. Cellular Retinol-Binding Protein 1

Effects of retinoids on prostate gland or prostate cell lines implicate retinoids in the regulation of prostate growth and suppression of prostate cancer development (185). Retinoids exert their effects through a variety of binding proteins including cellular retinol-binding protein (CRBP), retinol-binding proteins (RBP), cellular retinoic-acid-binding protein (CRABP), and two classes of nuclear proteins, i.e., retinoic acid receptors (RARs) and retinoic acid X receptors (RXRs) (186). *CRBP1* is postulated to promote apoptosis via its upregulation of all *trans*-retinoic acid (ATRA) synthesis. Therefore, loss of *CRBP1* could disrupt a retinoic-acid-mediated apoptosis pathway and hence support prostatic tumor progression (187). Low expression of *CRBP1* by promoter methylation has been associated with the malignant tumor tissues including prostate (188, 189). *CRBP1* promoter hypermethylation was selectively found in prostate cancer tissue, rare in BPHs or normal prostate tissues (25, 189, 190). Low expression and hypermethylation in *CRBP1* occur frequently in prostate tumors. However, data indicated that *CRBP1* hypermethylation is not an early event in tumorigenesis (189).

3.2.6. Multidrug Resistance 1 (MDR1/ABCB1)

Multidrug resistance 1 (MDR1) is a transmembrane calcium-dependent efflux pump to detoxify xenobiotics or induce multidrug resistance with GSTs. It is reported to be inactivated in prostate cancer, and some reports showed significantly high hypermethylation at *MDR1* promoter compared to BPH (30, 87, 90, 122, 191). A recent global methylation study showed 6.2- and 13.7-fold higher methylation at *MDR1* in AR-positive (LNCaP) and AR-negative prostate cancer cells (DU145 and PC3), respectively, compared to normal prostate epithelial cell lines (RWPE1) (57). However, Cho et al. showed no significant differences in frequency of *MDR1* methylation among normal ($N=20$), PIN ($N=25$), and prostate cancer tissues ($N=35$), while the prevalence of *MDR1* methylation was as high as 100% (121). Recent multigene methylation analyses showed that the frequency of methylation in *MDR1* gene in prostate cancer samples was 55.3 and 11.6% in BPH. Multigene methylation models, which contain *MDR1* and GSTs, may serve as a good biomarker for prostate cancer (192).

3.2.7. Endothelin B Receptor Gene (EDNRB)

Endothelin B receptor interacts with endothelins to regulate several critical biological processes and may induce cell death by apoptosis and inhibit tumor progression (193). Several studies reported that the *EDNRB* promoter is hypermethylated in a high proportion of prostate tumors and that much less frequency of methylation was found in normal tissues (30, 87, 194, 195). However, other studies found that *EDNRB* methylation frequencies in prostate tumors and paired normal were same, although a high proportion of tumors are methylated (88, 95, 196). Because a high methylation is present in normal and tumor tissues, methylation in *EDNRB* cannot be considered as a specific biomarker for prostate cancer.

3.2.8. EPH Receptor A7 (EPHA7)

Ephrins and EPHS are involved in embryonic development and play a key role for the differentiation of the nervous and vascular systems (197, 198). Their signaling pathway networks with the Wnt signaling pathway during embryogenesis, tissue regeneration, and carcinogenesis (199). Recent expression microarray data, which were profiling androgen-dependent and castrate-resistant cells, revealed that EPHA7 is downregulated in castrate-resistant cells (200). Silencing of *EPHA7* is reactivated by 5-aza treatment (198). These data are supported by a significant correlation between methylation and loss of expression of *EPHA7* (201). A recent report showed higher frequency of methylation of *EPHA7* promoter region in prostate tumor tissues than hyperplasias (42% vs. 19%) (198). A role of *EPHA7* methylation in progression of prostate cancer was confirmed by a positive association between hypermethylation and Gleason scores (198).

3.2.9. Tazarotene-Induced Gene 1

Tazarotene-induced gene 1 (*TIG1*) is frequently silenced in prostate tumors (202). This gene, also known as retinoid-acid-receptor-responsive 1 gene, was first identified as an RA-responsive gene (203). Several researchers reported that *TIG1* was methylated frequently in prostate tumors, but was not or barely low methylated in normal tissues or BPH (88, 122, 164, 183, 204, 205). Zhang et al. further found that the methylation of *TIG1* and *RARβ* was positively correlated. Therefore, it is possible that the methylation of the retinoid response gene *TIG1* occurred in response to the methylation and inactivation of *RARβ*. In addition, concordant hypermethylation of retinoid signaling genes, e.g., *RARβ* or *TIG1* (164), was observed.

Ellinger et al. analyzed the diagnostic and prognostic possibilities of methylation analysis in serum DNA of prostate cancer patients. They found hypermethylation in *TIG1* was more frequent in prostate cancer patients (10%) than in BPH (0%) and healthy individuals (0%) (88). Although the levels of hypermethylation frequency for specific genes are usually lower in serum or urine DNA than those in prostate tissues (Table 1), use of non-invasive biosamples may be worth it for the specific diagnosis of prostate cancer (87).

3.2.10. Aldehyde Dehydrogenase 1A2 and 1A3

Aldehyde dehydrogenases (*ALDH*s) are a group of $NAD(P)^+$-dependent enzymes involved in metabolism of wide variety of aliphatic and aromatic aldehydes (206). *ALDH1A2*, known as retinaldehyde dehydrogenases (RALDHs), and 1A3 are embryonically lethal in gene knockout mice and involved in retinaldehyde oxidation into retinoic acid (RA), a compound with prodifferentiation properties. Most prostate cancer patients show a decreased prostatic RA concentration, and altered retinoid metabolism has been noted in prostate cancer (207, 208). Kim et al. reported *ALDH1A2* promoter region was hypermethylated in primary prostate tumors, as compared with normal prostate specimens (209). Their results are supported by Touma et al., who observed a lower expression of *ALDH1A2* in all prostate tumor FFPE sections relative to normal prostate tissue on the same sections. Therefore, *ALDH1A2* is suggested as a tentative tumor suppressor gene in prostate cancer, and its alteration is suspected as an early event in prostate cancer. *ALDH1A3* was reported to be androgen responsive (210), and upregulation of *ALDH1A3* can increase the oxidation of retinal to RA. Shames et al. reported hypermethylation in the promoter region of *ALDH1A3* in prostate tumor (48). Recently, disulfiram, an inhibitor of *ALDH*s and demethylation agent, showed inhibition of prostate cancer cell growth (211). Thus, promoter methylation at *ALDH1A2* or *1A3* is a suspected biomarker for prostate cancer diagnosis or prevention.

3.3. Tumor Cell Invasion/Metastasis

Metastasis is an extremely complicated process, which occurs through a series of sequential steps that include the invasion, transport, adhesion at a distant site, and outgrowth into a secondary organ. Although metastases are the cause of 90% of human cancer mortality, little is known about the genetic and biochemical determinants of metastasis.

3.3.1. Adenomatous Polyposis Coli

The methylated adenomatous polyposis coli (*APC*) gene causes familial adenomatous polyposis, which is an inherited disorder characterized by extensive colon polyps and the development of colorectal cancer in early adulthood. The APC is involved in the Wnt signal transduction pathway (212). The APC complex is known to function as a gatekeeper in the cell, preventing the transcription of gene products that promote cell proliferation and survival rather than differentiation and apoptosis (213). Hypermethylation of *APC* implies silencing of this gatekeeper, making the cell vulnerable to further epigenetic and genetic changes and, thus, progression toward the development of invasive cancer.

APC promoter methylation is common in various human tumors, especially colon (214). Most studies found a prevalence of 14–100% in prostate cancer tissues but only 5–6% in noncancerous tissues (25, 29–31, 35, 36, 50, 51, 86, 89, 90, 93, 121, 122, 166, 184, 192, 204, 215, 216). Recent studies found that methylation in *APC* is associated with progression of prostate cancer (50, 51, 217). In two small cohorts of prostate cancer patients, a threefold statistically significantly increased HR for promoter methylation in *APC* has been reported among the patients who experienced *PSA* recurrence, metastasis, or death (50, 51). Richiardi et al. found that hypermethylation in the promoter of the *APC* gene is involved in prostate cancer progression using large survival analysis of two independent series of unselected prostate cancer patients (217). Rogers et al. reported somewhat low methylation frequency of *APC* in urine collected after DRE; however, overall, 100% of patients with biopsy-proven prostate cancer had at least one gene methylation among *APC*, *GSTP1*, and *EDNRB* in urine vs. 60% of those without evidence of prostate cancer on biopsy (195). A recent multiplex urine assay study for prostate cancer diagnosis (184) showed that the sensitivities of *APC* (52%) in the urine sediments were similar to those seen by other investigators, who demonstrated a similar sensitivity for *APC* (36).

3.3.2. CD44 (CD44)

CD44 is a transmembrane glycoprotein that is involved in signal transduction and cell–cell and cell–matrix interactions by serving as a receptor. It codes a lipid raft protein like *CAV1* or E-cadherin. Lipid rafts are also involved in angiogenesis and local invasion (19). The *CD44* expression in prostate tumor tissues is lower than ones in adjacent normal tissues. This low expression is correlated with *CD44* promoter methylation (22, 178). Gao et al. reported that decreased *CD44* expression is associated with Gleason score and the distant metastatic progression of prostate cancer (218). Therefore, *CD44* is considered as a metastasis suppressor gene. Furthermore, *CD44* expression and its promoter methylation may correlate with not only tumorigenesis but also progression of prostate cancer (219). However, there are inconsistent results for *CD44* promoter methylation in many reports (22, 28, 87, 95, 122, 178, 219, 220).

3.3.3. E-Cadherin (CDH1)

The E-cadherin (*CDH1*) belongs to the family of cell–cell adhesion molecules and one of the key proteins in the maintenance of cell differentiation and the normal architecture of epithelial tissues (221). DNA methylation-induced *CDH1* silencing was observed in prostate tumor and was associated with tumorigenesis, metastasis, and poor patient outcome (29). Treatment with the demethylating agent 5-aza restored E-cadherin expression in the E-cadherin-negative prostate cancer cell lines (222). The prevalence of methylation varies from 0 to 77% (22, 28–31, 35, 36, 45, 95, 122, 160, 178, 222, 223). The reason for the discrepancy among these studies may come from technical issues, e.g., different CpG targets, detection methods, and samples, but also tumor status issues. Li et al. reported that the overall methylation frequencies of E-cadherin promoter were high in advanced stage samples (70%) and low in early stage (33%) prostate tumors (222). In addition, a recent study reported that methylated and unmethylated E-cadherin gene expression is dominant in primary prostate cancer and bone metastasis, respectively (223). These data suggested that *CDH1* methylation might be a useful biomarker to assess progression of prostate cancer (222).

3.3.4. H-Cadherin (CDH13)

H-cadherin (*CDH13*) belongs to the cadherin family of cell surface glycoproteins responsible for selective cell recognition and adhesion (224). Like *CDH1*, previous reports suggested a role for *CDH13* in cancer invasion and metastasis in human cancers (29, 225, 226). Low expression by *CDH13* methylation has frequently been observed in various cancers (225), including prostate cancer (29, 45, 226). *CDH13* was known as a tumor suppressor gene because low expression of *CDH13* resulted in significant inhibition of tumor growth (227). However, data from animal study suggested that *CDH13* is not involved in the metastasis (228). Although the molecular and biological mechanisms underlying the functions of *CDH13* are unknown, several groups reported *CDH13* promoter methylation in prostate tumors (29, 226). However, Cho et al. reported that the frequency of *CDH13* promoter methylation in prostate cancer was not different from that in BPH tissues (53.6 and 53.3%, respectively) (122).

3.3.5. S100 Calcium-Binding Protein A2 (S100A2) and A6 (S100A6)

Although most S100 proteins are commonly upregulated in tumors and this is often associated with tumor progression, *S100A2* has been documented as a tumor suppressor in some cancers but as an oncogene in others (229). In the case of prostate cancer, Rehman et al. reported that *S100A2* is downregulated (230). *S100A2* methylation was seen in 94% of prostate tumor and 100% of cases of metastatic cancer. However, *S100A2* methylation was also seen in 75% of cases of nonmalignant tissues and in 100% of cases of BPH (25). One interesting fact was age-related increase in *S100A2* methylation levels. This age-related methylation of *S100A2* might be zone dependent because it was observed in a transition zone lesion, but not in a lesion from the peripheral zone (25).

S100A6 is coexpressed with *S100A2* in prostate tissue. *S100A6* methylation was absent in nonmalignant tissues and 100% in BPH tissues, whereas methylation was seen in 52% of prostate tumors. Loss of *S100A6* proteins is frequent in prostatic tumors (230).

3.3.6. Tissue Inhibitor of Metalloproteinase-2 and -3

MMPs are proteolytic enzymes that degrade the extracellular matrix and the basement membrane. High expressions of this enzyme have been associated with tumor growth, invasion, and tumor-induced angiogenesis (231). These pathways are controlled by the balance between the levels of the MMPs and tissue inhibitors of metalloproteinases (TIMPs) (232). Thus, TIMPs are called angiogenesis inhibitors.

TIMP-2 is one of the frequently investigated members of this family because of its involvement in cancer progression and metastasis in a variety of human cancers (233, 234). Pulukuri et al. observed that 25 (60%) of 42 prostate tumors were methylated in comparison with 5 (16%) of 32 normal prostate samples (235). These findings further supported that majority of the prostate cancer tissues have weak or no expression of *TIMP-2* when compared with BPH or normal prostate tissues (235). However, these results were not confirmed by a previous study (236). Ross et al. found that *TIMP-2* was expressed in a majority of prostate tumors and correlated with clinical stages and recurrence. *TIMP-2* expression appears to have a tumor-promoting role in prostate cancer and warrants further investigation (236).This was in contrary to the Pulukuri's study which indicated antitumor effects.

The roles of *TIMP-3* in cancer progression were investigated by several groups. High expression of *TIMP-3* reduces metastasis, induces apoptosis, increases drug sensitivity, and inhibits tumor growth (237–239). A low expression by promoter methylation of *TIMP-3* has been reported to be associated with poor outcomes (240). A recent global methylation study showed 12.08- and 22.3-fold higher methylation at *TIMP-3* in AR-positive (LNCaP) and AR-negative cells (DU145 or PC3), respectively, compared to normal prostate epithelial cell lines (RWPE1) (57). The promoter region of *TIMP-3* was found to be methylated in 97% of prostate tumors (25). However, other studies reported low (0%) and 6% frequencies of *TIMP-3* methylation (30, 56), while additional two studies found *TIMP-3* promoter methylation in 37 and 41% of urine sediments from prostate cancer patients (31, 36). As a diagnostic biomarker in urine DNA, value of *TIMP-3* may be limited due to low frequency of methylation in normal samples.

3.3.7. SRC Family Tyrosine Kinase (FYN)

The SRC family of kinases (SFKs) is the largest family of nonreceptor protein tyrosine kinases and is responsible for signal transduction during differentiation, adhesion, and migration. Aberrant SRC/SFK activity has been widely implicated in cancer development. Several lines of evidence indicate a role for SFKs in the development of prostate cancer, e.g., SFK overexpression in prostate cancer cell lines and tissues (241).

Posadas et al. reported overexpression of *FYN*, a member of SFK, in prostate cancer cell lines and tissues than in normal tissues (242). Sorensen et al. reported frequent aberrant methylation in the *FYN* promoter region in both prostate cancer cell lines and primary prostate tumors. In addition, methylation-induced silencing was confirmed by Western blot and RT-PCR results (243). Methylation at *FYN* promoter should be further investigated to be evaluated as a biomarker of prostate cancer.

3.3.8. Neutral Endopeptidase 24.11

Neutral endopeptidase 24.11 (*NEP*), one of cell surface peptidases, is expressed in prostate. This protein inactivates growth factors needed in the growth of castrate-resistant prostate cancer (244). Therefore, loss of *NEP* activates protein kinase B (Akt), which may accelerate prostate tumor growth (245). Several investigators reported hypermethylation in *NEP* promoter in prostate tumor tissues (87, 244, 246). Usmani et al. observed that methylation of the *NEP* promoter was present only in castrate-resistant prostate cancer cell lines not in androgen-dependent prostate cancer cell lines. Reactivation of *NEP* by demethylating agent 5-aza-2′-deoxycytidine shows that hypermethylation of *NEP* is associated with a loss of *NEP* expression in prostate tumor (244). Further studies are needed to elucidate the impact of *NEP* promoter methylation on the progression to castrate-resistant prostate cancer.

3.4. DNA Repair Genes

Although the specific causes of prostate cancer are not known, androgens, estrogens abnormalities, inflammation, and DNA repair capacity have been implicated. DNA is constantly damaged by endogenous oxygen free radicals and exogenous chemicals. DNA mutations are estimated to spontaneously occur 20,000–40,000 times every day (247, 248). The DNA repair process is important to the survival of cell; therefore, different repair pathways are available to reverse the different types of DNA damage. In fact, over 250 DNA repair enzymes participate in this process (249, 250). Defects in these DNA repair pathways may increase persistent mutations in daughter cell generations, genomic instability, and ultimately prostate cancer risk.

3.4.1. Methylguanine-Methyltransferase

DNA repair genes can be classified into several distinct pathways, including the direct reversal (DR) pathway. The only known enzyme in the DR pathway is methylguanine-methyltransferase (*MGMT*). *MGMT* transfers the alkyl group at the O^6 position of guanine to a cysteine residue within its active site, leading to the direct restoration of the natural chemical composition of DNA without the need for genomic reconstruction. Therefore, defective *MGMT* activity is associated with an increased mutation rate (251). Reports regarding *MGMT* methylation in prostate tumor tissues have been inconsistent.

While three studies reported a low frequency of *MGMT* promoter hypermethylation (0–2%) in prostate tumor tissues (29, 30, 56), others observed higher prevalence of hypermethylation (19–76%) (25, 31, 36, 37, 42, 93, 252). Two other groups reported 15 and 19% *MGMT* hypermethylation frequencies in urine sediment samples from prostate cancer patients, respectively (31, 36). These data suggest that *MGMT* promoter methylation can be a potential biomarker for early detection and surveillance of prostate cancer. However, larger studies will be necessary to resolve these inconsistent results.

4. Conclusions

Although a few large-scale genome-wide analyses of epigenetic variations are currently ongoing, most published studies are small scale with a retrospective design. Therefore, meta-analysis or large studies should be performed to obtain the complete extent and pattern of differential DNA methylation in the promoter region in the critical genes. Since epigenetic changes are involved in carcinogenesis and progression of prostate cancer, information of these epigenetic changes may provide clues for better diagnostic, prognostic, and predictive modalities than existing ones. The ultimate goals of these epigenetic studies are to improve patients' outcomes and enhance quality of life.

A number of clinical trials and therapies are targeting methylated genes. Unlike DNA somatic mutations, DNA methylations are reversible. Thus, hypermethylated tumor suppressor genes can be reactivated with drugs. Several demethylating agents such as 5-azacytidine (Vidaza) and 5-aza-2′-deoxycytidine (decitabine) have been approved as treatments for the myelodysplastic syndrome (MDS) and leukemia (253–255). Some MDS patients treated with 5-azacytidine showed a significant survival benefit (256). However, a major limitation of these therapies is their nonspecific target approach, which may induce unintended side effects. Therefore, not only tumor suppressor genes but also silenced oncogenes can be reactivated. Future studies should focus on developing drugs that can target specific genes.

References

1. Crawford, E. D. (2003) Epidemiology of prostate cancer, *Urology* 62, 3–12.
2. Jemal, A., Siegel, R., Xu, J., and Ward, E. (2010) Cancer statistics, 2010, *CA Cancer J Clin* 60, 277–300.
3. EMGT. (2009) http://www.egtm.eu/tumour_markers_in_prostate_cancer.htm,.
4. Baylin, S. B., and Herman, J. G. (2000) DNA hypermethylation in tumorigenesis: epigenetics joins genetics, *Trends Genet* 16, 168–174.
5. Smiraglia, D. J., and Plass, C. (2002) The study of aberrant methylation in cancer via restriction landmark genomic scanning, *Oncogene* 21, 5414–5426.
6. Rush, L. J., Dai, Z., Smiraglia, D. J., Gao, X., Wright, F. A., Fruhwald, M., Costello, J. F., Held, W. A., Yu, L., Krahe, R., Kolitz, J. E., Bloomfield, C. D., Caligiuri, M. A., and Plass, C. (2001) Novel methylation targets in de novo acute myeloid leukemia with prevalence of chromosome 11 loci, *Blood* 97, 3226–3233.
7. Costello, J. F., Fruhwald, M. C., Smiraglia, D. J., Rush, L. J., Robertson, G. P., Gao, X., Wright, F. A., Feramisco, J. D., Peltomaki, P., Lang, J. C., Schuller, D. E., Yu, L., Bloomfield, C. D., Caligiuri, M. A., Yates, A., Nishikawa, R., Su Huang, H., Petrelli, N. J., Zhang, X., O'Dorisio, M. S., Held, W. A., Cavenee, W. K., and Plass, C. (2000) Aberrant CpG-island methylation has non-random and tumour-type-specific patterns, *Nat Genet* 24, 132–138.
8. Baylin, S. B., Herman, J. G., Graff, J. R., Vertino, P. M., and Issa, J. P. (1998) Alterations in DNA methylation: a fundamental aspect of neoplasia, *Adv Cancer Res* 72, 141–196.
9. Di Croce, L., Raker, V. A., Corsaro, M., Fazi, F., Fanelli, M., Faretta, M., Fuks, F., Lo Coco, F., Kouzarides, T., Nervi, C., Minucci, S., and Pelicci, P. G. (2002) Methyltransferase recruitment and DNA hypermethylation of target promoters by an oncogenic transcription factor, *Science* 295, 1079–1082.
10. Yan, P. S., Shi, H., Rahmatpanah, F., Hsiau, T. H., Hsiau, A. H., Leu, Y. W., Liu, J. C., and Huang, T. H. (2003) Differential distribution of DNA methylation within the *RASSF1A* CpG island in breast cancer, *Cancer Res* 63, 6178–6186.
11. Graff, J. R., Herman, J. G., Myohanen, S., Baylin, S. B., and Vertino, P. M. (1997) Mapping patterns of CpG island methylation in normal and neoplastic cells implicates both upstream and downstream regions in de novo methylation, *J Biol Chem* 272, 22322–22329.
12. Esteller, M. (2000) Epigenetic lesions causing genetic lesions in human cancer: promoter hypermethylation of DNA repair genes, *Eur J Cancer* 36, 2294–2300.
13. Bachman, K. E., Herman, J. G., Corn, P. G., Merlo, A., Costello, J. F., Cavenee, W. K., Baylin, S. B., and Graff, J. R. (1999) Methylation-associated silencing of the tissue inhibitor of metalloproteinase-3 gene suggest a suppressor role in kidney, brain, and other human cancers, *Cancer Res* 59, 798–802.
14. Toyota, M., Ohe-Toyota, M., Ahuja, N., and Issa, J.-P. J. (2000) Distinct genetic profiles in colorectal tumors with or without the CpG island methylator phenotype, *PNAS* 97, 710–715.

15. Stirzaker, C., Millar, D. S., Paul, C. L., Warnecke, P. M., Harrison, J., Vincent, P. C., Frommer, M., and Clark, S. J. (1997) Extensive DNA methylation spanning the Rb promoter in retinoblastoma tumors, *Cancer Res* 57, 2229–2237.
16. Deng, G., Chen, A., Hong, J., Chae, H. S., and Kim, Y. S. (1999) Methylation of CpG in a small region of the hMLH1 promoter invariably correlates with the absence of gene expression, *Cancer Res* 59, 2029–2033.
17. Gonzalgo, M. L., Bender, C. M., You, E. H., Glendening, J. M., Flores, J. F., Walker, G. J., Hayward, N. K., Jones, P. A., and Fountain, J. W. (1997) Low frequency of *p16/CDKN2A* methylation in sporadic melanoma: comparative approaches for methylation analysis of primary tumors, *Cancer Res* 57, 5336–5347.
18. Gonzalez-Zulueta, M., Bender, C. M., Yang, A. S., Nguyen, T., Beart, R. W., Van Tornout, J. M., and Jones, P. A. (1995) Methylation of the 5′ CpG island of the p16/CDKN2 tumor suppressor gene in normal and transformed human tissues correlates with gene silencing, *Cancer Res* 55, 4531–4535.
19. Patra, S. K., and Bettuzzi, S. (2007) Epigenetic DNA-methylation regulation of genes coding for lipid raft-associated components: a role for raft proteins in cell transformation and cancer progression (review), *Oncol Rep* 17, 1279–1290.
20. Cui, J., Rohr, L. R., Swanson, G., Speights, V. O., Maxwell, T., and Brothman, A. R. (2001) Hypermethylation of the caveolin-1 gene promoter in prostate cancer, *Prostate* 46, 249–256.
21. Bachmann, N., Haeusler, J., Luedeke, M., Kuefer, R., Perner, S., Assum, G., Paiss, T., Hoegel, J., Vogel, W., and Maier, C. (2008) Expression changes of *CAV1* and EZH2, located on 7q31 approximately q36, are rarely related to genomic alterations in primary prostate carcinoma, *Cancer Genet Cytogenet* 182, 103–110.
22. Woodson, K., Hanson, J., and Tangrea, J. (2004) A survey of gene-specific methylation in human prostate cancer among black and white men, *Cancer Lett* 205, 181–188.
23. Karam, J. A., Lotan, Y., Roehrborn, C. G., Ashfaq, R., Karakiewicz, P. I., and Shariat, S. F. (2007) Caveolin-1 overexpression is associated with aggressive prostate cancer recurrence, *Prostate 67,* 614–622.
24. Di Vizio, D., Sotgia, F., Williams, T. M., Hassan, G. S., Capozza, F., Frank, P. G., Pestell, R. G., Loda, M., Freeman, M. R., and Lisanti, M. P. (2007) Caveolin-1 is required for the upregulation of fatty acid synthase (FASN), a tumor promoter, during prostate cancer progression, *Cancer Biol Ther* 6, 1263–1268.
25. Jeronimo, C., Henrique, R., Hoque, M. O., Mambo, E., Ribeiro, F. R., Varzim, G., Oliveira, J., Teixeira, M. R., Lopes, C., and Sidransky, D. (2004) A quantitative promoter methylation profile of prostate cancer, *Clin Cancer Res* 10, 8472–8478.
26. Konishi, N., Nakamura, M., Kishi, M., Nishimine, M., Ishida, E., and Shimada, K. (2002) Heterogeneous methylation and deletion patterns of the INK4a/ARF locus within prostate carcinomas, *Am J Pathol* 160, 1207–1214.
27. Nguyen, T. T., Nguyen, C. T., Gonzales, F. A., Nichols, P. W., Yu, M. C., and Jones, P. A. (2000) Analysis of cyclin-dependent kinase inhibitor expression and methylation patterns in human prostate cancers, *Prostate* 43, 233–242.
28. Schwarzenbach, H., Chun, F. K., Isbarn, H., Huland, H., and Pantel, K. (2010) Genomic profiling of cell-free DNA in blood and bone marrow of prostate cancer patients, *J Cancer Res Clin Oncol.*
29. Maruyama, R., Toyooka, S., Toyooka, K. O., Virmani, A. K., Zochbauer-Muller, S., Farinas, A. J., Minna, J. D., McConnell, J., Frenkel, E. P., and Gazdar, A. F. (2002) Aberrant promoter methylation profile of prostate cancers and its relationship to clinicopathological features, *Clin Cancer Res* 8, 514–519.
30. Yegnasubramanian, S., Kowalski, J., Gonzalgo, M. L., Zahurak, M., Piantadosi, S., Walsh, P. C., Bova, G. S., De Marzo, A. M., Isaacs, W. B., and Nelson, W. G. (2004) Hypermethylation of CpG islands in primary and metastatic human prostate cancer, *Cancer Res* 64, 1975–1986.
31. Hoque, M. O., Topaloglu, O., Begum, S., Henrique, R., Rosenbaum, E., Van Criekinge, W., Westra, W. H., and Sidransky, D. (2005) Quantitative methylation-specific polymerase chain reaction gene patterns in urine sediment distinguish prostate cancer patients from control subjects, *J Clin Oncol* 23, 6569–6575.
32. Gu, K., Mes-Masson, A. M., Gauthier, J., and Saad, F. (1998) Analysis of the p16 tumor suppressor gene in early-stage prostate cancer, *Mol Carcinog* 21, 164–170.
33. Herman, J. G., Merlo, A., Mao, L., Lapidus, R. G., Issa, J. P., Davidson, N. E., Sidransky, D., and Baylin, S. B. (1995) Inactivation of the CDKN2/p16/MTS1 gene is frequently associated with aberrant DNA methylation in all common human cancers, *Cancer Res* 55, 4525–4530.
34. Jarrard, D. F., Bova, G. S., Ewing, C. M., Pin, S. S., Nguyen, S. H., Baylin, S. B., Cairns, P.,

Sidransky, D., Herman, J. G., and Isaacs, W. B. (1997) Deletional, mutational, and methylation analyses of CDKN2 (p16/MTS1) in primary and metastatic prostate cancer, *Genes Chromosomes Cancer* 19, 90-96.

35. Florl, A. R., Steinhoff, C., Muller, M., Seifert, H. H., Hader, C., Engers, R., Ackermann, R., and Schulz, W. A. (2004) Coordinate hypermethylation at specific genes in prostate carcinoma precedes LINE-1 hypomethylation, *Br J Cancer* 91, 985–994.
36. Roupret, M., Hupertan, V., Yates, D. R., Catto, J. W., Rehman, I., Meuth, M., Ricci, S., Lacave, R., Cancel-Tassin, G., de la Taille, A., Rozet, F., Cathelineau, X., Vallancien, G., Hamdy, F. C., and Cussenot, O. (2007) Molecular detection of localized prostate cancer using quantitative methylation-specific PCR on urinary cells obtained following prostate massage, *Clin Cancer Res* 13, 1720–1725.
37. Higuchi, T., Nakamura, M., Shimada, K., Ishida, E., Hirao, K., and Konishi, N. (2008) HRK inactivation associated with promoter methylation and LOH in prostate cancer, *Prostate* 68, 105–113.
38. Nakamura, M., Watanabe, T., Klangby, U., Asker, C., Wiman, K., Yonekawa, Y., Kleihues, P., and Ohgaki, H. (2001) p14ARF deletion and methylation in genetic pathways to glioblastomas, *Brain Pathol* 11, 159–168.
39. Lin, H. H., Ke, H. L., Huang, S. P., Wu, W. J., Chen, Y. K., and Chang, L. L. (2009) Increase sensitivity in detecting superficial, low grade bladder cancer by combination analysis of hypermethylation of E-cadherin, p16, p14, *RASSF1A* genes in urine, *Urol Oncol.*
40. Chim, C. S., Chan, W. W., and Kwong, Y. L. (2008) Epigenetic dysregulation of the DAP kinase/p14/HDM2/p53/Apaf-1 apoptosis pathway in acute leukaemias, *J Clin Pathol* 61, 844–847.
41. Calmon, M. F., Colombo, J., Carvalho, F., Souza, F. P., Filho, J. F., Fukuyama, E. E., Camargo, A. A., Caballero, O. L., Tajara, E. H., Cordeiro, J. A., and Rahal, P. (2007) Methylation profile of genes *CDKN2A (p14* and *p16*), *DAPK1, CDH1,* and *ADAM23* in head and neck cancer, *Cancer Genet Cytogenet* 173, 31–37.
42. Konishi, N., Nakamura, M., Kishi, M., Nishimine, M., Ishida, E., and Shimada, K. (2002) DNA hypermethylation status of multiple genes in prostate adenocarcinomas, *Jpn J Cancer Res* 93, 767–773.
43. Yam, C. H., Fung, T. K., and Poon, R. Y. (2002) Cyclin A in cell cycle control and cancer, *Cell Mol Life Sci* 59, 1317–1326.
44. Yang, N., Eijsink, J. J., Lendvai, A., Volders, H. H., Klip, H., Buikema, H. J., van Hemel, B. M., Schuuring, E., van der Zee, A. G., and Wisman, G. B. (2009) Methylation markers for *CCNA1* and C13ORF18 are strongly associated with high-grade cervical intraepithelial neoplasia and cervical cancer in cervical scrapings, *Cancer Epidemiol Biomarkers Prev* 18, 3000–3007.
45. Padar, A., Sathyanarayana, U. G., Suzuki, M., Maruyama, R., Hsieh, J. T., Frenkel, E. P., Minna, J. D., and Gazdar, A. F. (2003) Inactivation of cyclin D2 gene in prostate cancers by aberrant promoter methylation, *Clin Cancer Res* 9, 4730–4734.
46. Aaltomaa, S., Eskelinen, M., and Lipponen, P. (1999) Expression of cyclin A and D proteins in prostate cancer and their relation to clinicopathological variables and patient survival, *Prostate* 38, 175–182.
47. Wegiel, B., Bjartell, A., Tuomela, J., Dizeyi, N., Tinzl, M., Helczynski, L., Nilsson, E., Otterbein, L. E., Harkonen, P., and Persson, J. L. (2008) Multiple cellular mechanisms related to cyclin A1 in prostate cancer invasion and metastasis, *J Natl Cancer Inst* 100, 1022–1036.
48. Shames, D. S., Girard, L., Gao, B., Sato, M., Lewis, C. M., Shivapurkar, N., Jiang, A., Perou, C. M., Kim, Y. H., Pollack, J. R., Fong, K. M., Lam, C. L., Wong, M., Shyr, Y., Nanda, R., Olopade, O. I., Gerald, W., Euhus, D. M., Shay, J. W., Gazdar, A. F., and Minna, J. D. (2006) A genome-wide screen for promoter methylation in lung cancer identifies novel methylation markers for multiple malignancies, *PLoS Med* 3, e486.
49. Henrique, R., Costa, V. L., Cerveira, N., Carvalho, A. L., Hoque, M. O., Ribeiro, F. R., Oliveira, J., Teixeira, M. R., Sidransky, D., and Jeronimo, C. (2006) Hypermethylation of Cyclin D2 is associated with loss of mRNA expression and tumor development in prostate cancer, *J Mol Med* 84, 911–918.
50. Henrique, R., Ribeiro, F. R., Fonseca, D., Hoque, M. O., Carvalho, A. L., Costa, V. L., Pinto, M., Oliveira, J., Teixeira, M. R., Sidransky, D., and Jeronimo, C. (2007) High promoter methylation levels of *APC* predict poor prognosis in sextant biopsies from prostate cancer patients, *Clin Cancer Res* 13, 6122–6129.
51. Rosenbaum, E., Hoque, M. O., Cohen, Y., Zahurak, M., Eisenberger, M. A., Epstein, J. I., Partin, A. W., and Sidransky, D. (2005) Promoter hypermethylation as an independent prognostic factor for relapse in patients with prostate cancer following radical prostatectomy, *Clin Cancer Res* 11, 8321–8325.

52. Mittag, F., Kuester, D., Vieth, M., Peters, B., Stolte, B., Roessner, A., and Schneider-Stock, R. (2006) *DAPK* promotor methylation is an early event in colorectal carcinogenesis, *Cancer Lett* 240, 69–75.
53. Cohen, O., Feinstein, E., and Kimchi, A. (1997) DAP-kinase is a Ca2+/calmodulin-dependent, cytoskeletal-associated protein kinase, with cell death-inducing functions that depend on its catalytic activity, *EMBO J* 16, 998–1008.
54. Chan, M. W., Chan, L. W., Tang, N. L., Tong, J. H., Lo, K. W., Lee, T. L., Cheung, H. Y., Wong, W. S., Chan, P. S., Lai, F. M., and To, K. F. (2002) Hypermethylation of multiple genes in tumor tissues and voided urine in urinary bladder cancer patients, *Clin Cancer Res* 8, 464–470.
55. Simpson, D. J., Clayton, R. N., and Farrell, W. E. (2002) Preferential loss of Death Associated Protein kinase expression in invasive pituitary tumours is associated with either CpG island methylation or homozygous deletion, *Oncogene* 21, 1217–1224.
56. Yamanaka, M., Watanabe, M., Yamada, Y., Takagi, A., Murata, T., Takahashi, H., Suzuki, H., Ito, H., Tsukino, H., Katoh, T., Sugimura, Y., and Shiraishi, T. (2003) Altered methylation of multiple genes in carcinogenesis of the prostate, *Int J Cancer* 106, 382–387.
57. Mishra, D. K., Chen, Z., Wu, Y., Sarkissyan, M., Koeffler, H. P., and Vadgama, J. V. (2010) Global methylation pattern of genes in androgen-sensitive and androgen-independent prostate cancer cells, *Mol Cancer Ther* 9, 33–45.
58. Carvalho, J. R., Filipe, L., Costa, V. L., Ribeiro, F. R., Martins, A. T., Teixeira, M. R., Jeronimo, C., and Henrique, R. (2010) Detailed analysis of expression and promoter methylation status of apoptosis-related genes in prostate cancer, *Apoptosis* 15, 956–965.
59. Michie, A. M., McCaig, A. M., Nakagawa, R., and Vukovic, M. (2010) Death-associated protein kinase (*DAPK*) and signal transduction: regulation in cancer, *FEBS J* 277, 74–80.
60. Verri, C., Roz, L., Conte, D., Liloglou, T., Livio, A., Vesin, A., Fabbri, A., Andriani, F., Brambilla, C., Tavecchio, L., Calarco, G., Calabro, E., Mancini, A., Tosi, D., Bossi, P., Field, J. K., Brambilla, E., and Sozzi, G. (2009) Fragile histidine triad gene inactivation in lung cancer: the European Early Lung Cancer project, *Am J Respir Crit Care Med* 179, 396–401.
61. Paulsson, K., An, Q., Moorman, A. V., Parker, H., Molloy, G., Davies, T., Griffiths, M., Ross, F. M., Irving, J., Harrison, C. J., Young, B. D., and Strefford, J. C. (2009) Methylation of tumour suppressor gene promoters in the presence and absence of transcriptional silencing in high hyperdiploid acute lymphoblastic leukaemia, *Br J Haematol* 144, 838–847.
62. Hong, F. Z., Wang, B., Li, H. M., and Liew, C. T. (2005) (Hypermethylation of fragile histidine triad gene and 3p14 allelic deletion in ovarian carcinomas), *Zhonghua Bing Li Xue Za Zhi* 34, 257–261.
63. Goldberg, M., Rummelt, C., Laerm, A., Helmbold, P., Holbach, L. M., and Ballhausen, W. G. (2006) Epigenetic silencing contributes to frequent loss of the fragile histidine triad tumour suppressor in basal cell carcinomas, *Br J Dermatol* 155, 1154–1158.
64. Neyaz, M. K., Kumar, R. S., Hussain, S., Naqvi, S. H., Kohaar, I., Thakur, N., Kashyap, V., Das, B. C., Husain, S. A., and Bharadwaj, M. (2008) Effect of aberrant promoter methylation of *FHIT* and *RASSF1A* genes on susceptibility to cervical cancer in a North Indian population, *Biomarkers* 13, 597–606.
65. Leal, M. F., Lima, E. M., Silva, P. N., Assumpcao, P. P., Calcagno, D. Q., Payao, S. L., Burbano, R. R., and Smith, M. A. (2007) Promoter hypermethylation of *CDH1*, *FHIT*, MTAP and PLAGL1 in gastric adenocarcinoma in individuals from Northern Brazil, *World J Gastroenterol* 13, 2568–2574.
66. Kvasha, S., Gordiyuk, V., Kondratov, A., Ugryn, D., Zgonnyk, Y. M., Rynditch, A. V., and Vozianov, A. F. (2008) Hypermethylation of the 5′CpG island of the *FHIT* gene in clear cell renal carcinomas, *Cancer Lett* 265, 250–257.
67. Kim, J. W., Cheng, Y., Liu, W., Li, T., Yegnasubramanian, S., Zheng, S. L., Xu, J., Isaacs, W. B., and Chang, B. L. (2009) Genetic and epigenetic inactivation of *LPL* gene in human prostate cancer, *Int J Cancer* 124, 734–738.
68. Sard, L., Accornero, P., Tornielli, S., Delia, D., Bunone, G., Campiglio, M., Colombo, M. P., Gramegna, M., Croce, C. M., Pierotti, M. A., and Sozzi, G. (1999) The tumor-suppressor gene *FHIT* is involved in the regulation of apoptosis and in cell cycle control, *Proc Natl Acad Sci USA* 96, 8489–8492.
69. Guo, Z., Johansson, S. L., Rhim Js., and Vishwanatha, J. K. (2000) Fragile histidine triad gene expression in primary prostate cancer and in an in vitro model, *Prostate* 43, 101–110.
70. Latil, A., Bieche, I., Fournier, G., Cussenot, O., Pesche, S., and Lidereau, R. (1998) Molecular analysis of the *FHIT* gene in human prostate cancer, *Oncogene* 16, 1863–1868.
71. Waha, A., Koch, A., Hartmann, W., Mack, H., Schramm, J., Sorensen, N., Berthold, F.,

Wiestler, O. D., and Pietsch, T. (2004) Analysis of HIC-1 methylation and transcription in human ependymomas, *Int J Cancer* 110, 542–549.

72. Tam, K. F., Liu, V. W., Liu, S. S., Tsang, P. C., Cheung, A. N., Yip, A. M., and Ngan, H. Y. (2007) Methylation profile in benign, borderline and malignant ovarian tumors, *J Cancer Res Clin Oncol* 133, 331–341.
73. Chopin, V., and Leprince, D. (2006) (Chromosome arm 17p13.3: could *HIC1* be the one?), *Med Sci (Paris)* 22, 54–61.
74. Chen, W. Y., Zeng, X., Carter, M. G., Morrell, C. N., Chiu Yen, R. W., Esteller, M., Watkins, D. N., Herman, J. G., Mankowski, J. L., and Baylin, S. B. (2003) Heterozygous disruption of *Hic1* predisposes mice to a gender-dependent spectrum of malignant tumors, *Nat Genet* 33, 197–202.
75. Chen, W., Cooper, T. K., Zahnow, C. A., Overholtzer, M., Zhao, Z., Ladanyi, M., Karp, J. E., Gokgoz, N., Wunder, J. S., Andrulis, I. L., Levine, A. J., Mankowski, J. L., and Baylin, S. B. (2004) Epigenetic and genetic loss of *Hic1* function accentuates the role of p53 in tumorigenesis, *Cancer Cell* 6, 387–398.
76. Kekeeva, T. V., Popova, O. P., Shegai, P. V., Alekseev, B., Adnreeva, I., Zaletaev, D. V., and Nemtsova, M. V. (2007) (Abberant methylation of p16, *HIC1*, N33 and *GSTP1* genes in tumor epitelium and tumor-associated stromal cells of prostate cancer), *Mol Biol (Mosk)* 41, 79–85.
77. Gallucci, M., Merola, R., Leonardo, C., De Carli, P., Farsetti, A., Sentinelli, S., Sperduti, I., Mottolese, M., Carlini, P., Vico, E., Simone, G., and Cianciulli, A. (2009) Genetic profile identification in clinically localized prostate carcinoma, *Urol Oncol* 27, 502–508.
78. Kioussi, C., Briata, P., Baek, S. H., Rose, D. W., Hamblet, N. S., Herman, T., Ohgi, K. A., Lin, C., Gleiberman, A., Wang, J., Brault, V., Ruiz-Lozano, P., Nguyen, H. D., Kemler, R., Glass, C. K., Wynshaw-Boris, A., and Rosenfeld, M. G. (2002) Identification of a Wnt/Dvl/beta-Catenin - > *Pitx2* pathway mediating cell-type-specific proliferation during development, *Cell* 111, 673–685.
79. Maier, S., Nimmrich, I., Koenig, T., Eppenberger-Castori, S., Bohlmann, I., Paradiso, A., Spyratos, F., Thomssen, C., Mueller, V., Nahrig, J., Schittulli, F., Kates, R., Lesche, R., Schwope, I., Kluth, A., Marx, A., Martens, J. W., Foekens, J. A., Schmitt, M., and Harbeck, N. (2007) DNA-methylation of the homeodomain transcription factor *PITX2* reliably predicts risk of distant disease recurrence in tamoxifen-treated, node-negative breast cancer patients-Technical and clinical validation in a multi-centre setting in collaboration with the European Organisation for Research and Treatment of Cancer (EORTC) PathoBiology group, *Eur J Cancer* 43, 1679–1686.
80. Harbeck, N., Nimmrich, I., Hartmann, A., Ross, J. S., Cufer, T., Grutzmann, R., Kristiansen, G., Paradiso, A., Hartmann, O., Margossian, A., Martens, J., Schwope, I., Lukas, A., Muller, V., Milde-Langosch, K., Nahrig, J., Foekens, J., Maier, S., Schmitt, M., and Lesche, R. (2008) Multicenter study using paraffin-embedded tumor tissue testing *PITX2* DNA methylation as a marker for outcome prediction in tamoxifen-treated, node-negative breast cancer patients, *J Clin Oncol* 26, 5036–5042.
81. Nimmrich, I., Sieuwerts, A. M., Meijer-van Gelder, M. E., Schwope, I., Bolt-de Vries, J., Harbeck, N., Koenig, T., Hartmann, O., Kluth, A., Dietrich, D., Magdolen, V., Portengen, H., Look, M. P., Klijn, J. G., Lesche, R., Schmitt, M., Maier, S., Foekens, J. A., and Martens, J. W. (2008) DNA hypermethylation of *PITX2* is a marker of poor prognosis in untreated lymph node-negative hormone receptor-positive breast cancer patients, *Breast Cancer Res Treat* 111, 429–437.
82. Weiss, G., Cottrell, S., Distler, J., Schatz, P., Kristiansen, G., Ittmann, M., Haefliger, C., Lesche, R., Hartmann, A., Corman, J., and Wheeler, T. (2009) DNA methylation of the *PITX2* gene promoter region is a strong independent prognostic marker of biochemical recurrence in patients with prostate cancer after radical prostatectomy, *J Urol* 181, 1678–1685.
83. Banez, L. L., Sun, L., van Leenders, G. J., Wheeler, T. M., Bangma, C. H., Freedland, S. J., Ittmann, M. M., Lark, A. L., Madden, J. F., Hartman, A., Weiss, G., and Castanos-Velez, E. (2010) Multicenter clinical validation of *PITX2* methylation as a prostate specific antigen recurrence predictor in patients with post-radical prostatectomy prostate cancer, *J Urol* 184, 149–156.
84. Vanaja, D. K., Ehrich, M., Van den Boom, D., Cheville, J. C., Karnes, R. J., Tindall, D. J., Cantor, C. R., and Young, C. Y. (2009) Hypermethylation of genes for diagnosis and risk stratification of prostate cancer, *Cancer Invest* 27, 549–560.
85. Hussain, S. P., and Harris, C. C. (2007) Inflammation and cancer: an ancient link with novel potentials, *Int J Cancer* 121, 2373–2380.

86. Bastian, P. J., Ellinger, J., Wellmann, A., Wernert, N., Heukamp, L. C., Muller, S. C., and von Ruecker, A. (2005) Diagnostic and prognostic information in prostate cancer with the help of a small set of hypermethylated gene loci, *Clin Cancer Res* 11, 4097–4106.
87. Bastian, P. J., Palapattu, G. S., Yegnasubramanian, S., Rogers, C. G., Lin, X., Mangold, L. A., Trock, B., Eisenberger, M. A., Partin, A. W., and Nelson, W. G. (2008) CpG island hypermethylation profile in the serum of men with clinically localized and hormone refractory metastatic prostate cancer, *J Urol* 179, 529-534; discussion 534–525.
88. Ellinger, J., Bastian, P. J., Jurgan, T., Biermann, K., Kahl, P., Heukamp, L. C., Wernert, N., Muller, S. C., and von Ruecker, A. (2008) CpG island hypermethylation at multiple gene sites in diagnosis and prognosis of prostate cancer, *Urology* 71, 161–167.
89. Bastian, P. J., Ellinger, J., Heukamp, L. C., Kahl, P., Muller, S. C., and von Rucker, A. (2007) Prognostic value of CpG island hypermethylation at *PTGS2*, RAR-beta, EDNRB, and other gene loci in patients undergoing radical prostatectomy, *Eur Urol* 51, 665-674; discussion 674.
90. Okegawa, T., Nutahara, K., and Higashihara, E. (2010) Association of circulating tumor cells with tumor-related methylated DNA in patients with hormone-refractory prostate cancer, *Int J Urol* 17, 466–475.
91. Kuzmin, I., Gillespie, J. W., Protopopov, A., Geil, L., Dreijerink, K., Yang, Y., Vocke, C. D., Duh, F. M., Zabarovsky, E., Minna, J. D., Rhim, J. S., Emmert-Buck, M. R., Linehan, W. M., and Lerman, M. I. (2002) The *RASSF1A* tumor suppressor gene is inactivated in prostate tumors and suppresses growth of prostate carcinoma cells, *Cancer Res* 62, 3498–3502.
92. Liu, L., Yoon, J. H., Dammann, R., and Pfeifer, G. P. (2002) Frequent hypermethylation of the *RASSF1A* gene in prostate cancer, *Oncogene* 21, 6835–6840.
93. Kang, G. H., Lee, S., Lee, H. J., and Hwang, K. S. (2004) Aberrant CpG island hypermethylation of multiple genes in prostate cancer and prostatic intraepithelial neoplasia, *J Pathol* 202, 233–240.
94. Kawamoto, K., Okino, S. T., Place, R. F., Urakami, S., Hirata, H., Kikuno, N., Kawakami, T., Tanaka, Y., Pookot, D., Chen, Z., Majid, S., Enokida, H., Nakagawa, M., and Dahiya, R. (2007) Epigenetic modifications of *RASSF1A* gene through chromatin remodeling in prostate cancer, *Clin Cancer Res* 13, 2541–2548.
95. Singal, R., Ferdinand, L., Reis, I. M., and Schlesselman, J. J. (2004) Methylation of multiple genes in prostate cancer and the relationship with clinicopathological features of disease, *Oncol Rep* 12, 631–637.
96. Aitchison, A., Warren, A., Neal, D., and Rabbitts, P. (2007) *RASSF1A* promoter methylation is frequently detected in both pre-malignant and non-malignant microdissected prostatic epithelial tissues, *Prostate* 67, 638–644.
97. Srinivas, S. R., Gopal, E., Zhuang, L., Itagaki, S., Martin, P. M., Fei, Y. J., Ganapathy, V., and Prasad, P. D. (2005) Cloning and functional identification of slc5a12 as a sodium-coupled low-affinity transporter for monocarboxylates (SMCT2), *Biochem J* 392, 655–664.
98. Kennedy, K. M., and Dewhirst, M. W. (2010) Tumor metabolism of lactate: the influence and therapeutic potential for MCT and CD147 regulation, *Future Oncol* 6, 127–148.
99. Ganapathy, V., Thangaraju, M., Gopal, E., Martin, P. M., Itagaki, S., Miyauchi, S., and Prasad, P. D. (2008) Sodium-coupled monocarboxylate transporters in normal tissues and in cancer, *AAPS J* 10, 193–199.
100. Schagdarsurengin, U., Gimm, O., Dralle, H., Hoang-Vu, C., and Dammann, R. (2006) CpG island methylation of tumor-related promoters occurs preferentially in undifferentiated carcinoma, *Thyroid* 16, 633–642.
101. Li, H., Myeroff, L., Smiraglia, D., Romero, M. F., Pretlow, T. P., Kasturi, L., Lutterbaugh, J., Rerko, R. M., Casey, G., Issa, J. P., Willis, J., Willson, J. K., Plass, C., and Markowitz, S. D. (2003) *SLC5A8*, a sodium transporter, is a tumor suppressor gene silenced by methylation in human colon aberrant crypt foci and cancers, *Proc Natl Acad Sci USA* 100, 8412–8417.
102. Park, J., Brena, RM., Gruidl, M., Zhou, J, Huang, T, Plass, C, and Tockman, MS. (2005) CpG island hypermethylation profiling of lung cancer using restriction landmark genomic scanning (RLGS) analysis., *Cancer Biomarkers* 1, 193–200.
103. Thangaraju, M., Gopal, E., Martin, P. M., Ananth, S., Smith, S. B., Prasad, P. D., Sterneck, E., and Ganapathy, V. (2006) *SLC5A8* triggers tumor cell apoptosis through pyruvate-dependent inhibition of histone deacetylases, *Cancer Res* 66, 11560–11564.
104. Dong, S. M., Lee, E. J., Jeon, E. S., Park, C. K., and Kim, K. M. (2005) Progressive methylation during the serrated neoplasia pathway of the colorectum, *Mod Pathol* 18, 170–178.
105. Ganapathy, V., Gopal, E., Miyauchi, S., and Prasad, P. D. (2005) Biological functions of

SLC5A8, a candidate tumour suppressor, *Biochem Soc Trans* 33, 237–240.

106. Hong, C., Maunakea, A., Jun, P., Bollen, A. W., Hodgson, J. G., Goldenberg, D. D., Weiss, W. A., and Costello, J. F. (2005) Shared epigenetic mechanisms in human and mouse gliomas inactivate expression of the growth suppressor *SLC5A8*, *Cancer Res* 65, 3617–3623.

107. Porra, V., Ferraro-Peyret, C., Durand, C., Selmi-Ruby, S., Giroud, H., Berger-Dutrieux, N., Decaussin, M., Peix, J. L., Bournaud, C., Orgiazzi, J., Borson-Chazot, F., Dante, R., and Rousset, B. (2005) Silencing of the tumor suppressor gene *SLC5A8* is associated with BRAF mutations in classical papillary thyroid carcinomas, *J Clin Endocrinol Metab* 90, 3028–3035.

108. Ueno, M., Toyota, M., Akino, K., Suzuki, H., Kusano, M., Satoh, A., Mita, H., Sasaki, Y., Nojima, M., Yanagihara, K., Hinoda, Y., Tokino, T., and Imai, K. (2004) Aberrant methylation and histone deacetylation associated with silencing of *SLC5A8* in gastric cancer, *Tumour Biol* 25, 134–140.

109. Hu, S., Liu, D., Tufano, R. P., Carson, K. A., Rosenbaum, E., Cohen, Y., Holt, E. H., Kiseljak-Vassiliades, K., Rhoden, K. J., Tolaney, S., Condouris, S., Tallini, G., Westra, W. H., Umbricht, C. B., Zeiger, M. A., Califano, J. A., Vasko, V., and Xing, M. (2006) Association of aberrant methylation of tumor suppressor genes with tumor aggressiveness and BRAF mutation in papillary thyroid cancer, *Int J Cancer* 119, 2322–2329.

110. Park, J. Y., Helm, J. F., Zheng, W., Ly, Q. P., Hodul, P. J., Centeno, B. A., and Malafa, M. P. (2008) Silencing of the candidate tumor suppressor gene solute carrier family 5 member 8 (*SLC5A8*) in human pancreatic cancer, *Pancreas* 36, e32–39.

111. Park, J. Y., Zheng, W., Kim, D., Cheng, J. Q., Kumar, N., Ahmad, N., and Pow-Sang, J. (2007) Candidate tumor suppressor gene *SLC5A8* is frequently down-regulated by promoter hypermethylation in prostate tumor, *Cancer Detect Prev* 31, 359–365.

112. Pinheiro, C., Reis, R. M., Ricardo, S., Longatto-Filho, A., Schmitt, F., and Baltazar, F. (2010) Expression of monocarboxylate transporters 1, 2, and 4 in human tumours and their association with CD147 and *CD44*, *J Biomed Biotechnol 2010*, 427694.

113. Weihe, E., and Eiden, L. E. (2000) Chemical neuroanatomy of the vesicular amine transporters, *FASEB J* 14, 2435–2449.

114. Kristiansen, G., Pilarsky, C., Wissmann, C., Kaiser, S., Bruemmendorf, T., Roepcke, S., Dahl, E., Hinzmann, B., Specht, T., Pervan, J., Stephan, C., Loening, S., Dietel, M., and Rosenthal, A. (2005) Expression profiling of microdissected matched prostate cancer samples reveals CD166/MEMD and CD24 as new prognostic markers for patient survival, *J Pathol* 205, 359–376.

115. Sorensen, K. D., Wild, P. J., Mortezavi, A., Adolf, K., Torring, N., Heeboll, S., Ulhoi, B. P., Ottosen, P., Sulser, T., Hermanns, T., Moch, H., Borre, M., Orntoft, T. F., and Dyrskjot, L. (2009) Genetic and epigenetic *SLC18A2* silencing in prostate cancer is an independent adverse predictor of biochemical recurrence after radical prostatectomy, *Clin Cancer Res* 15, 1400–1410.

116. Chang, B. L., Liu, W., Sun, J., Dimitrov, L., Li, T., Turner, A. R., Zheng, S. L., Isaacs, W. B., and Xu, J. (2007) Integration of somatic deletion analysis of prostate cancers and germline linkage analysis of prostate cancer families reveals two small consensus regions for prostate cancer genes at 8p, *Cancer Res* 67, 4098–4103.

117. Cheng, Y., Kim, J. W., Liu, W., Dunn, T. A., Luo, J., Loza, M. J., Kim, S. T., Zheng, S. L., Xu, J., Isaacs, W. B., and Chang, B. L. (2009) Genetic and epigenetic inactivation of *TNFRSF10C* in human prostate cancer, *Prostate* 69, 327–335.

118. Shivapurkar, N., Toyooka, S., Toyooka, K. O., Reddy, J., Miyajima, K., Suzuki, M., Shigematsu, H., Takahashi, T., Parikh, G., Pass, H. I., Chaudhary, P. M., and Gazdar, A. F. (2004) Aberrant methylation of trail decoy receptor genes is frequent in multiple tumor types, *Int J Cancer* 109, 786–792.

119. van Noesel, M. M., van Bezouw, S., Salomons, G. S., Voute, P. A., Pieters, R., Baylin, S. B., Herman, J. G., and Versteeg, R. (2002) Tumor-specific down-regulation of the tumor necrosis factor-related apoptosis-inducing ligand decoy receptors *DcR1* and DcR2 is associated with dense promoter hypermethylation, *Cancer Res* 62, 2157–2161.

120. Hornstein, M., Hoffmann, M. J., Alexa, A., Yamanaka, M., Muller, M., Jung, V., Rahnenfuhrer, J., and Schulz, W. A. (2008) Protein phosphatase and TRAIL receptor genes as new candidate tumor genes on chromosome 8p in prostate cancer, *Cancer Genomics Proteomics* 5, 123–136.

121. Cho, N. Y., Kim, J. H., Moon, K. C., and Kang, G. H. (2009) Genomic hypomethylation and CpG island hypermethylation in prostatic intraepithelial neoplasm, *Virchows Arch* 454, 17–23.

122. Cho, N. Y., Kim, B. H., Choi, M., Yoo, E. J., Moon, K. C., Cho, Y. M., Kim, D., and Kang,

G. H. (2007) Hypermethylation of CpG island loci and hypomethylation of LINE-1 and Alu repeats in prostate adenocarcinoma and their relationship to clinicopathological features, *J Pathol* 211, 269–277.

123. Barnabas, N., Xu, L., Savera, A., Hou, Z., and Barrack, E. R. (2010) Chromosome 8 markers of metastatic prostate cancer in African American men: Gain of the MIR151 gene and loss of the NKX3-1 gene, *Prostate.*

124. Ju, J. H., Maeng, J. S., Zemedkun, M., Ahronovitz, N., Mack, J. W., Ferretti, J. A., Gelmann, E. P., and Gruschus, J. M. (2006) Physical and functional interactions between the prostate suppressor homeoprotein *NKX3.1* and serum response factor, *J Mol Biol* 360, 989–999.

125. Shen, M. M., and Abate-Shen, C. (2010) Molecular genetics of prostate cancer: new prospects for old challenges, *Genes Dev* 24, 1967–2000.

126. Ouyang, X., DeWeese, T. L., Nelson, W. G., and Abate-Shen, C. (2005) Loss-of-function of *Nkx3.1* promotes increased oxidative damage in prostate carcinogenesis, *Cancer Res* 65, 6773–6779.

127. Bowen, C., Bubendorf, L., Voeller, H. J., Slack, R., Willi, N., Sauter, G., Gasser, T. C., Koivisto, P., Lack, E. E., Kononen, J., Kallioniemi, O. P., and Gelmann, E. P. (2000) Loss of *NKX3.1* expression in human prostate cancers correlates with tumor progression, *Cancer Res* 60, 6111–6115.

128. Gurel, B., Ali, T. Z., Montgomery, E. A., Begum, S., Hicks, J., Goggins, M., Eberhart, C. G., Clark, D. P., Bieberich, C. J., Epstein, J. I., and De Marzo, A. M. (2010) *NKX3.1* as a marker of prostatic origin in metastatic tumors, *Am J Surg Pathol* 34, 1097–1105.

129. Asatiani, E., Huang, W. X., Wang, A., Rodriguez Ortner, E., Cavalli, L. R., Haddad, B. R., and Gelmann, E. P. (2005) Deletion, methylation, and expression of the *NKX3.1* suppressor gene in primary human prostate cancer, *Cancer Res* 65, 1164–1173.

130. Lind, G. E., Skotheim, R. I., Fraga, M. F., Abeler, V. M., Henrique, R., Saatcioglu, F., Esteller, M., Teixeira, M. R., and Lothe, R. A. (2005) The loss of *NKX3.1* expression in testicular-and prostate-cancers is not caused by promoter hypermethylation, *Mol Cancer* 4, 8.

131. Chung, W., Kwabi-Addo, B., Ittmann, M., Jelinek, J., Shen, L., Yu, Y., and Issa, J. P. (2008) Identification of novel tumor markers in prostate, colon and breast cancer by unbiased methylation profiling, *PLoS One* 3, e2079.

132. Kwabi-Addo, B., Wang, S., Chung, W., Jelinek, J., Patierno, S. R., Wang, B. D., Andrawis, R., Lee, N. H., Apprey, V., Issa, J. P., and Ittmann, M. (2010) Identification of differentially methylated genes in normal prostate tissues from African American and Caucasian men, *Clin Cancer Res* 16, 3539–3547.

133. Reibenwein, J., Pils, D., Horak, P., Tomicek, B., Goldner, G., Worel, N., Elandt, K., and Krainer, M. (2007) Promoter hypermethylation of *GSTP1*, AR, and 14-3-3sigma in serum of prostate cancer patients and its clinical relevance, *Prostate* 67, 427–432.

134. Lodygin, D., and Hermeking, H. (2005) The role of epigenetic inactivation of 14-3-3sigma in human cancer, *Cell Res* 15, 237–246.

135. Henrique, R., Jeronimo, C., Hoque, M. O., Carvalho, A. L., Oliveira, J., Teixeira, M. R., Lopes, C., and Sidransky, D. (2005) Frequent 14-3-3 sigma promoter methylation in benign and malignant prostate lesions, *DNA Cell Biol* 24, 264–269.

136. Henderson, B. E., Ross, R. K., Pike, M. C., and Casagrande, J. T. (1982) Endogenous hormones as a major factor in human cancer, *Cancer Res* 42, 3232–3239.

137. Henderson, B. E., Ross, R. K., and Pike, M. C. (1991) Toward the primary prevention of cancer, *Science* 254, 1131–1138.

138. Ellem, S. J., and Risbridger, G. P. (2010) Aromatase and regulating the estrogen: androgen ratio in the prostate gland, *J Steroid Biochem Mol Biol* 118, 246-251.

139. Wang, Q., Li, W., Zhang, Y., Yuan, X., Xu, K., Yu, J., Chen, Z., Beroukhim, R., Wang, H., Lupien, M., Wu, T., Regan, M. M., Meyer, C. A., Carroll, J. S., Manrai, A. K., Janne, O. A., Balk, S. P., Mehra, R., Han, B., Chinnaiyan, A. M., Rubin, M. A., True, L., Fiorentino, M., Fiore, C., Loda, M., Kantoff, P. W., Liu, X. S., and Brown, M. (2009) Androgen receptor regulates a distinct transcription program in androgen-independent prostate cancer, *Cell* 138, 245p256.

140. Eder, I. E., Culig, Z., Ramoner, R., Thurnher, M., Putz, T., Nessler-Menardi, C., Tiefenthaler, M., Bartsch, G., and Klocker, H. (2000) Inhibition of LncaP prostate cancer cells by means of androgen receptor antisense oligonucleotides, *Cancer Gene Ther* 7, 997–1007.

141. Mitchell, S. H., Zhu, W., and Young, C. Y. (1999) Resveratrol inhibits the expression and function of the androgen receptor in LNCaP prostate cancer cells, *Cancer Res* 59, 5892–5895.

142. Tong, Q., Zeng, F., Lin, C., Zhao, J., and Lu, G. (2003) Growth inhibiting effects of antisense eukaryotic expression vector of proliferating cell nuclear antigen gene on human

bladder cancer cells, *Chin Med J (Engl)* 116, 1203–1206.

143. Heisler, L. E., Evangelou, A., Lew, A. M., Trachtenberg, J., Elsholtz, H. P., and Brown, T. J. (1997) Androgen-dependent cell cycle arrest and apoptotic death in PC-3 prostatic cell cultures expressing a full-length human androgen receptor, *Mol Cell Endocrinol* 126, 59–73.
144. Grossmann, M. E., Huang, H., and Tindall, D. J. (2001) Androgen receptor signaling in androgen-refractory prostate cancer, *J Natl Cancer Inst* 93, 1687–1697.
145. Jarrard, D. F., Kinoshita, H., Shi, Y., Sandefur, C., Hoff, D., Meisner, L. F., Chang, C., Herman, J. G., Isaacs, W. B., and Nassif, N. (1998) Methylation of the androgen receptor promoter CpG island is associated with loss of androgen receptor expression in prostate cancer cells, *Cancer Res* 58, 5310–5314.
146. Kinoshita, H., Shi, Y., Sandefur, C., Meisner, L. F., Chang, C., Choon, A., Reznikoff, C. R., Bova, G. S., Friedl, A., and Jarrard, D. F. (2000) Methylation of the androgen receptor minimal promoter silences transcription in human prostate cancer, *Cancer Res* 60, 3623–3630.
147. Sasaki, M., Tanaka, Y., Perinchery, G., Dharia, A., Kotcherguina, I., Fujimoto, S., and Dahiya, R. (2002) Methylation and inactivation of estrogen, progesterone, and androgen receptors in prostate cancer, *J Natl Cancer Inst* 94, 384–390.
148. Nakayama, T., Watanabe, M., Suzuki, H., Toyota, M., Sekita, N., Hirokawa, Y., Mizokami, A., Ito, H., Yatani, R., and Shiraishi, T. (2000) Epigenetic regulation of androgen receptor gene expression in human prostate cancers, *Lab Invest* 80, 1789–1796.
149. Schayek, H., Bentov, I., Sun, S., Plymate, S. R., and Werner, H. (2010) Progression to metastatic stage in a cellular model of prostate cancer is associated with methylation of the androgen receptor gene and transcriptional suppression of the insulin-like growth factor-I receptor gene, *Exp Cell Res* 316, 1479–1488.
150. Bosland, M. C. (2005) The role of estrogens in prostate carcinogenesis: a rationale for chemoprevention, *Rev Urol 7 Suppl* 3, S4–S10.
151. Li, L. C., Okino, S. T., and Dahiya, R. (2004) DNA methylation in prostate cancer, *Biochim Biophys Acta* 1704, 87–102.
152. Hobisch, A., Hittmair, A., Daxenbichler, G., Wille, S., Radmayr, C., Hobisch-Hagen, P., Bartsch, G., Klocker, H., and Culig, Z. (1997) Metastatic lesions from prostate cancer do not express oestrogen and progesterone receptors, *J Pathol* 182, 356–361.
153. Horvath, L. G., Henshall, S. M., Lee, C. S., Head, D. R., Quinn, D. I., Makela, S., Delprado, W., Golovsky, D., Brenner, P. C., O'Neill, G., Kooner, R., Stricker, P. D., Grygiel, J. J., Gustafsson, J. A., and Sutherland, R. L. (2001) Frequent loss of estrogen receptor-beta expression in prostate cancer, *Cancer Res* 61, 5331–5335.
154. Zhu, X., Leav, I., Leung, Y. K., Wu, M., Liu, Q., Gao, Y., McNeal, J. E., and Ho, S. M. (2004) Dynamic regulation of estrogen receptor-beta expression by DNA methylation during prostate cancer development and metastasis, *Am J Pathol* 164, 2003–2012.
155. Zhang, X., Leung, Y. K., and Ho, S. M. (2007) AP-2 regulates the transcription of estrogen receptor (ER)-beta by acting through a methylation hotspot of the 0N promoter in prostate cancer cells, *Oncogene* 26, 7346–7354.
156. Konishi, N., Nakaoka, S., Hiasa, Y., Kitahori, Y., Ohshima, M., Samma, S., and Okajima, E. (1993) Immunohistochemical evaluation of estrogen receptor status in benign prostatic hypertrophy and in prostate carcinoma and the relationship to efficacy of endocrine therapy, *Oncology* 50, 259–263.
157. Moriyama-Gonda, N., Shiina, H., Terashima, M., Satoh, K., and Igawa, M. (2008) Rationale and clinical implication of combined chemotherapy with cisplatin and oestrogen in prostate cancer: primary evidence based on methylation analysis of oestrogen receptor-alpha, *BJU Int* 101, 485–491.
158. Li, L. C., Chui, R., Nakajima, K., Oh, B. R., Au, H. C., and Dahiya, R. (2000) Frequent methylation of estrogen receptor in prostate cancer: correlation with tumor progression, *Cancer Res* 60, 702–706.
159. Leav, I., Lau, K. M., Adams, J. Y., McNeal, J. E., Taplin, M. E., Wang, J., Singh, H., and Ho, S. M. (2001) Comparative studies of the estrogen receptors beta and alpha and the androgen receptor in normal human prostate glands, dysplasia, and in primary and metastatic carcinoma, *Am J Pathol* 159, 79–92.
160. Yao, Q., He, X. S., Zhang, J. M., and He, J. (2006) (Promotor hypermethylation of E-cadherin, p16 and estrogen receptor in prostate carcinoma), *Zhonghua Nan Ke Xue* 12, 28–31.
161. Nojima, D., Li, L. C., Dharia, A., Perinchery, G., Ribeiro-Filho, L., Yen, T. S., and Dahiya, R. (2001) CpG hypermethylation of the promoter region inactivates the estrogen receptor-beta gene in patients with prostate carcinoma, *Cancer* 92, 2076–2083.
162. Hayashi, K., Yokozaki, H., Naka, K., Yasui, W., Lotan, R., and Tahara, E. (2001)

Overexpression of retinoic acid receptor beta induces growth arrest and apoptosis in oral cancer cell lines, *Jpn J Cancer Res* 92, 42–50.

163. Nakayama, T., Watanabe, M., Yamanaka, M., Hirokawa, Y., Suzuki, H., Ito, H., Yatani, R., and Shiraishi, T. (2001) The role of epigenetic modifications in retinoic acid receptor beta2 gene expression in human prostate cancers, *Lab Invest* 81, 1049–1057.
164. Zhang, J., Liu, L., and Pfeifer, G. P. (2004) Methylation of the retinoid response gene *TIG1* in prostate cancer correlates with methylation of the retinoic acid receptor beta gene, *Oncogene* 23, 2241–2249.
165. Zon, G., Barker, M. A., Kaur, P., Groshen, S., Jones, L. W., Imam, S. A., and Boyd, V. L. (2009) Formamide as a denaturant for bisulfite conversion of genomic DNA: Bisulfite sequencing of the GSTPi and *RARb*eta2 genes of 43 formalin-fixed paraffin-embedded prostate cancer specimens, *Anal Biochem* 392, 117–125.
166. Roupret, M., Hupertan, V., Catto, J. W., Yates, D. R., Rehman, I., Proctor, L. M., Phillips, J., Meuth, M., Cussenot, O., and Hamdy, F. C. (2008) Promoter hypermethylation in circulating blood cells identifies prostate cancer progression, *Int J Cancer* 122, 952–956.
167. Henrique, R., and Jeronimo, C. (2004) Molecular detection of prostate cancer: a role for *GSTP1* hypermethylation, *Eur Urol* 46, 660-669; discussion 669.
168. Nelson, C. P., Kidd, L. C., Sauvageot, J., Isaacs, W. B., De Marzo, A. M., Groopman, J. D., Nelson, W. G., and Kensler, T. W. (2001) Protection against 2-hydroxyamino-1-methyl-6-phenylimidazo(4,5-b)pyridine cytotoxicity and DNA adduct formation in human prostate by glutathione S-transferase P1, *Cancer Res* 61, 103–109.
169. Lee, W. H., Morton, R. A., Epstein, J. I., Brooks, J. D., Campbell, P. A., Bova, G. S., Hsieh, W. S., Isaacs, W. B., and Nelson, W. G. (1994) Cytidine methylation of regulatory sequences near the pi-class glutathione S-transferase gene accompanies human prostatic carcinogenesis, *Proc Natl Acad Sci USA* 91, 11733–11737.
170. Harden, S. V., Guo, Z., Epstein, J. I., and Sidransky, D. (2003) Quantitative *GSTP1* methylation clearly distinguishes benign prostatic tissue and limited prostate adenocarcinoma, *J Urol* 169, 1138–1142.
171. Cairns, P., Esteller, M., Herman, J. G., Schoenberg, M., Jeronimo, C., Sanchez-Cespedes, M., Chow, N. H., Grasso, M., Wu, L., Westra, W. B., and Sidransky, D. (2001) Molecular detection of prostate cancer in urine by *GSTP1* hypermethylation, *Clin Cancer Res* 7, 2727–2730.
172. Lee, W. H., Isaacs, W. B., Bova, G. S., and Nelson, W. G. (1997) CG island methylation changes near the *GSTP1* gene in prostatic carcinoma cells detected using the polymerase chain reaction: a new prostate cancer biomarker, *Cancer Epidemiol Biomarkers Prev* 6, 443–450.
173. Santourlidis, S., Florl, A., Ackermann, R., Wirtz, H. C., and Schulz, W. A. (1999) High frequency of alterations in DNA methylation in adenocarcinoma of the prostate, *Prostate* 39, 166–174.
174. Goessl, C., Krause, H., Muller, M., Heicappell, R., Schrader, M., Sachsinger, J., and Miller, K. (2000) Fluorescent methylation-specific polymerase chain reaction for DNA-based detection of prostate cancer in bodily fluids, *Cancer Res* 60, 5941–5945.
175. Jeronimo, C., Usadel, H., Henrique, R., Oliveira, J., Lopes, C., Nelson, W. G., and Sidransky, D. (2001) Quantitation of *GSTP1* methylation in non-neoplastic prostatic tissue and organ-confined prostate adenocarcinoma, *J Natl Cancer Inst* 93, 1747–1752.
176. Gonzalgo, M. L., Pavlovich, C. P., Lee, S. M., and Nelson, W. G. (2003) Prostate cancer detection by *GSTP1* methylation analysis of postbiopsy urine specimens, *Clin Cancer Res* 9, 2673–2677.
177. Jeronimo, C., Varzim, G., Henrique, R., Oliveira, J., Bento, M. J., Silva, C., Lopes, C., and Sidransky, D. (2002) I105V polymorphism and promoter methylation of the *GSTP1* gene in prostate adenocarcinoma, *Cancer Epidemiol Biomarkers Prev* 11, 445–450.
178. Woodson, K., Hayes, R., Wideroff, L., Villaruz, L., and Tangrea, J. (2003) Hypermethylation of *GSTP1*, *CD44*, and E-cadherin genes in prostate cancer among US Blacks and Whites, *Prostate* 55, 199–205.
179. Kollermann, J., Muller, M., Goessl, C., Krause, H., Helpap, B., Pantel, K., and Miller, K. (2003) Methylation-specific PCR for DNA-based detection of occult tumor cells in lymph nodes of prostate cancer patients, *Eur Urol* 44, 533–538.
180. Payne, S. R., Serth, J., Schostak, M., Kamradt, J., Strauss, A., Thelen, P., Model, F., Day, J. K., Liebenberg, V., Morotti, A., Yamamura, S., Lograsso, J., Sledziewski, A., and Semjonow, A. (2009) DNA methylation biomarkers of prostate cancer: confirmation of candidates and evidence urine is the most sensitive body fluid for non-invasive detection, *Prostate* 69, 1257–1269.

181. Suh, C. I., Shanafelt, T., May, D. J., Shroyer, K. R., Bobak, J. B., Crawford, E. D., Miller, G. J., Markham, N., and Glode, L. M. (2000) Comparison of telomerase activity and *GSTP1* promoter methylation in ejaculate as potential screening tests for prostate cancer, *Mol Cell Probes* 14, 211–217.
182. Goessl, C., Muller, M., Heicappell, R., Krause, H., and Miller, K. (2001) DNA-based detection of prostate cancer in blood, urine, and ejaculates, *Ann N Y Acad Sci* 945, 51–58.
183. Ellinger, J., Haan, K., Heukamp, L. C., Kahl, P., Buttner, R., Muller, S. C., von Ruecker, A., and Bastian, P. J. (2008) CpG island hypermethylation in cell-free serum DNA identifies patients with localized prostate cancer, *Prostate* 68, 42–49.
184. Vener, T., Derecho, C., Baden, J., Wang, H., Rajpurohit, Y., Skelton, J., Mehrotra, J., Varde, S., Chowdary, D., Stallings, W., Leibovich, B., Robin, H., Pelzer, A., Schafer, G., Auprich, M., Mannweiler, S., Amersdorfer, P., and Mazumder, A. (2008) Development of a multiplexed urine assay for prostate cancer diagnosis, *Clin Chem* 54, 874–882.
185. Pasquali, D., Rossi, V., Bellastella, G., Bellastella, A., and Sinisi, A. A. (2006) Natural and synthetic retinoids in prostate cancer, *Curr Pharm Des* 12, 1923–1929.
186. Bushue, N., and Wan, Y. J. (2010) Retinoid pathway and cancer therapeutics, *Adv Drug Deliv Rev*.
187. Murphy, T. M., Perry, A. S., and Lawler, M. (2008) The emergence of DNA methylation as a key modulator of aberrant cell death in prostate cancer, *Endocr Relat Cancer* 15, 11–25.
188. Esteller, M., Guo, M., Moreno, V., Peinado, M. A., Capella, G., Galm, O., Baylin, S. B., and Herman, J. G. (2002) Hypermethylation-associated Inactivation of the Cellular Retinol-Binding-Protein 1 Gene in Human Cancer, *Cancer Res* 62, 5902–5905.
189. Jeronimo, C., Henrique, R., Oliveira, J., Lobo, F., Pais, I., Teixeira, M. R., and Lopes, C. (2004) Aberrant cellular retinol binding protein 1 (*CRBP1*) gene expression and promoter methylation in prostate cancer, *J Clin Pathol* 57, 872–876.
190. Suzuki, M., Shigematsu, H., Shivapurkar, N., Reddy, J., Miyajima, K., Takahashi, T., Gazdar, A. F., and Frenkel, E. P. (2006) Methylation of apoptosis related genes in the pathogenesis and prognosis of prostate cancer, *Cancer Lett* 242, 222–230.
191. Enokida, H., Shiina, H., Igawa, M., Ogishima, T., Kawakami, T., Bassett, W. W., Anast, J. W., Li, L. C., Urakami, S., Terashima, M., Verma, M., Kawahara, M., Nakagawa, M., Kane, C. J., Carroll, P. R., and Dahiya, R. (2004) CpG hypermethylation of *MDR1* gene contributes to the pathogenesis and progression of human prostate cancer, *Cancer Res* 64, 5956–5962.
192. Enokida, H., Shiina, H., Urakami, S., Igawa, M., Ogishima, T., Li, L. C., Kawahara, M., Nakagawa, M., Kane, C. J., Carroll, P. R., and Dahiya, R. (2005) Multigene methylation analysis for detection and staging of prostate cancer, *Clin Cancer Res* 11, 6582–6588.
193. Knight, L. J., Burrage, J., Bujac, S. R., Haggerty, C., Graham, A., Gibson, N. J., Ellison, G., Growcott, J. W., Brooks, A. N., Hughes, A. M., Xinarianos, G., Nikolaidis, G., Field, J. K., and Liloglou, T. (2009) Epigenetic silencing of the endothelin-B receptor gene in non-small cell lung cancer, *Int J Oncol* 34, 465–471.
194. Nelson, J. B., Lee, W. H., Nguyen, S. H., Jarrard, D. F., Brooks, J. D., Magnuson, S. R., Opgenorth, T. J., Nelson, W. G., and Bova, G. S. (1997) Methylation of the 5′ CpG island of the endothelin B receptor gene is common in human prostate cancer, *Cancer Res* 57, 35–37.
195. Rogers, C. G., Gonzalgo, M. L., Yan, G., Bastian, P. J., Chan, D. Y., Nelson, W. G., and Pavlovich, C. P. (2006) High concordance of gene methylation in post-digital rectal examination and post-biopsy urine samples for prostate cancer detection, *J Urol* 176, 2280–2284.
196. Jeronimo, C., Henrique, R., Campos, P. F., Oliveira, J., Caballero, O. L., Lopes, C., and Sidransky, D. (2003) Endothelin B receptor gene hypermethylation in prostate adenocarcinoma, *J Clin Pathol* 56, 52–55.
197. Adams, R. H. (2002) Vascular patterning by Eph receptor tyrosine kinases and ephrins, *Semin Cell Dev Biol* 13, 55–60.
198. Guan, M., Xu, C., Zhang, F., and Ye, C. (2009) Aberrant methylation of *EphA7* in human prostate cancer and its relation to clinicopathologic features, *Int J Cancer* 124, 88–94.
199. Katoh, M. (2006) Comparative integromics on Eph family, *Int J Oncol* 28, 1243–1247.
200. Oudes, A. J., Roach, J. C., Walashek, L. S., Eichner, L. J., True, L. D., Vessella, R. L., and Liu, A. Y. (2005) Application of Affymetrix array and Massively Parallel Signature Sequencing for identification of genes involved in prostate cancer progression, *BMC Cancer* 5, 86.
201. Wang, J., Kataoka, H., Suzuki, M., Sato, N., Nakamura, R., Tao, H., Maruyama, K., Isogaki, J., Kanaoka, S., Ihara, M., Tanaka,

M., Kanamori, M., Nakamura, T., Shinmura, K., and Sugimura, H. (2005) Downregulation of *EphA7* by hypermethylation in colorectal cancer, *Oncogene* 24, 5637–5647.

202. Youssef, E. M., Chen, X. Q., Higuchi, E., Kondo, Y., Garcia-Manero, G., Lotan, R., and Issa, J. P. (2004) Hypermethylation and silencing of the putative tumor suppressor Tazarotene-induced gene 1 in human cancers, *Cancer Res* 64, 2411–2417.
203. Lotan, R. (2002) Is *TIG1* a new tumor suppressor in prostate cancer?, *J Natl Cancer Inst* 94, 469–470.
204. Tokumaru, Y., Harden, S. V., Sun, D. I., Yamashita, K., Epstein, J. I., and Sidransky, D. (2004) Optimal use of a panel of methylation markers with *GSTP1* hypermethylation in the diagnosis of prostate adenocarcinoma, *Clin Cancer Res* 10, 5518–5522.
205. Tokumaru, Y., Sun, D. I., Nomoto, S., Yamashita, K., and Sidransky, D. (2003) Re: Is *TIG1* a new tumor suppressor in prostate cancer?, *J Natl Cancer Inst* 95, 919–920.
206. Vasiliou, V., Pappa, A., and Estey, T. (2004) Role of human aldehyde dehydrogenases in endobiotic and xenobiotic metabolism, *Drug Metab Rev* 36, 279–299.
207. Pasquali, D., Thaller, C., and Eichele, G. (1996) Abnormal level of retinoic acid in prostate cancer tissues, *J Clin Endocrinol Metab* 81, 2186–2191.
208. Touma, S. E., Perner, S., Rubin, M. A., Nanus, D. M., and Gudas, L. J. (2009) Retinoid metabolism and *ALDH1A2* (RALDH2) expression are altered in the transgenic adenocarcinoma mouse prostate model, *Biochem Pharmacol* 78, 1127–1138.
209. Kim, H., Lapointe, J., Kaygusuz, G., Ong, D. E., Li, C., van de Rijn, M., Brooks, J. D., and Pollack, J. R. (2005) The retinoic acid synthesis gene *ALDH1a2* is a candidate tumor suppressor in prostate cancer, *Cancer Res* 65, 8118–8124.
210. Trasino, S. E., Harrison, E. H., and Wang, T. T. (2007) Androgen regulation of aldehyde dehydrogenase 1A3 (*ALDH1A3*) in the androgen-responsive human prostate cancer cell line LNCaP, *Exp Biol Med (Maywood)* 232, 762–771.
211. Lin, J., Haffner, M. C., Zhang, Y., Lee, B. H., Brennen, W. N., Britton, J., Kachhap, S. K., Shim, J. S., Liu, J. O., Nelson, W. G., Yegnasubra-manian, S., and Carducci, M. A. (2010) Disulfiram is a DNA demethylating agent and inhibits prostate cancer cell growth, *Prostate.*
212. Costa, V. L., Henrique, R., Ribeiro, F. R., Carvalho, J. R., Oliveira, J., Lobo, F., Teixeira, M. R., and Jeronimo, C. (2010) Epigenetic regulation of Wnt signaling pathway in urological cancer, *Epigenetics* 5, 343–351.
213. Baylin, S. B., and Ohm, J. E. (2006) Epigenetic gene silencing in cancer—a mechanism for early oncogenic pathway addiction?, *Nat Rev Cancer 6,* 107–116.
214. Lind, G. E., Thorstensen, L., Lovig, T., Meling, G. I., Hamelin, R., Rognum, T. O., Esteller, M., and Lothe, R. A. (2004) A CpG island hypermethylation profile of primary colorectal carcinomas and colon cancer cell lines, *Mol Cancer* 3, 28.
215. Bastian, P. J., Palapattu, G. S., Yegnasubramanian, S., Lin, X., Rogers, C. G., Mangold, L. A., Trock, B., Eisenberger, M., Partin, A. W., and Nelson, W. G. (2007) Prognostic value of preoperative serum cell-free circulating DNA in men with prostate cancer undergoing radical prostatectomy, *Clin Cancer Res* 13, 5361–5367.
216. Bastian, P. J., Yegnasubramanian, S., Palapattu, G. S., Rogers, C. G., Lin, X., De Marzo, A. M., and Nelson, W. G. (2004) Molecular biomarker in prostate cancer: the role of CpG island hypermethylation, *Eur Urol 46,* 698–708.
217. Richiardi, L., Fiano, V., Vizzini, L., De Marco, L., Delsedime, L., Akre, O., Tos, A. G., and Merletti, F. (2009) Promoter methylation in *APC*, RUNX3, and *GSTP1* and mortality in prostate cancer patients, *J Clin Oncol* 27, 3161–3168.
218. Gao, X., Porter, A. T., and Honn, K. V. (1997) Involvement of the multiple tumor suppressor genes and 12-lipoxygenase in human prostate cancer. Therapeutic implications, *Adv Exp Med Biol* 407, 41–53.
219. Kito, H., Suzuki, H., Ichikawa, T., Sekita, N., Kamiya, N., Akakura, K., Igarashi, T., Nakayama, T., Watanabe, M., Harigaya, K., and Ito, H. (2001) Hypermethylation of the *CD44* gene is associated with progression and metastasis of human prostate cancer, *Prostate* 49, 110–115.
220. Lou, W., Krill, D., Dhir, R., Becich, M. J., Dong, J. T., Frierson, H. F., Jr., Isaacs, W. B., Isaacs, J. T., and Gao, A. C. (1999) Methylation of the *CD44* metastasis suppressor gene in human prostate cancer, *Cancer Res* 59, 2329–2331.
221. Graziano, F., Humar, B., and Guilford, P. (2003) The role of the E-cadherin gene (*CDH1*) in diffuse gastric cancer susceptibility: from the laboratory to clinical practice, *Ann Oncol* 14, 1705–1713.
222. Li, L. C., Zhao, H., Nakajima, K., Oh, B. R., Ribeiro Filho, L. A., Carroll, P., and Dahiya, R. (2001) Methylation of the E-cadherin gene promoter correlates with progression of prostate cancer, *J Urol* 166, 705–709.

223. Saha, B., Kaur, P., Tsao-Wei, D., Naritoku, W. Y., Groshen, S., Datar, R. H., Jones, L. W., and Imam, S. A. (2008) Unmethylated E-cadherin gene expression is significantly associated with metastatic human prostate cancer cells in bone, *Prostate* 68, 1681–1688.

224. Riou, P., Saffroy, R., Comoy, J., Gross-Goupil, M., Thiery, J. P., Emile, J. F., Azoulay, D., Piatier-Tonneau, D., Lemoine, A., and Debuire, B. (2002) Investigation in liver tissues and cell lines of the transcription of 13 genes mapping to the 16q24 region that are frequently deleted in hepatocellular carcinoma, *Clin Cancer Res* 8, 3178–3186.

225. Toyooka, K. O., Toyooka, S., Virmani, A. K., Sathyanarayana, U. G., Euhus, D. M., Gilcrease, M., Minna, J. D., and Gazdar, A. F. (2001) Loss of expression and aberrant methylation of the *CDH13* (H-cadherin) gene in breast and lung carcinomas, *Cancer Res* 61, 4556–4560.

226. Alumkal, J. J., Zhang, Z., Humphreys, E. B., Bennett, C., Mangold, L. A., Carducci, M. A., Partin, A. W., Garrett-Mayer, E., DeMarzo, A. M., and Herman, J. G. (2008) Effect of DNA methylation on identification of aggressive prostate cancer, *Urology* 72, 1234–1239.

227. Lee, S. W. (1996) H-cadherin, a novel cadherin with growth inhibitory functions and diminished expression in human breast cancer, *Nat Med* 2, 776–782.

228. Mashimo, T., Watabe, M., Cuthbert, A. P., Newbold, R. F., Rinker-Schaeffer, C. W., Helfer, E., and Watabe, K. (1998) Human chromosome 16 suppresses metastasis but not tumorigenesis in rat prostatic tumor cells, *Cancer Res* 58, 4572–4576.

229. Salama, I., Malone, P. S., Mihaimeed, F., and Jones, J. L. (2008) A review of the S100 proteins in cancer, *Eur J Surg Oncol* 34, 357–364.

230. Rehman, I., Cross, S. S., Catto, J. W., Leiblich, A., Mukherjee, A., Azzouzi, A. R., Leung, H. Y., and Hamdy, F. C. (2005) Promoter hypermethylation of calcium binding proteins S100A6 and S100A2 in human prostate cancer, *Prostate* 65, 322–330.

231. Gokaslan, Z. L., Chintala, S. K., York, J. E., Boyapati, V., Jasti, S., Sawaya, R., Fuller, G., Wildrick, D. M., Nicolson, G. L., and Rao, J. S. (1998) Expression and role of matrix metalloproteinases MMP-2 and MMP-9 in human spinal column tumors, *Clin Exp Metastasis* 16, 721–728.

232. Gomez, D. E., Alonso, D. F., Yoshiji, H., and Thorgeirsson, U. P. (1997) Tissue inhibitors of metalloproteinases: structure, regulation and biological functions, *Eur J Cell Biol* 74, 111–122.

233. Imren, S., Kohn, D. B., Shimada, H., Blavier, L., and DeClerck, Y. A. (1996) Overexpression of tissue inhibitor of metalloproteinases-2 retroviral-mediated gene transfer in vivo inhibits tumor growth and invasion, *Cancer Res 56*, 2891–2895.

234. Mohanam, S., Wang, S. W., Rayford, A., Yamamoto, M., Sawaya, R., Nakajima, M., Liotta, L. A., Nicolson, G. L., Stetler-Stevenson, W. G., and Rao, J. S. (1995) Expression of tissue inhibitors of metalloproteinases: negative regulators of human glioblastoma invasion in vivo, *Clin Exp Metastasis* 13, 57–62.

235. Pulukuri, S. M., Patibandla, S., Patel, J., Estes, N., and Rao, J. S. (2007) Epigenetic inactivation of the tissue inhibitor of metalloproteinase-2 (TIMP-2) gene in human prostate tumors, *Oncogene* 26, 5229–5237.

236. Ross, J. S., Kaur, P., Sheehan, C. E., Fisher, H. A., Kaufman, R. A., Jr., and Kallakury, B. V. (2003) Prognostic significance of matrix metalloproteinase 2 and tissue inhibitor of metalloproteinase 2 expression in prostate cancer, *Mod Pathol* 16, 198–205.

237. Han, X., Zhang, H., Jia, M., Han, G., and Jiang, W. (2004) Expression of TIMP-3 gene by construction of a eukaryotic cell expression vector and its role in reduction of metastasis in a human breast cancer cell line, *Cell Mol Immunol* 1, 308–310.

238. Deng, X., Bhagat, S., Dong, Z., Mullins, C., Chinni, S. R., and Cher, M. (2006) Tissue inhibitor of metalloproteinase-3 induces apoptosis in prostate cancer cells and confers increased sensitivity to paclitaxel, *Eur J Cancer* 42, 3267–3273.

239. Finan, K. M., Hodge, G., Reynolds, A. M., Hodge, S., Holmes, M. D., Baker, A. H., and Reynolds, P. N. (2006) In vitro susceptibility to the pro-apoptotic effects of TIMP-3 gene delivery translates to greater in vivo efficacy versus gene delivery for TIMPs-1 or -2, *Lung Cancer* 53, 273–284.

240. Smith, E., De Young, N. J., Tian, Z. Q., Caruso, M., Ruszkiewicz, A. R., Liu, J. F., Jamieson, G. G., and Drew, P. A. (2008) Methylation of TIMP3 in esophageal squamous cell carcinoma, *World J Gastroenterol* 14, 203–210.

241. Fizazi, K. (2007) The role of Src in prostate cancer, *Ann Oncol* 18, 1765–1773.

242. Posadas, E. M., Al-Ahmadie, H., Robinson, V. L., Jagadeeswaran, R., Otto, K., Kasza, K. E., Tretiakov, M., Siddiqui, J., Pienta, K. J., Stadler, W. M., Rinker-Schaeffer, C., and Salgia, R. (2009) FYN is overexpressed in human prostate cancer, *BJU Int* 103, 171–177.

243. Sorensen, K. D., Borre, M., Orntoft, T. F., Dyrskjot, L., and Torring, N. (2008) Chromo-

somal deletion, promoter hypermethylation and downregulation of FYN in prostate cancer, *Int J Cancer* 122, 509–519.

244. Usmani, B. A., Shen, R., Janeczko, M., Papandreou, C. N., Lee, W. H., Nelson, W. G., Nelson, J. B., and Nanus, D. M. (2000) Methylation of the neutral endopeptidase gene promoter in human prostate cancers, *Clin Cancer Res* 6, 1664–1670.
245. Osman, I., Dai, J., Mikhail, M., Navarro, D., Taneja, S. S., Lee, P., Christos, P., Shen, R., and Nanus, D. M. (2006) Loss of neutral endopeptidase and activation of protein kinase B (Akt) is associated with prostate cancer progression, *Cancer* 107, 2628–2636.
246. Osman, I., Yee, H., Taneja, S. S., Levinson, B., Zeleniuch-Jacquotte, A., Chang, C., Nobert, C., and Nanus, D. M. (2004) Neutral endopeptidase protein expression and prognosis in localized prostate cancer, *Clin Cancer Res* 10, 4096–4100.
247. Friedberg, E. C. (2001) How nucleotide excision repair protects against cancer, *Nat Rev Cancer* 1, 22–33.
248. Mullaart, E., Lohman, P. H., Berends, F., and Vijg, J. (1990) DNA damage metabolism and aging, *Mutat Res* 237, 189–210.
249. Wood, R. D., Mitchell, M., Sgouros, J., and Lindahl, T. (2001) Human DNA repair genes, *Science* 291, 1284–1289.
250. Wood, R. D., Mitchell, M., and Lindahl, T. (2005) Human DNA repair genes, 2005, *Mutat Res* 577, 275–283.
251. Park, J. Y., Huang, Y., and Sellers, T. A. (2009) Single nucleotide polymorphisms in DNA repair genes and prostate cancer risk, *Methods Mol Biol* 471, 361–385.
252. Kim, J. I., Suh, J. T., Choi, K. U., Kang, H. J., Shin, D. H., Lee, I. S., Moon, T. Y., and Kim, W. T. (2009) Inactivation of O6-methylguanine-DNA methyltransferase in soft tissue sarcomas: association with K-ras mutations, *Hum Pathol* 40, 934–941.
253. Mack, G. S. (2006) Epigenetic cancer therapy makes headway, *J Natl Cancer Inst* 98, 1443–1444.
254. Muller, C. I., Ruter, B., Koeffler, H. P., and Lubbert, M. (2006) DNA hypermethylation of myeloid cells, a novel therapeutic target in MDS and AML, *Curr Pharm Biotechnol* 7, 315–321.
255. Oki, Y., Aoki, E., and Issa, J. P. (2007) Decitabine-bedside to bench, *Crit Rev Oncol Hematol* 61, 140–152.
256. Muller, A., and Florek, M. (2010) 5-Azacytidine/Azacitidine, *Recent Results Cancer Res* 184, 159–170.
257. Woodson, K., Gillespie, J., Hanson, J., Emmert-Buck, M., Phillips, J. M., Linehan, W. M., and Tangrea, J. A. (2004) Heterogeneous gene methylation patterns among pre-invasive and cancerous lesions of the prostate: a histopathologic study of whole mount prostate specimens, *Prostate* 60, 25–31.

Chapter 6

Epigenetics of Bladder Cancer

Wun-Jae Kim and Yong-June Kim

Abstract

Epigenetic changes are closely associated with tumor development and prognosis of bladder cancer, and its detection in specimens (tissue/body fluid) may be feasible and more sensitive than conventional methods. Additionally, the epigenetic changes are interesting from a clinical point of view because it may be possible to reverse epigenetic changes and restore the gene function. Epigenetic markers might therefore be more useful than conventional molecular markers for the detection, prediction of prognosis, and treatment of bladder cancer.

Key words: Bladder neoplasms, Detection, Epigenesis, Marker, Prognosis

1. Introduction

Bladder cancers comprise heterogeneous cell populations, and numerous factors are likely to be involved in dictating recurrence, progression, and patient survival. Many tumor markers for bladder cancer have been evaluated for use in detecting and monitoring bladder cancer tissue specimens, bladder washes, and urine specimens (1, 2). However, none of the biomarkers reported to date have shown sufficient sensitivity and specificity to detect the entire spectrum of bladder cancers in routine clinical practice. For these reasons, the role of epigenetic changes in regulating tumorigenesis is of particular interest. Recent progress in understanding epigenetic modification including DNA methylation, histone modifications, and microRNA (miRNA) has led to new opportunities for understanding, detection, treatment, and prevention of cancer. Moreover, the reversible nature of epigenetic aberrations has led to emergence of the promising field of epigenetic therapy. We herein

Ramona G. Dumitrescu and Mukesh Verma (eds.), *Cancer Epigenetics: Methods and Protocols*, Methods in Molecular Biology, vol. 863, DOI 10.1007/978-1-61779-612-8_6,

review the current knowledge on epigenetic issues in bladder cancer and discuss its implications for understanding the molecular basis and treatment of this disease.

2. Detection of Bladder Cancer

Currently, patients with bladder cancer are monitored for cancer recurrence or progression by periodic cystoscopy and urine cytology, the frequency of which varies depending on the risk factors associated with the disease (3–5). Although cystoscopic examination is the gold standard used to diagnose bladder cancer, it is costly, incurs substantial patient discomfort, and has variable sensitivity (3, 6). Moreover, the sensitivity of cytological analysis is low, especially for low-grade transitional cell carcinomas, and its accuracy is dependent on the pathologist's experience. Challenge for the clinician is the development of reasonable surveillance protocols that provide cost-effective as well as noninvasive monitoring. Because some epigenetic events occur early in the disease process, molecular diagnosis may facilitate detection before symptomatic or overt radiographic manifestations appear.

The presence of an abnormal methylation pattern can be easily detected in various biological fluids and tissues (7–22). Cancer detection using abnormal DNA methylation is quite powerful due to the inherent stability of DNA compared to RNA or proteins. It is also possible that these approaches might be used to discriminate one type of cancer from another because altered methylation patterns are often cancer specific (23–25). Several researchers investigating exfoliated urinary cells or tumor tissues revealed that detection of aberrant promoter methylation in tissue and urine was feasible and appeared to be more sensitive than conventional methods in bladder tumor (7–22) (Table 1). Recently, Hoque et al. (21) reported the potential of detecting DNA hypermethylation in voided urine and its promising role as a tumor marker for bladder cancer. In this study, a quantitative real-time PCR assay was introduced to examine urine sediment DNA obtained from 175 patients with bladder cancer and 94 age-matched control subjects for promoter hypermethylation of nine genes (*APC*, *p14^ARF^*, *CDH1*, *GSTP1*, *MGMT*, *CDKN2A*, *RARb2*, *RASSF1A*, and *TIM-3*). The combined methylation analysis of four genes (*CDKN2A*, *p14^ARF^*, *MGMT*, and *GSTP1*) displayed 69% sensitivity and 100% specificity. Similarly, Friedrich et al. (19) investigated DNA methylation of apoptosis-associated genes in urine sediments. Methylation was detected in 22% of the samples (8 of 37) for *DAPK*, 51% (18 of 37) for *TERT*, and 65% (24 of 37) for *BCL2*. The combined methylation analysis of three genes (*DAPK*, *BCL2*, and *TERT*) provided both high sensitivity (78%) and specificity (100%) for detection of bladder cancer.

Table 1
Detection of bladder cancer by DNA methylation

Methylation markers	Sensitivity (%)	Specificity (%)	Reference
Tissue			
CDH1	84 (43/51)	76	(7)
DBC1	52 (36/69)	N/A	(8)
p16^{INF4a}	60 (24/40)	N/A	(9)
RASSF1A	48 (19/40)	100	(10)
RASSF1A	60 (33/55)	100	(11)
RUNX3	73 (90/124)	100	(12)
SOX9	56 (57/101)	N/A	(15)
APC, RASSF1A, p14^{ARF}	100 (45/45)	100	(13)
APC, CDH1, CDH13, FHIT, RASSF1A	78 (76/98)	N/A	(16)
Dkk3, SFRP1, SFRP2, SFRP4, SFRP5, Wif1	77	67	(14)
SFRP1, SFRP2, SFRP4, SFRP5	62 (221/355)	N/A	(17)
LAMA3, LAMB3, LAMC2	55 (70/128)	N/A	(18)
Urine			
RASSF1A	50 (7/14)	100	(10)
APC, RASSF1A, p14^{ARF}	87 (39/45)	100	(13)
CDKN2A, GSTP1, MGMT, p14^{ARF}*,*	69	100	(21)
DAPK, BCL2, TERT	78 (29/37)	100	(19)
DAPK, RARß, CDH1, p16^{INF4a}	91 (20/22)	76	(20)
LAMA3, LAMB3, LAMC2	49 (35/71)	N/A	(18)
NID2, TWIST1	96 (46/48)	93	(22)

NA not available

In summary, modern techniques for DNA methylation profiling permit sensitive and quantitative detection of hypermethylated genes in all biological fluids and biopsy specimens. Using only an extension of the selected methylation marker panel might result in higher sensitivity and specificity in the methylation analysis of urine and tissue, therefore making this a promising, noninvasive diagnostic and monitoring tool for bladder cancer detection.

3. Prediction of Prognosis

Bladder cancer can be classified as nonmuscle invasive or muscle invasive tumor according to its histopathology and clinical behavior (3, 4). At present, 75% of bladder cancers are nonmuscle invasive, 20% are invasive, and up to 5% will have de novo metastasis (3, 4). It is estimated that 50–70% of patients with a nonmuscle invasive tumor have a recurrence or a new occurrence of transitional cell carcinoma within 5 years, whereas 5–20% progress to a more advanced stage (26). In other words, tumors with similar morphology

Table 2
Prediction of bladder cancer recurrence by DNA methylation status

Methylation markers	No.	F/U (months)	Clinical relevance	Reference
APAF-1, IGFBP-1	110	55	Higher recurrence rate in NMIBC and MIBC	(27)
*p14^ARF^*	27	N/A	Higher recurrence rate	(28)
TIMP-3	95	N/A	Lower recurrence rate in NMIBC	(29)
RUNX3	124	N/A	Higher recurrence rate	(12)
CDH1, DAPK, GSTP1, MLH1, MGMT, p16^INK4a^, VHL	55	N/A	Higher recurrence rate in NMIBC	(30)

F/U, follow-up; *NMIBC*, nonmuscle invasive bladder cancer; *MIBC*, muscle invasive bladder cancer; *NA*, not available

behave in different ways. Thus, it is a major clinical challenge to accurately differentiate those patients whose tumor will recur and/or progress after initial treatment from those without recurrence and/or progression.

Several investigators have shown a positive association between hypermethylation status of genes (e.g., *DAPK*, *p14^ARF^*, *TIMP-3*, and *RUNX3*) and high recurrence rate of bladder cancer, and some of these were independent predictive factors for bladder tumor recurrence (12, 27–30) (Table 2). Friedrich et al. (29) evaluated the methylation status of 20 cancer-associated genes in 105 consecutive patients with primary nonmuscle invasive bladder carcinoma. Among these genes, methylation status of six genes (*SOCS-1*, *STAT-1*, *BCL2*, *DAPK*, *TIMP-3*, *CDH1*) was associated with tumor recurrence (29). However, only *TIMP-3* showed a significant association with prolonged recurrence-free survival. More recently, *APAF-1* and *IGFBP-3* methylation levels were reported as independent prognostic markers for recurrence in nonmuscle invasive bladder cancers (27).

Regarding progression and survival, although only few data are available, the significant associations between hypermethylation of the promoter region and decreased survival in bladder cancer have been reported (15–18, 24, 31–33) (Table 3). Yates et al. (33) reported promising results using 17 gene promoters and 96 malignant urothelial samples. In their study, multivariate analysis revealed that the overall degree of methylation was more significantly associated with subsequent progression and death than the tumor stage. Furthermore, epigenetic predictive models developed using artificial intelligence techniques identified the presence and timing of tumor progression with 97% specificity and 75% sensitivity. In concordance with earlier findings, we evaluated the association between *RUNX3* inactivation and bladder cancers after a long-term

Table 3
Prediction of bladder cancer progression/survival by DNA methylation status

Methylation markers	No.	F/U (months)	Remarks	Reference
APC	38	16	Poor cancer-specific survival	(31)
LAMC2	128	N/A	Poor overall survival	(18)
p14^{ARF}	45	34	Poor overall survival	(32)
RUNX3	118	49	Higher progression rate and poor cancer-specific survival	(24)
SOX9	101	N/A	Poor overall survival	(15)
APC, CDH1, EDNRB, RASSF1A, TNFRSF25	96	N/A	Poor survival	(33)
CDH1, FHIT	98	N/A	Poor survival	(16)
SFRP1, SFRP2, SFRP4, SFRP5	355	N/A	Poor overall survival	(17)

F/U, follow-up; *NA*, not available

follow-up of this cohort (24). At the 50-month median follow-up period, multivariate Cox regression analyses revealed that *RUNX3* hypermethylation was the only strong predictor of bladder cancer progression. Moreover, *RUNX3 hypermethylation* was significantly associated with cancer-specific survival in bladder cancer. These findings confirmed the importance of the methylation marker as a strong prognostic tool for bladder cancer and suggest its potential usefulness from the clinical standpoint.

In summary, earlier reports consistently indicated that methylation of promoter regions are promising markers for prognosis in bladder cancer. However, numerous factors are involved in prognosis, and future studies including multivariate analyses with large numbers of patients and long-term follow-up are needed to confirm that the methylation status of genes is independent of other variables. The true value of methylation in predicting bladder cancer behavior will become identified when such focused research is completed.

4. Epigenetic Therapy

Inactivation of cancer-related genes by altered DNA methylation, histone, and chromatin modifications made us realize that silenced chromatin may represent a viable therapeutic target. The potential reversibility of DNA methylation patterns suggests that these are a viable target for the treatment of cancer. One specific goal of epigenetic therapy is to restore normal DNA methylation patterns and to prevent the cells from acquiring further methylation in DNA that could lead to silence genes crucial to normal cell function. Treating cancer with DNA methylase inhibitors or histone deacetylase (HDAC) inhibitors has, in a number of cases, been effective in reactivating tumor-suppressor genes, which in turn reduce cancer cell proliferation (34, 35). Therefore, a new therapeutic strategy called "epigenetic therapy" has been introduced in which drugs that can modify chromatin or DNA methylation patterns are used alone or in combination in order to enhance therapeutic outcomes (36). Several exciting clinical trials, such as combination of DNA methylation inhibitors and/or HDAC inhibitors, are currently under way to test the possibility of synergistic effects and dose reduction; however, further validation studies are necessary to confirm the essential values of epigenetic therapy. Such new therapeutic modalities in relation to bladder cancer and the discovery of new therapeutic targets which can awaken silenced genes should be promising for both urologists and bladder cancer patients in terms of improving the disease outcome in coming years.

5. Conclusions

It is clear from work of many laboratories that much has been discovered about the molecular events which underlie the appearance of promoter methylation and gene silencing in relation to bladder cancer detection, recurrence, progression, and survival but even more remain to be elucidated. Understanding of the epigenetic events that lead to urothelial tumorigenesis and progression is increasing, and this will allow clinicians to identify key epigenetic changes that can be targeted for detection, prediction, and therapy. Epigenetic markers in bladder cancer could be valuable tools for stratification of heterogeneous bladder cancer patient populations into risk groups which can be used to guide clinical decision-making, including observation vs. adjuvant therapy. Aberrant patterns of epigenetic modification could be in near future, crucial parameters in bladder cancer diagnosis, prognosis, and therapy.

References

1. Habuchi, T., Marberger, M., Droller, M.J., Hemstreet, G.P., Grossman, H.B., Schalken, J.A., Schmitz-Drager, B.J., Murphy, W.M., Bono, A.V., Goebell, P., Getzenberg, R.H., Hautmann, S.H., Messing, E., Fradet, Y., and Lokeshwar, V.B. (2005) Prognostic markers for bladder cancer: International Consensus Panel on bladder tumor markers. *Urology* 66, 64–74.
2. Liou, L.S. (2006) Urothelial cancer biomarkers for detection and surveillance. *Urology* 67, 25–33.
3. Babjuk, M., Oosterlinck, W., Sylvester, R., Kaasinen, E., Bohle, A., and Palou-Redorta, J. (2008) EAU guidelines on non-muscle-invasive urothelial carcinoma of the bladder. *Eur Urol* 54, 303–314.

4. Stenzl, A., Cowan, N.C., De Santis, M., Jakse, G., Kuczyk, M.A., Merseburger, A.S., Ribal, M.J., Sherif, A., and Witjes, J.A. (2009) The Updated EAU Guidelines on Muscle-Invasive and Metastatic Bladder Cancer. *Eur Urol*, 55, 815–825.
5. Sylvester, R.J., van der Meijden, A.P., Oosterlinck, W., Witjes, J.A., Bouffioux, C., Denis, L., Newling, D.W., and Kurth, K. (2006) Predicting recurrence and progression in individual patients with stage Ta T1 bladder cancer using EORTC risk tables: a combined analysis of 2596 patients from seven EORTC trials. *Eur Urol* 49, 466–465.
6. Kim, W.J. and Bae, S.C. (2008) Molecular biomarkers in urothelial bladder cancer. *Cancer Sci* 99, 646–652.
7. Ribeiro-Filho, L.A., Franks, J., Sasaki, M., Shiina, H., Li, L.C., Nojima, D., Arap, S., Carroll, P., Enokida, H., Nakagawa, M., Yonezawa, S., and Dahiya, R. (2002) CpG hypermethylation of promoter region and inactivation of E-cadherin gene in human bladder cancer. *Mol Carcinog* 34, 187–198.
8. Habuchi, T., Takahashi, T., Kakinuma, H., Wang, L., Tsuchiya, N., Satoh, S., Akao, T., Sato, K., Ogawa, O., Knowles, M.A., and Kato, T. (2001) Hypermethylation at 9q32-33 tumour suppressor region is age-related in normal urothelium and an early and frequent alteration in bladder cancer. *Oncogene* 20, 531–537.
9. Chang, L.L., Yeh, W.T., Yang, S.Y., Wu, W.J., and Huang, C.H. (2003) Genetic alterations of p16INK4a and p14ARF genes in human bladder cancer. *J Urol* 170, 595–600.
10. Chan, M.W., Chan, L.W., Tang, N.L., Lo, K.W., Tong, J.H., Chan, A.W., Cheung, H.Y., Wong, W.S., Chan, P.S., Lai, F.M., and To, K.F. (2003) Frequent hypermethylation of promoter region of RASSF1A in tumor tissues and voided urine of urinary bladder cancer patients. *Int J Cancer* 104, 611–616.
11. Lee, M.G., Kim, H.Y., Byun, D.S., Lee, S.J., Lee, C.H., Kim, J.I., Chang, S.G., and Chi, S.G. (2001) Frequent epigenetic inactivation of RASSF1A in human bladder carcinoma. *Cancer Res* 61, 6688–6692.
12. Kim, W.J., Kim, E.J., Jeong, P., Quan, C., Kim, J., Li, Q.L., Yang, J.O., Ito, Y., and Bae, S.C. (2005) RUNX3 inactivation by point mutations and aberrant DNA methylation in bladder tumors. *Cancer Res* 65, 9347–9354.
13. Dulaimi, E., Uzzo, R.G., Greenberg, R.E., Al-Saleem, T., and Cairns, P. (2004) Detection of bladder cancer in urine by a tumor suppressor gene hypermethylation panel. *Clin Cancer Res* 10, 1887–1893.
14. Urakami, S., Shiina, H., Enokida, H., Kawakami, T., Kawamoto, K., Hirata, H., Tanaka, Y., Kikuno, N., Nakagawa, M., Igawa, M., and Dahiya, R. (2006) Combination analysis of hypermethylated Wnt-antagonist family genes as a novel epigenetic biomarker panel for bladder cancer detection. *Clin Cancer Res* 12, 2109–2116.
15. Aleman, A., Adrien, L., Lopez-Serra, L., Cordon-Cardo, C., Esteller, M., Belbin, T.J., and Sanchez-Carbayo, M. (2008) Identification of DNA hypermethylation of SOX9 in association with bladder cancer progression using CpG microarrays. *Br J Cancer* 98, 466–473.
16. Maruyama, R., Toyooka, S., Toyooka, K.O., Harada, K., Virmani, A.K., Zochbauer-Muller, S., Farinas, A.J., Vakar-Lopez, F., Minna, J.D., Sagalowsky, A., Czerniak, B., and Gazdar, A.F. (2001) Aberrant promoter methylation profile of bladder cancer and its relationship to clinicopathological features. *Cancer Res* 61, 8659–8663.
17. Marsit, C.J., Karagas, M.R., Andrew, A., Liu, M., Danaee, H., Schned, A.R., Nelson, H.H., and Kelsey, K.T. (2005) Epigenetic inactivation of SFRP genes and TP53 alteration act jointly as markers of invasive bladder cancer. *Cancer Res* 65, 7081–7085.
18. Sathyanarayana, U.G., Maruyama, R., Padar, A., Suzuki, M., Bondaruk, J., Sagalowsky, A., Minna, J.D., Frenkel, E.P., Grossman, H.B., Czerniak, B., and Gazdar, A.F. (2004) Molecular detection of noninvasive and invasive bladder tumor tissues and exfoliated cells by aberrant promoter methylation of laminin-5 encoding genes. *Cancer Res* 64, 1425–1430.
19. Friedrich, M.G., Weisenberger, D.J., Cheng, J.C., Chandrasoma, S., Siegmund, K.D., Gonzalgo, M.L., Toma, M.I., Huland, H., Yoo, C., Tsai, Y.C., Nichols, P.W., Bochner, B.H., Jones, P.A., and Liang, G. (2004) Detection of methylated apoptosis-associated genes in urine sediments of bladder cancer patients. *Clin Cancer Res* 10, 7457–7465.
20. Chan, M.W., Chan, L.W., Tang, N.L., Tong, J.H., Lo, K.W., Lee, T.L., Cheung, H.Y., Wong, W.S., Chan, P.S., Lai, F.M., and To, K.F. (2002) Hypermethylation of multiple genes in tumor tissues and voided urine in urinary bladder cancer patients. *Clin Cancer Res* 8, 464–470.
21. Hoque, M.O., Begum, S., Topaloglu, O., Chatterjee, A., Rosenbaum, E., Van Criekinge,W., Westra, W.H., Schoenberg, M., Zahurak, M., Goodman, S.N., and Sidransky, D. (2006) Quantitation of promoter methylation of multiple genes in urine DNA and bladder cancer detection. *J Natl Cancer Inst* 98, 996–1004.

22. Renard, I., Joniau, S., van Cleynenbreugel, B., Collette, C., Naome, C., Vlassenbroeck, I., Nicolas, H., de Leval, J., Straub, J., Van Criekinge, W., Hamida, W., Hellel, M., Thomas, A., de Leval, L., Bierau, K., and Waltregny, D. (2010) Identification and Validation of the Methylated TWIST1 and NID2 Genes through Real-Time Methylation-Specific Polymerase Chain Reaction Assays for the Noninvasive Detection of Primary Bladder Cancer in Urine Samples. *Eur Urol* 58, 96–104.
23. Kim, W.J. and Kim, Y.J. (2009) Epigenetic biomarkers in urothelial bladder cancer. *Expert Rev Mol Diagn* 9, 259–269.
24. Kim, E.J., Kim, Y.J., Jeong, P., Ha, Y.S., Bae, S.C., and Kim, W.J. (2008) Methylation of the RUNX3 promoter as a potential prognostic marker for bladder tumor. *J Urol* 180, 1141–1145.
25. Hoque, M.O. (2009) DNA methylation changes in prostate cancer: current developments and future clinical implementation. *Expert Rev Mol Diagn* 9, 243–257.
26. Donat, S.M. (2003) Evaluation and follow-up strategies for superficial bladder cancer. *Urol Clin North Am* 30, 765–776.
27. Christoph, F., Weikert, S., Kempkensteffen, C., Krause, H., Schostak, M., Miller, K., and Schrader, M. (2006) Regularly methylated novel pro-apoptotic genes associated with recurrence in transitional cell carcinoma of the bladder. *Int J Cancer* 119, 1396–1402.
28. Dominguez, G., Carballido, J., Silva, J., Silva, J.M., Garcia, J.M., Menendez, J., Provencio, M., Espana, P., and Bonilla, F. (2002) p14ARF promoter hypermethylation in plasma DNA as an indicator of disease recurrence in bladder cancer patients. *Clin Cancer Res* 8, 980–985.
29. Friedrich, M.G., Chandrasoma, S., Siegmund, K.D., Weisenberger, D.J., Cheng, J.C., Toma, M.I., Huland, H., Jones, P.A., and Liang, G. (2005) Prognostic relevance of methylation markers in patients with non-muscle invasive bladder carcinoma. *Eur J Cancer* 41, 2769–2778.
30. Tada, Y., Wada, M., Taguchi, K., Mochida, Y., Kinugawa, N., Tsuneyoshi, M., Naito, S., and Kuwano, M. (2002) The association of death-associated protein kinase hypermethylation with early recurrence in superficial bladder cancers. *Cancer Res* 62, 4048–4053.
31. Ellinger, J., El Kassem, N., Heukamp, L.C., Matthews, S., Cubukluoz, F., Kahl, P., Perabo, F.G., Muller, S.C., von Ruecker, A., and Bastian, P.J. (2008) Hypermethylation of cell-free serum DNA indicates worse outcome in patients with bladder cancer. *J Urol* 179, 346–352.
32. Kawamoto, K., Enokida, H., Gotanda, T., Kubo, H., Nishiyama, K., Kawahara, M., and Nakagawa, M. (2006) p16INK4a and p14ARF methylation as a potential biomarker for human bladder cancer. *Biochem Biophys Res Commun* 339, 790–796.
33. Yates, D.R., Rehman, I., Abbod, M.F., Meuth, M., Cross, S.S., Linkens, D.A., Hamdy, F.C., and Catto, J.W. (2007) Promoter hypermethylation identifies progression risk in bladder cancer. *Clin Cancer Res* 13, 2046–2053.
34. Baylin, S.B., Herman, J.G., Graff, J.R., Vertino, P.M., and Issa, J.P. (1998) Alterations in DNA methylation: a fundamental aspect of neoplasia. *Adv Cancer Res* 72, 141–196.
35. Laird, P.W., Jackson-Grusby, L., Fazeli, A., Dickinson, S.L., Jung, W.E., Li, E., Weinberg, R.A., and Jaenisch, R. (1995) Suppression of intestinal neoplasia by DNA hypomethylation. *Cell* 81, 197–205.
36. Egger, G., Liang, G., Aparicio, A., and Jones, P.A. (2004) Epigenetics in human disease and prospects for epigenetic therapy. *Nature* 429, 457–463.

Chapter 7

Epigenetics in Myeloid Malignancies

Stefan Deneberg

Abstract

Myeloid hematological malignancies are among the epigenetically best characterized neoplasms. The comparatively low number of recurring balanced and unbalanced chromosomal abnormalities as well as common genetic mutations has enabled scientists to relate epigenetic states to these. The ease of accessing malignant cells through bone marrow aspiration has certainly contributed to the fast expansion of knowledge. Even so, the clinical and pathogenetic relevance of epigenetic changes is still not known, and the field will certainly evolve very fast with the development of new analytic techniques. The first example of successful epigenetic therapy is seen in myeloid malignancies, in the high-risk myelodysplastic syndromes (MDS) which are routinely treated with the demethylating agent azacytidine.

This chapter will concentrate on describing the epigenetic changes in acute myeloid leukemia (AML), chronic myeloid leukemia (CML) and MDS. An overview of clinical relevance and epigenetic therapeutic approaches is also made.

Key words: DNA methylation, Histone modifications, Acute myeloid leukemia, Chronic myeloid leukemia, Myelodysplastic syndromes

1. Introduction

In 1987, Stephen Baylin et al. reported that the 5′ region of the calcitonin gene had altered DNA methylation (1). This was the first report of gene-specific epigenetic dysregulation in hematopoietic malignancies of the myeloid lineage, soon to be followed by an ever increasing number of reports. The diagnostic and prognostic clinical use of the increasing body of knowledge about epigenetic changes in the myeloid malignancies has however not paralleled the development of molecular genomics. There are still, after almost 25 years of research, no clinically available, validated tests or incorporation of epigenetic profiles into the prognostic instruments

Ramona G. Dumitrescu and Mukesh Verma (eds.), *Cancer Epigenetics: Methods and Protocols*, Methods in Molecular Biology, vol. 863, DOI 10.1007/978-1-61779-612-8_7, © Springer Science+Business Media, LLC 2012

used in everyday hematological–oncological practice. One reason is likely the lack of standardization between laboratories with various techniques with varying sensitivity and specificity as well as a multitude of small studies with sometimes conflicting results. In the last few years, the emergence of more standardized, commercially available platforms will hopefully bring epigenetic testing to the clinic. In contrast to the lack of clinical diagnostic and prognostic applications, it is among hematological malignancies that the presumably epigenetically acting drugs have proven efficacious and gained Food and Drug Administration (FDA) and European Medicines Agency (EMEA) approval. The use of low-dose 5-azacytidine (VIDAZA) and decitabine (Dacogen) in high-risk myelodysplastic syndromes (MDS) and suberoylanilide hydroxamic acid (vorinostat, Zolinza) for cutaneous T-cell lymphoma has already helped a lot of patients and holds a promise for the whole field of epigenetic research. This chapter will outline the current knowledge about epigenetic changes in myeloid hematological malignancies.

2. Mutations Affecting the Epigenetic State in Myeloid Malignancies

In myeloid malignancies, a number of distinct mutations have been defined that are more or less common and possibly driving the malignant state. Some of these have direct epigenetic implications.

2.1. TET2

The *TET2* mutations, recently described in MDS, MPD, and acute myeloid leukemia (AML), are one of these epigenetic changes (2). The *TET* family of genes consists of three genes, *TET1*, *2*, and *3*. The founding member, *TET1*, was found as a translocation partner in AML, t(10;11)(q22;q23), hence the name "*T*ranslocation *E*leven *T*en" (3). Mutations have been found in the *TET2* gene in various myeloid malignancies with frequencies of 15–27% in MDS, 20–51% in CMML, 8–20% in MPD, 24–43% in secondary AML, and 12–20% in de novo AML (2). Mutations are found throughout the coding region and are in general inactivating. The normal function of the *TET1* gene product is to hydroxylate 5-methylcytosine residues to 5-hydroxymethylcytosine, and similar functions have been shown for *TET2* and *TET3* genes (4). This may facilitate a subsequent conversion back to cytosine by excision repair enzymes or an enzymatic process. Inactivation mutations in the gene would thus be expected to result in an increase in 5-methylcytosine, but this is currently not clear. In fact, a recently published study showed that 5-methylcytosine content as measured with the IlluminaHumanMethylation27K array was actually diminished in cells with low 5-hydroxymethylcytosine levels (4). This array however mainly interrogates promoter regions which may explain the discrepancy with another recent study where overall 5-methylcytosine content measured by mass spectrometry was increased in *TET2*-mutated samples (5). Further, *TET2* mutations and mutations in isocitrate dehydrogenase (*IDH*) 1 and 2 are mutually exclusive in AML but displayed similarities in gene expression and methylation patterns, implying that they are separate disease-driving mutations affecting similar pathways (5).

2.2. *DNMT3a*

Genome-wide sequencing studies have revealed mutations in the *DNMT3a* gene in 8% of MDS and 22% of AML cases, with a higher incidence in cytogenetically normal leukemias. Newly published data claim that these mutations do not influence methylation levels in AML cells but are associated with worse outcome. No mutations were found in other DNMTs (6). These data are intriguing, and further studies on this newly discovered mutation and its impact on the epigenetic machinery are eagerly anticipated.

3. Acute Myeloid Leukemia

3.1. Background

AML is the predominant type of acute leukemia in adults. The median age at diagnosis is 71 years. Most patients younger than 70 years of age receive intensive chemotherapy aimed at inducing a complete remission. To consolidate treatment, around 40% of patients below 60 years of age receive allogeneic stem cell transplantation, either in first remission or after successful treatment after relapse depending on individual risk stratification. Genetically, AML is one of the most studied types of neoplasias and among the first where genetic information was incorporated into clinical decision-making (7). Recurrent nonrandom translocations, inversions, and deletions are typically seen in all hematological malignancies including AML, some of which are characteristic of favorable outcome, for instance t(8;21), inv(16), and t(15;17) (7). A complex karyotype or certain deletions are poor prognostic signs (8, 9). Furthermore, molecular aberrations such as *nucleophosmin 1* mutations, FMS-like tyrosine kinase 3-internal tandem duplication (FLT3-ITD), CCAAT/enhancer-binding protein alpha (CEBPA), and mixed lineage leukemia (MLL) translocations have in recent years contributed to prognostic stratification (10) and also, in the case of FLT3-ITD, efforts of using targeted therapy (11). The application of epigenetic assays to the study of AML has resulted in the discovery of several novel tumor suppressor genes and increased understanding of the pathogenesis of the disease.

3.2. How to Define an Epigenetic "Normal" Reference

A point seldom considered in epigenetic discovery is the "denominator issue." When describing a promoter as "aberrantly methylated" or showing "aberrant repressive histone marks," one always compares the tissue of interest with some kind of normal tissue. When studying breast cancer, one often uses surgically removed ductal tissue adjacent to the tumor, allowing paired analyses both in regard to individual epigenetic changes and tissue type-specific changes. In hematological malignancies, especially leukemias, this is not so simple since there is no (or very little) adjacent unaffected tissue. The use of resting memory T-cells as reference is not appropriate when studying myeloid malignancies since the different lineage will affect your results greatly. Often one is left with using bone marrow or peripheral blood from healthy donors, introducing an interindividual bias. Worse, most of these healthy donors are medical students or lab associates who are quite young in contrast to most patients, also introducing a possible age-associated epigenetic bias (12). Many investigators use CD34-separated myeloid progenitors when studying myeloid leukemias or MDS. This may be fine as long as one is studying DNA methylation pattern changes during myeloid differentiation which are less pronounced than in lymphoid differentiation, especially in CpG islands in contrast to island shores (13). That is however not the case when it comes to histone modifications which change dramatically during myeloid differentiation (Lennartsson et al., manuscript in preparation). Hence, in the study of epigenetic aberrations in hematological neoplasms, there are several pitfalls in regard to what reference material is used. As a researcher and a reader, one has to relate to this when interpreting papers on the subject.

3.3. Aberrant DNA Methylation, Specific Mechanisms, and Correlation with AML Subtypes

Due to the relative ease of investigating DNA methylation with standard laboratory techniques and the obtainability of AML blasts of relatively high purity, there are a huge number of publications on the subject (14, 15). In contrast to molecular and karyotypical aberrations, there seems to be hundreds, if not thousands, of genes implicated as aberrantly methylated AML. Depending on methodology and the number of genes investigated, it seems that there are no cases of AML where aberrant DNA methylation is not a feature (16, 17). In line with this, there is evidence that the levels of DNMT1, DNMT3a, and DNMT3b are increased in blast cells of AML patients (18). Global hypomethylation was among the first described changes in AML (19). The reason for the apparent contradiction between global hypomethylation and increased gene-specific CpG island methylation is an issue that is not resolved. It has been suggested that alternate transcripts of *DNMT3b* lacking the catalytic domain may be responsible (20), but other studies counter that (21). Other explanations may be increased activity of DNA demethylases (22), folate deficiency, or the previously predominant view that the global hypomethylation is a passive process.

The cross talk between histone modifications and DNA methylation is also implicated. Loss of monoacetylation of H4Lys16 and trimethylation of H4Lys20 in leukemia cells correlate with DNA hypomethylation of Sat2, NBL2, and D4Z4 tandem repeat sequences (23).

There is no consensus regarding the connection between global DNA hypomethylation and the alleged proneoplastic events coupled with this, such as increased chromosome breakage, increased microsatellite instability (MSI), and concurrent defects in the mismatch repair system seen for instance in colon cancer (24). MSI is however not an uncommon finding in AML. The prevalence of MSI ranges from 20% to 30% and perhaps higher in therapy-related and secondary AML (25). The often associated promoter hypermethylation of MLH1 or MSH2 is however a rare event in itself with incidence ranging from 2 to 4% (26).

Numerous studies have investigated specific gene promoters for methylation in AML. A list of the most common recurring genes is supplied in Table 1. An interesting finding was the inverse correlation of age and the number of genes methylated found in one study, perhaps indicative of a different methylation pattern in de novo AML (27). On a genome-wide scale, a few studies have been published as to date showing high levels of CpG island hypermethylation nonrandomly distributed. Using restriction landmark genome scanning (RLGS), Rush et al. could show promoter methylation in 8.3% of CpG islands (28), nonrandomly distributed. No studies have however shown a stable correlation between DNA methylation patterns and the French-American British (FAB) histological AML subtypes, with the exception of FAB M3 acute promyelocytic leukemia (APL) (17). Recent genome-wide methylation analyses have confirmed that different methylation patterns exist among AML cases that can only partially be explained by distinctive molecular and cytogenetic subgroups. Figueroa et al. (17) conducted a large-scale DNA profiling study of 344 AML samples showing specific methylation profiles for each of the core-binding leukemias, t(8;21), t(15;17), and inv(16) as well as CCAAT/enhancer-binding protein alpha (CEBPA) mutation and silencing, as well as different profiles for NPM1-mutated cases. Cases harboring 11q23 translocations also clustered separately in this study, in line with other studies that have described a specific methylation profile for MLL-translocated AML, also elegantly shown by functional experiments by Alvarez et al. (29). The histone methyltransferase activity of MLL, a gene with multiple translocation partners in 5% of AML, may partially explain this (30, 31). Interestingly, MLL is also a common target for activating partial tandem mutations (PTD) with an incidence of 5–11% in cytogenetically normal AML (32). MLL-PTD mutants retain the functional C-terminal SET domain that has methyltransferase activity. This mutated form of MLL is a marker of poor prognosis and has been shown to

Table 1
Promoter methylation in AML in four studies using different methylation assays. The frequencies of methylated samples are given as percentages

References	Ekmekci et al. (105)	Kroeger et al. (106)	Galm et al. (46)	Herman et al. (61)
N examined	28	30	60	60
Method	*MSP* (%)	*Bseq/Bpyroseq* (%)	*MSP* (%)	*MSP* (%)
DAPK	61		5	
ER	44			
CDKN2B (p15)	43	47	32	88
SOCS1	39		45	
CDH1	18		13	
RARα	18			
p73	10		13	
CDH13		83		
OLIG2		77		
PGRA		72		
PGRB		70		
NOR1		63		
NPM2		63		
SLC26A4		30		
HIN1		23		
RARb2			20	
MGMT			5	
CDKN2A (p16)			3	0
TIMP-3			0	
RASSF1a			0	

MSP=methylation specific PCR Bseq/Bpyroseq=Bisulfite sequencina/pvrosequencing

upregulate certain Homeobox genes by an increase of H3/H4 acetylation (33), and is associated with a genome-wide increase in promoter methylation (34). Furthermore, the specific methylation pattern seen in APL, characterized by t(15;17), may be explained by the activity of the fusion protein PML-RARα which interacts with DNMTs and direct them to RARα targets, causing promoter DNA methylation and gene silencing (35). The oncoprotein PML-RARα has also been shown to interact with other epigenetically acting proteins such as HDACs and the Polycomb repressive complex

2 (36, 37). The first-line treatment for APL, pharmacological doses of all-*trans*-retinoic-acid (ATRA), dissociates the repressive complexes from the promoter, inducing reexpression of the silenced genes and concurrent differentiation of the APL cells (35). Similar mechanisms have also been suggested for another fusion protein, AML1-ETO, the product of t(8;21) that participates in a protein complex with RARα, recruiting DNMTs and HDACs inducing a repressive epigenetic state at these promoter sites (38). *EVI-1*, overexpressed in inv(3) AML, is associated with unfavorable outcome and has recently been shown to display a specific genome-wide DNA methylation signature and interact with DNMT3a and DNMT3b (39). In other tumor types, bivalent histone marks as well as Polycomb group-enriched promoters in embryonic stem cells have predisposed the promoter methylation patterns seen in cancer (40). There is some evidence that similar mechanisms are active in AML as shown for *CDKN2B* by Zangenberg and Paul et al. (41, 42). To summarize, some of the aberrant methylation patterns seen in AML have molecular explanations. However, identification of these as well as identifying which aberrations are driving the disease and which are only “passengers” remains a challenge.

In contrast to DNA methylation, histone modifications have been relatively little investigated in AML. On a genome-wide level, H3K9 trimethylation was investigated in AML patients and found decreased at promoter regions. Interestingly, an H3K9me3 pattern also predicted event-free survival in this group of AML patients (43). There was no apparent correlation between H3K9me3 and known cytogenetic aberrations.

4. Epigenetic Changes as Diagnostic and Prognostic Tools in AML

The clinical and pathological diagnosis of AML has never been a clinical problem. However, with improved therapy, the importance of determining minimal residual disease (MRD) as a sign of early relapses or need for intensified therapy has arisen. Traditionally, MRD has been evaluated by cytogenetic techniques and later by PCR-based technology utilizing clone-specific aberrations when present. Immunophenotyping by flow cytometry is also a simple, clinically useful procedure, however not as sensitive as PCR (44). There have been few studies investigating the feasibility of using epigenetic marks for MRD detection. Since the covalent methylation of DNA is considered a more stable epigenetic change than histone modifications, this is the more explored. Promoter methylation of *ERα* and *CDKN2B* was investigated in AML and ALL and found to correlate well with T-cell receptor/immunoglobulin MRD levels in ALL as well as with a high relapse risk in AML and ALL (45). The study used bone marrow samples as the source of DNA, but hopefully this technology can be adapted to use peripheral blood for early relapse detection analogous to chimerism detection after allogeneic stem cell transplantation. This is a promising practical application of epigenetic techniques in need of prospective clinical evaluation.

Regarding clinical prognostic use, several promoter methylated genes have been proposed as either heralding good or bad prognosis (16, 27, 46–49). However, most of these studies were made with small patient samples and using different methylation detection techniques, so their clinical usefulness as prognostic markers are preliminary. In recent years, studies using a test cohort with subsequent control and validation cohorts have been published. Figueroa et al. found a 15-gene methylation classifier independently predictive of overall survival in their genome-wide methylation study using the HELP assay (17), and Bullinger et al. used a similar approach but with different methodology (MALDI-TOF-MS) to find another validated set of genes predictive of overall survival (50). Alvarez et al. used Illumina GoldenGate Methylation arrays to corroborate previous findings of specific epigenetic signatures of balanced translocation AML cases as well as showing a univariate prognostic value of methylation of *DBC1* (deleted in bladder cancer 1), which however was lost in multivariate analysis (29). These three studies have shown how DNA methylation profiling can be used for prognostic; however, there is still a great need for prospective evaluation and standardized methodology.

5. Myelodysplastic Syndromes

5.1. Introduction

MDS is a group of heterogeneous clonal bone marrow disorders characterized by bone marrow failure with dysregulated apoptotic mechanisms and differentiation block but not always increased proliferation (51). It is mainly a disease of the elderly but occurs rarely even in children. Many MDS progress to AML, and the distinction between the diseases is set at a blast percentage of 20% in the bone marrow in the latest World Health Organization classification (52). The increasing knowledge of disease driving molecular and cytogenetic aberrations has resulted in a more complex classification of MDS, likely reflecting that these are actually different syndromes with a more or less common phenotype. This diversity hampers both clinical and preclinical studies of MDS since it is difficult to infer results from limited studies to the whole MDS population, and careful sample selection is obviously of paramount importance when studying MDS. This of course also applies to epigenetic studies where the last years have seen a formidable increase in the number of publications, in part due to the success of DNMT inhibitory therapy in MDS (53).

5.2. Epigenetic Changes in MDS

Several individual genes and pathways have been found to be epigenetically silenced in MDS by promoter DNA methylation, some found to be predictive in retrospective studies, such as *CDH1* (54), *CDH13*, *ER*, *NOR1*, *NPM2*, *OLIG2*, *CDKN2B*, *PGRA*, *PGRB*, and *RIL* (55). One of the most investigated genes is *CDKN2B* which is methylated in a large proportion of MDS cases, prevalence ranges from 15 to 80%, depending on sample selection and methodology (56). *CDKN2B* is a cyclin-dependent kinase inhibitor central for cell-cycle regulation. Methylation of *CDKN2B* has been linked to certain subtypes of MDS such as therapy-related MDS, deletion 5q and 7, and associate with poor prognosis (54, 57, 58). In contrast with *CDKN2B* and as opposed to many solid cancers including lymphoma, the frequency of methylation of *CDKN2A* (*p16*) is low in myeloid lineage neoplasms, underscoring that DNA methylation is not a random process but rather a disease, or perhaps lineage-specific event (59–61).

A recent genome-wide investigation using the HELP assay investigated the difference between de novo AML and MDS (62). Aberrant methylation in MDS and secondary AML was more frequent than in de novo AML and unsupervised clustering as well as principal component analysis of the methylation patterns easily distinguished between the diseases. This indicates that MDS and de novo AML are different entities epigenetically, an important point to consider. Furthermore, the same study showed an enrichment of WNT pathway genes that were hypermethylated in MDS compared to CD34+ cells. In another large study, utilizing the Illumina GoldenGate Methylation array, different risk groups of MDS were compared together with SNP array data (63). The principal findings showed that every MDS sample had aberrant promoter methylation and that the methylation levels increased with increasing severity of MDS through MDS-AML. Promoter methylation was much more common than chromosomal deletions and was found to cooperate in several samples where deletion of the FZD9 locus (a WNT receptor) on chromosome 7 was accompanied by promoter methylation of the remaining allele. These cases were also associated with the poorest clinical outcome. This finding demonstrates the possibility of cooperation between chromosomal deletions and epigenetic silencing. However, even if present in a few samples, there was no general correlation between complex cytogenetic abnormalities and promoter methylation, and the authors conclude that they appear as separate mechanistic processes.

5.3. A CpG Island Methylator Phenotype in MDS

The existence of a "CpG island methylator phenotype" (CIMP) has been shown to be a separate clinical and histopathological entity in colon cancer, characterized by hypermethylation of a number of well-defined genes including MSH1 and associated with

MSI and typical histopathological findings such as hyperplastic and mixed polyps and serrated adenomas mainly in the right part of the colon (64). The existence of a highly DNA-methylated CIMP in MDS has been suggested on the basis of independently poor outcome of MDS cases with hypermethylation of multiple genes (55). Outcome based on the average methylation levels of the ten genes implicated in this study was validated in two separate retrospective cohorts increasing the validity of the findings. However, in contrast with CIMP in colon cancer that is associated with typical histopathological findings, the suggested CIMP in MDS is independent of correlation to morphological, WHO, and IPSS classifications (55). The lack of correlations with specific subtypes of MDS and the absence of decisive functional studies still make it questionable if there is such a disease entity as the CIMP in MDS or if the increased methylation levels are secondary events to tumor progression in general. The latter does not preclude that genes silenced by methylation contribute to tumor aggressiveness and chemoresistance and thus may serve as potent clinical markers and potential targets of therapy; however, the jury is still out regarding the existence of CIMP in MDS.

5.4. Epigenetically Acting Therapy in MDS and AML

There has been tremendous hope for epigenetically acting therapeutic agents following the success of decitabine and azacytidine in high-risk MDS and AML following MDS (65). Several studies have explored the effects of decitabine and azacytidine in elderly with high-risk MDS and AML; however, often both de novo AML and AML following MDS have been included. Overall response rates have varied from 22% to over 50% with various dosing regimens and combinations (66). Many efforts have been made to find predictive markers for success of DNMT inhibitory therapy, but so far none has emerged as a stable predictor. There are some indications that demethylating therapy may be more effective in high-risk MDS with chromosome 7 abnormalities and/or chromosome 5 abnormalities (excluding del (5q) in MDS) (67, 68), but this finding could not be verified in a large retrospective study recently published (69). Lower baseline methylation levels have been suggested to vouch for a better effect of azacytidine (68). In a recent publication of a phase II trial of decitabine in elderly patients with previously untreated AML, responders to therapy had higher baseline values of miR-29b, a microRNA that targets DNMT3a and DNMT3b directly and DNMT1 through Sp1 (70) and thus lower the global DNA methylation levels. This view is however challenged in a recent publication that found no evidence that either global methylation levels or promoter methylation of specific tumor suppressor genes could predict response to azacytidine in combination with the histone deacetylase inhibitor entinostat (71).

A multitude of phase I and phase II studies have shown the efficacy of DNMT inhibition in MDS (72, 73). The two FDA-approved agents, 5-azacytidine and 5-aza-2 -deoxycytidine, were originally designed as cytosine analogues but later proved to inhibit DNMTs, likely have more modes of action than just pure demethylating activity (74). Also supporting this is the lack of correlation between demethylation of specific promoters and cell death (75) and that the pattern of gene activation only partially can be explained by promoter hypomethylation (76). However, as shown in the genome-wide study by Figueroa et al., there is a gross reduction of promoter methylation already at day 15 after treatment start with 5-azacytidine and entinostat, much earlier than blast clearance is expected (62). The slow response to treatment is seen both with decitabine and azacytidine treatment and does speak against pure cytotoxic effects which usually manifest itself by rapid blast clearance.

Histone deacetylase inhibitors (HDACi) have also been explored alone or in combination regimens for MDS and AML (77, 78). Phase I studies of vorinostat (SAHA) and MGCD0103 showed effect in a population with mainly MDS and AML patients and were well tolerated (79, 80). As with DNMT inhibitors, the mode of action of HDACi is not thought to be entirely dependent of epigenetic mechanisms. Even if gene reactivation has been shown, it seems that at least SAHA works through induction of reactive oxygen species (81).

6. Chronic Myeloid Leukemia

Chronic myeloid leukemia (CML) is a proliferative clonal disorder of hematopoietic stem cells that primarily affects the myeloid lineage. It shares clinical features with the myeloproliferative disorders essential thrombocythemia (ET), polycythemia vera (PCV), and primary myelofibrosis (PMF), such as elevated white blood cell and platelet counts and splenomegaly. The diagnosis is based on finding the Philadelphia chromosome translocation, t(9;22), fusing the BCR gene with ABL resulting in uncontrolled tyrosine kinase activity (82, 83). Recently, an activating mutation in another tyrosine kinase, JAK-2, was found to be present in 95–96% of PCV and in 50% of ET and PMF cases (84).

CML is characterized by an initial chronic phase of undefined duration. Unless treated, the disease sooner or later, with a median of 5–6 years, progresses to a blast crisis, sometimes preceded by an accelerated phase. Proliferation is increased in the chronic phase, and with disease progression, a maturation defect is added resulting in a blast increase in marrow and peripheral blood similar to acute leukemia (85). The principal treatment for many years has been cytoreductive treatment with hydroxyurea and later α-interferon and stem cell transplantation. In 2001, the tyrosine kinase inhibitor imatinib (Gleevec) was approved for treatment of chronic phase CML (86). It has revolutionized the treatment and prognosis of CML where long-term survival, but not cure, now can be achieved without stem cell transplantation. Several analogues are now reaching the market with increased potency and less sensitive to receptor mutations causing imatinib resistance.

6.1. Epigenetic Changes in CML

Many studies of DNA methylation status of individual genes have been conducted in CML, often comparing progressive stages of the disease. An almost unanimous finding is that promoter DNA methylation is increased with increasing stage of CML with an opposing pattern for repetitive DNA and also for cancer-testis antigens (87). This has been described for genes such as *HOXA5* and *HOXA4* (88), *TFAP2A* and *EBF2* (89), as well as a multitude of others (90–94). Furthermore, DNA methylation patterns in the major breakpoint cluster region (M-BCR) have been shown to correlate to the type of blast crisis, lymphoid, or myeloid. The possible causative effect of this finding has however not been examined (95). Another interesting observation is the coupling of overexpressed DNMT1, 3a, and 3b with increasing stage of CML (96). Intriguingly, one promoter (Pa) in the ABL part of the Philadelphia fusion chromosome defining CML is hypermethylated on disease progression (97). This methylation does however not seem to impact response to interferon treatment (98).

In contrast to AML and MDS, *CDKN2B* methylation is rarely seen, even on progression of CML to blast crisis (61).

6.2. Therapeutic Implications

The most common cause of resistance to tyrosine kinase inhibitor therapy in CML is mutations of the *BCR-ABL* gene. However, an epigenetic mechanism ofimatinib resistance has also been described (99). Methylation of the promoter of the proapoptotic BCL-2-interacting mediator (BIM) was coupled to lower expression. BIM levels were associated with lack of imatinib response in vivo and in vitro and reexpression after azacytidine treatment in cell line-restored response.

The effect of treatment of primary CML cells and CML cell lines with a tyrosine kinase inhibitor (AMN107, Novartis) was enhanced by combination with an HDAC inhibitor (LBH589, Novartis) as well as with SAHA (100). Also, LBH589 was reported as having in vitro apoptosis inducing effect on primary CML cells resistant to imatinib, including the *BCR-ABL* mutation T315I (101). An in vitro study by Lee et al. described an alternative mechanism of imatinib resistance in a cell line involving upregulation of class I and III HDACs and downregulation of HAT enzymes causing aberrant protein acetylation of the p53 protein among others (102). The imatinib-resistant cells were more sensitive to SAHA treatment, which may indicate that HDACs have other targets than histone proteins. A recent publication showed that imatinib in combination with various HDACi could induce apoptosis of CML stem cells who are not thought to be targeted by tyrosine kinase inhibitors alone (103). There are ongoing clinical phase I trials of various HDACi in combination with imatinib. Decitabine has also shown activity in CML of various stages with an overall response rate of 28–55% but with low rates of cytogenetic responses, in the range if 7–12% (104). Neither is in clinical use outside of studies.

7. Concluding Remark

The dysregulation of the epigenetic machinery in myeloid malignancies is a seemingly central characteristic, likely affecting every transformed cell in every patient. Even so, its role as a driver or passenger anomaly has not been established yet. The dynamics and relationship to the cell of origin of the respective tumor are just beginning to be explored. Nevertheless, epigenetic strategies for therapy, detection, and monitoring of myeloid neoplasms will certainly evolve and find its way to the clinical setting within the next decade.

References

1. Baylin, S. B., Fearon, E. R., Vogelstein, B., de Bustros, A., Sharkis, S. J., Burke, P. J., Staal, S. P., and Nelkin, B. D. (1987) Hypermethylation of the 5′ region of the calcitonin gene is a property of human lymphoid and acute myeloid malignancies, *Blood 70*, 412–417.
2. Bacher, U., Haferlach, C., Schnittger, S., Kohlmann, A., Kern, W., and Haferlach, T. (2010) Mutations of the TET2 and CBL genes: novel molecular markers in myeloid malignancies, *Ann Hematol 89*, 643–652.
3. Lorsbach, R. B., Moore, J., Mathew, S., Raimondi, S. C., Mukatira, S. T., and Downing, J. R. (2003) TET1, a member of a novel protein family, is fused to MLL in acute myeloid leukemia containing the t(10;11)(q22;q23), *Leukemia 17*, 637–641.
4. Ko, M., Huang, Y., Jankowska, A. M., Pape, U. J., Tahiliani, M., Bandukwala, H. S., An, J., Lamperti, E. D., Koh, K. P., Ganetzky, R., Liu, X. S., Aravind, L., Agarwal, S., Maciejewski, J. P., and Rao, A. (2010) Impaired hydroxylation of 5-methylcytosine in myeloid cancers with mutant TET2, *Nature 468*, 839–843.
5. Figueroa, M. E., Abdel-Wahab, O., Lu, C., Ward, P. S., Patel, J., Shih, A., Li, Y., Bhagwat, N., Vasanthakumar, A., Fernandez, H. F., Tallman, M. S., Sun, Z., Wolniak, K., Peeters, J. K., Liu, W., Choe, S. E., Fantin, V. R., Paietta, E., Lowenberg, B., Licht, J. D., Godley, L. A., Delwel, R., Valk, P. J., Thompson, C. B., Levine, R. L., and Melnick, A. (2010) Leukemic IDH1 and IDH2 mutations result in a hypermethylation phenotype, disrupt TET2 function, and impair hematopoietic differentiation, *Cancer Cell 18*, 553–567.
6. Ley, T. J., Ding, L., Walter, M. J., McLellan, M. D., Lamprecht, T., Larson, D. E., Kandoth, C., Payton, J. E., Baty, J., Welch, J., Harris, C. C., Lichti, C. F., Townsend, R. R., Fulton, R. S., Dooling, D. J., Koboldt, D. C., Schmidt, H., Zhang, Q., Osborne, J. R., Lin, L., O'Laughlin, M., McMichael, J. F., Delehaunty, K. D., McGrath, S. D., Fulton, L. A., Magrini, V. J., Vickery, T. L., Hundal, J., Cook, L. L., Conyers, J. J., Swift, G. W., Reed, J. P.,

Alldredge, P. A., Wylie, T., Walker, J., Kalicki, J., Watson, M. A., Heath, S., Shannon, W. D., Varghese, N., Nagarajan, R., Westervelt, P., Tomasson, M. H., Link, D. C., Graubert, T. A., DiPersio, J. F., Mardis, E. R., and Wilson, R. K. (2010) DNMT3A mutations in acute myeloid leukemia, *N Engl J Med 363*, 2424–2433.

7. Walker, H., Smith, F. J., and Betts, D. R. (1994) Cytogenetics in acute myeloid leukaemia, *Blood Rev 8*, 30–36.

8. Mrozek, K., Heerema, N. A., and Bloomfield, C. D. (2004) Cytogenetics in acute leukemia, *Blood Rev 18*, 115–136.

9. Grimwade, D., Walker, H., Oliver, F., Wheatley, K., Harrison, C., Harrison, G., Rees, J., Hann, I., Stevens, R., Burnett, A., and Goldstone, A. (1998) The importance of diagnostic cytogenetics on outcome in AML: analysis of 1,612 patients entered into the MRC AML 10 trial. The Medical Research Council Adult and Children's Leukaemia Working Parties, *Blood 92*, 2322–2333.

10. Dohner, K. and Dohner, H. (2008) Molecular characterization of acute myeloid leukemia, *Haematologica 93*, 976–982.

11. Sanz, M., Burnett, A., Lo-Coco, F., and Lowenberg, B. (2009) FLT3 inhibition as a targeted therapy for acute myeloid leukemia, *Curr Opin Oncol 21*, 594–600.

12. Christensen, B. C., Houseman, E. A., Marsit, C. J., Zheng, S., Wrensch, M. R., Wiemels, J. L., Nelson, H. H., Karagas, M. R., Padbury, J. F., Bueno, R., Sugarbaker, D. J., Yeh, R. F., Wiencke, J. K., and Kelsey, K. T. (2009) Aging and environmental exposures alter tissue-specific DNA methylation dependent upon CpG island context, *PLoS Genet 5*, e1000602.

13. Ji, H., Ehrlich, L. I., Seita, J., Murakami, P., Doi, A., Lindau, P., Lee, H., Aryee, M. J., Irizarry, R. A., Kim, K., Rossi, D. J., Inlay, M. A., Serwold, T., Karsunky, H., Ho, L., Daley, G. Q., Weissman, I. L., and Feinberg, A. P. (2010) Comprehensive methylome map of lineage commitment from haematopoietic progenitors, *Nature 467*, 338–342.

14. Plass, C., Oakes, C., Blum, W., and Marcucci, G. (2008) Epigenetics in acute myeloid leukemia, *Semin Oncol 35*, 378–387.

15. Mahmud, M. and Stebbing, J. (2010) Epigenetic modifications in AML and MDS, *Leuk Res 34*, 139–140.

16. Deneberg, S., Grovdal, M., Karimi, M., Jansson, M., Nahi, H., Corbacioglu, A., Gaidzik, V., Dohner, K., Paul, C., Ekstrom, T. J., Hellstrom-Lindberg, E., and Lehmann, S. (2010) Gene-specific and global methylation patterns predict outcome in patients with acute myeloid leukemia, *Leukemia 24*, 932–941.

17. Figueroa, M. E., Lugthart, S., Li, Y., Erpelinck-Verschueren, C., Deng, X., Christos, P. J., Schifano, E., Booth, J., van Putten, W., Skrabanek, L., Campagne, F., Mazumdar, M., Greally, J. M., Valk, P. J., Lowenberg, B., Delwel, R., and Melnick, A. (2010) DNA methylation signatures identify biologically distinct subtypes in acute myeloid leukemia, *Cancer Cell 17*, 13–27.

18. Melki, J. R., Warnecke, P., Vincent, P. C., and Clark, S. J. (1998) Increased DNA methyltransferase expression in leukaemia, *Leukemia 12*, 311–316.

19. Gama-Sosa, M. A., Slagel, V. A., Trewyn, R. W., Oxenhandler, R., Kuo, K. C., Gehrke, C. W., and Ehrlich, M. (1983) The 5-methylcytosine content of DNA from human tumors, *Nucleic Acids Res 11*, 6883–6894.

20. Ostler, K. R., Davis, E. M., Payne, S. L., Gosalia, B. B., Exposito-Cespedes, J., Le Beau, M. M., and Godley, L. A. (2007) Cancer cells express aberrant DNMT3B transcripts encoding truncated proteins, *Oncogene 26*, 5553–5563.

21. Ehrlich, M., Woods, C. B., Yu, M. C., Dubeau, L., Yang, F., Campan, M., Weisenberger, D. J., Long, T., Youn, B., Fiala, E. S., and Laird, P. W. (2006) Quantitative analysis of associations between DNA hypermethylation, hypomethylation, and DNMT RNA levels in ovarian tumors, *Oncogene 25*, 2636–2645.

22. Jost, J. P., Oakeley, E. J., Zhu, B., Benjamin, D., Thiry, S., Siegmann, M., and Jost, Y. C. (2001) 5-Methylcytosine DNA glycosylase participates in the genome-wide loss of DNA methylation occurring during mouse myoblast differentiation, *Nucleic Acids Res 29*, 4452–4461.

23. Fraga, M. F., Ballestar, E., Villar-Garea, A., Boix-Chornet, M., Espada, J., Schotta, G., Bonaldi, T., Haydon, C., Ropero, S., Petrie, K., Iyer, N. G., Perez-Rosado, A., Calvo, E., Lopez, J. A., Cano, A., Calasanz, M. J., Colomer, D., Piris, M. A., Ahn, N., Imhof, A., Caldas, C., Jenuwein, T., and Esteller, M. (2005) Loss of acetylation at Lys16 and trimethylation at Lys20 of histone H4 is a common hallmark of human cancer, *Nat Genet 37*, 391–400.

24. Boland, C. R. and Goel, A. (2010) Microsatellite instability in colorectal cancer, *Gastroenterology 138*, 2073-2087 e2073.

25. Nomdedeu, J. F., Perea, G., Estivill, C., Lasa, A., Carnicer, M. J., Brunet, S., Aventin, A., and Sierra, J. (2005) Microsatellite instability

is not an uncommon finding in adult de novo acute myeloid leukemia, *Ann Hematol 84*, 368–375.

26. Seedhouse, C. H., Das-Gupta, E. P., and Russell, N. H. (2003) Methylation of the hMLH1 promoter and its association with microsatellite instability in acute myeloid leukemia, *Leukemia 17*, 83–88.
27. Toyota, M., Kopecky, K. J., Toyota, M. O., Jair, K. W., Willman, C. L., and Issa, J. P. (2001) Methylation profiling in acute myeloid leukemia, *Blood 97*, 2823–2829.
28. Rush, L. J., Dai, Z., Smiraglia, D. J., Gao, X., Wright, F. A., Fruhwald, M., Costello, J. F., Held, W. A., Yu, L., Krahe, R., Kolitz, J. E., Bloomfield, C. D., Caligiuri, M. A., and Plass, C. (2001) Novel methylation targets in de novo acute myeloid leukemia with prevalence of chromosome 11 loci, *Blood 97*, 3226–3233.
29. Alvarez, S., Suela, J., Valencia, A., Fernandez, A., Wunderlich, M., Agirre, X., Prosper, F., Martin-Subero, J. I., Maiques, A., Acquadro, F., Rodriguez Perales, S., Calasanz, M. J., Roman-Gomez, J., Siebert, R., Mulloy, J. C., Cervera, J., Sanz, M. A., Esteller, M., and Cigudosa, J. C. (2010) DNA methylation profiles and their relationship with cytogenetic status in adult acute myeloid leukemia, *PLoS One 5*, e12197.
30. Krivtsov, A. V., Feng, Z., Lemieux, M. E., Faber, J., Vempati, S., Sinha, A. U., Xia, X., Jesneck, J., Bracken, A. P., Silverman, L. B., Kutok, J. L., Kung, A. L., and Armstrong, S. A. (2008) H3K79 methylation profiles define murine and human MLL-AF4 leukemias, *Cancer Cell 14*, 355–368.
31. Rohrs, S., Dirks, W. G., Meyer, C., Marschalek, R., Scherr, M., Slany, R., Wallace, A., Drexler, H. G., and Quentmeier, H. (2009) Hypomethylation and expression of BEX2, IGSF4 and TIMP3 indicative of MLL translocations in acute myeloid leukemia, *Mol Cancer 8*, 86.
32. Gaidzik, V. and Dohner, K. (2008) Prognostic implications of gene mutations in acute myeloid leukemia with normal cytogenetics, *Semin Oncol 35*, 346–355.
33. Dorrance, A. M., Liu, S., Yuan, W., Becknell, B., Arnoczky, K. J., Guimond, M., Strout, M. P., Feng, L., Nakamura, T., Yu, L., Rush, L. J., Weinstein, M., Leone, G., Wu, L., Ferketich, A., Whitman, S. P., Marcucci, G., and Caligiuri, M. A. (2006) Mll partial tandem duplication induces aberrant Hox expression in vivo via specific epigenetic alterations, *J Clin Invest 116*, 2707–2716.
34. Whitman, S. P., Hackanson, B., Liyanarachchi, S., Liu, S., Rush, L. J., Maharry, K., Margeson, D., Davuluri, R., Wen, J., Witte, T., Yu, L., Liu, C., Bloomfield, C. D., Marcucci, G., Plass, C., and Caligiuri, M. A. (2008) DNA hypermethylation and epigenetic silencing of the tumor suppressor gene, SLC5A8, in acute myeloid leukemia with the MLL partial tandem duplication, *Blood 112*, 2013–2016.
35. Di Croce, L., Raker, V. A., Corsaro, M., Fazi, F., Fanelli, M., Faretta, M., Fuks, F., Lo Coco, F., Kouzarides, T., Nervi, C., Minucci, S., and Pelicci, P. G. (2002) Methyltransferase recruitment and DNA hypermethylation of target promoters by an oncogenic transcription factor, *Science 295*, 1079–1082.
36. Grignani, F., De Matteis, S., Nervi, C., Tomassoni, L., Gelmetti, V., Cioce, M., Fanelli, M., Ruthardt, M., Ferrara, F. F., Zamir, I., Seiser, C., Lazar, M. A., Minucci, S., and Pelicci, P. G. (1998) Fusion proteins of the retinoic acid receptor-alpha recruit histone deacetylase in promyelocytic leukaemia, *Nature 391*, 815–818.
37. Villa, R., Pasini, D., Gutierrez, A., Morey, L., Occhionorelli, M., Vire, E., Nomdedeu, J. F., Jenuwein, T., Pelicci, P. G., Minucci, S., Fuks, F., Helin, K., and Di Croce, L. (2007) Role of the polycomb repressive complex 2 in acute promyelocytic leukemia, *Cancer Cell 11*, 513–525.
38. Fazi, F., Zardo, G., Gelmetti, V., Travaglini, L., Ciolfi, A., Di Croce, L., Rosa, A., Bozzoni, I., Grignani, F., Lo-Coco, F., Pelicci, P. G., and Nervi, C. (2007) Heterochromatic gene repression of the retinoic acid pathway in acute myeloid leukemia, *Blood 109*, 4432–4440.
39. Lugthart, S., Figueroa, M. E., Bindels, E., Skrabanek, L., Valk, P. J., Li, Y., Meyer, S., Erpelinck-Verschueren, C., Greally, J., Lowenberg, B., Melnick, A., and Delwel, R. (2010) Aberrant DNA hypermethylation signature in acute myeloid leukemia directed by EVI1, *Blood.*
40. Ohm, J. E., McGarvey, K. M., Yu, X., Cheng, L., Schuebel, K. E., Cope, L., Mohammad, H. P., Chen, W., Daniel, V. C., Yu, W., Berman, D. M., Jenuwein, T., Pruitt, K., Sharkis, S. J., Watkins, D. N., Herman, J. G., and Baylin, S. B. (2007) A stem cell-like chromatin pattern may predispose tumor suppressor genes to DNA hypermethylation and heritable silencing, *Nat Genet 39*, 237–242.
41. Paul, T. A., Bies, J., Small, D., and Wolff, L. (2010) Signatures of polycomb repression and reduced H3K4 trimethylation are associated with p15INK4b DNA methylation in AML, *Blood 115*, 3098–3108.
42. Zangenberg, M., Grubach, L., Aggerholm, A., Silkjaer, T., Juhl-Christensen, C., Nyvold,

C. G., Kjeldsen, E., Ommen, H. B., and Hokland, P. (2009) The combined expression of HOXA4 and MEIS1 is an independent prognostic factor in patients with AML, *Eur J Haematol 83*, 439–448.

43. Muller-Tidow, C., Klein, H. U., Hascher, A., Isken, F., Tickenbrock, L., Thoennissen, N., Agrawal-Singh, S., Tschanter, P., Disselhoff, C., Wang, Y., Becker, A., Thiede, C., Ehninger, G., Zur Stadt, U., Koschmieder, S., Seidl, M., Muller, F. U., Schmitz, W., Schlenke, P., McClelland, M., Berdel, W. E., Dugas, M., and Serve, H. (2010) Profiling of histone H3 lysine 9 trimethylation levels predicts transcription factor activity and survival in acute myeloid leukemia, *Blood 116*, 3564–3571.
44. Grimwade, D., Vyas, P., and Freeman, S. (2010) Assessment of minimal residual disease in acute myeloid leukemia, *Curr Opin Oncol 22*, 656–663.
45. Agrawal, S., Unterberg, M., Koschmieder, S., Stadt, U., Brunnberg, U., Verbeek, W., Buchner, T., Berdel, W. E., Serve, H., and Muller-Tidow, C. (2007) DNA methylation of tumor suppressor genes in clinical remission predicts the relapse risk in acute myeloid leukemia, *Cancer Res 67*, 1370–1377.
46. Galm, O., Wilop, S., Luders, C., Jost, E., Gehbauer, G., Herman, J. G., and Osieka, R. (2005) Clinical implications of aberrant DNA methylation patterns in acute myelogenous leukemia, *Ann Hematol 84 Suppl 1*, 39–46.
47. Hess, C. J., Errami, A., Berkhof, J., Denkers, F., Ossenkoppele, G. J., Nygren, A. O., Schuurhuis, G. J., and Waisfisz, Q. (2008) Concurrent methylation of promoters from tumor associated genes predicts outcome in acute myeloid leukemia, *Leuk Lymphoma 49*, 1132–1141.
48. Li, Q., Kopecky, K. J., Mohan, A., Willman, C. L., Appelbaum, F. R., Weick, J. K., and Issa, J. P. (1999) Estrogen receptor methylation is associated with improved survival in adult acute myeloid leukemia, *Clin Cancer Res 5*, 1077–1084.
49. Shimamoto, T., Ohyashiki, J. H., and Ohyashiki, K. (2005) Methylation of p15(INK4b) and E-cadherin genes is independently correlated with poor prognosis in acute myeloid leukemia, *Leuk Res 29*, 653–659.
50. Bullinger, L., Ehrich, M., Dohner, K., Schlenk, R. F., Dohner, H., Nelson, M. R., and van den Boom, D. (2010) Quantitative DNA methylation predicts survival in adult acute myeloid leukemia, *Blood 115*, 636–642.
51. Tormo, M., Marugan, I., and Calabuig, M. (2010) Myelodysplastic syndromes: an update on molecular pathology, *Clin Transl Oncol 12*, 652–661.
52. Vardiman, J. W., Harris, N. L., and Brunning, R. D. (2002) The World Health Organization (WHO) classification of the myeloid neoplasms, *Blood 100*, 2292–2302.
53. Issa, J. P. (2010) Epigenetic changes in the myelodysplastic syndrome, *Hematol Oncol Clin North Am 24*, 317–330.
54. Grovdal, M., Khan, R., Aggerholm, A., Antunovic, P., Astermark, J., Bernell, P., Engstrom, L. M., Kjeldsen, L., Linder, O., Nilsson, L., Olsson, A., Wallvik, J., Tangen, J. M., Oberg, G., Jacobsen, S. E., Hokland, P., Porwit, A., and Hellstrom-Lindberg, E. (2007) Negative effect of DNA hypermethylation on the outcome of intensive chemotherapy in older patients with high-risk myelodysplastic syndromes and acute myeloid leukemia following myelodysplastic syndrome, *Clin Cancer Res 13*, 7107–7112.
55. Shen, L., Kantarjian, H., Guo, Y., Lin, E., Shan, J., Huang, X., Berry, D., Ahmed, S., Zhu, W., Pierce, S., Kondo, Y., Oki, Y., Jelinek, J., Saba, H., Estey, E., and Issa, J. P. (2010) DNA methylation predicts survival and response to therapy in patients with myelodysplastic syndromes, *J Clin Oncol 28*, 605–613.
56. Rosu-Myles, M. and Wolff, L. (2008) p15Ink4b: dual function in myelopoiesis and inactivation in myeloid disease, *Blood Cells Mol Dis 40*, 406–409.
57. Aggerholm, A., Holm, M. S., Guldberg, P., Olesen, L. H., and Hokland, P. (2006) Promoter hypermethylation of p15INK4B, HIC1, CDH1, and ER is frequent in myelodysplastic syndrome and predicts poor prognosis in early-stage patients, *Eur J Haematol 76*, 23–32.
58. Au, W. Y., Fung, A., Man, C., Ma, S. K., Wan, T. S., Liang, R., and Kwong, Y. L. (2003) Aberrant p15 gene promoter methylation in therapy-related myelodysplastic syndrome and acute myeloid leukaemia: clinicopathological and karyotypic associations, *Br J Haematol 120*, 1062–1065.
59. Uchida, T., Kinoshita, T., Nagai, H., Nakahara, Y., Saito, H., Hotta, T., and Murate, T. (1997) Hypermethylation of the p15INK4B gene in myelodysplastic syndromes, *Blood 90*, 1403–1409.
60. Quesnel, B., Guillerm, G., Vereecque, R., Wattel, E., Preudhomme, C., Bauters, F., Vanrumbeke, M., and Fenaux, P. (1998) Methylation of the p15(INK4b) gene in myelodysplastic syndromes is frequent and acquired during disease progression, *Blood 91*, 2985–2990.

61. Herman, J. G., Civin, C. I., Issa, J. P., Collector, M. I., Sharkis, S. J., and Baylin, S. B. (1997) Distinct patterns of inactivation of p15INK4B and p16INK4A characterize the major types of hematological malignancies, *Cancer Res 57*, 837–841.
62. Figueroa, M. E., Skrabanek, L., Li, Y., Jiemjit, A., Fandy, T. E., Paietta, E., Fernandez, H., Tallman, M. S., Greally, J. M., Carraway, H., Licht, J. D., Gore, S. D., and Melnick, A. (2009) MDS and secondary AML display unique patterns and abundance of aberrant DNA methylation, *Blood 114*, 3448–3458.
63. Jiang, Y., Dunbar, A., Gondek, L. P., Mohan, S., Rataul, M., O'Keefe, C., Sekeres, M., Saunthararajah, Y., and Maciejewski, J. P. (2009) Aberrant DNA methylation is a dominant mechanism in MDS progression to AML, *Blood 113*, 1315–1325.
64. Kondo, Y. and Issa, J. P. (2004) Epigenetic changes in colorectal cancer, *Cancer Metastasis Rev 23*, 29–39.
65. Fenaux, P., Mufti, G. J., Hellstrom-Lindberg, E., Santini, V., Gattermann, N., Germing, U., Sanz, G., List, A. F., Gore, S., Seymour, J. F., Dombret, H., Backstrom, J., Zimmerman, L., McKenzie, D., Beach, C. L., and Silverman, L. R. (2010) Azacitidine prolongs overall survival compared with conventional care regimens in elderly patients with low bone marrow blast count acute myeloid leukemia, *J Clin Oncol 28*, 562–569.
66. Cashen, A. F., Schiller, G. J., O'Donnell, M. R., and DiPersio, J. F. (2010) Multicenter, phase II study of decitabine for the first-line treatment of older patients with acute myeloid leukemia, *J Clin Oncol 28*, 556–561.
67. Ravandi, F., Issa, J. P., Garcia-Manero, G., O'Brien, S., Pierce, S., Shan, J., Borthakur, G., Verstovsek, S., Faderl, S., Cortes, J., and Kantarjian, H. (2009) Superior outcome with hypomethylating therapy in patients with acute myeloid leukemia and high-risk myelodysplastic syndrome and chromosome 5 and 7 abnormalities, *Cancer 115*, 5746–5751.
68. Raj, K., John, A., Ho, A., Chronis, C., Khan, S., Samuel, J., Pomplun, S., Thomas, N. S., and Mufti, G. J. (2007) CDKN2B methylation status and isolated chromosome 7 abnormalities predict responses to treatment with 5-azacytidine, *Leukemia 21*, 1937–1944.
69. Itzykson, R., Thepot, S., Quesnel, B., Dreyfus, F., Beyne-Rauzy, O., Turlure, P., Vey, N., Recher, C., Dartigeas, C., Legros, L., Delaunay, J., Salanoubat, C., Visanica, S., Stamatoullas, A., Isnard, F., Marfaing-Koka, A., de Botton, S., Chelghoum, Y., Taksin, A. L., Plantier, I., Ame, S., Boehrer, S., Gardin, C., Beach, C. L., Ades, L., and Fenaux, P. (2011) Prognostic factors of response and overall survival in 282 higher-risk myelodysplastic syndromes treated with azacitidine, *Blood 117*, 403–411.
70. Blum, W., Garzon, R., Klisovic, R. B., Schwind, S., Walker, A., Geyer, S., Liu, S., Havelange, V., Becker, H., Schaaf, L., Mickle, J., Devine, H., Kefauver, C., Devine, S. M., Chan, K. K., Heerema, N. A., Bloomfield, C. D., Grever, M. R., Byrd, J. C., Villalona-Calero, M., Croce, C. M., and Marcucci, G. (2010) Clinical response and miR-29b predictive significance in older AML patients treated with a 10-day schedule of decitabine, *Proc Natl Acad Sci U S A 107*, 7473–7478.
71. Fandy, T. E., Herman, J. G., Kerns, P., Jiemjit, A., Sugar, E. A., Choi, S. H., Yang, A. S., Aucott, T., Dauses, T., Odchimar-Reissig, R., Licht, J., McConnell, M. J., Nasrallah, C., Kim, M. K., Zhang, W., Sun, Y., Murgo, A., Espinoza-Delgado, I., Oteiza, K., Owoeye, I., Silverman, L. R., Gore, S. D., and Carraway, H. E. (2009) Early epigenetic changes and DNA damage do not predict clinical response in an overlapping schedule of 5-azacytidine and entinostat in patients with myeloid malignancies, *Blood 114*, 2764–2773.
72. Fenaux, P. and Ades, L. (2009) Review of azacitidine trials in Intermediate-2-and High-risk myelodysplastic syndromes, *Leuk Res 33 Suppl 2*, S7–11.
73. Keating, G. M. (2009) Azacitidine: a review of its use in higher-risk myelodysplastic syndromes/acute myeloid leukaemia, *Drugs 69*, 2501-2518.
74. Hollenbach, P. W., Nguyen, A. N., Brady, H., Williams, M., Ning, Y., Richard, N., Krushel, L., Aukerman, S. L., Heise, C., and MacBeth, K. J. (2010) A comparison of azacitidine and decitabine activities in acute myeloid leukemia cell lines, *PLoS One 5*, e9001.
75. Xiong, J. and Epstein, R. J. (2009) Growth inhibition of human cancer cells by 5-aza-2 - deoxycytidine does not correlate with its effects on INK4a/ARF expression or initial promoter methylation status, *Mol Cancer Ther 8*, 779–785.
76. Flotho, C., Claus, R., Batz, C., Schneider, M., Sandrock, I., Ihde, S., Plass, C., Niemeyer, C. M., and Lubbert, M. (2009) The DNA methyltransferase inhibitors azacitidine, decitabine and zebularine exert differential effects on cancer gene expression in acute myeloid leukemia cells, *Leukemia 23*, 1019–1028.
77. Kuendgen, A., Schmid, M., Schlenk, R., Knipp, S., Hildebrandt, B., Steidl, C., Germing, U., Haas, R., Dohner, H., and

Gattermann, N. (2006) The histone deacetylase (HDAC) inhibitor valproic acid as monotherapy or in combination with all-trans retinoic acid in patients with acute myeloid leukemia, *Cancer 106*, 112–119.

78. Prebet, T. and Vey, N. (2010) Vorinostat in acute myeloid leukemia and myelodysplastic syndromes, *Expert Opin Investig Drugs 20*, 287–295.
79. Garcia-Manero, G., Assouline, S., Cortes, J., Estrov, Z., Kantarjian, H., Yang, H., Newsome, W. M., Miller, W. H., Rousseau, C., Kalita, A., Bonfils, C., Dubay, M., Patterson, T. A., Li, Z., Besterman, J. M., Reid, G., Laille, E., Martell, R. E., and Minden, M. (2008) Phase 1 study of the oral isotype specific histone deacetylase inhibitor MGCD0103 in leukemia, *Blood 112*, 981–989.
80. Garcia-Manero, G., Yang, H., Bueso-Ramos, C., Ferrajoli, A., Cortes, J., Wierda, W. G., Faderl, S., Koller, C., Morris, G., Rosner, G., Loboda, A., Fantin, V. R., Randolph, S. S., Hardwick, J. S., Reilly, J. F., Chen, C., Ricker, J. L., Secrist, J. P., Richon, V. M., Frankel, S. R., and Kantarjian, H. M. (2008) Phase 1 study of the histone deacetylase inhibitor vorinostat (suberoylanilide hydroxamic acid [SAHA]) in patients with advanced leukemias and myelodysplastic syndromes, *Blood 111*, 1060–1066.
81. Ungerstedt, J. S., Sowa, Y., Xu, W. S., Shao, Y., Dokmanovic, M., Perez, G., Ngo, L., Holmgren, A., Jiang, X., and Marks, P. A. (2005) Role of thioredoxin in the response of normal and transformed cells to histone deacetylase inhibitors, *Proceedings of the National Academy of Sciences of the United States of America 102*, 673–678.
82. Barnes, D. J. and Melo, J. V. (2002) Cytogenetic and molecular genetic aspects of chronic myeloid leukaemia, *Acta Haematol 108*, 180–202.
83. Druker, B. J., O'Brien, S. G., Cortes, J., and Radich, J. (2002) Chronic myelogenous leukemia, *Hematology Am Soc Hematol Educ Program 2002*, 111–135.
84. Tefferi, A. and Gilliland, D. G. (2005) The JAK2V617F tyrosine kinase mutation in myeloproliferative disorders: status report and immediate implications for disease classification and diagnosis, *Mayo Clin Proc 80*, 947–958.
85. Sawyers, C. L. (1999) Chronic myeloid leukemia, *N Engl J Med 340*, 1330–1340.
86. Hochhaus, A. (2008) First-Line management of CML: a state of the art review, *J Natl Compr Canc Netw 6 Suppl 2*, S1–S10.
87. Roman-Gomez, J., Jimenez-Velasco, A., Agirre, X., Castillejo, J. A., Navarro, G., San Jose-Eneriz, E., Garate, L., Cordeu, L., Cervantes, F., Prosper, F., Heiniger, A., and Torres, A. (2008) Repetitive DNA hypomethylation in the advanced phase of chronic myeloid leukemia, *Leuk Res 32*, 487-490.
88. Strathdee, G., Holyoake, T. L., Sim, A., Parker, A., Oscier, D. G., Melo, J. V., Meyer, S., Eden, T., Dickinson, A. M., Mountford, J. C., Jorgensen, H. G., Soutar, R., and Brown, R. (2007) Inactivation of HOXA genes by hypermethylation in myeloid and lymphoid malignancy is frequent and associated with poor prognosis, *Clin Cancer Res 13*, 5048–5055.
89. Dunwell, T., Hesson, L., Rauch, T. A., Wang, L., Clark, R. E., Dallol, A., Gentle, D., Catchpoole, D., Maher, E. R., Pfeifer, G. P., and Latif, F. (2010) A genome-wide screen identifies frequently methylated genes in haematological and epithelial cancers, *Mol Cancer 9*, 44.
90. Chim, C. S., Wong, K. Y., Leung, C. Y., Chung, L. P., Hui, P. K., Chan, S. Y., and Yu, L. Epigenetic inactivation of the hsa-miR-203 in haematological malignancies, *J Cell Mol Med*.
91. Chim, C. S., Wong, K. Y., Qi, Y., Loong, F., Lam, W. L., Wong, L. G., Jin, D. Y., Costello, J. F., and Liang, R. (2010) Epigenetic inactivation of the miR-34a in hematological malignancies, *Carcinogenesis 31*, 745–750.
92. Strathdee, G., Ferguson, S., Sim, A., and Brown, R. DNA methylation does not regulate JUNB expression in CML: comment on "Downregulation of JUNB mRNA expression in advanced phase chronic myelogenous leukemia" by Hoshino et al. [Leuk. Res. 33 (2009) 1361-1366], *Leuk Res 34*, 685–686.
93. Uhm, K. O., Lee, E. S., Lee, Y. M., Park, J. S., Kim, S. J., Kim, B. S., Kim, H. S., and Park, S. H. (2009) Differential methylation pattern of ID4, SFRP1, and SHP1 between acute myeloid leukemia and chronic myeloid leukemia, *J Korean Med Sci 24*, 493–497.
94. Wang, Y. L., Qian, J., Lin, J., Yao, D. M., Qian, Z., Zhu, Z. H., and Li, J. Y. (2010) Methylation status of DDIT3 gene in chronic myeloid leukemia, *J Exp Clin Cancer Res 29*, 54.
95. Ohyashiki, J. H., Ohyashiki, K., Kawakubo, K., Tauchi, T., Shimamoto, T., and Toyama, K. (1993) The methylation status of the major breakpoint cluster region in human leukemia cells, including Philadelphia chromosome-positive cells, is linked to the lineage of hematopoietic cells, *Leukemia 7*, 801–807.

96. Mizuno, S., Chijiwa, T., Okamura, T., Akashi, K., Fukumaki, Y., Niho, Y., and Sasaki, H. (2001) Expression of DNA methyltransferases DNMT1, 3A, and 3B in normal hematopoiesis and in acute and chronic myelogenous leukemia, *Blood 97*, 1172–1179.
97. Asimakopoulos, F. A., Shteper, P. J., Krichevsky, S., Fibach, E., Polliack, A., Rachmilewitz, E., Ben-Neriah, Y., and Ben-Yehuda, D. (1999) ABL1 methylation is a distinct molecular event associated with clonal evolution of chronic myeloid leukemia, *Blood 94*, 2452–2460.
98. Issa, J. P., Kantarjian, H., Mohan, A., O'Brien, S., Cortes, J., Pierce, S., and Talpaz, M. (1999) Methylation of the ABL1 promoter in chronic myelogenous leukemia: lack of prognostic significance, *Blood 93*, 2075–2080.
99. San Jose-Eneriz, E., Agirre, X., Jimenez-Velasco, A., Cordeu, L., Martin, V., Arqueros, V., Garate, L., Fresquet, V., Cervantes, F., Martinez-Climent, J. A., Heiniger, A., Torres, A., Prosper, F., and Roman-Gomez, J. (2009) Epigenetic down-regulation of BIM expression is associated with reduced optimal responses to imatinib treatment in chronic myeloid leukaemia, *Eur J Cancer 45*, 1877–1889.
100. Fiskus, W., Wang, Y., Joshi, R., Rao, R., Yang, Y., Chen, J., Kolhe, R., Balusu, R., Eaton, K., Lee, P., Ustun, C., Jillella, A., Buser, C. A., Peiper, S., and Bhalla, K. (2008) Cotreatment with vorinostat enhances activity of MK-0457 (VX-680) against acute and chronic myelogenous leukemia cells, *Clin Cancer Res 14*, 6106–6115.
101. Bixby, D. and Talpaz, M. (2009) Mechanisms of resistance to tyrosine kinase inhibitors in chronic myeloid leukemia and recent therapeutic strategies to overcome resistance, *Hematology Am Soc Hematol Educ Program 2009*, 461–476.
102. Lee, S. M., Bae, J. H., Kim, M. J., Lee, H. S., Lee, M. K., Chung, B. S., Kim, D. W., Kang, C. D., and Kim, S. H. (2007) Bcr-Abl-independent imatinib-resistant K562 cells show aberrant protein acetylation and increased sensitivity to histone deacetylase inhibitors, *J Pharmacol Exp Ther 322*, 1084–1092.
103. Zhang, B., Strauss, A. C., Chu, S., Li, M., Ho, Y., Shiang, K. D., Snyder, D. S., Huettner, C. S., Shultz, L., Holyoake, T., and Bhatia, R. (2010) Effective targeting of quiescent chronic myelogenous leukemia stem cells by histone deacetylase inhibitors in combination with imatinib mesylate, *Cancer Cell 17*, 427–442.
104. Kantarjian, H. M., O'Brien, S., Cortes, J., Giles, F. J., Faderl, S., Issa, J. P., Garcia-Manero, G., Rios, M. B., Shan, J., Andreeff, M., Keating, M., and Talpaz, M. (2003) Results of decitabine (5-aza-2'deoxycytidine) therapy in 130 patients with chronic myelogenous leukemia, *Cancer 98*, 522–528.
105. Ekmekci, C. G., Gutierrez, M. I., Siraj, A. K., Ozbek, U., and Bhatia, K. (2004) Aberrant methylation of multiple tumor suppressor genes in acute myeloid leukemia, *Am J Hematol 77*, 233–240.
106. Kroeger, H., Jelinek, J., Estecio, M. R., He, R., Kondo, K., Chung, W., Zhang, L., Shen, L., Kantarjian, H. M., Bueso-Ramos, C. E., and Issa, J. P. (2008) Aberrant CpG island methylation in acute myeloid leukemia is accentuated at relapse, *Blood 112*, 1366-1373.

Chapter 8

The Epigenetics of Brain Tumors

Adrian M. Dubuc, Stephen Mack, Alexander Unterberger, Paul A. Northcott, and Michael D. Taylor

Abstract

Glioblastoma, medulloblastoma, and ependymoma represent molecularly and clinically diverse forms of adult and pediatric brain tumors. While each tumor displays genetic, transcriptional, and cytogenetic heterogeneity, the epigenome of these tumors has only recently emerged as a major field of interest. Here, we describe advances in our understanding of the epigenetics of brain tumors, focusing on DNA methylation, histone modifications, and microRNA deregulation which contribute to the pathogenesis of these diseases.

Key words: Medulloblastoma, Ependymoma, Glioblastoma, Promoter hypermethylation, Global hypomethylation, Differentiation, MicroRNAs

1. Introduction

Brain tumors are among the most devastating forms of cancer and an indiscriminate killer of men, women, and children of all ages. Each year, over 30,000 individuals across North America alone are diagnosed with a malignant or benign tumor (1). While nearly 100 central nervous system (CNS) tumors exist, these tumors are stratified based on age of the patient, histology, and growth. Our ability to treat this disease varies dramatically depending on the tumor type; the overall 5-year survival rate following diagnosis of a primary malignant brain tumor is ~30% (1).

Of adult tumors, glioblastoma multiforme (GBM) represents 50% of all gliomas (20% of all adult brain tumors) and is attributed as the most aggressive form of the disease (2). Surgical resection remains quite difficult due to the diffuse nature of tumor cells and local invasion/infiltration, resulting in poor overall outcomes. Standard treatment protocols have remained relatively unchanged since their

Ramona G. Dumitrescu and Mukesh Verma (eds.), *Cancer Epigenetics: Methods and Protocols*, Methods in Molecular Biology, vol. 863, DOI 10.1007/978-1-61779-612-8_8, © Springer Science+Business Media, LLC 2012

inception and involve aggressive radio- and chemotherapeutic treatment following surgery (3).

Similarly, medulloblastoma and ependymoma are among the most devastating pediatric brain tumors. Medulloblastoma represents the most common pediatric malignant brain tumor which has shown major improvements in cure rates over the last decade (4). However, survivors often suffer from serious adverse effects and cognitive delays as a result of damaging nature of treatment (4). While rarer, ependymoma treatment is plagued by a vastly different problem. Currently, there exists no effective chemotherapeutics hindering our ability to adequately treat this disease (5).

Given the limitations of current treatment protocols for both adult and pediatric brain tumors, new methods are needed to effectively combat these forms of cancer. This will likely require a greater understanding of the underlying molecular biology of brain tumors.

While the field of neuro-oncology has been revolutionized through the advent of improved surgical techniques and advances in genomic technologies, our understandings of the epigenetics remains quite poor. The importance of epigenetic processes has been demonstrated in the CNS where cell-specific and spatiotemporal DNA methylation patterns and histone marks appear to regulate differentiation (6). Epigenetic deregulation is now understood to represent one of the hallmarks of cancer (7, 8), synergizing with genetic events or acting single-handedly (9). Here, we aim at presenting an understanding of the current knowledge of epigenetic changes that occur in major adult and pediatric forms of brain tumors, emphasizing the most important findings and discussing future directions.

2. Glioblastoma

GBM (WHO grade IV) is among the most aggressive and frequent forms of adult brain tumor, with a very poor survival rate (10) and an incidence of 3.05 new cases per 100,000 population in the United States (11). It typically occurs in adults at a median age of 64 years (11), but can manifest at any age as a primary GBM occurring de novo or as a secondary event which occurs as a progression of malignant transformation from lower grade tumors. The current life expectancy of patients with GBM is seen to be 14.6 months through current methods of multimodal therapy, with total resection and a combination of chemo- and radiotherapy (12).

It is understood that primary and secondary GBMs arise from both of genetic and epigenetic causations, displaying largely divergent cytogenetic, genetic, and transcriptional profiles. While secondary GBMs undergo an accumulation of genetic events, including *TP53* inactivation (13, 14), loss of heterozygosity (LOH) of chromosome

19q (13) or 10q (15), and amplification of *MDM4* (16), to progress from lower grades to a grade IV GBM, primary GBMs undergo a largely different set of genetic changes. These include amplification of *EGFR* (17, 18) and inactivation of *CDKN2* (19), *PI3K-R1* (20), and *NF1* (21).

The epigenetic causes of glioblastoma have come under increased investigation in recent years. DNA methylation has been proposed to serve as a potential mutagen, where methylated cytosines deaminate to thymine (22). This mutational event, in combination with insufficient repair of guanine methylation by O^6-methylguanine-DNA methyltransferase (*MGMT*), is believed to contribute to *TP53* mutations in glioblastoma (23, 24). Epigenetic characteristic of glioblastoma includes global hypomethylation, with regional, punctate hypermethylation, and altered expression of the epigenetic machinery ultimately resulting in increased genomic instability, activation of oncogenes, and silencing of tumor suppressor genes.

DNA hypomethylation in GBMs is in part explained by a correlating decrease in expression of de novo DNA methyltransferase *DNMT3b* (25). This global change in methylation leads to reactivation and remobilization of repeat elements satellite 2, D4Z4 and Alu elements (26), resulting in increased copy number alterations of genomic regions in proximity to these elements (26). By contrast, tumor-specific DNA hypermethylation has predominantly been examined in the context of promoter hypermethylation and gene silencing. These findings affect both our understanding of tumor initiation/progression and, most importantly, can predict drug response such as the methylation status of *MGMT*. MGMT reverses alkylation at the O^6 position of guanine, allowing the cell to repair cross-linked DNA. Initial studies demonstrated promoter hypermethylation (27) and gene silencing (28, 29) of *MGMT* in a subset of GBMs suggesting susceptibility to alkylation agents due to the epigenetic inactivation of their repair machinery (30–32). Thirty-percent (30%) of patients with GBM shown to be lacking expression of *MGMT* (29), respond favorably to alkylating agents, carmustine (33) or temozolomide (34), with improved outcome relative to patients with unmethylated *MGMT*.

Candidate gene approaches have demonstrated the hypermethylation of notable genes in GBMs including tumor suppressor genes *RB* (35), *HIC1* (36), *CDKN2A* (36–38), *p14* (39), *PTEN* (40, 41), and *p53/p73* (42), apoptosis machinery *RASSF1A* (43) and *CASP8* (44), the suppressor of cytokine-signaling (SOCS) family 1 (45), 2, and 3 (46, 47), as well as members of the Wnt-signaling pathway, *SFRP1*, *SFRP2*, and *NKD2* (48). Promoter hypomethylation also clearly plays a role in the reexpression of normally silenced genes, including *CD133* (49), as well as *MMP9* and *IL8* (50).

Perhaps the greatest advances in our understanding of the DNA methylation contributions to gliomagenesis is derived from The Cancer Genome Atlas (TCGA) project (http://cancergenome.nih.gov/). Using a large cohort of nearly 300 GBMs, DNA methylation arrays tiling 27,000 CpG sites identified a highly methylated subset of GBMs, indicative of a CpG island methylator phenotype (GBM-CIMP) (51). Interestingly, GBM-CIMP tumors appear to cooperate with specific genetic events, displaying distinct copy number alterations and genetic mutations (51). There are clear and distinct clinical characteristics of GBM-CIMP +ve tumors, which occur in younger (~30–40) patients and display significantly better survival rates than GBM-CIMP-negative tumors within the proneural group (51).

The coiling of DNA into histone units also plays an important role in the epigenome and is impacted in GBMs. Posttranslational modifications to histones can positively and negatively regulate access of transcription factors to DNA, providing an additional level of transcriptional complexity. Expression of histone remodeling complex gene *BMI1* (52), *EZH2* (53), as well as class II and IV HDACs (54) was found to be altered in a subset of human GBMs. These alterations have a significant impact on gene expression by causing a change in the overall chromatin structure, as observed in the overall histone H3 acetylation seen in GBM (54). Subsequently, HDAC inhibitors have been used for treatment of GBMs and have seen some success as a sensitizing agent for radiotherapy (55) and chemotherapy (56, 57).

MicroRNA (miR) posttranscriptional regulation of gene expression also serves as an epigenetic mechanism. miRNAs (miRs) have been linked to cancer initiation, maintenance, and progression, inhibiting differentiation of tumor cells and promoting proliferation (58). Specifically, in GBMs, miR-21 was shown to be upregulated, affecting downstream target and tumor suppressor genes: *TP53*, *TGF-β* (59), *TIMP3* (60), and *PTEN* (61). Notable miRNAs with cancer(GBM)-specific expression changes include the upregulation of miR-26a, involved in development and proliferation of glioblastoma (62) and silencing of miR-124, a cell cycle regulator and neuronal differentiator (63, 64); miR-128, a glioma proliferation inhibitor (65); and miR-451, an inhibitor of invasion (66). While research into miRs deregulation in gliomas is still in its infancy, anti-miR therapies have been suggested as putative viable targets for therapy, although this remains to be seen.

Future directions of research into the epigenome of GBM involve a comprehensive examination of the GBM epigenome. This should include a comprehensive sequencing of all the changes in CG methylation in the GBM epigenome (as compared to normal tissue), as well as known activating/inhibitory histone modifications throughout the genome and changes in miR expression. This information, combined with our current knowledge of the

GBM transcriptome, would provide researchers with a complete picture of all the epigenetics changes affording for the development of novel therapeutics, as well as adaption of existing strategies for treatment of this cancer.

3. Medulloblastoma

Medulloblastoma (WHO grade IV), a pediatric brain tumor of the cerebella, is the most common solid pediatric malignancy and a highly aggressive cancer (67) which often (~33%) presents with leptomeningeal dissemination (68). Improvements in clinical treatment have resulted in the amelioration of 5-year survival rate to approximately 70% (69); however, current treatment protocols result in significant cognitive problems for survivors (4). At a histological level, medulloblastomas display morphological heterogeneity leading to the following classification: classic (73%), desmoplastic (10%), extensively nodular (<1%), and large cell and anaplastic (17%) (4), the latter being associates with poor outcome (70).

Studies on the cytogenetic and underlying molecular signature of this disease have revealed the heterogeneous nature of medulloblastoma. We now understand medulloblastoma consists of at least four intrinsic subgroups—WNT, sonic hedgehog (SHH), group C, and group D (71–73)—that display vastly divergent genetic and expression attributes, resulting in distinct clinical characteristics (74) and permitted further stratification of high-risk and standard-risk patients (4). These subgroups demonstrate distinct pathway activities with wingless signaling pathway (WNT) and SHH pathways, characterizing two of the four molecular subgroups, named after these molecular features. These aberrant signaling pathways have been heavily investigated, resulting in a greater understanding of signaling in the pathogenic state and facilitating the creation of SHH-target pharmacological inhibitors (75). Despite our knowledge of the genetic and molecular landscape, the epigenetic contributions remain very poorly characterized.

While medulloblastoma epigenetics has been pursued for nearly 20 years, initial techniques examined gross DNA methylation levels across the epigenome, lacking the ability to pinpoint specific changes (76). Advances in molecular biology techniques led to restriction landmark genomic screening (RLGS) studies which, while both time consuming and difficult to analyze (77), provided the first link between genetic and epigenetic synergy (78) identifying DNA hypermethylation on chromosome 17p11.2, a region frequently deleted in 30–50% of medulloblastoma (73). This technique was also used to identify novel candidates putatively implicated in tumorigenesis, such as the cell cycle regulators $p15^{INK4B}$

and $p16^{INK4A}$ (79). Identification of gene-specific silencing led to a flurry of candidate gene investigations noting methylation-induced silencing of apoptotic machinery (80), and tumor suppressor genes *RASSF1A* (81) and *HIC1* (82, 83). Currently, there are approximately ~30 genes known to be silenced by DNA methylation in the medulloblastoma epigenome. However, perhaps the most striking observation of epigenetic deregulation was reported in 2007 in which Pfister et al. (84) report a statistically significant relationship between a strong methylator phenotype and poor outcome (84), demonstrating the clinical importance of describing specific epigenetic changes. These findings are recapitulated in a mouse model, where reduction of DNA methylation levels or treatment with broad spectrum demethylases results in statistically significant improvements in the latency of medulloblastoma formation and overall survival (85).

Currently, there exists a dramatic shift from candidate gene towards epigenome-wide, array-based research. Various existent methodologies have each some advantages and limitations. One such method involves the use of chemical inhibitors of epigenetic processes, such as decitabine (DAC), a cytosine analogue, in trying to force reexpression of silenced genes. The chemical structure of DAC does not permit methylation at the 5 position, thus incorporation into DNA, via cell division, causes widespread demethylation (86). Using DAC incorporation into medulloblastoma cell lines, array-based transcriptional profiling revealed the reexpression of *S100* family genes (87), highly suggestive of gene regulation by hypermethylation. A similar strategy was also used to detect *COL1A2* (88) and *SPINT2* (89), a member of the HGF/MET-signaling pathway which importantly can be targeted by pharmacological inhibitors (90). While providing useful candidates for further investigation, DAC studies are limited by a high rate of false positive associated with secondary effects and cytotoxicity of the drug, as well as a restriction to in vitro cultures. By contrast, other techniques such as aPRIMES (84) and DAMD (91) permit the detection of hypermethylation in primary tumor by relying on the inherent properties of methylated vs. unmethylated DNA to identify sample-to-sample variation. These studies detected silencing of developmental genes *ZIC2* (84) and *PTCH1* (91) among others. Ultimately, large cohort studies detailing methylation in primary medulloblastoma samples have yet to be completed, and these findings would add considerable clarity to our current understanding of the medulloblastoma DNA methylome.

Aberrant microRNA (miRNA) expression is also known to be an important contributor to the epigenetic instability of medulloblastoma. Our understanding of miRNA in medulloblastoma is limited. However, initial reports, following the identification of miRNA deregulation in other brain tumors, linked overexpression of *CDK6* to decreased levels of miR-124 (92). Genome-wide investigations initially detailed miRNA changes in Hh-signaling (SHH-subgroup) murine medulloblastoma (93). A comparison of high vs. low *Gli1* expression revealed 34 miRNA differentially regulated and forming an Hh-miRNA signature. It appears that downregulation of miR-126b, miR-324-5p, and miR-326 in MB permits for deregulation of Hh-signaling and results in increased proliferation of tumor cells (93). Using this dataset, the authors then proceeded to examine cancer-specific miRNA changes by investigating expression differences between normal cerebella (fetal, adult) and medulloblastoma tissue (94) of a set of 250 miRNAs. There appeared to be more miRNA downregulated in medulloblastoma vs. normal cerebellar tissue. The group did identify a smaller subset of miRNA upregulated in MB, including the onco-miR 17-92, implicated in leukemia and lung adenocarcinomas (94). Two simultaneous investigations further characterized the specific role of miR17-92 upregulation (95, 96). Both human genetic and mouse models clearly demonstrate the upregulation of this miR cluster specifically in the SHH-subgroup, and this results in increased mitogenic signaling (95). Most recently, miRNA across all MB subgroups was interrogated revealing distinct expression patterns in WNT, SHH, and group C tumors (97). Further understanding of microRNA deregulation in this disease may help in understanding the cell of origin of medulloblastoma subgroups and provide us with novel pharmacological targets.

Histone-mediated silencing represents perhaps the most intriguing and least understood level of epigenetic control in medulloblastoma. The most striking evidence for a histone-mediated role in the initiation or progression of this disease stems from genetic work which has demonstrated targeted homozygous deletions and subclonal amplifications of histone methyltransferases and demethylases (98). These include deletions of *EHMT1*, *SMYD4*, *L3MBTL2*, *L3MBTL3*, and *SCML2* as well as focal amplifications of *JMJD2C*, *JMJD2B*, and *MYST3* (98). Interestingly, there appears to be a specific convergence on the ninth lysine residue on histone 3 (H3K9). Staining of H3K9-dimethylation revealed an absence of this chromatin mark in 41% of 62 medulloblastomas profiled on a tissue microarray (98). Candidate gene approaches have begun to point towards histone modifications, and not other transcriptional mechanisms, governing control of aberrant expression in medulloblastoma, such as H3K27me3 silencing, *NEURL1* inhibiting apoptosis, and uncoupling Notch regulation (99). Additionally, increased histone acetylation appears to mediate transcriptional activation observed in targeting important Hh genes such as Gli1 (100). Ultimately, there is no technology that effectively allows us to interrogate histone marks in primary tumors. This limitation has resulted in significant delays in our understanding and characterization of these events.

To date, no large-scale epigenetic studies have been performed addressing the medulloblastoma DNA methylome. Array-based tools can now comprehensively examine over 400,000 CpG sites located across CpG islands, CpG island shores, and untranslated regions (UTRs). Given the vast knowledge of the medulloblastoma transcriptome and genome, a large-scale investigation would provide us with a clear understanding of this disease.

4. Ependymoma

Ependymoma is a clinically and genetically heterogeneous tumor of the CNS. It arises nearly anywhere in the CNS including the supratentorial region comprising the parenchyma of the cerebral hemispheres, the posterior fossa encompassing the cerebellum and brain stem, and the spinal cord (101). Ninety percent (90%) of childhood ependymomas occur intracranially, with two-thirds of cases arising within the posterior fossa (101). This is in contrast to most adult ependymomas, which tend to present within the spinal cord. The clinical behavior of ependymoma also varies. While some patients experience a relentless course with multiple recurrences, others harbor slow-growing variants capable of recurring up to 15 years after the initial treatment (102). The 5-year survival rate ranges from 39 to 64%, with a 5-year progression free survival rate of 23–45% (102).

In the past, deciphering the genetic basis of ependymoma has been difficult, plagued by small sample numbers and the use of low-resolution microarray technologies. To add to these difficulties, there are no appropriate cell lines and animal models of ependymoma. These studies have identified the most common chromosomal aberrations in ependymoma to involve losses of chromosome 1p, 3, 6q, 9p, 10q, 13q, 16p, 17, 21, and 22q and gains of 1q, 4q, 5, 7, 8, 9q, 12q, and 20 (103). A consistent finding in many of these studies is that up to 50% of tumors arising within the posterior fossa exhibit a balanced genomic profile (102). This was observed in a recent report, which examined 206 ependymomas by high-resolution Affymetrix 500K SNP arrays (104). Here, Johnson et al. (104) generated the first mouse model of ependymoma, and provided evidence that the cell of origin of ependymoma arises within the radial glial cell lineage. Indeed, genome-wide copy number studies have led to breakthroughs in ependymoma genetics; however, the epigenetic basis of this disease, particularly at a genome-wide scale, remains poorly understood.

To this date, nearly all ependymoma epigenetic studies have focused on analyzing the promoter methylation status in selected candidate genes. These genes have been chosen based upon location within known regions of chromosomal loss in ependymoma and/or frequent methylation in other cancer types. *RASSF1A* has been reported to be the most frequently hypermethylated tumor suppressor gene in ependymoma with an incidence of 86% (30/35) and present universally in all histological subtypes, ages, and anatomical locations (105). Given the observation of LOH at chromosome 17p13.3 (106) in ependymoma, others have investigated the promoter methylation status of *HIC-1* (107, 108). Waha et al. (107) identified *HIC-1* promoter hypermethylation in 83% (43/52) of ependymomas with a significant enrichment in tumors arising in pediatric intracranial ependymomas. Another frequently reported chromosomal abnormality in supratentorial ependymomas is focal chromosome 9p loss, encompassing the *CDKN2A/p16INK4a* locus (102, 104). In a large study of 152 cases, Rousseau et al. (109) identified *CDKN2A* promoter hypermethylation in 21% (26/123) of cases, along with promoter methylation of neighboring tumor suppressor genes *CDKN2B* and *p14ARF*, in 32% (23/71) and 21% (23/108) of cases, respectively. Given the positive therapeutic response in GBM patients harboring *MGMT* promoter methylation, this gene has also been analyzed in several ependymoma cohorts (108, 110–112). In 142 cases, Koos et al. (110) identified *MGMT* promoter hypermethylation in 27% (39/142) of ependymomas, arising primarily in nonanaplastic histological variants. Others have reported, less frequently methylated genes in ependymoma including *BLU*, *GSTP1*, *DAPK*, *FHIT*, *MGMT*, *MCJ*, *RARB*, *TIMP3*, *THBS1*, *TP73*, and a family of TRAIL-pathway-related genes *CASP8*, *TFRSF10C*, and *TFRSF10D* (5).

In addition to the accumulation of methylation at CpG island promoters, cancer genomes also exhibit global hypomethylation largely at repetitive regions. In a recent report, Xie et al. (113) developed a novel genome-wide approach to survey ALU repeat sequences and applied this technique to six pediatric intracranial ependymomas. Here, they identified many differentially methylated CpG sites associated with tumor aggressiveness and recurrence. Interestingly, they found that differentially methylated CpG sites were enriched in sequences with low CpG density flanking, rather than within, ALU repeats. This may represent a more general cancer phenomenon with yet unknown biological significance.

Candidate gene approaches have limited our understanding of the epigenetic mechanisms important in ependymoma development. Further, the contribution of these genes to tumorigenesis remains unclear due to the lack of appropriate mouse models and cell lines. As genome-wide epigenetic approaches continue to emerge, in surveying areas such as DNA methylation and histone modification, application of these technologies to large ependymoma tumor studies will provide important insight into the molecular underpinnings of this disease.

5. Conclusion

Large investigations, with high-resolution techniques, have allowed us to gain greater insight into the underlying epigenetic signature of glioblastoma. The knowledge we have gained has enabled us to improve stratification of this disease based on the presence or absence of epigenetic events, such as the DNA hypermethylation of MGMT, which directly influences treatment options. In addition, epigenome-wide investigations have allowed us to further subdivide the distinct transcriptional/genetic tumor subgroups, which may aid in determining which patients require more aggressive treatment.

While our understanding of the epigenetic events affecting other CNS tumors is not as robust, increased knowledge of the epigenetic pathways and machinery aberrantly silenced in medulloblastoma and ependymoma may lead to targeted therapies aimed at repairing specific molecular functions. Finally, the dynamic and reversible nature of epigenetic changes makes this area of research an attractive target for pharmacological inhibitors. Currently, no clinical trials exist evaluating pharmacologically mediated demethylation therapies on CNS tumor growth; however, as our understanding of the epigenome increases, these may represent suitable avenues for future investigations.

References

1. CBTRUS. (2010) 2010 CBTRUS Statistical Report, in *Central Brain Tumour Registry of the United States.*
2. Ang, C., Gulot, M.C., Ramanakumar, A.V., Roberge, D., and Kavan, P. (2010) Clinical Significance of molecular biomarkers in glioblastoma. *Can J Neurol Sci* 37, 625–630.
3. Nishikawa, R. (2010) Standard therapy for glioblastoma - a review of where we are. *Neurol Med Chir* 50, 713–719.
4. Ellison, D. (2010) Childhood medulloblastoma: novel approaches to the classification of a heterogeneous disease. *Acta Neuropathol* 120, 305–316.
5. Mack, S.C. and Taylor, M.D. (2009) The genetic and epigenetic basis of ependymoma. *Childs Nerv Syst* 25, 1195–1201.
6. Christophersen, N.S. and Helin, K. (2010) Epigenetic Control of embryonic stem cell fate. *J Exp Med* 25, 2287–2295.
7. Baylin, S.B. and Ohm, J.E. (2006) Epigenetic gene silencing in cancer - a mechanism for early oncogenic pathway addiction. *Nat Rev Cancer* 6, 107–116.
8. Jones, P.A. and Baylin, S.B. (2002) The fundamental role of epigenetic events in cancer. *Nat Rev Cancer* 3, 415–428.
9. Garinis, G.A., Patrinos, G.P., Spanakis, N.E., and Menounos, P.G. (2002) DNA hypermethylation: when tumour suppressor genes go silent. *Hum Genet* 111, 115–127.
10. Louis, D.N., Ohgaki, H., Wiestler, O.D., Cavenee, W.K., Burger, P.C., Jouvet, A., Scheithauer, B.W., and Kleihues, P. (2007) The 2007 WHO classification of tumours of the central nervous system. *Acta Neuropathol* 114, 97–109.
11. Schwartzbaum, J.A., Fisher, J.L., Aldape, K.D., and Wrensch, M. (2006) Epidemiology and molecular pathology of glioma. *Nat Clin Pract Neurol* 2, 494–503; quiz 491 p following 516.
12. Stupp, R., Mason, W.P., van den Bent, M. J., Weller, M., Fisher, B., Taphoorn, M. J., Belanger, K., Brandes, A.A., Marosi, C., Bogdahn, U., Curschmann, J., Janzer, R. C., Ludwin, S. K., Gorlia, T., Allgeier, A., Lacombe, D., Cairncross, J. G., Eisenhauer,

E., and Mirimanoff, R. O. (2005) Radiotherapy plus concomitant and adjuvant temozolomide for glioblastoma. *N Engl J Med* 352, 987–996.

13. Benjamin, R., Capparella, J., and Brown, A. (2003) Classification of glioblastoma multiforme in adults by molecular genetics. *Cancer J* 9, 82–90.
14. Louis, D. N. (1997) A molecular genetic model of astrocytoma histopathology. *Brain Pathol* 7, 755–764.
15. Bostrom, J., Cobbers, J. M., Wolter, M., Tabatabai, G., Weber, R. G., Lichter, P., Collins, V. P., and Reifenberger, G. (1998) Mutation of the PTEN (MMACl) tumor suppressor gene in a subset of glioblastomas but not in meningiomas with loss of chromosome arm 10q. *Cancer Res* 58, 29–33.
16. Riemenschneider, M. J., Buschges, R., Wolter, M., Reifenberger, J., Bostrom, J., Kraus, J. A., Schlegel, U., and Reifenberger, G. (1999) Amplification and overexpression of the MDM4 (MDMX) gene from 1q32 in a subset of malignant gliomas without TP53 mutation or MDM2 amplification. *Cancer Res* 59, 6091–6096.
17. Collins, V. P. (2002) Cellular mechanisms targeted during astrocytoma progression. *Cancer Lett* 188, 1–7.
18. von Deimling, A., Louis, D. N., and Wiestler, O. D. (1995) Molecular pathways in the formation of gliomas. *Glia* 15, 328–338.
19. Schmidt, E. E., Ichimura, K., Reifenberger, G., and Collins, V. P. (1994) CDKN2 (p16/MTSl) gene deletion or CDK4 amplification occurs in the majority of glioblastomas. *Cancer Res* 54, 6321–6324.
20. Sancho-Martinez, I., and Martin-Villalba, A. (2009) Tyrosine phosphorylation and CD95: a FAScinating switch. *Cell Cycle* 8, 838–842.
21. Zhu, Y., Guignard, F., Zhao, D., Liu, L., Burns, D. K., Mason, R. P., Messing, A., and Parada, L. F. (2005) Early inactivation of p53 tumor suppressor gene cooperating with NFl loss induces malignant astrocytoma. *Cancer Cell* 8, 119–130.
22. Duncan, B. K., and Miller, J. H. (1980) Mutagenic deamination of cytosine residues in DNA. *Nature* 287, 560–561.
23. Bentivegna, S.S., and Bresnick, E. (1994) Inhibition of human O6-methylguanine-DNA methyltransferase by 5-methylcytosine. *Cancer Res* 54, 327–329.
24. Nakamura, M., Watanabe, T., Yonekawa, Y., Kleihues, P., and Ohgaki, H. (2001) Promoter methylation of the DNA repair gene MGMT in astrocytomas is frequently associated with G:C → A:T mutations of the TP53 tumor suppressor gene. *Carcinogenesis* 22, 1715–1719.
25. Fanelli, M., Caprodossi, S., Ricci-Vitiani, L., Porcellini, A., Tomassoni-Ardori, F., Amatori, S., Andreoni, F., Magnani, M., De Maria, R., Santoni, A., Minucci, S., and Pelicci, P.G. (2008) Loss of pericentromeric DNA methylation pattern in human glioblastoma is associated with altered DNA methyltransferases expression and involves the stem cell compartment. *Oncogene* 27, 358–365.
26. Cadieux, B., Ching, T.T., VandenBerg, S.R., and Costello, J.F. (2006) Genome-wide hypomethylation in human glioblastomas associated with specific copy number alteration, methylenetetrahydrofolate reductase allele status, and increased proliferation. *Cancer Res* 66, 8469–8476.
27. Qian, X.C., and Brent, T.P. (1997) Methylation hot spots in the 5 flanking region denote silencing of the O6-methylguanine-DNA methyltransferase gene. *Cancer Res* 57, 3672–3677.
28. Silber, J.R., Mueller, B.A., Ewers, T.G., and Berger, M.S. (1993) Comparison of O6-methylguanine-DNA methyltransferase activity in brain tumors and adjacent normal brain. *Cancer Res* 53, 3416–3420.
29. Silber, J. R., Bobola, M. S., Ghatan, S., Blank, A., Kolstoe, D. D., and Berger, M. S. (1998) O6-methylguanine-DNA methyltransferase activity in adult gliomas: relation to patient and tumor characteristics. *Cancer Res* 58, 1068–1073.
30. Belanich, M., Pastor, M., Randall, T., Guerra, D., Kibitel, J., Alas, L., Li, B., Citron, M., Wasserman, P., White, A., Eyre, H., Jaeckle, K., Schulman, S., Rector, D., Prados, M., Coons, S., Shapiro, W., and Yarosh, D. (1996) Retrospective study of the correlation between the DNA repair protein alkyltransferase and survival of brain tumor patients treated with carmustine. *Cancer Res* 56, 783–788.
31. Jaeckle, K.A., Eyre, H.J., Townsend, J.J., Schulman, S., Knudson, H.M., Belanich, M., Yarosh, D.B., Bearman, S.I., Giroux, D. J. and Schold, S.C. (1998) Correlation of tumor O6 methylguanine-DNA methyltransferase levels with survival of malignant astrocytoma patients treated with bis-chloroethylnitrosourea: a Southwest Oncology Group study. *J Clin Oncol* 16, 3310–3315.
32. Silber, J.R., Blank, A., Bobola, M.S., Ghatan, S., Kolstoe, D.D., and Berger, M.S. (1999) O6-methylguanine-DNA methyltransferase-deficient phenotype in human gliomas: frequency and time to tumor progression after alkylating agent-based chemotherapy. *Clin Cancer Res* 5, 807–814.

33. Esteller, M., Garcia-Foncillas, J., Andion, E., Goodman, S.N., Hidalgo, O.F., Vanaclocha, V., Baylin, S. B., and Herman, J. G. (2000) Inactivation of the DNA-repair gene MGMT and the clinical response of gliomas to alkylating agents. *N Engl J Med* 343, 1350–1354.
34. Hegi, M.E., Diserens, A.C., Gorlia, T., Hamou, M.F., de Tribolet, N., Weller, M., Kros, J.M., Hainfellner, J.A., Mason, W., Mariani, L., Bromberg, J.E., Hau, P., Mirimanoff, R.O., Cairncross, J.G., Janzer, R.C., and Stupp, R. (2005) MGMT gene silencing and benefit from temozolomide in glioblastoma. *N Engl J Med* 352, 997–1003.
35. Nakamura, M., Yonekawa, Y., Kleihues, P., and Ohgaki, H. (2001) Promoter hypermethylation of the RB1 gene in glioblastomas. *Lab Invest* 81, 77–82.
36. Li, Q., Jedlicka, A., Ahuja, N., Gibbons, M.C., Baylin, S.B., Burger, P. C., and Issa, J. P. (1998) Concordant methylation of the ER and N33 genes in glioblastoma multiforme. *Oncogene* 16, 3197–3202.
37. Costello, J.F., Berger, M.S., Huang, H.S., and Cavenee, W.K. (1996) Silencing of p16/CDKN2 expression in human gliomas by methylation and chromatin condensation. *Cancer Res* 56, 2405–2410.
38. Park, S.H., Jung, K.C., Ro, J.Y., Kang, G.H. and Khang, S.K. (2000) 5 CpG island methylation of p16 is associated with absence of p16 expression in glioblastomas. *J Korean Med Sci* 15, 555–559.
39. Nakamura, M., Watanabe, T., Klangby, U., Asker, C., Wiman, K., Yonekawa, Y., Kleihues, P., and Ohgaki, H. (2001) p14ARF deletion and methylation in genetic pathways to glioblastomas. *Brain Pathol* 11, 159–168.
40. Baeza, N., Weller, M., Yonekawa, Y., Kleihues, P., and Ohgaki, H. (2003) PTEN methylation and expression in glioblastomas. *Acta Neuropathol* 106, 479–485.
41. Wiencke, J. K., Zheng, S., Jelluma, N., Tihan, T., Vandenberg, S., Tamguney, T., Baumber, R., Parsons, R., Lamborn, K.R., Berger, M.S., Wrensch, M.R., Haas-Kogan, D.A., and Stokoe, D. (2007) Methylation of the PTEN promoter defines low-grade gliomas and secondary glioblastoma. *Neuro Oncol* 9, 271–279.
42. Watanabe, T., Huang, H., Nakamura, M., Wischhusen, J., Weller, M., Kleihues, P., and Ohgaki, H. (2002) Methylation of the p73 gene in gliomas. *Acta Neuropathol* 104, 357–362.
43. Horiguchi, K., Tomizawa, Y., Tosaka, M., Ishiuchi, S., Kurihara, H., Mori, M., and Saito, N. (2003) Epigenetic inactivation of RASSF1A candidate tumor suppressor gene at 3p21.3 in brain tumors. *Oncogene* 22, 7862–7865.
44. Martinez, R., Setien, F., Voelter, C., Casado, S., Quesada, M. P., Schackert, G., and Esteller, M. (2007) CpG island promoter hypermethylation of the pro-apoptotic gene caspase-8 is a common hallmark of relapsed glioblastoma multiforme. *Carcinogenesis* 28, 1264–1268.
45. Zhou, H., Miki, R., Eeva, M., Fike, F.M., Seligson, D., Yang, L., Yoshimura, A., Teitell, M.A., Jamieson, C.A., and Cacalano, N.A. (2007) Reciprocal regulation of SOCS 1 and SOCS3 enhances resistance to ionizing radiation in glioblastoma multiforme. *Clin Cancer Res* 13, 2344–2353.
46. Martini, M., Pallini, R., Luongo, G., Cenci, T., Lucantoni, C., and Larocca, L.M. (2008) Prognostic relevance of SOCS3 hypermethylation in patients with glioblastoma multiforme. *Int J Cancer* 123, 2955–2960.
47. Teofili, L., Martini, M., Cenci, T., Guidi, F., Torti, L., Giona, F., Foa, R., Leone, G., and Larocca, L. M. (2008) Epigenetic alteration of SOCS family members is a possible pathogenetic mechanism in JAK2 wild type myeloproliferative diseases. *Int J Cancer* 123, 1586–1592.
48. Gotze, S., Wolter, M., Reifenberger, G., Muller, O., and Sievers, S. (2010) Frequent promoter hypermethylation of Wnt pathway inhibitor genes in malignant astrocytic gliomas. *Int J Cancer* 126, 2584–2593.
49. Tabu, K., Sasai, K., Kimura, T., Wang, L., Aoyanagi, E., Kohsaka, S., Tanino, M., Nishihara, H., and Tanaka, S. (2008) Promoter hypomethylation regulates CD133 expression in human gliomas. *Cell Res* 18, 1037–1046.
50. Martinez, R., Martin-Subero, J. I., Rohde, V., Kirsch, M., Alaminos, M., Fernandez, A. F., Ropero, S., Schackert, G., and Esteller, M. (2009) A microarray-based DNA methylation study of glioblastoma multiforme. *Epigenetics* 4, 255–264.
51. Noushmehr, H., Welsenberger, D.J., Diefes, K., Phillips, H.S., Pujara, K., et al. (2010) Identification of a CpG island methylator phenotype that defines a distinct subgroup of gliomas. *Cancer Cell* 17, 510-522.
52. Abdouh, M., Facchino, S., Chatoo, W., Balasingam, V., Ferreira, J., and Bernier, G. (2009) BMI1 sustains human glioblastoma multiforme stem cell renewal. *J Neurosci* 29, 8884–8896.
53. Lee, J., Son, M. J., Woolard, K., Donin, N.M., Li, A., Cheng, C.H., Kotliarova, S., Kotliarov, Y., Walling, J., Ahn, S., Kim, M., Totonchy,

M., Cusack, T., Ene, C., Ma, H., Su, Q., Zenklusen, J.C., Zhang, W., Maric, D., and Fine, H.A. (2008) Epigenetic-mediated dysfunction of the bone morphogenetic protein pathway inhibits differentiation of glioblastoma-initiating cells. *Cancer Cell* 13, 69–80.

54. Lucio-Eterovic, A.K., Cortez, M.A., Valera, E.T., Motta, F.J., Queiroz, R.G., Machado, H.R., Carlotti, C.G., Jr., Neder, L., Scrideli, C.A., and Tone, L.G. (2008) Differential expression of 12 histone deacetylase (HDAC) genes in astrocytomas and normal brain tissue: class II and IV are hypoexpressed in glioblastomas. *BMC Cancer 8*, 243.
55. Kim, J.H., Shin, J.H., and Kim, I.H. (2004) Susceptibility and radiosensitization of human glioblastoma cells to trichostatin A, a histone deacetylase inhibitor. *Int J Radiat Oncol Biol Phys* 59, 1174–1180.
56. Kim, M.S., Blake, M., Baek, J.H., Kohlhagen, G., Pommier, Y., and Carrier, F. (2003) Inhibition of histone deacetylase increases cytotoxicity to anticancer drugs targeting DNA. *Cancer Res* 63, 7291–7300.
57. Egler, V., Korur, S., Failly, M., Boulay, J.L., Imber, R., Lino, M.M., and Merlo, A. (2008) Histone deacetylase inhibition and blockade of the glycolytic pathway synergistically induce glioblastoma cell death. *Clin Cancer Res* 14, 3132–3140.
58. Lu, J., Getz, G., Miska, E.A., Alvarez-Saavedra, E., Lamb, J., Peck, D., Sweet-Cordero, A., Ebert, B. L., Mak, R. H., Ferrando, A. A., Downing, J. R., Jacks, T., Horvitz, H. R., and Golub, T. R. (2005) MicroRNA expression profiles classify human cancers. *Nature* 435, 834–838.
59. Ciafre, S.A., Galardi, S., Mangiola, A., Ferracin, M., Liu, C.G., Sabatino, G., Negrini, M., Maira, G., Croce, C.M., and Farace, M.G. (2005) Extensive modulation of a set of microRNAs in primary glioblastoma. *Biochem Biophys Res Commun* 334, 1351–1358.
60. Gabriely, G., Wurdinger, T., Kesari, S., Esau, C.C., Burchard, J., Linsley, P.S., and Krichevsky, A.M. (2008) MicroRNA 21 promotes glioma invasion by targeting matrix metalloproteinase regulators. *Mol Cell Biol* 28, 5369–5380.
61. Papagiannakopoulos, T., Shapiro, A., and Kosik, K.S. (2008) MicroRNA-21 targets a network of key tumor-suppressive pathways in glioblastoma cells. *Cancer Res* 68, 8164–8172.
62. Kim, H., Huang, W., Jiang, X., Pennicooke, B., Park, P.J., and Johnson, M.D. (2010) Integrative genome analysis reveals an oncomir/oncogene cluster regulating glioblastoma survivorship. *Proc Natl Acad Sci USA* 107, 2183–2188.
63. Silber, J., Lim, D.A., Petritsch, C., Persson, A.I., Maunakea, A.K., Yu, M., Vandenberg, S.R., Ginzinger, D.G., James, C.D., Costello, J.F., Bergers, G., Weiss, W.A., Alvarez-Buylla, A., and Hodgson, J.G. (2008) miR-124 and miR-137 inhibit proliferation of glioblastoma multiforme cells and induce differentiation of brain tumor stem cells. *BMC Med* 6, 14.
64. Visvanathan, J., Lee, S., Lee, B., Lee, J.W., and Lee, S.K. (2007) The microRNA miR-124 antagonizes the anti-neural REST/SCP1 pathway during embryonic CNS development. *Genes Dev* 21, 744–749.
65. Godlewski, J., Nowicki, M.O., Bronisz, A., Williams, S., Otsuki, A., Nuovo, G., Raychaudhury, A., Newton, H.B., Chiocca, E. A., and Lawler, S. (2008) Targeting of the Bmi-1 oncogene/stem cell renewal factor by microRNA-128 inhibits glioma proliferation and self-renewal. *Cancer Res* 68, 9125–9130.
66. Godlewski, J., Nowicki, M.O., Bronisz, A., Nuovo, G., Palatini, J., De Lay, M., Van Brocklyn, J., Ostrowski, M.C., Chiocca, E.A., and Lawler, S.E. (2010) MicroRNA-451 regulates LKB1/AMPK signaling and allows adaptation to metabolic stress in glioma cells. *Mol Cell* 37, 620–632.
67. Dubuc, A.M., Northcott, P.A., Mack, S., Witt, H., Pfister, S., et al. (2010) The genetics of pediatric brain tumors. *Curr Neurol Neurosci Rep* 10, 215–223.
68. MacDonald, T. (2008) Aggressive Infantile embryonal tumours. *J Child Neurol* 23, 1195–1204.
69. Pfaffe, E., Remke, M., Sturm, D., Benner, A., Witt, H. et al. (2010) TP53 Mutation is Frequently Associated with CTNNB1 Mutation or MYCN Amplification and is Compatible with Long-Term Survival in Medulloblastoma. *J Clin Oncol* 28, 5188–5196.
70. Massimino, M., Giangaspero, F., Garrè, M.L., Gandola, L., Poggi, G., Biassoni, V., Gatta, G., Rukowski, S. (2010) Childhood medulloblastoma. *Crit Rev Oncol Hematol* 79, 65–83.
71. Thompson, M.C., Fuller, C., Hogg, T.L., Dalton, J., Finkelstein, D., et al.(2006) Genomics Identifies Medulloblastoma Subgroups That Are Enriched for Specific Genetic Alterations. *J Clin Oncol* 24, 1924–1931.
72. Kool, M., Koster, J., Bunt, J., Hasselt, N.E., Lakeman, A., et al.(2008) Integrated Genomics Identifies Five Medulloblastoma Subtypes with Distinct Genetic Profiles,

Pathway Signatures and Clinicopathological Features. *PLoS One* 3, e3088.

73. Northcott, P.A., Korshunov, A., Witt, H., Hielscher, T., Eberhart, C.G., et al. (2010) Medulloblastoma Comprises Four Distinct Molecular Variants, *J Clin Oncol 29*, 1408–1414.
74. Pfister, S.M., Korshunov, A., Kool, M., Hasselbatt, M., Eberhart, C.G., et al. (2010) Molecular diagnostics of CNS embryonal tumours. *Acta Neuropathol* 120, 553–566.
75. Low, J.A. and de Sauvage, F. (2010) Clinical Experience with Hedgehog Pathway Inhibitors, *J Clin Oncol* 28, 5321–5326.
76. Flatau, E., Bogenmann, E., and Jones, P.A. (1983) Variable 5-methylcytosine levels in Human Tumours Cell Lines and Fresh Pediatric Explants. *Cancer Res* 43, 4901–4905.
77. Smiraglia, D.J., Fruhwald, M., Costello, J.F., McCormick, S.P., Dai, Z. et al. (1999) A New Tool for the Rapid Cloning of Amplified and Hypermethylated Human DNA Sequences from Restriction Landmark Genome Scanning Gels. *Genomics* 58, 254–262.
78. Fruwald, M.C., O'Dorisio, D.M., Dai, Z., Rush, L.J., Krahe, R., et al. (2001) Aberrant Hypermethylation of the Major Breakpoint ClusterRegionin17p11.2inMedulloblastomas but not Supratentorial PNETs. *Genes Chromosomes Cancer* 30, 38–47.
79. Fruwald, M.C., O'Dorisio, D.M., Dai, Z., Tanner, S.M., Balster, D.A. et al.(2001) Aberrant promoter methylation of previously unidentified target genes is a common abnormality in medulloblastoma - Implications for tumour biology and potential clinical utility. *Oncogene* 20, 5033–5042.
80. Zuzak, T.J., Steinhoff, D.F., Sutton, L.N., Phillips, P.C., Eggert, A. et al. (2002) Loss of caspase-8 mRNA expression is common in childhood primitive neuroectodermal brain tumour/medulloblastoma. *Eur J Cancer* 38, 83–91.
81. Harada, K., Toyooka, S., Maitra, A., Maruyama, R., Toyooka, K.O., et al. (2002) Aberrant promoter methylation and silencing of RASSF1A gene in pediatric tumor and cell lines. *Oncogene* 21, 4345–4349.
82. Rood, B.R., Zhang, H., Weitman, D.M. and Cogen, P.H. (2002) Hypermethylation of HIC1 and 17p allelic loss in medulloblastoma. *Cancer Res* 62, 3794–3797.
83. Lusher, M.E., Lindsey, J., Latif, F., Pearson, A.D., Ellison, D.W. et al. (2002) Biallelic epigenetic inactivation of the RASSF1A tumour suppressor gene in medulloblastoma development. *Cancer Res* 62, 5906–5911.
84. Pfister, S., Schlaeger, C., Mendrzyk, F., Wittmann, A., Benner, A. et al. (2007) Array-based profiling of reference-independent methylation status (aPRIMES) identifies frequent promoter methylation and consecutive downregulation of ZIC2 in pediatric medulloblastoma. *Nucleic Acids Res* 35, e51.
85. Ecke, I., Petry, F., Rosenberger, A., Tauber, S., Monkemeyer, S. et al. (2009) Antitumour effect of combined 5-aza-cytidine and valproic acid treatment on rhabdomyosarcoma and medulloblastoma in pth mutant mice. *Cancer Res* 69, 887–895.
86. Suzuki, H., Gabrielson, E., Chen, W., Anbazhagan, R., van Engeland, M., et al. (2002) A genomic screen for genes upregulated by demethylation and histone deacetylase inhibition in human colorectal cancer. *Nature Genetics* 31, 141–149.
87. Lindsey, J.C., Lusher, M., Anderton, J.A., Gilbertson, R.J., Ellison, D.W. et al. (2007) Epigenetic deregulation of multiple S100 family gene family members by differential hypomethylation and hypermethylation events in medulloblastoma. *Br J Cancer* 97, 267–274.
88. Anderton, J.A., Lindsey, J., Lusher, M.E., Gilberston, R.J., Bailey, S. et al. (2008) Global analysis of the medulloblastoma epigenome identifies disease-subgroup-specific inactivation of COL1A2. *Neuro Oncol* 10, 981–994.
89. Kongkham, P.N., Northcott, P., Ra, Y.S., Nakahara, Y., Mainprize, T.G. et al. (2008) An epigenetic genome-wide screen identifies SPINT2 a novel tumour suppressor gene in pediatric medulloblastoma. *Cancer Res* 68, 9945–9953.
90. Cecchi, F., Rabe, D.C., and Bottaro, D. (2010) Targeting the HGF/MET signalling pathway in cancer. *Eur J Cancer* 46, 1260–1270.
91. Diede, S.J., Guenthoer, J., Geng, L.N., Mahoney, S.E. and Marotta, M. et al. (2010) DNA methylation of developmental genes in pediatric medulloblastoma identified by denaturation analysis of methylation differences. *Proc Natl Acad Sci* 107, 234–239.
92. Pierson, J., Hostager, B., Fan, R. and Vibhakar, R. (2008) Regulation of cyclin dependent kinase 6 by microRNA 124 in medulloblastoma. *J Neurooncol* 90, 1–7.
93. Ferretti, E., De Smaele, E., Miele, E., Laneve, P., Po, A. et al. (2008) Concerted microRNA control of Hedgehog signalling in cerebellar neuronal progenitor and tumour cells. *EMBO Journal* 27, 2616–2627.
94. Ferretti, E., De Smaele, E., Po, A., Di Marcotullio, L., Tosi, E. et al. (2009)

MicroRNA profiling in human medulloblastoma. *Int J Cancer* 124, 568–577.

95. Northcott, P.A., Fernandez, L.A., Hagan, J.P., Ellison, D.W., Grajkowska, W. et al. (2009) The miR-17/92 Polycistron is Up-Regulated in Sonic Hedgehog Driven Medulloblastoma and Induced by N-Myc in Sonic Hedgehog-Treated Cerebellar Neural Precursors. *Cancer Res* 69, 3249–3255.
96. Uziel, T., Karginov, F.V., Xie, S., Parker, J.S., Wang, Y.D. et al. (2009) The mir17-92 cluster collaborates with Sonic Hedgehog pathway in Medulloblastoma. *PNAS* 106, 2812–2817.
97. Cho, J.Y., Tsherniak, A., Tamayo, P., Santagata, S., Ligon, A. et al. (2010) Integrative Genomic Analysis of Medulloblastoma Identifies a Molecular Subgroup That Drives Poor Clinical Outcome. *J Clin Oncol* 29, 1424–1430.
98. Northcott, P.A., Nakahara, Y., Wu, X., Feuk, F., Ellison, D.W. et al. (2009) Multiple recurrent genetic events converge on control of histone lysine methylation in medulloblastoma. *Nature Genetics* 41, 465-472.
99. Teider, N., Scott, D., Neiss, A., Weeraratne, D., Amani, V.M. et al. (2010) Neuralized1 causes apoptosis and downregulates Notch target genes in medulloblastoma. *Neuro Oncol* 12, 1244–1256.
100. Canettieri, G., Di Marcotullio, M.L., Greco, A., Coni, S., Antonucci, L. et al. (2010) Histone deacetylase and Cullin3-REN(KCTD11) ubiquitin ligase interplay regulates Hedgehog signalling through Gli1 acetylation. *Nat Cell Biol* 12, 132–142.
101. Kilday, J.P., Ruman, R., Dyer, S., Ridley, L., Lowe, J., Coyle, B., and Grundy, R. (2009) Paediatric Ependymoma: Biological Perspectives. *Mol Cancer Res* 7, 27–31.
102. Korshunov, A., Witt, H., Hielscher, T., Benner, A., Remke, M., et al. (2010) Molecular staging of intracranial ependymoma in children and adults. *J Clin Oncol.* 28, 3182–3190.
103. Mack, S.C. and Taylor, M.D. (2009) The genetic and epigenetic basis of ependymoma. *Childs Nerv Syst* 25, 1195–1201.
104. Johnson, R.A., Wright, K., Poppleton, H., Mohankumar, K.M., Finkelstein, D. et al. (2010) Cross-species genomics matches driver mutations and cell compartments to model ependymoma. *Nature* 466, 632–636.
105. Hamilton, D.W., Lusher, M.E., Lindsey, J.C., Ellison, D.W., and Clifford, S.C. (2005) Epigenetic inactivation of the RASSF1A tumour suppressor gene in ependymoma. *Cancer letters* 227, 75–81.
106. von Haken, M.S., White, E.C., Daneshvar-Shyesther, L., Sih, S., Choi, E., et al. (1996) Molecular genetic analysis of chromo- some arm17p and chromosome arm22qDNAsequences in sporadic pediatric ependymomas, *Genes Chromosomes Cancer* 17, 37–44.
107. Waha, A., Koch, A., Hartmann, W., Mack, H., Schramm, J., et al. (2004) Analysis of HIC-1 methylation and transcription in human ependymomas. *Int J Cancer* 110, 542–549.
108. Modena, P., Lualdi, E., Facchinetti, F., Veltman, J., Reid, J.F., et al. (2006) Identification of tumor-specific molecular signatures in intracranial ependymoma and association with clinical characteristics. *J Clin Oncol* 24, 5223–5233.
109. Rousseau, E., Ruchoux, M.M., Scaravilli, F., Chapon, S.F., Vinchon, M. et al. (2003) CDKN2A, CDKN2B and p14ARF are frequently and differentially methylated in ependymal tumours. *Neuropathology and Applied Neurobiology* 14, 574–583.
110. Koos, B., Peetz-Dienhart, S., Riesmeier, B, Fruhwald, M.C., and Hasselblatt, M. (2010) O(6)-methylguanine-DNA methyltransferase (MGMT) promoter methylation is significantly less frequent in ependymal tumours as compared to malignant astrocytic gliomas. *Neuropathology and Applied Neurobiology* 36, 356–358.
111. Alonso, M.E., Bello, M.J., Gonzalez-Gomez, P., Arjona, D., de Campos, J.M., et al. (2004) Aberrant CpG island methylation of multiple genes in ependymal tumors. *J Neuro-oncol* 67, 159–165.
112. Sardi, I., Cetica, V., Massimino, M., Buccoliero, A.M., Giunti, L., et al. (2009) Promoter methylation and expression analysis of MGMT in advanced pediatric brain tumors. *Oncol Rep* 22, 773-779.
113. Xie, H., Wang, M., Bonaldo, M., Veena, R., Stellpflug, W., et al. (2010) Epigenomic analysis of Alu repeats in human ependymomas, *PNAS* 107, 6952-6957.

Chapter 9

DNA Methylation Changes in Cervical Cancers

Qiang Lu, Dehua Ma, and Shuping Zhao

Abstract

Cervical carcinoma is one of the major causes of death in women worldwide. It is difficult to foresee a dramatic increase in cure rate even with the most optimal combination of cytotoxic drugs, surgery, and radiation; therefore, testing of molecular targeted therapies against this malignancy is highly desirable. Cervical cancer is a multistep process with accumulation of genetic and epigenetic alterations in regulatory genes, leading to activation of oncogenes and inactivation or loss of tumor suppressor genes (TSGs). In the last decade, in addition to genetic alterations, epigenetic inactivation of TSGs by promoter hypermethylation has been recognized as an important and alternative mechanism in tumorigenesis. In cervical cancer, epigenetic alterations can affect the expression of papillomavirus as well as host genes in relation to stages representing the multistep process of carcinogenesis. Here we discuss these epigenetic alterations in cervical cancer focusing on DNA methylation.

Key words: Cervical cancer, DNA methylation, Histone modifications, Human papillomaviruses, Cervical intraepithelial neoplasia

1. Introduction

Cervical cancer is the second most common malignant neoplasm in women, in terms of both incidence and mortality rates worldwide (1). It takes the lives of more than 250,000 women each year globally, particularly in underresourced areas of low-, middle-, and high-income countries (2). The majority of cervical carcinomas are squamous cell carcinomas (SCCs), whereas adenocarcinomas (AC) account for the remaining 15–20% of cases. Presently, the principal treatment for cervical cancer is the radical hysterectomy. Patients with advanced stages are mainly treated with combined radiotherapy and chemotherapy or radiotherapy alone (3). However, the survival rate has not improved with current treatment for patients

Ramona G. Dumitrescu and Mukesh Verma (eds.), *Cancer Epigenetics: Methods and Protocols*, Methods in Molecular Biology, vol. 863, DOI 10.1007/978-1-61779-612-8_9, © Springer Science+Business Media, LLC 2012

with recurrent or distant metastatic cervical cancer (4). Furthermore, if cancer cells are resistant to radiation and chemotherapy, the therapeutic efficacy is limited (5). Therefore, it is necessary for the development of more effective and novel treatment. The diagnosis and treatment of this disease can have a profound impact on the quality of patients' lives.

Aberrant DNA methylation has been shown to play important roles during multistage carcinogenesis in various human organs. Overall DNA hypomethylation and regional DNA hypermethylation are commonly observed in human cancers of various organs (6–8). Furthermore, accumulating evidence suggests that aberrant DNA methylation is involved even in the early and precancerous stages of human carcinogenesis (9, 10). Precancerous conditions showing aberrant DNA methylation may rapidly progress and generate more malignant cancers (11, 12). Recent studies on cervical carcinoma have also demonstrated that epigenetic changes may play a role in the development of cervical cancer (13–16), which indicates that DNA methylation may be useful as a marker for early detection or predicting the risk of cancer precursors.

2. Methylation Changes of HPV

Human papillomavirus (HPV) is a member of the Papovaviridae family of virus. They consist of a 72-capsomere capsid containing the viral genome. Each capsomere is composed of two viral proteins: L1 and L2. The HPV genome consists of approximately 8,000 base pairs in length and is a double-stranded DNA molecule. All of the proteins are encoded in one of the two strands of the viral DNA and so are all read in the same direction. Due to the overlapping nature of the open reading frames (ORFs) that encode these proteins, alternative splicing is necessary for the gene expression. The genome can be divided into three regions: the long control region (LCR) without coding potential, the region of early proteins (E1–E8), and the region of late proteins (L1 and L2).

HPV classification is predicted on DNA sequence homology. At least 200 types of HPV have been identified, and these have been classified into 16 groups (17). Genital HPVs are classified according to their potential to induce malignant transformation as follows: high-risk types (16, 18, 31, 33, 35, 39, 45, 51, 52, 56, 58, 59, 68, 73, and 82), probable high-risk types (26, 53, and 66), and low-risk types (6, 11, 40, 42, 43, 44, 54, 61, 70, 72, 81, and CP6108) (18). Epidemiological and laboratory data suggest that the presence of specific HPV subtypes and the integration of their HPV DNA into the genome are important factors in the development of cervical neoplasia. Among high-risk strains, HPV 16 and 18 are those most closely associated with cervical carcinoma and are found in >50% and 20% of SCCs, respectively (19).

Infection with oncogenic HPV has been demonstrated to be the most significant risk factor in the etiology of cervical cancer (19–21) and its precursor lesion, cervical intraepithelial neoplasia (22–24). The carcinogenic role of HPV lies mainly on the E6 and E7 oncoproteins which initiate dysregulation of cellular proliferation and apoptotic mechanisms at well-defined targets. The primary targets are p53 and retinoblastoma (Rb) tumor suppressor proteins, respectively. The life cycle of HPV is dependent on cellular replication machinery and the differentiation of squamous epithelium. The association of the HPV genome and the cellular DNA replication machinery is mediated by El viral protein. Expression of E6 and E7 genes, which are highly related to the progression of cervical neoplasia, is controlled by the upstream LCR where the promoter and enhancers driving viral transcription are located. The role of E6 protein is to switch off apoptotic defense activated by genomic instability arising in consequence of E7-induced cell cycle activation. The early papillomaviral protein E2 mediates a negative feedback on E6/E7 expression through the E2 binding elements of the LCR. During HPV DNA integration, the viral genome usually breaks in the E1/E2 region. The break generally leads to loss of the E1 and E2 regions. Loss of E2 function results in overexpression of E6/E7. Overexpression of E6/E7, meanwhile, has been observed to lead to malignant transformation of host cells and to tumor formation (25). HPV viral integration into host genome DNA is associated with progression from polyclonal to monoclonal status in cervical intraepithelial neoplasia (CIN), and these events play a fundamental role in the progression from low- to high-grade cervical neoplasia (26).

Although HPV infection is necessary for the development of cervical cancer, its presence alone is insufficient to cause cervical cancer. The molecular mechanism responsible for the inefficiency of HPV-initiated cervical carcinogenesis remains elusive (27). Genetic changes with resultant genomic instability have long been recognized as an important mechanism for cervical carcinogenesis (13, 28). Reports of DNA methylation in cervical cancer and precancerous lesions support a role for this phenomenon in cervical cancer development (15, 16, 29).

The role of DNA hypermethylation in HPV genome has of late been the subject of study. Kalantari et al. have studied LI and LCR regions by bisulfite modification in 115 clinical samples. They found high heterogeneity in methylation status in different patients' samples and even in different samples of the same patient. The methylation frequency of L1 was 30% and lower in other positions, particularly at a C_pG site located in the linker between two nucleosomes positioned over HPV-16 enhancer and promoter. However, methylation at most sites was higher in carcinomas than in dysplasia, and maybe it is related to the tandem repetition and chromosomal integration that occurs in invasive lesions (30). Turan et al. performed a study to assess the status of the HPV-18 genome, and they found that HPV-18 L1 was mostly unmethylated in asymptomatic infections and infections with precancerous lesions. In contrast, L1 sequences were strongly methylated in all cervical carcinomas (31). Sushma et al. performed a study in two HPV-18 cervical cancer cell lines, Hela and C4-1, and clinical samples. They found that there was also clonal heterogeneity in the methylation status of the different regions analyzed. There was complete or partial methylation, respectively, of the HPV enhancer in three of the six cancers and lack of methylation in the eight samples from asymptomatic patients. The promoter sequences were methylated in three of the six cancers and four of the six smears (32). HPV DNA methylation patterns appear to influence viral transcription in vitro. Highly methylated regions of the HPV viral upstream regulatory region lead to inactive transcription in vitro, which can decrease viral proliferation.

DNA methylation status has an important effect on diagnosing, treating, and evaluating the prognosis of cervical cancers. It will be of major interest to analyze HPV oncogene expression in cervical tumors before and after treatment of patients with DNA methylation.

3. DNA Hypermethylation

Many studies described the importance of DNA methylation in human cancers and focused on regions of the genome that might have functional significance resulting from the extinction of gene activity. DNA methylation is a frequent epigenetic event in many human cancers (33, 34). Several studies have indicated that methylation is essential for normal development (35), long-term silencing of certain genes, such as inactivated X chromosome and imprinted genes (36).

Aberrant DNA methylation may play roles in carcinogenesis as a result of (a) increased gene mutagenicity due to deamination of 5-methylcytosine to thymine; (b) possible association of aberrant DNA methylation with genetic instability; and (c) silencing of tumor-related genes through DNA methylation on CpG islands in cooperation with histone modification. During carcinogenesis, tumor suppressor genes (TSGs) are inactivated by genetic changes including gene mutations, deletions, and genomic rearrangements. However, in many human cancers, these genes are also frequently silenced by epigenetic alterations (37, 38).

Cervical cancer is the second most commonly diagnosed cancer and the third leading cause of cancer death in women worldwide (39). In addition to HPV infection, the well-known critical event in the malignant transformation and immortalization of cervical epithelial cells, other factors, such as inactivation of tumor suppressors, are involved in the multistage pathogenesis of cervical cancer (40). There are numerous reports demonstrating that abnormal promoter hypermethylation leads to silencing or diminished expression of TSGs in cervical carcinoma.

3.1. Apoptosis-Related Genes

During the pathogenesis of cancers, apoptosis-related genes play an important role. It has been established that the suppression of apoptosis contributes to carcinogenesis and carcinoma progression and promoting resistance to immune-based cytotoxicity (41). It is evident that alterations in the apoptotic pathways are intimately involved in a variety of disease processes, including cancer (41–43). So the identification of abnormal points in the apoptotic pathway would potentially bring in new therapeutic opportunities where conventional cancer treatments fail. Studies analyzing apoptosis-related genes that can be inactivated by methylation in cervical cancer are limited.

3.1.1. DAPK

Death-associated protein kinase (*DAPK*) was first identified by Kimchi in 1995. *DAPK* gene is located in 9q34.1. *DAPK* is an actin-associated, calcium/calmodulin-dependent enzyme with serine/threonine kinase activity (44, 45). *DAPK* suppresses tumor growth and metastasis by increasing the occurrence of apoptosis in vivo and therefore has been characterized as a TSG (46). *DAPK* is a proapoptotic gene and participates in various apoptotic systems. *DAPK* acts as a tumor suppressor, and its inactivation by promoter hypermethylation has been frequently observed in various human cancers. A large number of studies have consistently demonstrated the hypermethylated state of this gene in cervical cancer. Therefore, it may serve as a marker for detection of this malignancy. Moreover, *DAPK* promoter methylation is more prominent in SCC than in AC of the uterine cervix (14, 47–52).

3.1.2. P53

P53 is the first TSG linked to apoptosis. As a transcription factor, *p53* can detect DNA damage and subsequently arrest cells in the G1 phase of the cell cycle and allow for DNA repairing. The *p53* pathway response to stresses can disrupt the fidelity of cell division and DNA replication. It has become evident that the mutation of *p53* can disrupt the apoptosis pathway in the majority of human tumors (53, 54). However, the *p53* pathway can be aberrantly methylated in some of their components. *P73*, a member of the *p53* family, represents a critical alternative mechanism for inactivation of *TAP73* gene via CpG island hypermethylation in cervical cancer. *TAP73* is also involved in cellular response to DNA damage induced by radiation and chemotherapeutic agents. When *TAP73* is overexpressed in cells, it can trigger *p53*-independent apoptosis by activating transcription of *p53*-responsive genes, such as *p21*, *Mdm2*, *Bax*, and *GADD45*, and inhibits cell growth in a *p53*-like manner by inducing apoptosis (55, 56).

3.1.3. hTERT

Activation of telomerase, the enzyme that synthesizes the telomere ends of linear chromosomes, has been implicated in human cell immortalization and cancer cell pathogenesis (57). The expression pattern of human telomerase reverse transcriptase (*hTERT*), the telomerase catalytic subunit, is correlated with telomerase activity. The promoter region of the *hTERT* gene is located in a CpG island and therefore may be regulated by DNA methylation (57). Studies on *hTERT* expression in cervical cancer have revealed that 0–33% of normal cervices exhibited *hTERT* mRNA expression, whereas 80–100% of cervical cancers showed *hTERT* expression (58–61). Despite it is expected that hypermethylation decreases gene expression, a study showed a correlation between reduced expression and catalytic subunit activity with demethylation (62). This may explain what was found with regard to better prognosis of patients with cervical cancer whose tumors lack *hTERT* methylation. *hTERT* methylation may be of prognostic significance in ovarian and cervical cancers (63).

3.1.4. DCR

TNF-related apoptosis-inducing ligand (*TRAIL*) is a natural potent anticancer agent that preferentially induces apoptosis in cancer cells and is not toxic to normal cells (64). *TRAIL* is known to bind to four different receptors, two proapoptotic (*DR4* and *DR5*), and two potentially anti-apoptotic receptors lacking death domains (*DcR1* and *DcR2*). Decoy receptors *DcR1* and *DcR2* are the members of the tumor necrosis factor receptor superfamily which may act as oncogenes because of their postulated anti-apoptotic effects (65, 66). *DcR1* and *DcR2* can be the target for abnormal methylation that leads to their silencing. One study confirmed that aberrant methylation of *DcR1* or *DcR2* was present in 100% of cervical cancer, suggesting that cervical cancer cells, by downregulating decoy receptor expression, obtain a growth advantage (67).

3.2. Cell Cycle-Related Genes

It is well established that normal cell cycle progression needs the cell's ability to translate extracellular signals such as those produced by growth factor receptor stimulation and the extracellular matrices to efficiently replicate DNA and divide. The regulation of the cell cycle requires a number of players, including cyclin-dependent kinases and their binding partners along with natural inhibitory molecules such as *p16*, *Rb*, and *p15* (40, 68).

3.2.1. P16

Located on chromosome 9p21, *p16* was first reported as a novel tumor suppress gene in 1994, acting as a negative regulator of the cell cycle (69). Mutation in *p16* leads to loss and confusion of the regulation of cell division, induces abnormal multiplication of the cells, and causes tumor formation (70). *P16* specifically compete with *cyclin D1* control *CDK4*, inhibiting the kinase activity of both, so that cells cannot be fast through the G1/S transition. *P16* gene has been one of the most widely studied in cervical cancer (71, 72).

Loss of expression of *p16* gene, often associated with aberrant methylation, is a frequent alteration in many types of human neoplasia (73, 74). The alteration in *p16* methylation is the earliest step of cervical cancer. The TSG $p16^{INK4A}$ is overexpressed in almost all high-risk HPV cervical cancer and precancerous lesions specimens (75). Another study was performed to evaluate the pattern of aberrant methylation during the multistage pathogenesis of cervical cancers. It was found that p16 methylation rate was over 20%, and there was no association of aberrant methylation with other risk factors including papillomavirus infection, smoking history, or hormone use (71).

3.3. Cell Signaling Pathway Genes

3.3.1. RASSF1A

The *RAS* association domain family 1 (*RASSF1*) gene has two main variants (*RASSF1A* and *RASSF1C*), which are transcribed from distinct promoters. Aberrant promoter hypermethylation and subsequent decrease in expression is a frequently detected epigenetic alteration in several malignancies including cervical cancer. *RASSF1A* protein is actively involved in microtubule regulation, genomic stability maintenance, cell cycle regulation, apoptosis modulation, cell motility, and invasion control and may act as a negative *Ras* effector inhibiting cell growth and inducing cell death (76–84). Studies in patients with cervical cancer have demonstrated its silencing by methylation in up to 30% of tumors (85–88). *RASSF1A* promoter hypermethylation was found in HPV-negative but not in HPV-positive cervical cancer cell lines (86). In agreement with the findings in the cell lines, the primary cervical tumors harboring HPV has a low frequency in *RASSF1A* promoter hypermethylation. This low frequency can be refined by the histological type; it is more frequent in AC than in SCC (85, 89, 90). These studies suggest that HPV and *RASSF1A* may be involved in the same tumorigenic pathway.

3.3.2. APC

The TSG adenomatous polyposis coli (*APC*) located on human chromosome 5p21–22 acts as an antagonist of the Wnt signaling pathway, leading to proteolytic degradation of β-catenin. The Wnt signaling pathway is known to play key roles during development and in maintaining homeostasis in many adult tissues. Its aberrant activation is associated with cancers in many tissues such as breast, colon, pancreas, skin, and liver (91–95). In the absence of Wnt stimulation, β-catenin enters the nucleus and associates with LEF/TCF transcription factors, leading to the transcription of Wnt target genes such as *cyclin D1*, *Myc*, and *TCF-1*. It has been established that mutational or epigenetic inactivation of *APC* contributes to uncontrolled proliferation in many tumor types (96, 97). *APC* can be inactivated by promoter hypermethylation in cervical, ovarian, and endometrial cancers (98). And further studies revealed that APC promoter hypermethylation is frequent in adenocarcinoma and seems incidental in SCC of cervical cancers (47, 48, 52).

3.3.3. PTEN

PTEN, a protein tyrosine phosphatase with homology to tensin, is a tumor suppressor gene located on chromosome 10q23 (99). Alterations of this gene have been identified in many cancers (100). As a tumor suppressor gene, *PTEN* plays a significant role in inhibiting phosphatidylinositol 3-kinase (*PI3K*) pathway and its downstream functions, including activation of Akt/protein kinase B, cell survival, and cell proliferation through anchorage of the cell cycle that, in some cases, is accompanied by apoptosis (101, 102). In the absence of *PTEN* gene, the increased PI3-kinase signaling may promote uncoordinated G1 cell cycle progression, allowing cells to bypass the normal signaling processes regulated by growth factors and the cell cycle checkpoints, thereby leading to tumorigenesis (103). Reduced or lost expression of *PTEN* has been reported in many tumors, such as breast cancer (104), lung cancer, glioblastoma, melanoma, prostate cancer, etc. (105). Hypermethylation of *PTEN* seems to be a late event in cervical carcinogenesis, as low-grade SIL and high-grade SIL lesions have unmethylated *PTEN* gene (106). But patients with recurrent or fatal cervical cancer had significantly higher percentage of methylation at this locus than those without evidence of recurrence (107). Thus, *PTEN* appears to have prognostic significance and may serve as predictor of disease-free survival.

3.4. DNA Repair

Alkylating agents alkylate guanine bases can lead to DNA mutations and apoptosis induction unless repaired. The major pathway of repair involves the transfer of the alkyl group from the DNA to a cysteine acceptor site in the protein *O*(6)-alkylguanine-DNA alkyltransferase (*AGT*) (108). *AGT*, also known as *O*(6)-methylguanine-DNA methyltransferase (*MGMT*), is the DNA repair protein responsible for removing alkylation adducts from the *O*(6)-position of guanine in DNA (109). This could speculate that lack of *MGMT* enzymatic activity may result in multiple mutations and promotes carcinogenesis. However, lack of its expression produces opposite effects for development and progression. Tumors acquire a mutator phenotype characterized by generation of transition point mutations in key genes such as *p53* and *K-ras*, but reduced *MGMT* activity renders tumors more sensitive to the killing by alkylating drugs because the activity of *MGMT* protein can be responsible for chemoresistance against alkylating chemotherapeutic agents (110). Low expression of *MGMT* may be related to the abnormal methylation of promoter (111). *MGMT* silencing might be a mechanism of tumorigenesis (112). *MGMT* expression is tumor type specific. Its expression is low in brain and malignant melanomas and high in ovarian and breast tumors (113–115). There is scarce information about the role of *MGMT* gene in cervical cancer. A number of studies have analyzed the frequency of *MGMT* promoter hypermethylation, which varies from 5 to 81% (14, 71, 88, 116). It should be noted that promoter methylation of other DNA repair genes such as *hMLH1* and *FANC* are also rare events in cervical carcinogenesis (50, 88, 106, 117, 118).

3.5. Additional Genes with Different Functions

3.5.1. CDH1

E-cadherin is one of the major constituents of cell adhesion complexes in epithelial cells (119, 120). It is a 97-kDa transmembrane glycoprotein encoded by the *E-cadherin* gene (*CDH1*) located on chromosome 16q22.1. It plays important roles in the establishment of adherent-type junctions by mediating calcium-dependent cellular interactions and is thought to be a tumor suppressor. Partial or total loss of *E-cadherin* expression occurs in the majority of human carcinomas including cervical cancer (121). Besides its role in physical cell-cell adhesions, *E-cadherin* is also thought to be involved in intracellular signaling in normal epithelial cells since downregulation of this molecule in epithelial cells is frequently associated with tumor formation and differentiation (122). Aberrant hypermethylation of CpG islands in *CDH1* promoter regions is associated with suppressed transcriptional activity, and it is frequently found in invasive cervical cancer, particularly in SCC histologic type (14, 48, 49). The CDH1 can be detected in serum samples of invasive cervical cancer patients, and promoter hypermethylation can indicate an increased risk for relapse (123, 124).

3.5.2. FHIT

The fragile histidine triad gene (*FHIT*) is a putative tumor suppressor and belongs to the histidine triad superfamily of nucleotide-binding proteins. It is located at the fragile site locus *FRA3B* on chromosome 3p14.2, a region of the genome which shows LOH in a variety of cancers. The abnormality in structure and function of the suppressor gene is obviously associated with the pathogenesis of some tumors, such as esophageal, head and neck, lung, gastric, breast, cervical carcinomas, and precancerous and cancerous lesions (125–131). In cervical cancer, *FHIT* promoter hypermethylation correlates inversely with *FHIT* gene expression and has been detected in up to 75% of cervical carcinomas (132–134). These findings support that *FHIT* promoter hypermethylation has a significant oncogenic effect in cervical carcinogenesis. Further study suggesting that hypermethylation of this gene has been associated with loss of expression and advanced stages of cervical carcinoma, suggesting its participation in disease progression (132).

3.5.3. RAR-β2

Retinoic acid receptor beta (*RAR-β2*) binds retinoic acid, the biologically active form of vitamin A, which mediates cellular signaling in embryonic morphogenesis, cell growth, and differentiation. *RAR-β2* limits growth of many cell types by regulating its target gene expression. Reduction or lack of *RAR-β2* gene expression has been detected in various malignancies (135). Loss of its expression due to promoter hypermethylation was first detected in colon and breast cancers. In cervical cancer, the *RAR-β2* gene is of particular interest because retinoic acid inhibits transformation of human keratinocytes by HPV-16 and leads to regression of moderate cervical dysplasia (136, 137). CpG methylation of the 5′ region of *RAR-β2* gene contributes to gene silencing also in cervical carcinogenesis. Frequency of *RAR-β2* methylation progressively increases from 11% in low grade to 29% in high-grade lesions and from 33% to 63% in invasive cancers (14, 15, 116, 138), suggesting that this abnormality is an early event in multistage cervical carcinogenesis.

3.5.4. HIC1

HIC1 is a zinc finger transcription factor that is transcriptionally silenced by promoter methylation in several types of human cancer (139–141). Homozygous disruption of *HIC1* impairs development and results in embryonic and perinatal lethality in mice, while heterozygous mice develop many different spontaneous malignant tumors including a predominance of epithelial cancers in males and lymphomas and sarcomas in females suggesting that this gene acts as a TSG. The complete loss of *HIC1* function in heterozygous mice appears to involve dense methylation of the remaining wild-type allele promoter (142). It has been found that the *HIC1* gene is downregulated in many cervical cancer cell lines and re-expressed upon treatment with a demethylating drug (15). In primary cervical tumors, its methylation rate varies between 18 and 45% (14, 47). It has recently been shown that its loss of function accentuates the tumorigenic effect of loss of *p53* (143). These results suggest that the tumor suppressor role of *HIC1* and its inactivation by promoter methylation in cervical cancer may be a critical epigenetic change in tumor development.

3.5.5. TSLC1

The tumor suppressor gene in lung cancer-1 (*TSLC1*) located on the chromosomal region 11q23.2 is abrogated or markedly reduced in a number of human cancer tissues and cell lines, including lung, prostate, breast, cervical, esophageal, and pancreatic cancers (16, 144–148). The *IGSF4/TSLC1* gene codes for an immunoglobulin-like intercellular adhesion molecule which mediates homophilic or heterophilic interactions in a calcium-independent pathway. It was first identified as a TSG in lung cancer, and silencing can derive from loss of heterozygosity or promoter hypermethylation (149). It was demonstrated also in cervical cancer that its silencing can be a result of LOH due to promoter hypermethylation. It has been shown that normal epithelium and CIN I lesions are free of methylation at *IGSF4*, whereas methylation rate in CIN III is 35%, which increases to 58 and 65% in invasive tumors (106, 150). These data demonstrate that *IGSF4* may play an important role in cervical cancer development.

3.5.6. SYK

The spleen tyrosine kinase (*Syk*) gene was originally cloned from porcine cDNA by Japanese scholars Taniguchi et al. (151). It encodes a kind of nonreceptor tyrosine kinase. *Syk* is one of the two members of the *Syk* family (*Syk* and *ZAP-70*), which is widely expressed in multiple cell types (152–156). The *Syk* protein contains 629-amino acid residues and is comprised of a kinase domain and two SH2 domains: SH2 (N) and SH2 (C), in tandem (157). Loss of *Syk* expression has been reported with malignant phenotypes such as increased motility and invasion (158). Emerging evidence indicates that wild-type *Syk* suppresses cell growth, and it may thus act as a tumor suppressor (159, 160). In cervical cancer, *Syk* mRNA expression decreases and is frequently lost throughout the progression of cervical carcinoma. Hypermethylation in the *Syk* promoter correlates with loss of *Syk* mRNA expression in human cervical carcinoma and is likely the mechanism underlying this loss. These data suggest that epigenetic inactivation of *Syk* may contribute to the development or/and progression of cervical carcinoma (161).

4. DNA Hypomethylation

In human cancers, global DNA hypomethylation leads to genomic instability; affects repeated DNA sequences, tissue-specific genes, and proto-oncogenes; or causes loss of imprinting with a biallelic expression, just as in case of *H19* and *IGF2* (162). Further, the level of DNA hypomethylation increases with tumor progression (163, 164). The main mechanisms set forward in attempting to explain cancer causation by hypomethylation are chromosome instability and reactivation of transposable elements and/or inappropriate gene activation. Global genomic and gene-specific epigenetic changes were found in cervical cancer. The first evidence for global DNA hypomethylation in cervical neoplastic tissues was provided by [3H)-*S*-adenosylmethionine incorporation assay (164). As expected, the extent of 3H-methyl group incorporation was increased threefold and sevenfold in the DNA from cervical dysplasia and cancer as compared to DNA from normal cervices, and the degree of DNA hypomethylation increases with the grade of cervical neoplasia (164). These findings were confirmed using a computer-assisted assay based on quantitative analysis of DNA methylation in individual interphase nuclei by immunolabelling with anti-5-methylcytosine antibodies. Progressive hypomethylation was observed in dysplastic and cancer cells as compared to normal controls (165). These data, along with observations of gene promoter hypermethylation of a number of genes during preinvasive to invasive stages of cervical cancer, suggest that both phenomena are coincident during carcinogenesis of the cervical cancer.

5. Histone Modification

Histone modifications are strongly associated with formation of nucleosome structure and are closely linked to CpG island methylation by interacting with methyl-CpG-binding proteins (MBDs) and DNA methyltransferases (DNMTs). Modifications include methylation, acetylation, and phosphorylation at specific positions of the histone tails (166). While histone methylation causes either activation or repression of gene transcription, histone hypoacetylation mediated by histone deacetylases leads mostly to unwinding of DNA, accessibility for transcriptional factors, and subsequent repression of gene transcription (167, 168). During the tumorigenic process, cancer cells lose the histone H4 isoforms monoacetylated and trimethylated predominantly at Lys16 and Lys20 residues, respectively. This event is associated with hypomethylation of DNA repetitive sequences, a hallmark of cancer cells (169). In cervical cancer, phosphorylated and acetylated forms of histone H3 in cytologic smears show a marked association of histone H3 modifications with progression of the disease from CIN I to CIN II and CIN III (170).

6. Future Perspectives

In developed countries, cytologic screening has contributed to a reduction in cervical cancer incidence and mortality (171–173). Although individual cytologic screens are insensitive, repeated testing beginning at an early age permits detection of precursors such as cervical intraepithelial neoplasia III (CIN III) prior to invasion. This process is inefficient and costly. However, it has prompted efforts to develop highly sensitive screening approaches that can be performed at more widely spaced intervals (174). Current cervical screening strategies, particularly those combined with HPV test, have very good negative predictive values, i.e., an oncogenic process can be excluded with great certainty. However, the positive predictive values are moderate since only some women with diagnostic findings of oncologic significance will develop invasive cervical cancer if left untreated. Thus, novel screening alternatives are needed for improving the prediction of oncogenic progression, reducing the ratio of surgical excisions with no oncogenic significance in histology, and determining the stages of cervical carcinogenesis. It has been realized that genetic and epigenetic alterations are present at the earliest steps of the malignant progression of cervix uteri. This led to testing the presence of these abnormalities, such as *p16* expression alteration (175, 176), for earlier diagnosis. A large number of studies looking at the methylation states of TSGs have uncovered that some genes are hypermethylated in preinvasive lesions. Thus, developing a panel of methylation markers may therefore have value in early detection of cancer precursors, increase in safety reassurances for women who are candidates for less frequent screens, and prediction of outcomes of women infected with carcinogenic HPV infections (177).

In the therapeutics, transcriptional therapy is very promising in cancer treatment and is being extensively evaluated. Although ample experimental evidence supports the development of drugs that target the epigenome via inhibition of DNA methylation or histone modification as cancer therapy, clinical results are pending to date. Unlike genetic changes, the aberrant DNA methylation and histone modifications of neoplastic cells are reversible, suggesting strategies to revert these epigenetic alterations via pharmacological manipulation. Consequently, some of the most promising epigenome-modifying agents which are two main classes of epigenetic drugs, methylation inhibitors and *HDAC* inhibitors, are currently in clinical trials for the treatment of cancer. However, it is too early to evaluate their efficacy.

7. Conclusion

Epigenetic changes have been reported in many cancers and are now recognized to be at least as common as genetic changes. Aberrant methylation of cytosine located within the dinucleotide CpG is by far the best-categorized epigenetic change. The cancer cell genome shows global hypomethylation as well as regional promoter hypermethylation of several TSGs. In cervical cancer, a number of epigenetic alterations occurring during all stages of cervical carcinogenesis in both HPV and host cellular genomes have been identified. These include global DNA hypomethylation, hypermethylation of key TSGs, and histone modifications. Moreover, epigenetic abnormalities occur very early in the carcinogenic process, and they can potentially serve as molecular markers for early detection. Thus, identification of a set of genes hypermethylated in cytologic smears could offer novel means for clinical screening. Assessment of hypermethylated genes in primary tumor or in serum DNA may serve as a prognostic factor or as a means of predicting response to radiation, chemotherapy, and transcriptional agents. Therefore, the reversible nature of epigenetic changes constitutes an attractive target for transcriptional therapies. DNA methylation and histone deacetylase inhibitors can reactivate expression of TSGs and induce histone hyperacetylation in the tumors of patients with cervical cancer. But further investigations and clinical trials are needed to prove and integrate epigenetic pathway-modulating agents.

References

1. Singh, M., Tyagi, S., Bhui, K., Prasad, S., and Shukla, Y. (2010) Regulation of cell growth through cell cycle arrest and apoptosis in HPV 16 positive human cervical cancer cells by tea polyphenols. *Invest New Drugs* 28, 216–224.
2. Cain, J.M., Ngan, H., Garland, S., and Wright, T. (2009) Control of cervical cancer: women's options and rights. *Int J Gynaecol Obstet* 106, 141–143
3. Moore, D.H. (2006) Cervical cancer. *Obstet Gynecol* 107, 1152–1161.

4. Petignat, P. and Roy, M. (2007) Diagnosis and management of cervical cancer. *BMJ* 335, 765–768.
5. Cadron, I., Van Gorp, T., Amant, F., Leunen, K., Neven, P., and Vergote, I. (2007) Chemotherapy for recurrent cervical cancer. *Gynecol Oncol* 107, S113–S118.
6. Baylin, S.B., and Ohm, J.E. (2006) Epigenetic gene silencing in cancer - a mechanism for early oncogenic pathway addiction? *Nat Rev Cancer* 6, 107–116.
7. Egger, G., Liang, G., Aparicio, A., and Jones, P.A. (2004) Epigenetics in human disease and prospects for epigenetic therapy. *Nature* 429, 457–463.
8. Jones, P.A. and Baylin, S.B. (2002) The fundamental role of epigenetic events in cancer. *Nat Rev Genet* 3, 415–428.
9. Eguchi, K., Kanai, Y., Kobayashi, K., and Hirohashi, S. (1997) DNA hypermethylation at the D17S5 locus in non-small cell lung cancers: its association with smoking history. *Cancer Res* 57, 4913–4915.
10. Kanai, Y., Ushijima, S., Ochiai, A., Eguchi, K., Hui, A., and Hirohashi, S. (1998) DNA hypermethylation at the D17S5 locus is associated with gastric carcinogenesis. *Cancer Lett* 122, 135–141.
11. Arai, E., Kanai, Y., Ushijima, S., Fujimoto, H., Mukai, K., and Hirohashi, S. (2006) Regional DNA hypermethylation and DNA methyltransferase (DNMT) 1 protein overexpression in both renal tumors and corresponding nontumorous renal tissues. *Int J Cancer* 119, 288–296.
12. Kanai, Y., Ushijima, S., Tsuda, H., Sakamoto, M., Sugimura, T., and Hirohashi, S. (1996) Aberrant DNA methylation on chromosome 16 is an early event in hepatocarcinogenesis. *Jpn J Cancer Res* 87, 1210–1217.
13. Sova, P., Feng, Q., Geiss, G., Wood, T., Strauss, R., Rudolf, V., Lieber, A., and Kiviat, N. (2006) Discovery of novel methylation biomarkers in cervical carcinoma by global demethylation and microarray analysis. *Cancer Epidemiol Biomarkers Prev* 15, 114–123
14. Narayan, G., Arias-Pulido, H., Koul, S., Vargas, H., Zhang, F.F., Villella, J., Schneider, A., Terry, M.B., Mansukhani, M., and Murty, V.V. (2003) Frequent promoter methylation of CDH1, DAPK, RARB, and HIC1 genes in carcinoma of cervix uteri: its relationship to clinical outcome. *Mol Cancer* 2, 24.
15. Feng, Q., Balasubramanian, A., Hawes, S.E., Toure, P., Sow, P.S., Dem, A., Dembele, B., Critchlow, C.W., Xi, L., Lu, H., et al. (2005a) Detection of hypermethylated genes in women with and without cervical neoplasia. *J Natl Cancer Inst* 97, 273–282.
16. Steenbergen, R.D., Kramer, D., Braakhuis, B.J., Stern, P.L., Verheijen, R.H., Meijer, C.J., and Snijders, P.J. (2004) TSLC1 gene silencing in cervical cancer cell lines and cervical neoplasia. J Natl Cancer Inst *96*, 294–305.
17. zur Hausen, H. (1999) Papillomaviruses in human cancers. *Proc Assoc Am Physicians* 111, 581–587
18. Munoz, N., Bosch, F.X., de Sanjose, S., Herrero, R., Castellsague, X., Shah, K.V., Snijders, P.J., and Meijer, C.J. (2003) Epidemiologic classification of human papillomavirus types associated with cervical cancer. *N Engl J Med* 348, 518–527.
19. Walboomers, J.M., Jacobs, M.V., Manos, M.M., Bosch, F.X., Kummer, J.A., Shah, K.V., Snijders, P.J., Peto, J., Meijer, C.J., and Munoz, N. (1999) Human papillomavirus is a necessary cause of invasive cervical cancer worldwide. *J Pathol* 189, 12–19.
20. Bosch, F.X., Manos, M.M., Munoz, N., Sherman, M., Jansen, A.M., Peto, J., Schiffman, M.H., Moreno, V., Kurman, R., and Shah, K.V. (1995). Prevalence of human papillomavirus in cervical cancer: a worldwide perspective. International biological study on cervical cancer (IBSCC) Study Group. *J Natl Cancer Inst* 87, 796–802.
21. Franco, E.L. (1996). Epidemiology of anogenital warts and cancer. *Obstet Gynecol Clin North Am* 23, 597–623.
22. Ho, G.Y., Burk, R.D., Klein, S., Kadish, A.S., Chang, C.J., Palan, P., Basu, J., Tachezy, R., Lewis, R., and Romney, S. (1995) Persistent genital human papillomavirus infection as a risk factor for persistent cervical dysplasia. *J Natl Cancer Inst* 87, 1365–1371.
23. Ho, G.Y., Bierman, R., Beardsley, L., Chang, C.J., and Burk, R.D. (1998). Natural history of cervicovaginal papillomavirus infection in young women. *N Engl J Med* 338, 423–428.
24. Ho, G.Y., Palan, P.R., Basu, J., Romney, S.L., Kadish, A.S., Mikhail, M., Wassertheil-Smoller, S., Runowicz, C., and Burk, R.D. (1998) Viral characteristics of human papillomavirus infection and antioxidant levels as risk factors for cervical dysplasia. *Int J Cancer* 78, 594–599.
25. Doorbar, J., Ely, S., Sterling, J., McLean, C., and Crawford, L. (1991) Specific interaction between HPV-16 E1-E4 and cytokeratins results in collapse of the epithelial cell intermediate filament network. *Nature* 352, 824–827.
26. Ueda, Y., Enomoto, T., Miyatake, T., Ozaki, K., Yoshizaki, T., Kanao, H., Ueno, Y., Nakashima, R., Shroyer, K.R., and Murata, Y. (2003) Monoclonal expansion with integration

of high-risk type human papillomaviruses is an initial step for cervical carcinogenesis: association of clonal status and human papillomavirus infection with clinical outcome in cervical intraepithelial neoplasia. *Lab Invest* 83, 1517–1527.

27. Harris, C.P., Lu, X.Y., Narayan, G., Singh, B., Murty, V.V., and Rao, P.H. (2003). Comprehensive molecular cytogenetic characterization of cervical cancer cell lines. *Genes Chromosomes Cancer* 36, 233–241.
28. Atkin, N.B. and Baker, M.C. (1997) DNA ploidy of cervical intraepithelial neoplasia (CIN). *Cancer Genet Cytogenet* 94, 151–152.
29. Lai, H.C., Lin, Y.W., Huang, T.H., Yan, P., Huang, R.L., Wang, H.C., Liu, J., Chan, M.W., Chu, T.Y., Sun, C.A., et al. (2008) Identification of novel DNA methylation markers in cervical cancer. *Int J Cancer* 123, 161–167.
30. Kalantari, M., Calleja-Macias, I.E., Tewari, D., Hagmar, B., Lie, K., Barrera-Saldana, H.A., Wiley, D.J., and Bernard, H.U. (2004) Conserved methylation patterns of human papillomavirus type 16 DNA in asymptomatic infection and cervical neoplasia. *J Virol* 78, 12762–12772.
31. Turan, T., Kalantari, M., Calleja-Macias, I.E., Cubie, H.A., Cuschieri, K., Villa, L.L., Skomedal, H., Barrera-Saldana, H.A., and Bernard, H.U. (2006) Methylation of the human papillomavirus-18L1 gene: a biomarker of neoplastic progression? *Virology* 349, 175–183.
32. Badal, S., Badal, V., Calleja-Macias, I.E., Kalantari, M., Chuang, L.S., Li, B.F., and Bernard, H.U. (2004) The human papillomavirus-18 genome is efficiently targeted by cellular DNA methylation. *Virology* 324, 483–492.
33. Baylin, S.B., Herman, J.G., Graff, J.R., Vertino, P.M., and Issa, J.P. (1998) Alterations in DNA methylation: a fundamental aspect of neoplasia. *Adv Cancer Res* 72, 141–196.
34. Costello, J.F., Fruhwald, M.C., Smiraglia, D.J., Rush, L.J., Robertson, G.P., Gao, X., Wright, F.A., Feramisco, J.D., Peltomaki, P., Lang, J.C., et al. (2000) Aberrant CpG-island methylation has non-random and tumour-type-specific patterns. *Nat Genet* 24, 132–138.
35. Li, E., Bestor, T.H. and Jaenisch, R. (1992). Targeted mutation of the DNA methyltransferase gene results in embryonic lethality. *Cell* 69, 915–926.
36. Bird, A.P. and Wolffe, A.P. (1999) Methylation-induced repression—belts, braces, and chromatin. *Cell* 99, 451–454.
37. Baylin, S.B. (2002) Mechanisms underlying epigenetically mediated gene silencing in cancer. Semin *Cancer Biol* 12, 331–337.
38. Feinberg, A.P. and Tycko, B. (2004) The history of cancer epigenetics. *Nat Rev Cancer* 4, 143–153.
39. Underwood, S.M., Ramsay-Johnson, E., Dean, A., Russ, J., and Ivalis, R. (2009) Expanding the scope of nursing research in low resource and middle resource countries, regions, and states focused on cervical cancer prevention, early detection, and control. *J Natl Black Nurses Assoc* 20, 42–54.
40. Duenas-Gonzalez, A., Lizano, M., Candelaria, M., Cetina, L., Arce, C., and Cervera, E. (2005) Epigenetics of cervical cancer. An overview and therapeutic perspectives. *Mol Cancer* 4, 38.
41. Thompson, C.B. (1995) Apoptosis in the pathogenesis and treatment of disease. *Science* 267, 1456–1462.
42. Wyllie, A.H., Kerr, J.F., and Currie, A.R. (1980) Cell death: the significance of apoptosis. *Int Rev Cytol* 68, 251–306.
43. Sen, S. and D'Incalci, M. (1992). Apoptosis. Biochemical events and relevance to cancer chemotherapy. *FEBS Lett* 307, 122–127.
44. Deiss, L.P., Feinstein, E., Berissi, H., Cohen, O., and Kimchi, A. (1995) Identification of a novel serine/threonine kinase and a novel 15-kD protein as potential mediators of the gamma interferon-induced cell death. *Genes Dev* 9, 15–30.
45. Cohen, O., Feinstein, E., and Kimchi, A. (1997) DAP-kinase is a Ca2+/calmodulin-dependent, cytoskeletal-associated protein kinase, with cell death-inducing functions that depend on its catalytic activity. *EMBO J* 16, 998–1008.
46. Inbal, B., Cohen, O., Polak-Charcon, S., Kopolovic, J., Vadai, E., Eisenbach, L., and Kimchi, A. (1997) DAP kinase links the control of apoptosis to metastasis. *Nature* 390, 180–184.
47. Dong, S.M., Kim, H.S., Rha, S.H., and Sidransky, D. (2001) Promoter hypermethylation of multiple genes in carcinoma of the uterine cervix. *Clin Cancer Res* 7, 1982–1986.
48. Kang, S., Kim, J.W., Kang, G.H., Lee, S., Park, N.H., Song, Y.S., Park, S.Y., Kang, S.B., and Lee, H.P. (2006) Comparison of DNA hypermethylation patterns in different types of uterine cancer: cervical squamous cell carcinoma, cervical adenocarcinoma and endometrial adenocarcinoma. *Int J Cancer* 118, 2168–2171.

49. Shivapurkar, N., Sherman, M.E., Stastny, V., Echebiri, C., Rader, J.S., Nayar, R., Bonfiglio, T.A., Gazdar, A.F., and Wang, S.S. (2007) Evaluation of candidate methylation markers to detect cervical neoplasia. *Gynecol Oncol* 107, 549–553.
50. Wisman, G.B., Nijhuis, E.R., Hoque, M.O., Reesink-Peters, N., Koning, A.J., Volders, H.H., Buikema, H.J., Boezen, H.M., Hollema, H., Schuuring, E., et al. (2006) Assessment of gene promoter hypermethylation for detection of cervical neoplasia. *Int J Cancer* 119, 1908–1914.
51. Yang, H.J., Liu, V.W., Wang, Y., Chan, K.Y., Tsang, P.C., Khoo, U.S., Cheung, A.N., and Ngan, H.Y. (2004) Detection of hypermethylated genes in tumor and plasma of cervical cancer patients. *Gynecol Oncol* 93, 435–440.
52. Henken, F.E., Wilting, S.M., Overmeer, R.M., van Rietschoten, J.G., Nygren, A.O., Errami, A., Schouten, J.P., Meijer, C.J., Snijders, P.J., and Steenbergen, R.D. (2007) Sequential gene promoter methylation during HPV-induced cervical carcinogenesis. *Br J Cancer* 97, 1457–1464.
53. Vousden, K.H. (2000). p53: death star. *Cell* 103, 691–694.
54. Harris, S.L. and Levine, A.J. (2005) The p53 pathway: positive and negative feedback loops. *Oncogene* 24, 2899–2908.
55. Yang, A., Kaghad, M., Wang, Y., Gillett, E., Fleming, M.D., Dotsch, V., Andrews, N.C., Caput, D., and McKeon, F. (1998) p63, a p53 homolog at 3q27-29, encodes multiple products with transactivating, death-inducing, and dominant-negative activities. *Mol Cell* 2, 305–316.
56. Zhu, J., Jiang, J., Zhou, W., and Chen, X. (1998) The potential tumor suppressor p73 differentially regulates cellular p53 target genes. *Cancer Res* 58, 5061–5065.
57. Widschwendter, A., Muller, H.M., Hubalek, M.M., Wiedemair, A., Fiegl, H., Goebel, G., Mueller-Holzner, E., Marth, C., and Widschwendter, M. (2004) Methylation status and expression of human telomerase reverse transcriptase in ovarian and cervical cancer. *Gynecol Oncol* 93, 407–416.
58. Snijders, P.J., van Duin, M., Walboomers, J.M., Steenbergen, R.D., Risse, E.K., Helmerhorst, T.J., Verheijen, R.H., and Meijer, C.J. (1998) Telomerase activity exclusively in cervical carcinomas and a subset of cervical intraepithelial neoplasia grade III lesions: strong association with elevated messenger RNA levels of its catalytic subunit and high-risk human papillomavirus DNA. *Cancer Res* 58, 3812–3818.
59. Nakano, K., Watney, E., and McDougall, J.K. (1998) Telomerase activity and expression of telomerase RNA component and telomerase catalytic subunit gene in cervical cancer. *Am J Pathol* 153, 857–864.
60. Takakura, M., Kyo, S., Kanaya, T., Tanaka, M., and Inoue, M. (1998) Expression of human telomerase subunits and correlation with telomerase activity in cervical cancer. *Cancer Res* 58, 1558–1561.
61. Wisman, G.B., Knol, A.J., Helder, M.N., Krans, M., de Vries, E.G., Hollema, H., de Jong, S., and van der Zee, A.G. (2001) Telomerase in relation to clinicopathologic prognostic factors and survival in cervical cancer. *Int J Cancer* 91, 658–664.
62. Guilleret, I. and Benhattar, J. (2003) Demethylation of the human telomerase catalytic subunit (hTERT) gene promoter reduced hTERT expression and telomerase activity and shortened telomeres. *Exp Cell Res* 289, 326–334.
63. Widschwendter, A., Muller, H.M., Hubalek, M.M., Wiedemair, A., Fiegl, H., Goebel, G., Mueller-Holzner, E., Marth, C., and Widschwendter, M. (2004) Methylation status and expression of human telomerase reverse transcriptase in ovarian and cervical cancer. *Gynecol Oncol* 93, 407–416.
64. Szliszka, E. and Krol, W. (2011) The role of dietary polyphenols in tumor necrosis factor-related apoptosis inducing ligand (TRAIL)-induced apoptosis for cancer chemoprevention. *Eur J Cancer Prev* 20, 63–69.
65. Ashkenazi, A. and Dixit, V.M. (1999) Apoptosis control by death and decoy receptors. *Curr Opin Cell Biol* 11, 255–260.
66. Ozoren, N. and El-Deiry, W.S. (2003) Cell surface Death Receptor signaling in normal and cancer cells. *Semin Cancer Biol* 13, 135–147.
67. Shivapurkar, N., Toyooka, S., Toyooka, K.O., Reddy, J., Miyajima, K., Suzuki, M., Shigematsu, H., Takahashi, T., Parikh, G., Pass, H.I., et al. (2004) Aberrant methylation of trail decoy receptor genes is frequent in multiple tumor types. *Int J Cancer* 109, 786–792.
68. Nakashima, R., Fujita, M., Enomoto, T., Haba, T., Yoshino, K., Wada, H., Kurachi, H., Sasaki, M., Wakasa, K., Inoue, M., et al. (1999) Alteration of p16 and p15 genes in human uterine tumours. *Br J Cancer* 80, 458–467.
69. Bressac-de Paillerets, B. (1994) [Discovery of a new gene frequently inactivated in human cancers: protein p16, a cell cycle regulator]. *Bull Cancer* 81, 853–856.

70. Nuovo, G.J., Plaia, T.W., Belinsky, S.A., Baylin, S.B., and Herman, J.G. (1999) In situ detection of the hypermethylation-induced inactivation of the p16 gene as an early event in oncogenesis. *Proc Natl Acad Sci U S A* 96, 12754–12759.
71. Virmani, A.K., Muller, C., Rathi, A., Zoechbauer-Mueller, S., Mathis, M., and Gazdar, A.F. (2001).Aberrant methylation during cervical carcinogenesis. *Clin Cancer Res* 7, 584–589.
72. Lea, J.S., Coleman, R., Kurien, A., Schorge, J.O., Miller, D.S., Minna, J.D., and Muller, C.Y. (2004) Aberrant p16 methylation is a biomarker for tobacco exposure in cervical squamous cell carcinogenesis. *Am J Obstet Gynecol* 190, 674–679.
73. Merlo, A., Herman, J.G., Mao, L., Lee, D.J., Gabrielson, E., Burger, P.C., Baylin, S.B., and Sidransky, D. (1995) 5 CpG island methylation is associated with transcriptional silencing of the tumour suppressor p16/CDKN2/MTS1 in human cancers. *Nat Med* 1, 686–692.
74. Otterson, G.A., Khleif, S.N., Chen, W., Coxon, A.B., and Kaye, F.J. (1995) CDKN2 gene silencing in lung cancer by DNA hypermethylation and kinetics of p16INK4 protein induction by 5-aza 2 deoxycytidine. *Oncogene* 11, 1211–1216.
75. Ishikawa, M., Fujii, T., Saito, M., Nindl, I., Ono, A., Kubushiro, K., Tsukazaki, K., Mukai, M., and Nozawa, S. (2006) Overexpression of p16 INK4a as an indicator for human papillomavirus oncogenic activity in cervical squamous neoplasia. *Int J Gynecol Cancer* 16, 347–353.
76. Donninger, H., Vos, M.D., and Clark, G.J. (2007) The RASSF1A tumor suppressor. *J Cell Sci* 120, 3163–3172.
77. Liu, L., Tommasi, S., Lee, D.H., Dammann, R., and Pfeifer, G.P. (2003) Control of microtubule stability by the RASSF1A tumor suppressor. *Oncogene* 22, 8125–8136.
78. Vos, M.D., Martinez, A., Elam, C., Dallol, A., Taylor, B.J., Latif, F., and Clark, G.J. (2004) A role for the RASSF1A tumor suppressor in the regulation of tubulin polymerization and genomic stability. *Cancer Res* 64, 4244–4250.
79. Shivakumar, L., Minna, J., Sakamaki, T., Pestell, R., and White, M.A. (2002) The RASSF1A tumor suppressor blocks cell cycle progression and inhibits cyclin D1 accumulation. *Mol Cell Biol* 22, 4309–4318.
80. Whang, Y.M., Kim, Y.H., Kim, J.S., and Yoo, Y.D. (2005) RASSF1A suppresses the c-Jun-NH2-kinase pathway and inhibits cell cycle progression. *Cancer Res* 65, 3682–3690.
81. Vos, M.D., Ellis, C.A., Bell, A., Birrer, M.J., and Clark, G.J. (2000) Ras uses the novel tumor suppressor RASSF1 as an effector to mediate apoptosis. *J Biol Chem* 275, 35669–35672.
82. Vos, M.D., Dallol, A., Eckfeld, K., Allen, N.P., Donninger, H., Hesson, L.B., Calvisi, D., Latif, F., and Clark, G.J. (2006) The RASSF1A tumor suppressor activates Bax via MOAP-1. *J Biol Chem* 281, 4557–4563.
83. Matallanas, D., Romano, D., Yee, K., Meissl, K., Kucerova, L., Piazzolla, D., Baccarini, M., Vass, J.K., Kolch, W., and O'Neill, E. (2007) RASSF1A elicits apoptosis through an MST2 pathway directing proapoptotic transcription by the p73 tumor suppressor protein. *Mol Cell* 27, 962–975.
84. Dallol, A., Agathanggelou, A., Tommasi, S., Pfeifer, G.P., Maher, E.R., and Latif, F. (2005) Involvement of the RASSF1A tumor suppressor gene in controlling cell migration. *Cancer Res* 65, 7653–7659.
85. Cohen, Y., Singer, G., Lavie, O., Dong, S.M., Beller, U., and Sidransky, D. (2003) The RASSF1A tumor suppressor gene is commonly inactivated in adenocarcinoma of the uterine cervix. *Clin Cancer Res* 9, 2981–2984.
86. Kuzmin, I., Liu, L., Dammann, R., Geil, L., Stanbridge, E.J., Wilczynski, S.P., Lerman, M.I., and Pfeifer, G.P. (2003) Inactivation of RAS association domain family 1A gene in cervical carcinomas and the role of human papillomavirus infection. *Cancer Res* 63, 1888–1893.
87. Yu, M.Y., Tong, J.H., Chan, P.K., Lee, T.L., Chan, M.W., Chan, A.W., Lo, K.W., and To, K.F. (2003) Hypermethylation of the tumor suppressor gene RASSFIA and frequent concomitant loss of heterozygosity at 3p21 in cervical cancers. *Int J Cancer* 105, 204–209.
88. Kang, S., Kim, J.W., Kang, G.H., Park, N.H., Song, Y.S., Kang, S.B., and Lee, H.P. (2005) Polymorphism in folate- and methionine-metabolizing enzyme and aberrant CpG island hypermethylation in uterine cervical cancer. *Gynecol Oncol* 96, 173–180.
89. Kang, S., Kim, H.S., Seo, S.S., Park, S.Y., Sidransky, D., and Dong, S.M. (2007) Inverse correlation between RASSF1A hypermethylation, KRAS and BRAF mutations in cervical adenocarcinoma. *Gynecol Oncol* 105, 662–666.
90. Lai, H.C., Lin, Y.W., Chang, C.C., Wang, H.C., Chu, T.W., Yu, M.H., and Chu, T.Y. (2007) Hypermethylation of two consecutive

tumor suppressor genes, BLU and RASSF1A, located at 3p21.3 in cervical neoplasias. *Gynecol Oncol* 104, 629–635.

91. Matsuda, Y., Schlange, T., Oakeley, E.J., Boulay, A., and Hynes, N.E. (2009) WNT signaling enhances breast cancer cell motility and blockade of the WNT pathway by sFRP1 suppresses MDA-MB-231 xenograft growth. *Breast Cancer Res* 11, R32.
92. Deng, Y.H., Pu, X.X., Huang, M.J., Xiao, J., Zhou, J.M., Lin, T.Y., and Lin, E.H. (2010) 5-Fluorouracil upregulates the activity of Wnt signaling pathway in CD133-positive colon cancer stem-like cells. *Chin J Cancer* 29, 810–815.
93. Hamada, F. (2009). [Wnt signaling and cancer]. *Kaibogaku Zasshi* 84, 111–112.
94. Takigawa, Y. and Brown, A.M. (2008) Wnt signaling in liver cancer. *Curr Drug Targets* 9, 1013–1024.
95. Katoh, M. (2005). WNT/PCP signaling pathway and human cancer (review). *Oncol Rep* 14, 1583–1588.
96. Samowitz, W.S., Slattery, M.L., Sweeney, C., Herrick, J., Wolff, R.K., and Albertsen, H. (2007) APC mutations and other genetic and epigenetic changes in colon cancer. *Mol Cancer Res* 5, 165–170.
97. Sarrio, D., Moreno-Bueno, G., Hardisson, D., Sanchez-Estevez, C., Guo, M., Herman, J.G., Gamallo, C., Esteller, M., and Palacios, J. (2003) Epigenetic and genetic alterations of APC and CDH1 genes in lobular breast cancer: relationships with abnormal E-cadherin and catenin expression and microsatellite instability. *Int J Cancer* 106, 208–215.
98. Yang, H.J., Liu, V.W., Wang, Y., Tsang, P.C., and Ngan, H.Y. (2006) Differential DNA methylation profiles in gynecological cancers and correlation with clinico-pathological data. *BMC Cancer* 6, 212.
99. Lynch, E.D., Ostermeyer, E.A., Lee, M.K., Arena, J.F., Ji, H., Dann, J., Swisshelm, K., Suchard, D., MacLeod, P.M., Kvinnsland, S., et al. (1997) Inherited mutations in PTEN that are associated with breast cancer, Cowden disease, and juvenile polyposis. *Am J Hum Genet* 61, 1254–1260.
100. Li, L. and Ross, A.H. (2007). Why is PTEN an important tumor suppressor? *J Cell Biochem* 102, 1368–1374.
101. Ramaswamy, S., Nakamura, N., Vazquez, F., Batt, D.B., Perera, S., Roberts, T.M., and Sellers, W.R. (1999) Regulation of G1 progression by the PTEN tumor suppressor protein is linked to inhibition of the phosphatidylinositol 3-kinase/Akt pathway. *Proc Natl Acad Sci U S A* 96, 2110–2115.
102. Tamura, M., Gu, J., Takino, T., and Yamada, K.M. (1999). Tumor suppressor PTEN inhibition of cell invasion, migration, and growth: differential involvement of focal adhesion kinase and p130Cas. *Cancer Res* 59, 442–449.
103. Li, D.M. and Sun, H. (1998) PTEN/MMAC1/TEP1 suppresses the tumorigenicity and induces G1 cell cycle arrest in human glioblastoma cells. *Proc Natl Acad Sci U S A* 95, 15406–15411.
104. Rhei, E., Kang, L., Bogomolniy, F., Federici, M.G., Borgen, P.I., and Boyd, J. (1997). Mutation analysis of the putative tumor suppressor gene PTEN/MMAC1 in primary breast carcinomas. *Cancer Res* 57, 3657–3659.
105. Teng, D.H., Hu, R., Lin, H., Davis, T., Iliev, D., Frye, C., Swedlund, B., Hansen, K.L., Vinson, V.L., Gumpper, K.L., et al. (1997) MMAC1/PTEN mutations in primary tumor specimens and tumor cell lines. *Cancer Res* 57, 5221–5225.
106. Gustafson, K.S., Furth, E.E., Heitjan, D.F., Fansler, Z.B., and Clark, D.P. (2004) DNA methylation profiling of cervical squamous intraepithelial lesions using liquid-based cytology specimens: an approach that utilizes receiver-operating characteristic analysis. *Cancer* 102, 259–268.
107. Cheung, T.H., Lo, K.W., Yim, S.F., Chan, L.K., Heung, M.S., Chan, C.S., Cheung, A.Y., Chung, T.K., and Wong, Y.F. (2004) Epigenetic and genetic alternation of PTEN in cervical neoplasm. *Gynecol Oncol* 93, 621–627.
108. Pegg, A.E. and Byers, T.L. (1992) Repair of DNA containing O6-alkylguanine. *FASEB J* 6, 2302–2310.
109. Jacinto, F.V. and Esteller, M. (2007) MGMT hypermethylation: a prognostic foe, a predictive friend. *DNA Repair (Amst)* 6, 1155–1160.
110. Esteller, M. and Herman, J.G. (2004) Generating mutations but providing chemosensitivity: the role of O6-methylguanine DNA methyltransferase in human cancer. *Oncogene* 23, 1–8.
111. Zochbauer-Muller, S., Fong, K.M., Virmani, A.K., Geradts, J., Gazdar, A.F., and Minna, J.D. (2001) Aberrant promoter methylation of multiple genes in non-small cell lung cancers. *Cancer Res* 61, 249–255.
112. Oh, K., Redston, M., and Odze, R.D. (2005) Support for hMLH1 and MGMT silencing as a mechanism of tumorigenesis in the hyperplastic-adenoma-carcinoma (serrated) carcinogenic

pathway in the colon. *Hum Pathol* 36, 101–111.

113. Preuss, I., Haas, S., Eichhorn, U., Eberhagen, I., Kaufmann, M., Beck, T., Eibl, R.H., Dall, P., Bauknecht, T., Hengstler, J., et al. (1996) Activity of the DNA repair protein O6-methylguanine-DNA methyltransferase in human tumor and corresponding normal tissue. *Cancer Detect Prev* 20, 130–136.
114. Hengstler, J.G., Tanner, B., Moller, L., Meinert, R., and Kaina, B. (1999) Activity of O(6)-methylguanine-DNA methyltransferase in relation to p53 status and therapeutic response in ovarian cancer. *Int J Cancer* 84, 388–395.
115. Margison, G.P., Povey, A.C., Kaina, B., and Santibanez Koref, M.F. (2003) Variability and regulation of O6-alkylguanine-DNA alkyltransferase. *Carcinogenesis* 24, 625–635.
116. Zambrano, P., Segura-Pacheco, B., Perez-Cardenas, E., Cetina, L., Revilla-Vazquez, A., Taja-Chayeb, L., Chavez-Blanco, A., Angeles, E., Cabrera, G., Sandoval, K., et al. (2005) A phase I study of hydralazine to demethylate and reactivate the expression of tumor suppressor genes. *BMC Cancer* 5, 44.
117. Narayan, G., Arias-Pulido, H., Nandula, S.V., Basso, K., Sugirtharaj, D.D., Vargas, H., Mansukhani, M., Villella, J., Meyer, L., Schneider, A., et al. (2004) Promoter hypermethylation of FANCF: disruption of Fanconi Anemia-BRCA pathway in cervical cancer. *Cancer Res* 64, 2994–2997.
118. Widschwendter, A., Gattringer, C., Ivarsson, L., Fiegl, H., Schneitter, A., Ramoni, A., Muller, H.M., Wiedemair, A., Jerabek, S., Muller-Holzner, E., et al. (2004) Analysis of aberrant DNA methylation and human papillomavirus DNA in cervicovaginal specimens to detect invasive cervical cancer and its precursors. *Clin Cancer Res* 10, 3396–3400.
119. Gumbiner, B.M. (2005) Regulation of cadherin-mediated adhesion in morphogenesis. *Nat Rev Mol Cell Biol* 6, 622–634.
120. Koriyama, C., Akiba, S., Itoh, T., Sueyoshi, K., Minakami, Y., Corvalan, A., Yonezawa, S., and Eizuru, Y. (2007) E-cadherin and beta-catenin expression in Epstein-Barr virus-associated gastric carcinoma and their prognostic significance. *World J Gastroenterol* 13, 3925–3931.
121. Branca, M., Giorgi, C., Ciotti, M., Santini, D., Di Bonito, L., Costa, S., Benedetto, A., Bonifacio, D., Di Bonito, P., Paba, P., et al. (2006) Down-regulation of E-cadherin is closely associated with progression of cervical intraepithelial neoplasia (CIN), but not with high-risk human papillomavirus (HPV) or disease outcome in cervical cancer. *Eur J Gynaecol Oncol* 27, 215–223.
122. Cavallaro, U. and Christofori, G. (2004) Cell adhesion and signalling by cadherins and Ig-CAMs in cancer. *Nat Rev Cancer* 4, 118–132.
123. Ren, C.C., Miao, X.H., Yang, B., Zhao, L., Sun, R., and Song, W.Q. (2006) Methylation status of the fragile histidine triad and E-cadherin genes in plasma of cervical cancer patients. *Int J Gynecol Cancer* 16, 1862–1867.
124. Widschwendter, A., Ivarsson, L., Blassnig, A., Muller, H.M., Fiegl, H., Wiedemair, A., Muller-Holzner, E., Goebel, G., Marth, C., and Widschwendter, M. (2004). CDH1 and CDH13 methylation in serum is an independent prognostic marker in cervical cancer patients. *Int J Cancer* 109, 163–166.
125. Hendricks, D.T., Taylor, R., Reed, M., and Birrer, M.J. (1997) FHIT gene expression in human ovarian, endometrial, and cervical cancer cell lines. *Cancer Res* 57, 2112–2115.
126. Birrer, M.J., Hendricks, D., Farley, J., Sundborg, M.J., Bonome, T., Walts, M.J., and Geradts, J. (1999) Abnormal Fhit expression in malignant and premalignant lesions of the cervix. *Cancer Res* 59, 5270–5274.
127. Tsao, I. and Atramentova, L.A. (2009) [Genetic and epigenetic changes of FHIT gene in patients with esophageal cancer]. *Tsitol Genet* 43, 40–44.
128. Pavelic, K., Krizanac, S., Cacev, T., Hadzija, M.P., Radosevic, S., Crnic, I., Levanat, S., and Kapitanovic, S. (2001) Aberration of FHIT gene is associated with increased tumor proliferation and decreased apoptosis-clinical evidence in lung and head and neck carcinomas. *Mol Med* 7, 442–453.
129. Wang, X., Yuan, L., Zheng, H., Liu, J., Huang, X., Wu, L., Yuan, H., and Zhao, J. (2009) [Expression of FHIT Protein in Lung Cancer by Cell Array.]. *Zhongguo Fei Ai Za Zhi* 12, 131–134.
130. Li, Y.Z. and Zhao, P. (2009). [Expressions of cyclinB1, FHIT and Ki-67 in 336 gastric carcinoma patients and their clinicopathologic significance]. *Zhonghua Yi Xue Za Zhi* 89, 2337–2341.
131. Syeed, N., Husain, S.A., Sameer, A.S., Chowdhri, N.A., and Siddiqi, M.A. (2011) Mutational and promoter hypermethylation status of FHIT gene in breast cancer patients of Kashmir. *Mutat Res* 707, 1–8.
132. Wu, Q., Shi, H., Suo, Z., and Nesland, J.M. (2003) 5′-CpG island methylation of the FHIT gene is associated with reduced protein

expression and higher clinical stage in cervical carcinomas. *Ultrastruct Pathol* 27, 417–422.

133. Wistuba, II, Montellano, F.D., Milchgrub, S., Virmani, A.K., Behrens, C., Chen, H., Ahmadian, M., Nowak, J.A., Muller, C., Minna, J.D., et al. (1997) Deletions of chromosome 3p are frequent and early events in the pathogenesis of uterine cervical carcinoma. *Cancer Res* 57, 3154–3158.
134. Larson, A.A., Kern, S., Curtiss, S., Gordon, R., Cavenee, W.K., and Hampton, G.M. (1997) High resolution analysis of chromosome 3p alterations in cervical carcinoma. *Cancer Res* 57, 4082–4090.
135. Widschwendter, M., Berger, J., Hermann, M., Muller, H.M., Amberger, A., Zeschnigk, M., Widschwendter, A., Abendstein, B., Zeimet, A.G., Daxenbichler, G., et al. (2000) Methylation and silencing of the retinoic acid receptor-beta2 gene in breast cancer. *J Natl Cancer Inst* 92, 826–832.
136. Khan, M.A., Jenkins, G.R., Tolleson, W.H., Creek, K.E., and Pirisi, L. (1993) Retinoic acid inhibition of human papillomavirus type 16-mediated transformation of human keratinocytes. *Cancer Res* 53, 905–909.
137. Meyskens, F.L., Jr., Surwit, E., Moon, T.E., Childers, J.M., Davis, J.R., Dorr, R.T., Johnson, C.S., and Alberts, D.S. (1994) Enhancement of regression of cervical intraepithelial neoplasia II (moderate dysplasia) with topically applied all-trans-retinoic acid: a randomized trial. *J Natl Cancer Inst* 86, 539–543.
138. Ivanova, T., Petrenko, A., Gritsko, T., Vinokourova, S., Eshilev, E., Kobzeva, V., Kisseljov, F., and Kisseljova, N. (2002) Methylation and silencing of the retinoic acid receptor-beta 2 gene in cervical cancer. *BMC Cancer* 2, 4.
139. Pehlivan, S., Artac, M., Sever, T., Bozcuk, H., Kilincarslan, C., and Pehlivan, M. (2010). Gene methylation of SFRP2, P16, DAPK1, HIC1, and MGMT and KRAS mutations in sporadic colorectal cancer. *Cancer Genet Cytogenet* 201, 128–132.
140. Kekeeva, T.V., Popova, O.P., Shegai, P.V., Alekseev, B., Adnreeva, I., Zaletaev, D.V., and Nemtsova, M.V. (2007) [Abberant methylation of p16, HIC1, N33 and GSTP1 genes in tumor epithelium and tumor-associated stromal cells of prostate cancer]. *Mol Biol (Mosk)* 41, 79–85.
141. Rathi, A., Virmani, A.K., Harada, K., Timmons, C.F., Miyajima, K., Hay, R.J., Mastrangelo, D., Maitra, A., Tomlinson, G.E., and Gazdar, A.F. (2003) Aberrant methylation of the HIC1 promoter is a frequent event in specific pediatric neoplasms. *Clin Cancer Res* 9, 3674–3678.
142. Chen, W.Y., Zeng, X., Carter, M.G., Morrell, C.N., Chiu Yen, R.W., Esteller, M., Watkins, D.N., Herman, J.G., Mankowski, J.L., and Baylin, S.B. (2003) Heterozygous disruption of Hic1 predisposes mice to a gender-dependent spectrum of malignant tumors. *Nat Genet* 33, 197–202.
143. Chen, W., Cooper, T.K., Zahnow, C.A., Overholtzer, M., Zhao, Z., Ladanyi, M., Karp, J.E., Gokgoz, N., Wunder, J.S., Andrulis, I.L., et al. (2004) Epigenetic and genetic loss of Hic1 function accentuates the role of p53 in tumorigenesis. *Cancer Cell* 6, 387–398.
144. Kuramochi, M., Fukuhara, H., Nobukuni, T., Kanbe, T., Maruyama, T., Ghosh, H.P., Pletcher, M., Isomura, M., Onizuka, M., Kitamura, T., et al. (2001) TSLC1 is a tumor-suppressor gene in human non-small-cell lung cancer. *Nat Genet* 27, 427–430.
145. Fukuhara, H., Kuramochi, M., Fukami, T., Kasahara, K., Furuhata, M., Nobukuni, T., Maruyama, T., Isogai, K., Sekiya, T., Shuin, T., et al. (2002) Promoter methylation of TSLC1 and tumor suppression by its gene product in human prostate cancer. *Jpn J Cancer Res* 93, 605–609.
146. Allinen, M., Peri, L., Kujala, S., Lahti-Domenici, J., Outila, K., Karppinen, S.M., Launonen, V., and Winqvist, R. (2002) Analysis of 11q21-24 loss of heterozygosity candidate target genes in breast cancer: indications of TSLC1 promoter hypermethylation. *Genes Chromosomes Cancer* 34, 384–389.
147. Ito, T., Shimada, Y., Hashimoto, Y., Kaganoi, J., Kan, T., Watanabe, G., Murakami, Y., and Imamura, M. (2003) Involvement of TSLC1 in progression of esophageal squamous cell carcinoma. *Cancer Res* 63, 6320–6326.
148. Jansen, M., Fukushima, N., Rosty, C., Walter, K., Altink, R., Heek, T.V., Hruban, R., Offerhaus, J.G., and Goggins, M. (2002) Aberrant methylation of the 5 CpG island of TSLC1 is common in pancreatic ductal adenocarcinoma and is first manifest in high-grade PanINs. *Cancer Biol Ther* 1, 293–296.
149. Watabe, K., Ito, A., Koma, Y.I., and Kitamura, Y. (2003) IGSF4: a new intercellular adhesion molecule that is called by three names, TSLC1, SgIGSF and SynCAM, by virtue of its diverse function. *Histol Histopathol* 18, 1321–1329.
150. Li, J., Zhang, Z., Bidder, M., Funk, M.C., Nguyen, L., Goodfellow, P.J., and Rader, J.S. (2005) IGSF4 promoter methylation and expression silencing in human cervical cancer. *Gynecol Oncol* 96, 150–158.

151. Taniguchi, T., Kobayashi, T., Kondo, J., Takahashi, K., Nakamura, H., Suzuki, J., Nagai, K., Yamada, T., Nakamura, S., and Yamamura, H. (1991) Molecular cloning of a porcine gene syk that encodes a 72-kDa protein-tyrosine kinase showing high susceptibility to proteolysis. *J Biol Chem* 266, 15790–15796.
152. Coopman, P.J., Do, M.T., Barth, M., Bowden, E.T., Hayes, A.J., Basyuk, E., Blancato, J.K., Vezza, P.R., McLeskey, S.W., Mangeat, P.H., et al. (2000) The Syk tyrosine kinase suppresses malignant growth of human breast cancer cells. *Nature* 406, 742–747.
153. Ulanova, M., Puttagunta, L., Marcet-Palacios, M., Duszyk, M., Steinhoff, U., Duta, F., Kim, M.K., Indik, Z.K., Schreiber, A.D., and Befus, A.D. (2005) Syk tyrosine kinase participates in beta1-integrin signaling and inflammatory responses in airway epithelial cells. *Am J Physiol Lung Cell Mol Physiol* 288, L497–507.
154. Yamada, T., Fujieda, S., Yanagi, S., Yamamura, H., Inatome, R., Sunaga, H., and Saito, H. (2001) Protein-tyrosine kinase Syk expressed in human nasal fibroblasts and its effect on RANTES production. *J Immunol* 166, 538–543.
155. Inatome, R., Yanagi, S., Takano, T., and Yamamura, H. (2001) A critical role for Syk in endothelial cell proliferation and migration. *Biochem Biophys Res Commun* 286, 195–199.
156. Yuan, Y., Wang, J., Li, J., Wang, L., Li, M., Yang, Z., Zhang, C., and Dai, J.L. (2006) Frequent epigenetic inactivation of spleen tyrosine kinase gene in human hepatocellular carcinoma. *Clin Cancer Res* 12, 6687–6695.
157. Turner, M., Schweighoffer, E., Colucci, F., Di Santo, J.P., and Tybulewicz, V.L. (2000) Tyrosine kinase SYK: essential functions for immunoreceptor signalling. *Immunol Today* 21, 148–154.
158. Brumbaugh, K.M., Binstadt, B.A., Billadeau, D.D., Schoon, R.A., Dick, C.J., Ten, R.M., and Leibson, P.J. (1997) Functional role for Syk tyrosine kinase in natural killer cell-mediated natural cytotoxicity. *J Exp Med* 186, 1965–1974.
159. Yuan, Y., Mendez, R., Sahin, A., and Dai, J.L. (2001) Hypermethylation leads to silencing of the SYK gene in human breast cancer. *Cancer Res* 61, 5558–5561.
160. Toyama, T., Iwase, H., Yamashita, H., Hara, Y., Omoto, Y., Sugiura, H., Zhang, Z., and Fujii, Y. (2003) Reduced expression of the Syk gene is correlated with poor prognosis in human breast cancer. *Cancer Lett* 189, 97–102.
161. Zhao, S., Sun, G., Tony, P.W., Ma, D., and Zhao, C. (2011) Expression and methylation status of the Syk gene in cervical carcinoma. *Arch Gynecol Obstet.* 283, 1113–1119.
162. Douc-Rasy, S., Barrois, M., Fogel, S., Ahomadegbe, J.C., Stehelin, D., Coll, J., and Riou, G. (1996) High incidence of loss of heterozygosity and abnormal imprinting of H19 and IGF2 genes in invasive cervical carcinomas. Uncoupling of H19 and IGF2 expression and biallelic hypomethylation of H19. *Oncogene* 12, 423–430.
163. Gama-Sosa, M.A., Slagel, V.A., Trewyn, R.W., Oxenhandler, R., Kuo, K.C., Gehrke, C.W., and Ehrlich, M. (1983) The 5-methylcytosine content of DNA from human tumors. *Nucleic Acids Res* 11, 6883–6894.
164. Kim, Y.I., Giuliano, A., Hatch, K.D., Schneider, A., Nour, M.A., Dallal, G.E., Selhub, J., and Mason, J.B. (1994) Global DNA hypomethylation increases progressively in cervical dysplasia and carcinoma. *Cancer* 74, 893–899.
165. de Capoa, A., Musolino, A., Della Rosa, S., Caiafa, P., Mariani, L., Del Nonno, F., Vocaturo, A., Donnorso, R.P., Niveleau, A., and Grappelli, C. (2003) DNA demethylation is directly related to tumour progression: evidence in normal, pre-malignant and malignant cells from uterine cervix samples. *Oncol Rep* 10, 545–549.
166. Mathers, J.C. (2008) Session 2: Personalised nutrition. Epigenomics: a basis for understanding individual differences? *Proc Nutr Soc* 67, 390–394.
167. Kristjuhan, A., Walker, J., Suka, N., Grunstein, M., Roberts, D., Cairns, B.R., and Svejstrup, J.Q. (2002) Transcriptional inhibition of genes with severe histone h3 hypoacetylation in the coding region. *Mol Cell* 10, 925–933.
168. Du, T.T. and Huang, Q.H. (2007) [The roles of histone lysine methylation in epigenetic regulation]. *Yi Chuan* 29, 387–392.
169. Fraga, M.F., Ballestar, E., Villar-Garea, A., Boix-Chornet, M., Espada, J., Schotta, G., Bonaldi, T., Haydon, C., Ropero, S., Petrie, K., et al. (2005) Loss of acetylation at Lys16 and trimethylation at Lys20 of histone H4 is a common hallmark of human cancer. *Nat Genet* 37, 391–400.
170. Anton, M., Horky, M., Kuchtickova, S., Vojtesek, B., and Blaha, O. (2004) Immunohistochemical detection of acetylation and phosphorylation of histone H3 in cervical smears. *Ceska Gynekol* 69, 3–6.
171. Pisani, P., Bray, F., and Parkin, D.M. (2002) Estimates of the world-wide prevalence of cancer for 25 sites in the adult population. *Int J Cancer* 97, 72–81.

172. Wang, S.S., Sherman, M.E., Hildesheim, A., Lacey, J.V., Jr., and Devesa, S. (2004) Cervical adenocarcinoma and squamous cell carcinoma incidence trends among white women and black women in the United States for 1976-2000. *Cancer* 100, 1035–1044.
173. Kulasingam, S.L., Hughes, J.P., Kiviat, N.B., Mao, C., Weiss, N.S., Kuypers, J.M., and Koutsky, L.A. (2002) Evaluation of human papillomavirus testing in primary screening for cervical abnormalities: comparison of sensitivity, specificity, and frequency of referral. *JAMA* 288, 1749–1757.
174. Bulkmans, N.W., Berkhof, J., Bulk, S., Bleeker, M.C., van Kemenade, F.J., Rozendaal, L., Snijders, P.J., and Meijer, C.J. (2007) High-risk HPV type-specific clearance rates in cervical screening. *Br J Cancer* 96, 1419–1424.
175. Nieh, S., Chen, S.F., Chu, T.Y., Lai, H.C., Lin, Y.S., Fu, E., and Gau, C.H. (2005) Is p16(INK4A) expression more useful than human papillomavirus test to determine the outcome of atypical squamous cells of undetermined significance-categorized Pap smear? A comparative analysis using abnormal cervical smears with follow-up biopsies. *Gynecol Oncol* 97, 35–40.
176. Kalof, A.N., Evans, M.F., Simmons-Arnold, L., Beatty, B.G., and Cooper, K. (2005) p16INK4A immunoexpression and HPV in situ hybridization signal patterns: potential markers of high-grade cervical intraepithelial neoplasia. *Am J Surg Pathol* 29, 674-679.
177. Laird, P.W. (2003) The power and the promise of DNA methylation markers. *Nat Rev Cancer* 3, 253-266.

Chapter 10

Epigenetics of Colon Cancer

Sharad Khare and Mukesh Verma

Abstract

Accumulation of genetic and epigenetic alterations transforms normal colonic epithelial cells to adenocarcinoma cells. Genetic alterations include mutations in tumor suppressor genes and oncogenes, whereas epigenetic mechanisms are defined as heritable alterations in gene expression that is independent of changes in the primary DNA sequence. Role of epigenetic mechanisms in development and maintenance of organ- and tissue-specific gene expression is now realized. Disturbances in epigenetic landscape can lead to malignant cellular makeover, and these heritable changes are maintained through various cycles of cell division that renders cells to have discrete identity with similar genetic information. Epigenetic alterations in colorectal cancer (CRC) that transform colonic epithelial cells into adenocarcinoma cells include aberrant DNA methylation, chromatin modifications, and noncoding RNAs, especially microRNA expression. CpG island DNA methylation and aberrant methylation of genes drive the initiation and progression of CRC. Histone modifications impinge on chromatin structure and gene expression and thus play an important role in gene silencing in CRC. DNA hypermethylation also leads to downregulation and inappropriate expression of certain microRNAs that act like tumor suppressor genes. Determining the causes and roles of epigenetic instability in CRC pathogenesis will lead to effective prevention and therapeutic strategies for patients with CRC. Epigenetic drugs that underscore the reversible nature of epigenetic events have led the possibility of epigenetic therapy as a treatment option in CRC.

Key words: Aberrant crypt foci, Colorectal cancer, CpG (cytosine-guanine), CpG island methylator phenotype, DNA methyltransferases, MicroRNA, Microsatellite instability, Mismatch repair

1. Introduction

Epigenetics is defined as the inheritance of information based on gene expression levels as opposed to genetics, which refers to information inherited on the basis of gene sequences. Epigenetic alterations play a major role in the initiation and progression of colorectal cancers (CRCs). Even in the hereditary CRCs, cancer progression is the result of the progressive accumulation of both genetic and epigenetic alterations. Two most common inherited colon cancer

Ramona G. Dumitrescu and Mukesh Verma (eds.), *Cancer Epigenetics: Methods and Protocols*, Methods in Molecular Biology, vol. 863, DOI 10.1007/978-1-61779-612-8_10,

syndromes, hereditary nonpolyposis colorectal cancer (HNPCC) and familial adenomatous polyposis (FAP), are caused by germ line mutations in mismatch repair (MMR) genes and the adenomatous polyposis coli (*APC*) gene, respectively. Inactivation of *APC* gene plays a rate-limiting role in majority of sporadic CRCs (1). Epigenetic silencing of *APC* through promoter hypermethylation has also been reported in a number sporadic CRC (2). Conversely, in HNPCC, a subset of CRC caused by inactivation of MMR system with a characteristic signature mutation called microsatellite instability (MSI) and therefore CRCs are classified as MSI-high (MSI-H), MSI-low (MSI-L), or MSI-stable (MSS). This occurs either through the aberrant CpG island methylation of *MLH1* (3) or point mutations in *MLH1* and *MSH2* genes (4) that normally regulate DNA conformity. A subset of sporadic CRCs has a specific phenotype named CIMP (CpG island methylator phenotype) with a high percentage of aberrantly methylated gene promoters (5). In patients with metastatic and MSS carcinomas, CpG island methylation and CIMP-positive are associated with worse prognosis (6). Thus, on the basis of methylation phenotype, CRCs can also be classified into five different groups: (1) CIMP-high, MSI-H, and *BRAF* mutation; (2) CIMP-high, MSI-L or MSS, and *BRAF* mutation; (3) CIMP-low, MSI-L or MSS, and *KRAS* mutation; (4) CIMP-negative and MSS; and (5) CIMP-negative, MSI-H (Lynch syndrome) (7). Each type has its own clinical and morphological features and prognostic factors that could have an incredible impact on prevention, management, and treatment of CRC.

2. Epigenetic Mechanisms in Colorectal Cancer

2.1. DNA Methylation

Epigenetic instability appears to be a common phenomenon in CRC. Stable DNA methylation pattern established during development is maintained throughout the genome. In cancers, however, several CpG (cytosine-guanine) islands become aberrantly methylated. CpG islands (CpG-rich 0.3–2-kb stretches of DNA) present in the 5′ regions of >50% genes in an unmethylated state often encompass the promoter and transcription start site of the gene that is recognized by DNA methyltransferase (DNMTs). Expression levels and activities of DNMTs and DNA methylases maintain the DNA methylation patterns in normal tissues. Aberrant methylation of these sites can be accompanied by transcriptional repression (8). A variety of tumor suppressor genes such as *Rb*, *CDKN2A/p16*, *MGMT*, *p14*^{ARF}, and *HLTF* are aberrantly methylated in CRC (5). Aberrant methylation of *CDKN2A/p16* is found in 40% of CRC. Furthermore, methylation of genes *HLTF*, *SLC5A8*, *SFRP2*, and *MGMT* at aberrant crypt foci (ACF) stage demonstrates that aberrant promoter methylation is occurring early in the adenoma sequence (9–11). However, it is not known whether aberrant methylation is a primary rather than a secondary event in the progression of CRC.

DNA hypermethylation augments silencing of tumor suppressor genes, whereas DNA hypomethylation activates proto-oncogenes and genomic instability. During tumorigenesis, DNA hypomethylation occurs at various genomic sequences. Chromosomal rearrangement and translocation of retrotransposons due to genomic instability is initiated by DNA hypomethylation. Loss of imprinting (LOI) of *IGF2* gene, an increased risk of CRC, is due to DNA hypomethylation (12).

A distinct group of colorectal tumors with CIMP have high proportion of aberrantly methylated gene promoters. However, the mechanisms causing CIMP tumor type is not clearly understood, but *BRAF* V600E mutation is commonly found in this subclass of colorectal tumors (13). This pathway in part overlaps with sporadic MSI tumors due to *MLH1* hypermethylation that results in loss of MMR function. ACF is considered the initial lesion of CIMP pathway. However, adenoma-carcinoma sequence involves hyperplastic ACF instead of dysplastic ACF with aberrant Wnt signaling. Methylated promoters of *MGMT*, *HLTF*, *SLC5A8*, *MINT1*, and *SFRP2* during ACF stage; *MLH1* promoter hypermethylation during the development of serrated adenoma; and finally methylated *TSP1* and *TIMP3* drive the progression of CIMP tumors (5).

DNA methylation imparts a direct inhibition between promoters and transcription factors such as *NFkB*, *E2F*, *CREB*, and *AP-2* (14). Alternatively, methylation silences transcriptional activity by regulating chromatin structure that involves recruitment of methyl-binding proteins and histone deacetylases. Transcriptional silencing followed by DNA methylation is mediated by recruitment of methyl-binding proteins MBD2, MBD3, and MeCP2. These proteins recognize methylated sequences and recruit histone deacetylases that induce changes in chromatin structure, which ultimately hinder the access of transcription factors to the promoter (15). These modifications tend to regulate the chromatin state in a transcriptionally active or repressed state. It is not clearly understood whether changes in methylation state of histone proteins precede changes in overall methylation or DNA methylation precedes alterations in histones and chromatin structure.

2.2. Histone Modifications

Another important epigenetic mechanism related to gene silencing in normal and cancer cells is the interaction of DNA methylation and histone modifications (16). Histone proteins assemble with DNA in nucleosomes that function as transcriptional regulators. The amino-terminal tails of histones undergo a variety of posttranscriptional covalent modifications including methylation, acetylation, and phosphorylation on specific residues (17). Different combinations of histone tail modifications influence transcription by affecting chromatin structure (14). Acetylation of lysine residues on histone H3 and H4 leads to the formation of open chromatin structure with transcriptional activation, whereas methylation of lysine leads to transcriptional activation or repression depending upon which residue is modified. Trimethylation of lysine 4 on histone H3 is a marker of transcriptional activation, whereas trimethylation of lysine 9 and 27 on histone H3 represents transcriptional repression. Similarly, acetylation of histone 3 at lysine 9 and 18, acetylation of histone 4 at lysine 12, dimethylation of histone 4 at arginine 3, and histone 3 at lysine 4 regulate chromatin in a transcriptionally active or repressed state. Phosphorylation on serine 10 and acetylation on lysine 14 of histone H3 has antagonistic effect on lysine 9 methylation of histone H3, leading to gene activation. In CRC, reduced acetylation and methylation of histone H3 at lysine 9 and 4, respectively, and increased methylation at lysine 9 in the promoter regions of *p16*, *MLH1*, and *MGMT* are associated with silencing of these genes (5).

2.3. Noncoding MicroRNAs

miRNAs are endogenous noncoding RNAs (20–22 nucleotides) that inhibit translation by base pairing to the 3′ untranslated region of messenger RNAs (mRNAs) (18). It is predicted that human genome may contain up to 1,000 miRNAs, and up to one-third of human mRNAs are regulated by miRNAs (18). Each miRNA can target hundreds of mRNAs, whereas many miRNAs can regulate a single mRNA to control expression level of each protein-coding gene (18). miRNAs act as either tumor suppressors or oncogenes depending upon the target mRNA, and thus overexpression and underexpression of miRNAs lead to downregulation of tumor suppressor genes and upregulation of oncogenes, respectively. miRNA expression profile is strongly associated with tumorigenesis. Changes in miRNA expression are achieved through several mechanisms including epigenetic alterations. An extensive analysis of genomic sequences of miRNA genes has shown that nearly half of them are associated with CpG islands (19). miRNA upregulation or downregulation may play a role in CRC, but the mechanisms involved in this process are still unclear. miRNA gene promoter sequences contain numerous p53 binding sites, an important tumor suppressor gene whose activity is lost in colorectal tumors (20).

miRNA-127, a tumor suppressor miRNA, is silenced in cancer by DNA methylation of its promoter and thus a primary target for epigenetic therapy via demethylating agents and HDAC inhibitors (21). Decreased expression of miRNAs 124a, let-7a-3, 10a, and 342 in CRCs is directly related to the increased methylation because these miRNA genes are located near a CpG island (22). The miRNA-342 increases apoptosis and has a tumor suppressor-like effect that is lost by increased methylation. *CDK6* and *Rb* are important targets of miRNA 124-a (22), whereas miRNA let-7a-3 targets *Ras*, a known human oncogene (23). Downregulation of miRNA-10a leads the inhibition on *HOXA3* and *HOXD10* translation (24).

The members of miRNA-34 family are considered as tumor suppressors. In fact, decreased levels of miRNA-34 have been reported in CRC, and one underlying mechanism appears to be CpG island methylation (25). miRNA-34b/c is found to be epigenetically silenced in many colon cancer cell lines and primary CRC tumors. Treatment with demethylating agents restores expression of miRNA-34b/c and inhibits tumor motility and metastasis (25). Lymph node metastasis of CRC demonstrated downregulation of miRNA-148a, miRNA-9, and miRNA-34b/c due to CpG island hypermethylation. Similarly, regaining miRNA function by demethylating agents resulted in inhibition of tumor growth and metastasis (26).

3. Epigenetic Cancer Therapy

Genetic mutations that are inherited through DNA replication are irreversible. However, epigenetic alterations are reversible. This phenomenon established the use of DNMT inhibitors as a smart concept for cancer therapy (27). The cytosine analogues 5-azacytidine (azacytidine) and 2′-deoxy-5-azacytidine (decitabine) are pharmacological inhibitors of DNMT and are currently being developed as drugs for epigenetic cancer therapy (28). The mechanism of demethylation involves covalent trapping and subsequent depletion of DNMTs. A recent study in colon cancer cells also demonstrated that their mode of action is not limited to DNA methylation and tRNA hypomethylation might contribute to patient responses (29). In cancer cell culture studies including colon cancer, both drugs reduce cytosine methylation, although the effectiveness can vary between cell lines. Recent studies have also shown that demethylation of colon carcinoma cells HCT-116 led to reduced c-Met expression and decreased signaling (30). Though DNMT inhibitors are not currently used in CRC, both drugs have received Food and Drug Administration approval for the treatment of myelodsplastic syndrome, a preleukemic bone marrow disease (31, 32).

4. Folate and Colorectal Cancer Risk

Epidemiological studies have suggested an inverse relationship of folate status with the risk of CRC (33). In these studies, folate status was assessed by dietary folate intake or by the measurement of blood folate levels. Since folate is a source of methyl group, the potential of folate exposure to alter DNA methylation is subject of many previous studies. Several studies indicate a 20–40% reduction in the risk of CRC with the highest dietary folate supplementation (34, 35). However, a well-designed folate prevention trial demonstrated no reduction in polyp formation, but an actual increase in more advanced colonic lesions was observed (36). The animal studies also demonstrated that excess folate supplementation may increase CRC risk and accelerate CRC progression if it is provided after neoplastic foci are established in the colorectum (37).

5. Methods in Measuring Epigenetic Changes

Considerable advances have been made in determining alterations in methylation, histones, and miRNA profiling (38). Methylation can be measured for specific genes or at genome level by methyl light technique (39). This PCR-based high-throughput method uses small amounts of input DNA (20 ng/sequence vs. 500 ng–1 μg for the analysis of total DNA 5-methylcytosine). Another popular method of methylation profiling is called methylation-specific multiplex ligation-dependent probe amplification assay (MS-MLPA) (40). MS-MLPA, a modification of the conventional MLPA assay, allows for the simultaneous detection of changes in methylation status as well as copy number changes of approximately 41 different DNA sequences in a single reaction requiring only 20 ng of human DNA. Microarray-based approaches are used to determine miRNA profiling. RNA (containing miRNA) is extracted from tissues using the mirVana miRNA isolation kit (Applied Biosystems), quantified and assessed for quality (41). miRNA profile is analyzed by the TaqMan Human MicroRNA Array Set v3.0 (Applied Biosystems). The array provides accurate quantification of 742 human miRNAs that includes three TaqMan MicroRNA Assay endogenous controls to aid in data normalization and one TaqMan MicroRNA Assay not related to humans as a negative control. This method has been successfully used for miRNA profiling of formalin-fixed tissue and serum- or plasma-extracted RNA (42). The extraction and analysis of miRNA is technically easier than mRNA analysis because the miRNA is subject to much less degradation due to its small size. For histone analysis, ChIP-on-chip and ChIP-seq method (using Illumina platform) is very common (38). Special attention should be paid to the purity and specificity of monoclonal antibodies, which are raised against specific modifications of histones (43).

6. Conclusion

Epigenetic alterations, especially aberrant DNA methylation, are becoming increasingly recognized as a causal mechanism in CRC. Histone modifications accompany DNA hypermethylation changes in CRC and likely establish a complex network to maintain gene silencing. Continued investigation into the role of epigenetic mechanisms in miRNA expression in CRC is likely to yield important information on new potential targets for therapy.

References

1. Miyaki, M., Konishi, M., Kikuchi-Yanoshita, R., Enomoto, M., Igari, T., Tanaka, K., Muraoka, M., Takahashi, H., Amada, Y., Fukayama, M., and et al. (1994) Characteristics of somatic mutation of the adenomatous polyposis coli gene in colorectal tumors. *Cancer Res* 54, 3011–3020.
2. Esteller, M., Sparks, A., Toyota, M., Sanchez-Cespedes, M., Capella, G., Peinado, M. A., Gonzalez, S., Tarafa, G., Sidransky, D., Meltzer, S. J., Baylin, S. B., and Herman, J. G. (2000) Analysis of adenomatous polyposis coli promoter hypermethylation in human cancer. *Cancer Res* 60, 4366–4371.
3. Veigl, M. L., Kasturi, L., Olechnowicz, J., Ma, A. H., Lutterbaugh, J. D., Periyasamy, S., Li, G. M., Drummond, J., Modrich, P. L., Sedwick, W. D., and Markowitz, S. D. (1998) Biallelic inactivation of hMLH1 by epigenetic gene silencing, a novel mechanism causing human MSI cancers. *Proc Natl Acad Sci U S A* 95, 8698–8702.
4. Alemayehu, A., Sebova, K., and Fridrichova, I. (2008) Redundant DNA methylation in colorectal cancers of Lynch-syndrome patients. *Genes Chromosomes Cancer* 47, 906–914.
5. Grady, W. M. and Carethers, J. M. (2008) Genomic and epigenetic instability in colorectal cancer pathogenesis. *Gastroenterology* 135, 1079–1099.
6. Ogino, S., Meyerhardt, J. A., Kawasaki, T., Clark, J. W., Ryan, D. P., Kulke, M. H., Enzinger, P. C., Wolpin, B. M., Loda, M., and Fuchs, C. S. (2007) CpG island methylation, response to combination chemotherapy, and patient survival in advanced microsatellite stable colorectal carcinoma. *Virchows Arch* 450, 529–537.
7. Jass, J. R. (2007) Classification of colorectal cancer based on correlation of clinical, morphological and molecular features. *Histopathology* 50, 113–130.
8. Baylin, S. B. and Herman, J. G. (2000) DNA hypermethylation in tumorigenesis: epigenetics joins genetics. *Trends Genet* 16, 168–174.
9. Li, H., Myeroff, L., Smiraglia, D., Romero, M. F., Pretlow, T. P., Kasturi, L., Lutterbaugh, J., Rerko, R. M., Casey, G., Issa, J. P., Willis, J., Willson, J. K., Plass, C., and Markowitz, S. D. (2003) SLC5A8, a sodium transporter, is a tumor suppressor gene silenced by methylation in human colon aberrant crypt foci and cancers. *Proc Natl Acad Sci U S A* 100, 8412–8417.
10. Chan, A. O., Broaddus, R. R., Houlihan, P. S., Issa, J. P., Hamilton, S. R., and Rashid, A. (2002) CpG island methylation in aberrant crypt foci of the colorectum. *Am J Pathol* 160, 1823–1830.
11. Moinova, H. R., Chen, W. D., Shen, L., Smiraglia, D., Olechnowicz, J., Ravi, L., Kasturi, L., Myeroff, L., Plass, C., Parsons, R., Minna, J., Willson, J. K., Green, S. B., Issa, J. P., and Markowitz, S. D. (2002) HLTF gene silencing in human colon cancer. *Proc Natl Acad Sci U S A* 99, 4562–4567.
12. Timp, W., Levchenko, A., and Feinberg, A. P. (2009) A new link between epigenetic progenitor lesions in cancer and the dynamics of signal transduction. *Cell Cycle* 8, 383–390.
13. Weisenberger, D. J., Siegmund, K. D., Campan, M., Young, J., Long, T. I., Faasse, M. A., Kang, G. H., Widschwendter, M., Weener, D., Buchanan, D., Koh, H., Simms, L., Barker, M., Leggett, B., Levine, J., Kim, M., French, A. J., Thibodeau, S. N., Jass, J., Haile, R., and Laird, P. W. (2006) CpG island methylator phenotype underlies sporadic microsatellite instability and is tightly associated with BRAF mutation in colorectal cancer. *Nat Genet* 38, 787–793.
14. Kondo, Y. and Issa, J. P. (2004) Epigenetic changes in colorectal cancer. *Cancer Metastasis Rev* 23, 29–39.

15. Deng, G., Chen, A., Pong, E., and Kim, Y. S. (2001) Methylation in hMLH1 promoter interferes with its binding to transcription factor CBF and inhibits gene expression. *Oncogene* 20, 7120–7127.
16. Bird, A. P. and Wolffe, A. P. (1999) Methylation-induced repression--belts, braces, and chromatin. *Cell* 99, 451–454.
17. Jenuwein, T. and Allis, C. D. (2001) Translating the histone code. *Science* 293, 1074–1080.
18. Zamore, P. D. and Haley, B. (2005) Ribo-gnome: the big world of small RNAs. *Science* 309, 1519–1524.
19. Weber, B., Stresemann, C., Brueckner, B., and Lyko, F. (2007) Methylation of human microRNA genes in normal and neoplastic cells. *Cell Cycle* 6, 1001–1005.
20. Xi, Y., Shalgi, R., Fodstad, O., Pilpel, Y., and Ju, J. (2006) Differentially regulated micro-RNAs and actively translated messenger RNA transcripts by tumor suppressor p53 in colon cancer. *Clin Cancer Res* 12, 2014–2024.
21. Lujambio, A. and Esteller, M. (2007) CpG island hypermethylation of tumor suppressor microRNAs in human cancer. *Cell Cycle* 6, 1455–1459.
22. Yang, L., Belaguli, N., and Berger, D. H. (2009) MicroRNA and colorectal cancer. *World J Surg* 33, 638–646.
23. Akao, Y., Nakagawa, Y., and Naoe, T. (2006) let-7 microRNA functions as a potential growth suppressor in human colon cancer cells. *Biol Pharm Bull* 29, 903–906.
24. Han, L., Witmer, P. D., Casey, E., Valle, D., and Sukumar, S. (2007) DNA methylation regulates MicroRNA expression. *Cancer Biol Ther* 6, 1284–1288.
25. Faber, C., Kirchner, T., and Hlubek, F. (2009) The impact of microRNAs on colorectal cancer. *Virchows Arch* 454, 359–367.
26. Lujambio, A., Calin, G. A., Villanueva, A., Ropero, S., Sanchez-Cespedes, M., Blanco, D., Montuenga, L. M., Rossi, S., Nicoloso, M. S., Faller, W. J., Gallagher, W. M., Eccles, S. A., Croce, C. M., and Esteller, M. (2008) A microRNA DNA methylation signature for human cancer metastasis. *Proc Natl Acad Sci U S A* 105, 13556–13561.
27. Lyko, F. and Brown, R. (2005) DNA methyltransferase inhibitors and the development of epigenetic cancer therapies. *J Natl Cancer Inst* 97, 1498–1506.
28. Issa, J. P. and Kantarjian, H. M. (2009) Targeting DNA methylation. *Clin Cancer Res* 15, 3938–3946.
29. Schaefer, M., Hagemann, S., Hanna, K., and Lyko, F. (2009) Azacytidine inhibits RNA methylation at DNMT2 target sites in human cancer cell lines. *Cancer Res* 69, 8127–8132.
30. Weber, B., Kimhi, S., Howard, G., Eden, A., and Lyko, F. (2010) Demethylation of a LINE-1 antisense promoter in the cMet locus impairs Met signalling through induction of illegitimate transcription. *Oncogene* 29, 5775–5784.
31. Silverman, L. R., Demakos, E. P., Peterson, B. L., Kornblith, A. B., Holland, J. C., Odchimar-Reissig, R., Stone, R. M., Nelson, D., Powell, B. L., DeCastro, C. M., Ellerton, J., Larson, R. A., Schiffer, C. A., and Holland, J. F. (2002) Randomized controlled trial of azacitidine in patients with the myelodysplastic syndrome: a study of the cancer and leukemia group B. *J Clin Oncol* 20, 2429–2440.
32. Kantarjian, H., Issa, J. P., Rosenfeld, C. S., Bennett, J. M., Albitar, M., DiPersio, J., Klimek, V., Slack, J., de Castro, C., Ravandi, F., Helmer, R., 3rd, Shen, L., Nimer, S. D., Leavitt, R., Raza, A., and Saba, H. (2006) Decitabine improves patient outcomes in myelodysplastic syndromes: results of a phase III randomized study. *Cancer* 106, 1794–1803.
33. Kim, Y. I. (2004) Folate and DNA methylation: a mechanistic link between folate deficiency and colorectal cancer? *Cancer Epidemiol Biomarkers Prev* 13, 511–519.
34. Kim, Y. I. (2003) Role of folate in colon cancer development and progression. *J Nutr* 133, 3731S-3739S.
35. Giovannucci, E. (2002) Epidemiologic studies of folate and colorectal neoplasia: a review. *J Nutr* 132, 2350S–2355S.
36. Cole, B. F., Baron, J. A., Sandler, R. S., Haile, R. W., Ahnen, D. J., Bresalier, R. S., McKeown-Eyssen, G., Summers, R. W., Rothstein, R. I., Burke, C. A., Snover, D. C., Church, T. R., Allen, J. I., Robertson, D. J., Beck, G. J., Bond, J. H., Byers, T., Mandel, J. S., Mott, L. A., Pearson, L. H., Barry, E. L., Rees, J. R., Marcon, N., Saibil, F., Ueland, P. M., and Greenberg, E. R. (2007) Folic acid for the prevention of colorectal adenomas: a randomized clinical trial. *JAMA* 297, 2351–2359.
37. Kim, Y. I. (2004) Will mandatory folic acid fortification prevent or promote cancer? *Am J Clin Nutr* 80, 1123–1128.
38. Kumar, D. and Verma, M. (2009) Methods in cancer epigenetics and epidemiology. *Methods Mol Biol* 471, 273–288.
39. Noushmehr, H., Weisenberger, D. J., Diefes, K., Phillips, H. S., Pujara, K., Berman, B. P., Pan, F., Pelloski, C. E., Sulman, E. P., Bhat, K. P., Verhaak, R. G., Hoadley, K. A., Hayes, D. N., Perou, C. M., Schmidt, H. K., Ding, L.,

Wilson, R. K., Van Den Berg, D., Shen, H., Bengtsson, H., Neuvial, P., Cope, L. M., Buckley, J., Herman, J. G., Baylin, S. B., Laird, P. W., and Aldape, K. Identification of a CpG island methylator phenotype that defines a distinct subgroup of glioma. *Cancer Cell* 17, 510–522.

40. Stephen, J. K., Chen, K. M., Shah, V., Havard, S., Kapke, A., Lu, M., Benninger, M. S., and Worsham, M. J. (2010) DNA hypermethylation markers of poor outcome in laryngeal cancer. *Clin Epigenetics* 1, 61–69.

41. Hoefig, K. P., Thorns, C., Roehle, A., Kaehler, C., Wesche, K. O., Repsilber, D., Branke, B., Thiere, M., Feller, A. C., and Merz, H. (2008) Unlocking pathology archives for microRNA-profiling. *Anticancer Res* 28, 119–123.

42. Chen, C., Ridzon, D. A., Broomer, A. J., Zhou, Z., Lee, D. H., Nguyen, J. T., Barbisin, M., Xu, N. L., Mahuvakar, V. R., Andersen, M. R., Lao, K. Q., Livak, K. J., and Guegler, K. J. (2005) Real-time quantification of microRNAs by stem-loop RT-PCR. *Nucleic Acids Res* 33, e179.

43. Zhang, Z. and Pugh, B. F. (2011) High-resolution genome-wide mapping of the primary structure of chromatin. *Cell* 144, 175–186.

Chapter 11

Promoter Methylation in Head and Neck Tumorigenesis

Josena K. Stephen, Kang Mei Chen, Shaleta Havard, Glynis Harris, and Maria J. Worsham

Abstract

In addition to genetic alterations of gains and losses, epigenetic events of promoter methylation appear to further undermine a destabilized genomic repertoire in squamous head and neck carcinoma (HNSCC). This chapter provides an overview of frequently methylated tumor suppressor genes in benign head and neck papillomas, primary HNSCC tumors, and HNSCC cell lines and their relevance as epigenetic markers in head and neck tumorigenesis.

Key words: Head and neck cancer, Benign, Cell lines, Malignant, Primary tumors, Promoter methylation

1. Introduction

Head and neck squamous cell carcinoma (HNSCC) is one of the most prevalent cancers in the world with over 500,000 cases diagnosed annually. In the United States alone, it accounts for nearly 3.2% of all newly diagnosed cancers (1). Not only one of the most ubiquitous, HNSCC is also one of most lethal cancers responsible for 2.1% of all cancer deaths in the United States and is noted as the sixth most common malignant disease worldwide (1). HNSCC carries a high mortality rate despite advances in chemotherapy and radiation therapies. This is due mainly to the highly heterogeneous nature of the disease, both morphologically and genetically. A current shortcoming in the prognosis and treatment of HNSCC is a lack of methods and large study cohorts to adequately address the etiologic complexity and diversity of the disease.

Ramona G. Dumitrescu and Mukesh Verma (eds.), *Cancer Epigenetics: Methods and Protocols*, Methods in Molecular Biology, vol. 863, DOI 10.1007/978-1-61779-612-8_11, © Springer Science+Business Media, LLC 2012

The study of human disease has focused primarily on genetic mechanisms. Dispelling the belief that the only way to treat such conditions is by fixing or replacing damaged genes, scientists are instead focusing on the field of epigenetics, the study of changes in gene silencing that occur without changing the DNA sequence. Many types of epigenetic processes have been identified—they include DNA methylation, histone acetylation, phosphorylation, ubiquitylation, and sumoylation. These processes are natural and essential to many organism functions, but if they occur improperly, there can be major adverse health and behavioral effects.

Epigenetic regulation is central to the biological function of all cells. Perhaps the best known epigenetic process, in part because it has been the easiest to study with existing technology, is DNA methylation. This is the addition or removal of a methyl group (CH_3) at cytosine bases. Hypermethylation is a well-described DNA modification that has been implicated in normal mammalian development (2, 3), imprinting (4), and X chromosome inactivation (5). However, recent studies have identified hypermethylation as a probable cause in the development of various cancers (6–8). Aberrant methylation by DNA-methyltransferases in the CpG islands of a gene's promoter region can lead to transcriptional repression akin to other abnormalities such as a point mutation or deletion (9). Gene transcriptional inactivation via hypermethylation at the CpG islands within the promoter regions is an important mechanism (10). This anomalous hypermethylation has been noted in a variety of tumor suppressor genes (TSGs), whose inactivation can lead many cells down the tumorigenesis continuum (10–12). In many cancers, aberrant DNA methylation of so-called CpG islands, CpG-rich sequences frequently associated with promoters or first exons, is associated with the inappropriate transcriptional silencing of critical genes (13–15). These DNA methylation events represent an important tumor-specific marker occurring early in tumor progression and one that can be easily detected by PCR-based methods in a manner that is minimally invasive to the patient.

Studies of sequential molecular alterations and genetic progression of preinvasive HNSCC have not been clearly defined. A tissue field of somatic genetic alterations precedes the histopathological phenotypic changes of carcinoma (16). Genomic changes could be of potential use in the diagnosis and prognosis of preinvasive HNSCC lesions and as markers for cancer risk assessment. Allelic imbalances at chromosomal loci at 3p, 9p, 11q, 13q, and 17p have been reported as early events in head and neck carcinogenesis (17–21). However, gene silencing via hypermethylation is still a relatively new idea in the development of HNSCC, and little is known about the contribution of epigenetics to the development of neoplasia, its transformation, progression, and recurrence in HNSCC. Therefore, epigenetic events of promoter hypermethylation are emerging as one of the most promising molecular strategies for cancer detection and represent an important tumor-specific marker occurring early in tumor progression.

2. DNA Methylation in HNSCC

Numerous tumor suppressor genes have been implicated as targets for methylation in other cancers (13–15). Promoter hypermethylation of genes in HNSCC has been reported for *p16*, *p14*, *DAPK*, *RASSF1A* (22–28), *RARβ2* (29–31), *MGMT*, a DNA repair gene that functions to remove mutagenic (O^6-guanine) adducts from DNA (32), and *E-cadherin*, a Ca^{2+}-dependent cell adhesion molecule that functions in cell–cell adhesion, cell polarity, and morphogenesis (33).

Historically, the molecular pathogenesis of cancer has been teased out one gene at a time. The development of several new high-throughput analytical methods for the analysis of DNA, mRNA, and proteins within a cell (34–37) has permitted a more detailed molecular characterization of the cancer genome. In HNSCC, recent comprehensive high-throughput methods from our group and others have underscored the contribution of both genetic (38–40) and epigenetic events (28, 41–45), often working together (46), in the development and progression of HNSCC. In HNSCC, methylation of *p16*, *RARβ*, and *MGMT* suggested early events, with incidences of methylation in HNSCC cell lines and primary tumors being similar (29, 45–48).

Aberrant DNA methylation patterns in HNSCC have served as powerful diagnostic, prognostic, and risk assessment biomarkers. Promoter hypermethylation pattern of the *p16*, *MGMT*, *GSTP1*, and *DAPK* genes has been used as molecular markers for cancer cell detection in the paired serum DNA, and almost half of the HNSCC patients with methylated tumors were found to display these epigenetic changes in the paired serum (28).

2.1. HNSCC Cell Lines

The majority of published epigenetic data in HNSCC comes from methylation specific PCR (MSP) following bisulfite treatment (49). The success of MSP has been attributed to its increased sensitivity; however, it generally relies on a preselected number of genes, assessed one gene at a time, as opposed to high-throughput microarray-based methylation analysis (50) and multi-candidate gene applications (46). Recently, using a multi-candidate gene approach, the methylation-specific multiplex ligation-dependent probe amplification (MS-MLPA) assay (Fig. 1) (46, 51), we identified nine genes, *TIMP3*, *APC*, *KLK10*, *TP73*, *CDH13*, *IGSF4*, *FHIT*, *ESR1*, and *DAPK1*, that were aberrantly methylated in paired HNSCC primary

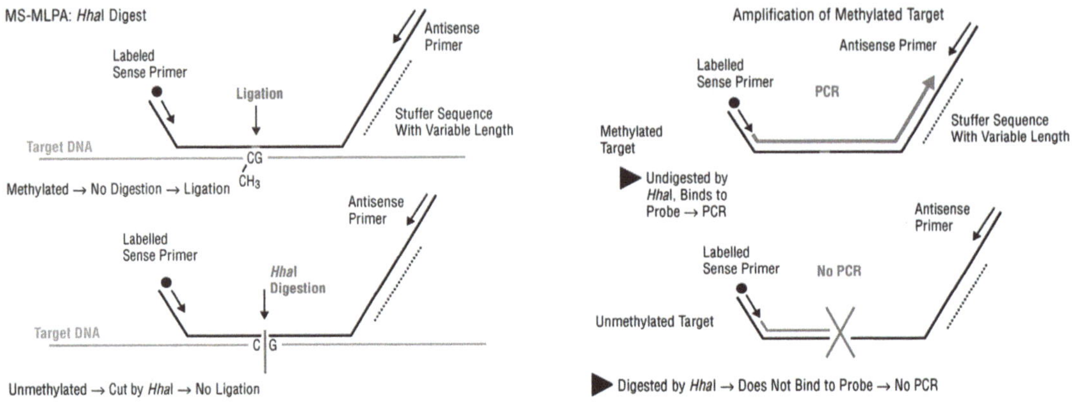

Fig. 1. Methylation-specific multiplex ligation-dependent probe amplification (MS-MLPA) with and without HhaI. CH_3 indicates methyl group; *PCR*, polymerase chain reaction (46).

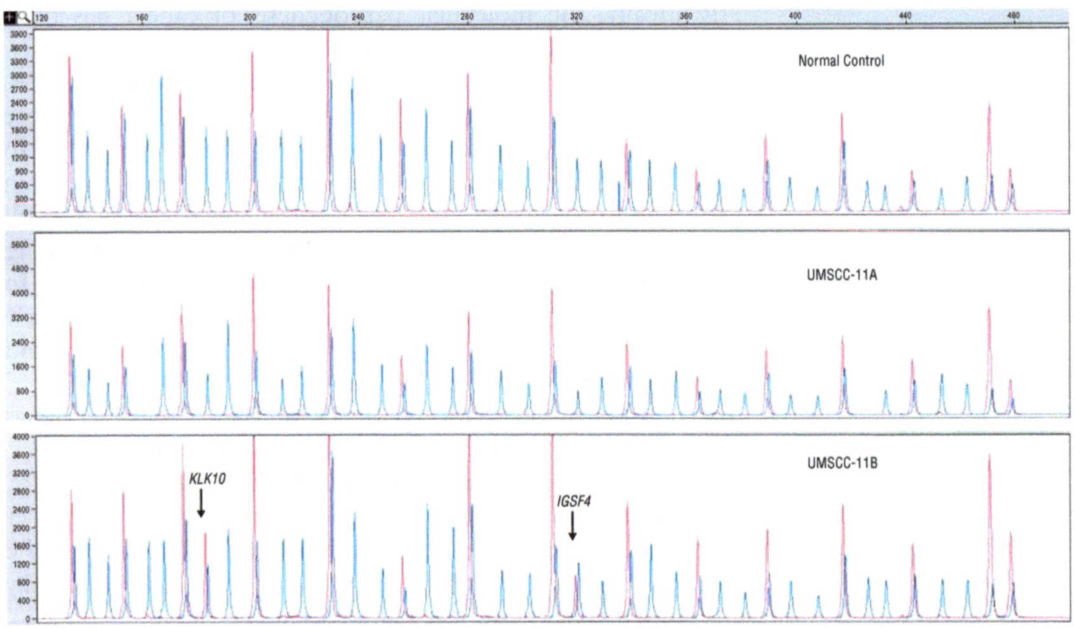

Fig. 2. Multiplex ligation-dependent probe amplification peaks with (*red*) and without (*blue*) *HhaI* for the normal DNA, UMSCC-11A, and UMSCC-11B (46).

(A) and recurrent or metastatic (B) UMSCC-11A/11B, UMSCC-17A/17B, and UMSCC-81A/81B cell lines (Figs. 2–4) (46).

The most frequently hypermethylated genes were *APC* and *IGSF4* observed in 3/6 cell lines, and *TP73* and *DAPK1* observed in 2/6. In recurrent/metastatic cell lines, promoter hypermethylation of *KLK10*, *IGSF4*, *TIMP3*, *FHIT* and *TP73* were a disease progression event, indicating complete abrogation of tumor suppressor function for *KLK10*, *IGSF4*, and *TIMP3*, and gene silencing of one of two copies of *TP73*. Hypermethylation of *IGSF4*,

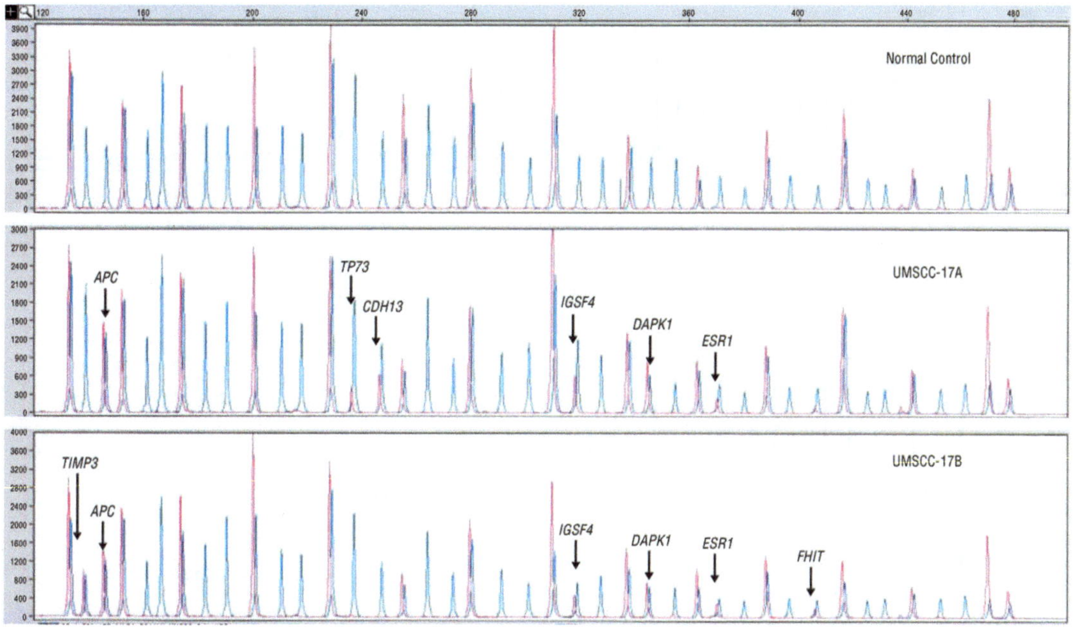

Fig. 3. Multiplex ligation-dependent probe amplification peaks with (*red*) and without (*blue*) *Hha*I for the normal DNA, UMSCC-17A, and UMSCC-17B (46).

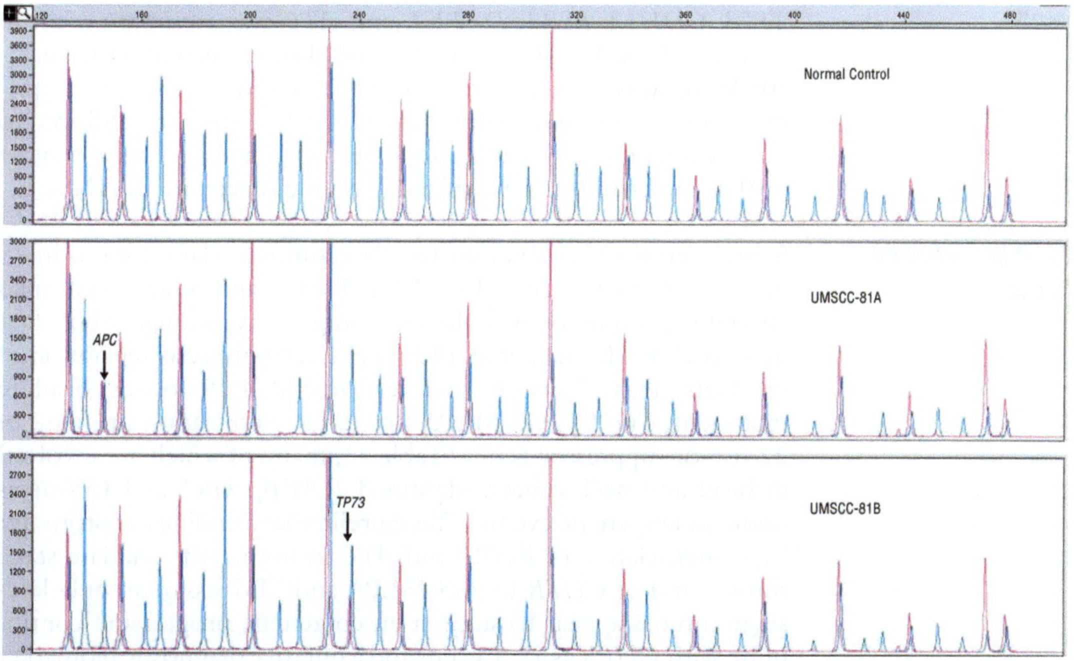

Fig. 4. Multiplex ligation-dependent probe amplification peaks with (*red*) and without (*blue*) *Hha*I for the normal DNA, UMSCC-81A, and UMSCC-81B (46).

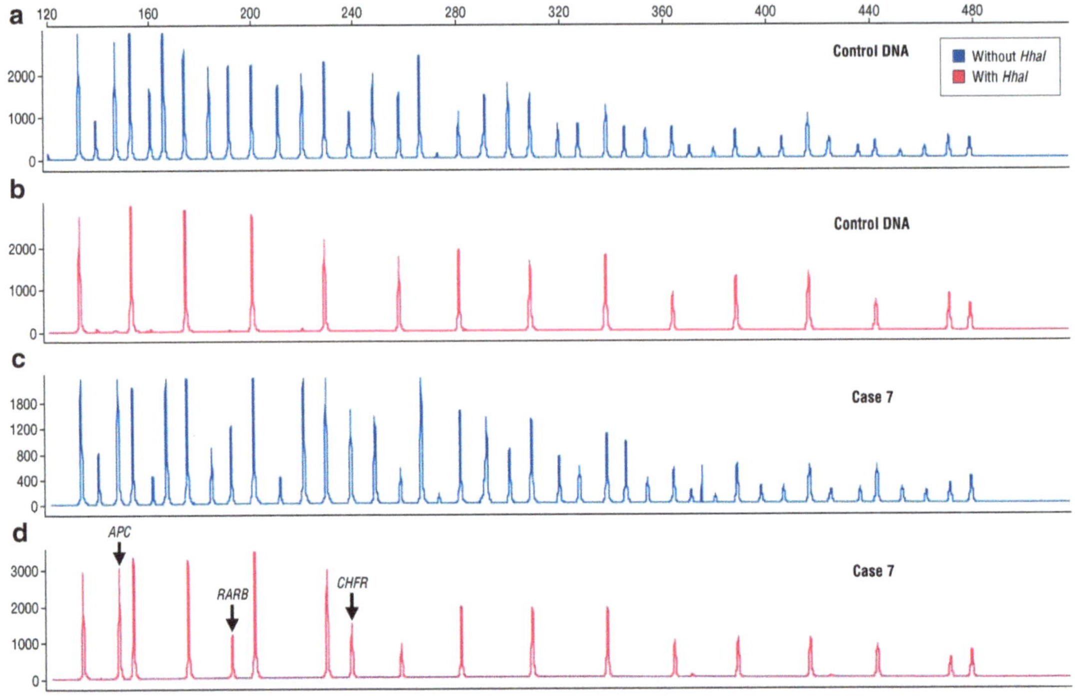

Fig. 5. Methylation-specific multiplex ligation-dependent probe amplification probe mix without (**a**, **c**) and with (**b**, **d**) *HhaI* enzyme. Fifteen peaks are seen in the control DNA sample (**b**). The methylation peaks in case 7 (**d**) that are not present in the control DNA (**b**) represent promoter hypermethylation of *APC*, *RARB*, and *CHFR* (29).

TP73, *CDH13*, *ESR1*, *DAPK1*, and *APC* was a primary event in UMSCC-17A (Fig. 3). Gene silencing through promoter hypermethylation was observed in 5/6 cell lines and contributed to primary and progressive events in HNSCC (46). In addition to genetic alterations of gains and losses, epigenetic events appear to further undermine a destabilized genomic repertoire in HNSCC.

2.2. Primary HNSCC Tissue

Subsequently (29), we evaluated aberrant methylation status in 28 primary HNSCC using MS-MLPA (Figs. 5 and 6) and confirmed aberrant promoter methylation using conventional MSP first described by Herman et al. (49) (gel electrophoresis separation of products, Figs. 7 and 8, and real-time PCR following bisulfite treatment, Fig. 9). MS-MLPA promoter methylation profiling of 22 tumor suppressor genes (Table 1), many of which are involved in head and neck cancer, identified *RARβ*, *APC*, and *CHFR* as frequent epigenetic events. These preliminary findings of promoter hypermethylation of *RARβ* and *APC* in both early- and late-stage tumors and of *CHFR* by MS-MLPA and MSP assays in only late-stage tumors appear to suggest an epigenetic progression continuum, with *CHFR* as a late event and a putative diagnostic biomarker for late-stage disease. The alterations of *RARβ*, *APC*, and *CHFR* via DNA hypermethylation have several implications in HNSCC.

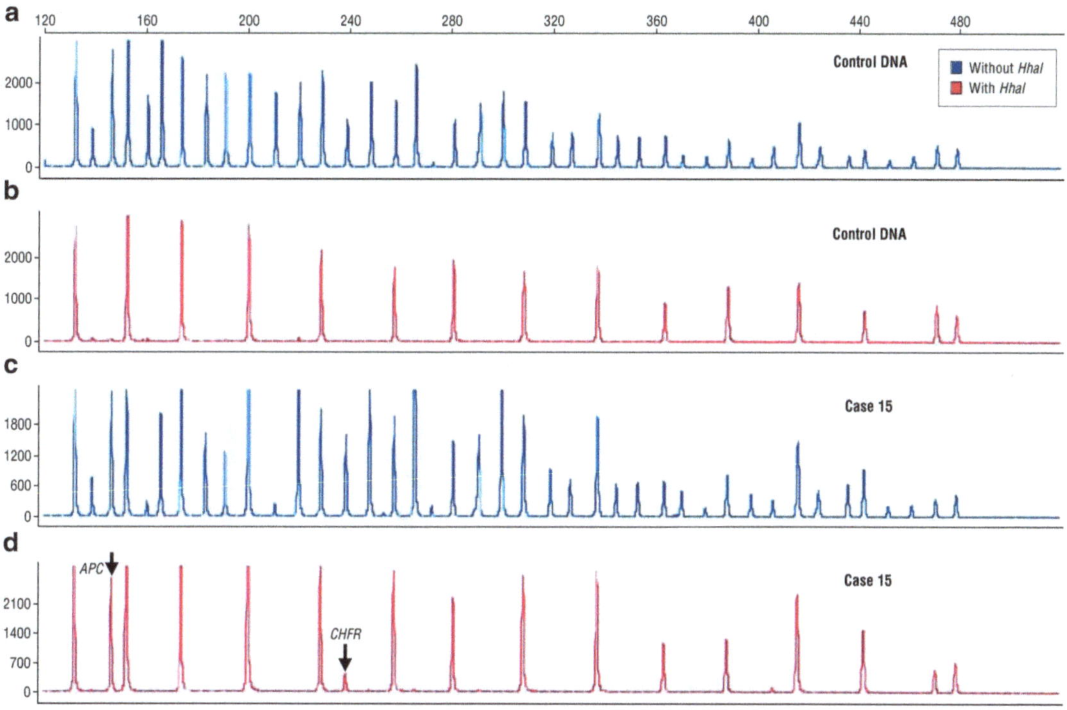

Fig. 6. Methylation-specific multiplex ligation-dependent probe amplification probe mix without (**a**, **c**) and with (**b**, **d**) *Hha*I enzyme in the control DNA and DNA from case 15. Methylation of *APC* and *CHFR* is seen in case 15 with *Hha*I digestion (**d**) (29).

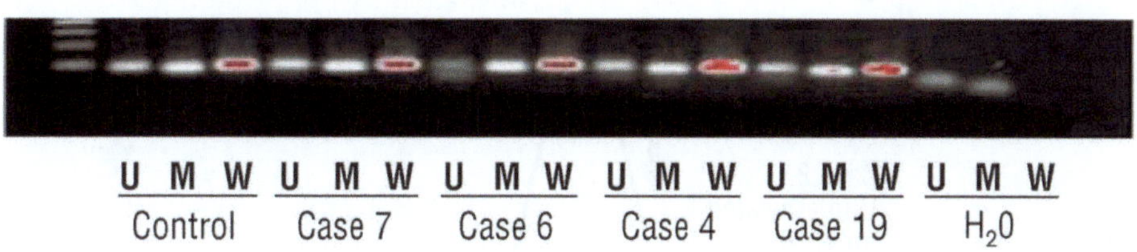

Fig. 7. Gel electrophoresis methylation-specific polymerase chain reaction results for *RARB*. Note the presence of the 84-bp methylation (M) band and the unmethylated (U) 94-bp product in cases 4, 6, 7, and 19; the latter indicates an admixture of normal and tumor cells. *H_2O* indicates water; *W*, wild types (29).

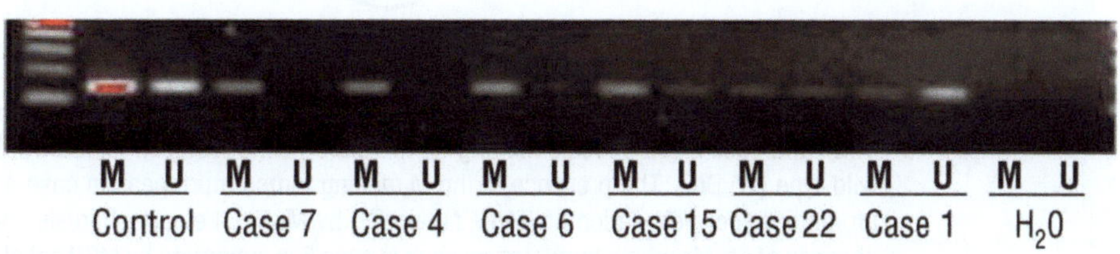

Fig. 8. Gel electrophoresis methylation-specific polymerase chain reaction results for *CHFR*. Note the presence of the 155-bp methylation (M) band in cases 1, 4, 6, 7, 15, and 22 and the unmethylated (U) 155-bp product in cases 1, 15, and 22; the latter indicates an admixture of normal and tumor cells. *H_2O* indicates water (29).

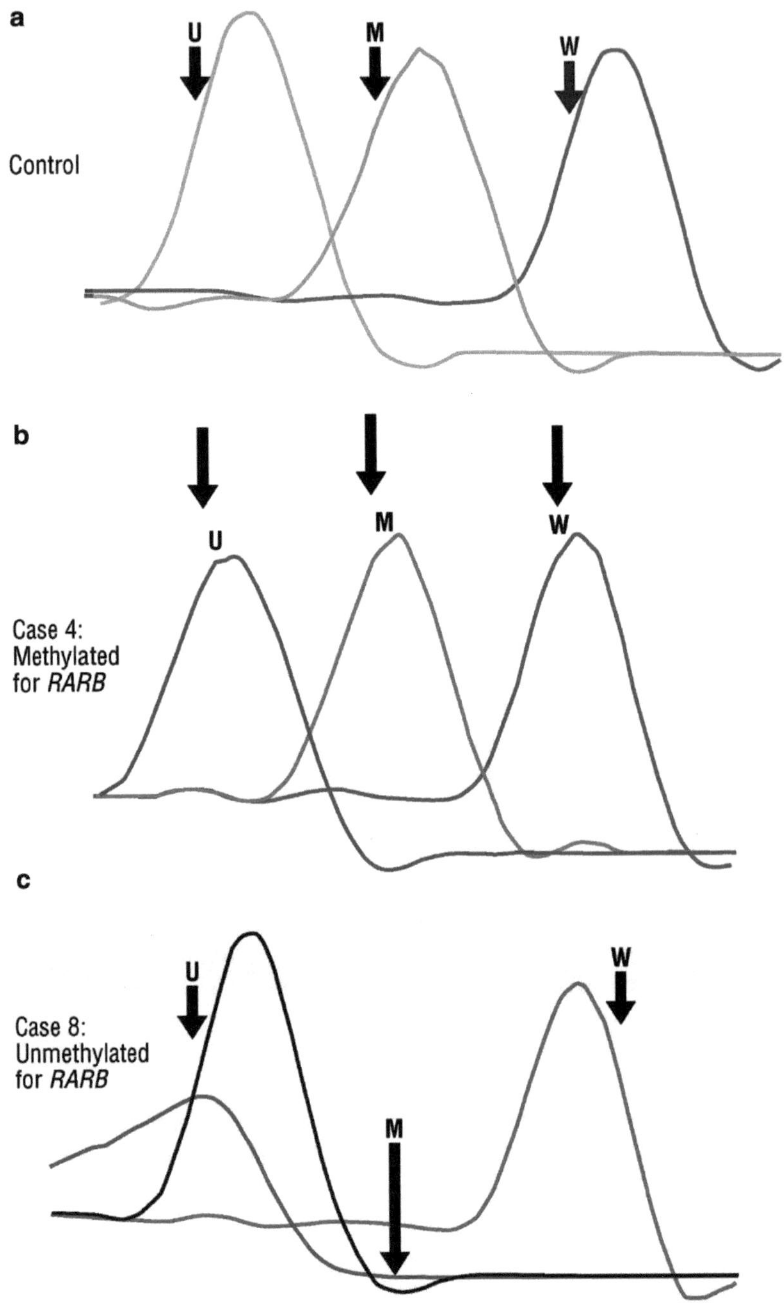

Fig. 9. Real-time polymerase chain reaction (PCR) with methylation-specific PCR (MSP) for methylated (M) and unmethylated (U) primers for *RARB* for the control specimen (**a**), case 4 (**b**), and case 8 (**c**). Specific melting temperature peaks are seen for control U, M, and wild-type (W) DNA. The presence of the M melting temperature peak in case 4 indicates promoter hypermethylation of *RARB*, supported by MSP gel electrophoresis (Fig. 4). The absence of an *M* melting temperature peak in case 8 is supported by MSP gel electrophoresis and MS multiplex ligation-dependent probe amplification (29).

Table 1
Methylation-specific MLPA probe panel (ME001)

#	Gene probe	Chrom loc	#	Gene probe	Chrom loc	#	Gene probe	Chrom loc
1	***TP73***	01p36		*CDK6*	07q21.3		*PAH*	12q23
2	***CASP8***	02q22.3	12	***CDKN2A***	09p21	21	***CHFR***	12q24.33
3	***VHL***	03p25.3	13	***CDKN2B***	09p21	22	***BRCA2***	13q12.3
4	***RARB***	03p24	14	***DAPK1***	09q34.1		*BRCA2*	13q12.3
5	[a]***MLH1***	03p21.1		*AI651963*	10p14		*MLH3*	14q24.3
6	***MLH1***	03p21.1		*CREM*	10p12.1		*TSC2*	16p13.3
	CTNNB1	03p22	15	***PTEN***	10q23.3		*CDH1*	16q22.1
7	[a]***RASSF1***	03p21.3	16	***CD44***	11p12	23	***CDH13***	16q24.2
8	***RASSF1***	03p21.3	17	***GSTP1***	11q13	24	***HIC1***	17p13.3
9	***FHIT***	03p14.2	18	***ATM***	11q23	25	***BRCA1***	17q21
	CASR	03q21	19	***IGSF4***	11q23		*BCL2*	18q21.3
10	***APC***	05q21		*TNFRSF1A*	12p13		*KLK3*	19q13
11	***ESR1***	06q25.1		*TNFRSF7*	12p13	26	***TIMP3***	22q12.3
	PARK2	06q26	20	***CDKN1B***	12q13.1			

Bolded = probes with *Hha*I site ($n = 26$ probes)
[a] Genes with multiple probes in the promoter region

Decreased expression of *RARβ* has been associated with increased keratinizing squamous differentiation in HNSCC cells and pharmacological doses of retinoid ATRA (9-*cis*-RA) induced RARβ in HNSCC cells, resulting in restoration of a more normal differentiation (52). More importantly, $RAR\beta_2$ silencing by promoter hypermethylation was shown to be an early event in head and neck carcinogenesis, and 5-aza-CdR restored $RAR\beta_2$ inducibility by ATRA in most cell lines (53). The examination of the prevalence and pattern of *CHFR* inactivation in human tumors found CpG methylation-dependent silencing of CHFR expression in 40% of primary colorectal cancers, 53% of colorectal adenomas, and 30% of primary HNSCC (54). We reported *CHFR* as a solely late stage 4 event, occurring in 7/28 HNSCC (29), suggesting a role for *CHFR* in tumor progression with potential utility as a biomarker of late-stage disease. Treatment with the methyltransferase inhibitor 5-aza-2′-deoxycytidine induced reexpression of CHFR (54). Additionally, because cancer cells that lack CHFR expression have been shown to be more susceptible to the microtubule inhibitor Taxol (54), silencing of *CHFR* by methylation can serve as a marker for predicting sensitivity to particular chemotherapeutic agents.

APC (adenomatous polyposis coli), a tumor suppressor gene, was originally implicated in colon cancer. Promoter hypermethylation of *APC* has been reported in 25% of oral cancers (55) and in Barrett's metaplasia and dysplasia (56). In our primary HNSCC cohort (29), *APC*, like *RARβ*, was hypermethylated in early- and late-stage tumors, suggesting DNA methylation of *APC* and *RARβ* as earlier epigenetic events, when compared to *CHFR*. Validation of these findings in larger HNSCC cohorts would further support these genes as relevant epigenetic biomarkers of cancer therapy given the reversible nature of epigenetic gene silencing.

3. Delineating an Epigenetic Continuum in HNSCC

A tissue field of somatic genetic alterations precedes the histopathological phenotypic changes of carcinoma (16). Genomic changes could be of potential use in the diagnosis and prognosis of HNSCC lesions and as markers for cancer risk assessment. Studies of sequential molecular alterations and genetic progression of preinvasive HNSCC have not been clearly defined. A few studies have shown recurring alterations of chromosome 9p21 in the early stages of HNSCC (17–19). However, gene silencing via hypermethylation is still a relatively new idea in the development of HNSCC, and little is known about the contribution of epigenetics to the development of neoplasia, its transformation, progression, and recurrence in HNSCC.

4. Benign Papillomas

Papillomas are benign neoplasms of epithelium on a connective tissue core (57). They can involve the nose and sinuses (sinonasal papillomas—SP) as well as the respiratory tract (respiratory papillomatosis—RP) to include the larynx, trachea, and bronchi. Both SP and RP have a tendency to recur. Recurrent respiratory (laryngeal) papillomatosis (RRP) is an extremely rare condition (58). Inverted SP are associated with invasive squamous cell carcinoma (SCC) (59), and a small percentage of RRP cases also progress to malignancy (60).

Human papilloma virus (HPV) is frequently associated with sinonasal (61, 62) and laryngeal (63–65) papillomas. Most HPV-positive cases of SP are of the inverted type (66). Benign papillomas are preferentially associated with the low-risk HPV types 6 and 11, whereas their malignant counterparts are exclusively positive for HPV-16 DNA (67). Studies on HPV typing in benign laryngeal papillomas have demonstrated an association of HPV-11 with a more aggressive course of the disease (68, 69). HPV infection in inverted papillomas (70) and in particular HPV-11 infection in RRP (71) may be an early event in a multistep process of malignant transformation.

5. Sinonasal Papillomas

Sinonasal papillomas have been categorized histologically as inverted, fungiform (exophytic), and cylindrical cell papillomas (72). Inverted papillomas are the most commonly occurring sinonasal papillomas followed by exophytic (59). Inverted papillomas are benign, rare sinonasal lesions well known for their local recurrence, invasiveness, and predisposition for malignant transformation. Recurrence rates vary widely, ranging from 6 to 33%, despite management by different surgical treatment options (73). Malignant transformation occurs in 7–10% of cases (59, 74). Morphology is not useful in determining if a lesion will recur or acquire malignant changes. A general belief is that once excised, and in the absence of malignancy in the excised specimen, a recurrence is unlikely to convert to malignancy (75).

Benign inverted papillomas were reported as monoclonal but lacking common genetic alterations associated with squamous head and neck cancer (75). Therefore, we evaluated seven patients with primary and recurrent sinonasal papillomas for aberrant promoter methylation status using MS-MLPA and confirmed aberrant methylation using conventional MSP. We found all seven cases had at least one epigenetic event of aberrant DNA hypermethylation with 10 of the 22 methylation-prone genes being methylated (Table 2). Commonly methylated genes included *CDKN2B*, *CDKN2A*, *TP73*, and *ESR1*. The *CDKN2B* gene, detected by MS-MLPA (Fig. 10), was a consistent target of aberrant methylation and was confirmed by MSP (Fig. 11). Recurrent biopsies from two inverted papilloma cases had common epigenetic events: aberrant methylation of *CDKN2B* and *DAPK1* in case 1 and *CDKN2B* in case 2, underscoring monoclonality for these lesions (76). Inactivation of the *CDKN2B* and *CDKN2A* genes at the genomic and epigenetic level is a frequent event in human oral SCCs (77) and in HNSCC (39, 46, 78). *TP73* and *ESR1* were aberrantly methylated in two of the seven cases. *TP73* is involved in cell cycle regulation and can activate TP53-responsive proteins, inhibit cell growth, and induce apoptosis (79). We have reported *TP73* hypermethylation in HNSCC to be a primary as well as a disease progression event (46). *ESR1* has metastasis suppressor properties in breast cancer cells (80), suggesting a tumor suppressor role (81). *ESR1* is methylated in Barrett's metaplastic and dysplastic samples as well as in some

Table 2
Clinical characteristics of cohort with MS-MLPA results

	Biopsies	Location	*TIMP3*	*APC*	*CDKN2A*	*MLH1*	*CDKN2B*	*TP73*	*FANCD2*	*DAPK1*	*ESR1*	*GSTP1*
Case 1—IP	1—[reference]	Nasal	M			M	M	M	M	M		
	2–10 months	Ethmoid and nasal maxillary-block 3					M			M	M	
	2–10 months	Ethmoid and nasal maxillary-block 4					M					
Case 2—IP	1—[reference]	Nasal cavity					M					
	2–6 months	Ethmoid sinus			M		M	M				M
Case 3—IP	1—[reference]	Ethmoid sinus					M					
Case 4—IP/EP	1—[reference]	Nasal mucosa					M				M	
Case 5—IP/EP	1—[reference]	Nasal vestibule					M					
Case 6—EP	1—[reference]	Frontal sinus			M		M					
Case 7—EP	1—[reference]	Nasal cavity		M								
		Total	1/7	1/7	2/7	1/7	6/7	2/7	1/7	1/7	2/7	1/7

EP exophytic papilloma; *IP/EP* inverted and exophytic papilloma; *IP* inverted papilloma; *M* methylated (76)

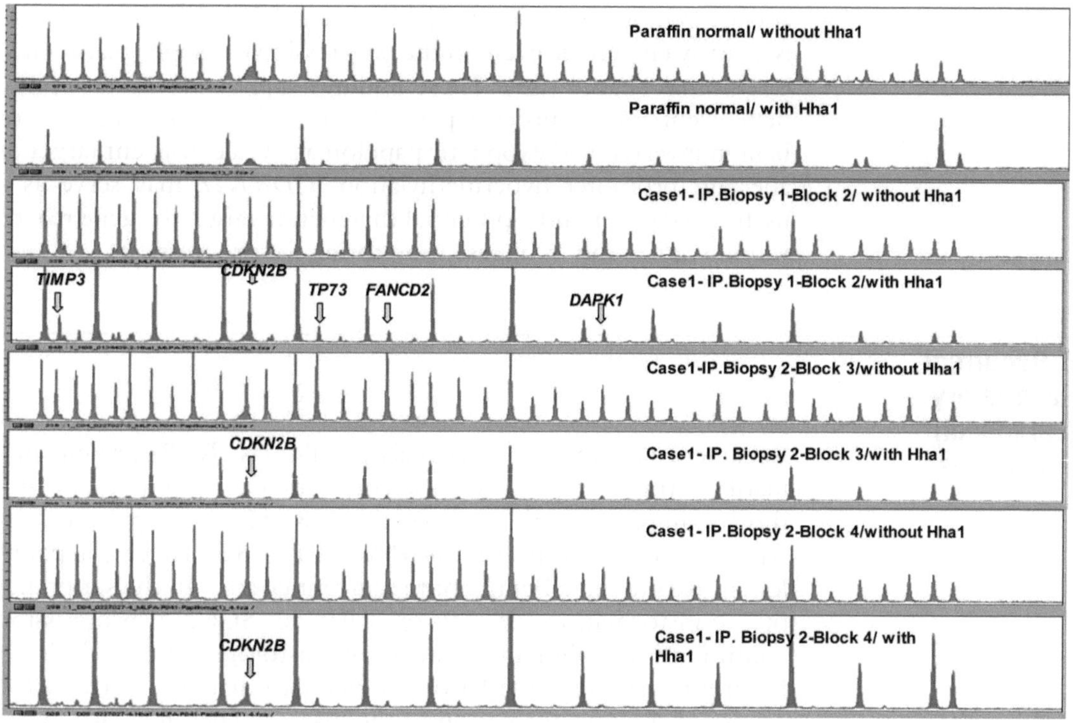

Fig. 10. MS-MLPA probe mix with and without *HhaI* enzyme (DNA sequencer—ABI 3130). Results for case 1—biopsy 1 block 2 and biopsy 2 blocks 3 and 4. Note 15 peaks in the control DNA sample with *HhaI*. Presence of a peak in biopsies 1 and 2 (blocks 3 and 4) not present in the control DNA is that of aberrantly methylated *CDKN2B* gene (76).

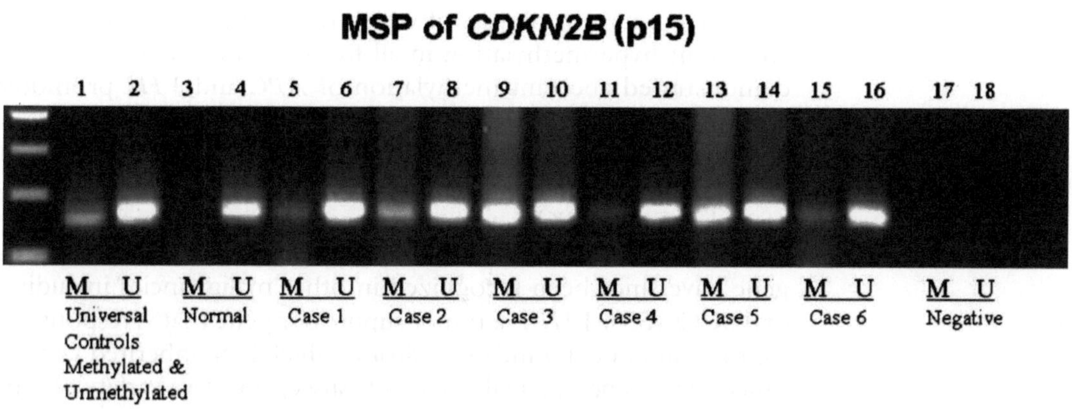

Fig. 11. Methylation-specific PCR (MSP) confirmation of aberrant methylation detected by MS-MLPA for *CDKN2B*. *Lane 1*: universal methylated control; *Lane 2*: universal unmethylated control; *Lanes 3 and 4*: normal control, note presence of only unmethylated PCR product; *Lanes 5–16* span cases 1–6. Note presence of methylated and unmethylated product, the latter indicating admixture of normal and papilloma cells; *Lanes 17 and 18*: negative control (76).

adenocarcinoma samples, suggesting that DNA hypermethylation is an early epigenetic event in the progression of esophageal adenocarcinomas (EAC) (56). These findings support a role for epigenetic events of promoter hypermethylation in the pathogenesis of benign inverted and exophytic papillomas. As a consistent target of aberrant promoter hypermethylation, *CDKN2B* may serve as a useful biomarker and a potential therapeutic target for gene reactivation studies and in disease monitoring for progression.

6. Recurrent Respiratory (Laryngeal) Papillomas

Recurrent respiratory (laryngeal) papillomas (RRP) present primarily as tiny warts on the vocal cords and can be potentially life-threatening due to airway obstruction (58). Human papillomavirus types 6 and 11 account for 80–90% of RRP (82). Laryngeal papillomas usually run a benign but recurrent course. In the spontaneous transformation of RP or RRP to SCC, a progression continuum to malignancy may not be histologically and clinically apparent, making these lesions difficult to diagnose early in the course of the transformation of the disease. Therefore, we investigated alterations in DNA methylation in recurrent biopsies from patients with RRP to assess the contribution of promoter methylation-mediated epigenetic events in RRP tumorigenesis. Samples from 15 subjects who had 1–6 subsequent biopsies were interrogated by MS-MLPA. Aberrant methylation of *CDKN2B* and *APC* genes were most frequent, occurring in 8 of 14 cases, with dissimilar epigenetic events in the remaining cases (Table 3). There were five cases that had at least one abnormally methylated gene in a recurrent biopsy, of which the *CDKN2B* gene showed consistent hypermethylation in all five cases (Table 4). One case demonstrated aberrant methylation of *APC* and *VHL* promoter regions in all three biopsies.

In precancerous oral tissues (78), aberrant methylation of *CDKN2B* has been implicated as an early event in the pathogenesis of oral lesions. *APC* is a tumor suppressor gene originally implicated in colon cancer. Genetic and epigenetic alterations in this gene have since been recognized in other malignancies including oral SCCs (55). *VHL* is a tumor suppressor gene that is responsible for the von Hippel–Lindau syndrome which is an inherited familial cancer syndrome that makes patients susceptible to a variety of cancers, malignant and benign. It has been found that treatment of methylated *VHL* tumors with a demethylating agent results in reexpression of the *VHL* transcripts (83). Persistence of the same aberrantly methylated gene in 36% of multiple recurrent biopsies (5/14) in our study supports a monoclonal origin for RRP and

Table 3
RRP case summary and methylation status

	Patient no.														
	1[a]	2[a]	3[a]	4[b]	5[a]	6[c]	7[b]	8[a]	9[a]	10[a]	11[b]	12[b]	13[b]	14[a]	15[a]
No. of biopsies	7	6	2	6	4	2	4	2	2	3	3	3	5	2	2
TIMP3[d]							M			M	M	M	M		
APC[d]			M	M	M		M	M					M	M	M
CDKN2A[d]				M	M		M				M	M		M	
MLH1					M		M								
KLK10										M		M			M
MEN1				M											
CDKN2B[d]		M		M	M		M			M	M	M	M		
VHL[d]			M	M							M	M	M		
TP73				M							M		M		
FANCD2				M											
BRCA2	M			M											
IGSF4				M			M								
RASSF1														M	
DAPK1[d]				M					M			M	M		
HIC1[d]				M	M			M			M				
ESR1		M										M			
CDKN1B										M					
BRCA1									M	M					
GSTP1[d]				M	M		M		M						

M methylated
[a] Cases with dissimilar epigenetic events in multiple biopsy specimens
[b] Cases with similar epigenetic events in multiple biopsy specimens
[c] Cases with absence of M genes
[d] Commonly M genes (present in >3 cases)
(48)

permits the tracing of an epigenetic continuum, implicating key tumor suppressor genes in RRP. The high frequency of epigenetic events points to the utilization of gene silencing mechanisms as one of the driving forces behind the growth of recurrent laryngeal papillomas (48).

Table 4
Epigenetically linked recurrent laryngeal papilloma cases

Patient No.	Biopsy	*APC*	*CDKN2B*	*VHL*	*TP73*	*GSTP1*
4	1—[reference]		M			
	2 (10 months)		M		M	
	3 (30 months)		M		M	
7	1—[reference]	M	M			M
	2 (3 months)		M			
	3 (6 months)	M	M			M
11	1—[reference]		M			
	2 (15 months)		M			
12	1—[reference]		M			
	2 (14 months)		M			
13	1—[reference]	M		M		
	2 (1 month)	M	M	M		
	3 (3 months)	M	M	M		

M methylated
(48)

7. Conclusion

Epigenetic events of promoter hypermethylation are emerging as one of the most promising molecular strategies for cancer detection and represent an important tumor-specific marker occurring early in tumor progression.

Acknowledgments

This work was supported by NIH DE 15990 (MJW).

References

1. Jemal, A., Tiwari, R.C., Murray, T., Ghafoor, A., Samuels, A., Ward, E., et al. (2004) Cancer statistics, 2004. *CA Cancer J Clin* 54, 8–29.
2. Costello, J.F.and Plass, C. (2001) Methylation matters. *J Med Genet* 38, 285–303.
3. Li, E., Bestor, T.H., and Jaenisch, R. (1992) Targeted mutation of the DNA methyltransferase gene results in embryonic lethality. *Cell* 69, 915–926.
4. Li, E., Beard, C., and Jaenisch, R. (1993) Role for DNA methylation in genomic imprinting. *Nature* 366, 362–365.
5. Pfeifer, G.P., Tanguay, R.L., Steigerwald, S.D., and Riggs, A.D. (1990) In vivo footprint and methylation analysis by PCR-aided genomic sequencing: comparison of active and inactive X chromosomal DNA at the CpG island and promoter of human PGK-1. *Genes Dev* 4, 1277–1287.

6. Costello, J.F., Fruhwald, M.C., Smiraglia, D.J., Rush, L.J., Robertson, G.P., Gao, X., et al. (2000) Aberrant CpG-island methylation has non-random and tumour-type-specific patterns. *Nat Genet* 24, 132–138.
7. Issa, J.P., Vertino, P.M., Wu, J., Sazawal, S., Celano, P., Nelkin, B.D., et al. (1993) Increased cytosine DNA-methyltransferase activity during colon cancer progression. *J Natl Cancer Inst* 85, 1235–1240.
8. Lin, S.Y., Yeh, K.T., Chen, W.T., Chen, H.C., Chen, S.T., and Chang, J.G. (2004) Promoter CpG methylation of caveolin-1 in sporadic colorectal cancer. *Anticancer Res* 24, 1645–1650.
9. Smiraglia, D.J., Smith, L.T., Lang, J.C., Rush, L.J., Dai, Z., Schuller, D.E., et al. (2003) Differential targets of CpG island hypermethylation in primary and metastatic head and neck squamous cell carcinoma (HNSCC). *J Med Genet* 40, 25–33.
10. Baylin, S.B., Herman, J.G., Graff, J.R., Vertino, P.M., and Issa, J.P. (1998) Alterations in DNA methylation: a fundamental aspect of neoplasia. *Adv Cancer Res* 72, 141–196.
11. Jones, P.A. and Laird, P.W. (1999) Cancer epigenetics comes of age. *Nat Genet* 21, 163–167.
12. Chan, M.F., Liang, G., and Jones, P.A. (2000) Relationship between transcription and DNA methylation. *Curr Top Microbiol Immunol* 249, 75–86.
13. Cairns, P. (2004) Detection of promoter hypermethylation of tumor suppressor genes in urine from kidney cancer patients. *Ann N Y Acad Sci* 1022, 40–43.
14. Kim, H., Kwon, Y.M., Kim, J.S., Lee, H., Park, J.H., Shim, Y.M., et al. (2004) Tumor-specific methylation in bronchial lavage for the early detection of non-small-cell lung cancer. *J Clin Oncol* 22, 2363–2370.
15. Roman-Gomez, J., Jimenez-Velasco, A., Castillejo, J.A., Agirre, X., Barrios, M., Navarro, G., et al. (2004) Promoter hypermethylation of cancer-related genes: a strong independent prognostic factor in acute lymphoblastic leukemia. *Blood* 104, 2492–2498.
16. Sanz-Ortega, J., Saez, M.C., Sierra, E., Torres, A., Balibrea, J.L., Hernando, F., et al. (2001) 3p21, 5q21, and 9p21 allelic deletions are frequently found in normal bronchial cells adjacent to non-small-cell lung cancer, while they are unusual in patients with no evidence of malignancy. *J Pathol* 195, 429–434.
17. Yoo, W.J., Cho, S.H., Lee, Y.S., Park, G.S., Kim, M.S., Kim, B.K., et al. (2004) Loss of heterozygosity on chromosomes 3p,8p,9p and 17p in the progression of squamous cell carcinoma of the larynx. *J Korean Med Sci* 19, 345–351.
18. Sanz-Ortega, J., Valor, C., Saez, M.C., Ortega, L., Sierra, E., Poch, J., et al. (2003) 3p21, 5q21, 9p21 and 17p13 allelic deletions accumulate in the dysplastic spectrum of laryngeal carcinogenesis and precede malignant transformation. *Histol Histopathol* 18, 1053–1057.
19. Papadimitrakopoulou, V.A., Izzo, J., Mao, L., Keck, J., Hamilton, D., Shin, D.M., et al. (2001) Cyclin D1 and p16 alterations in advanced premalignant lesions of the upper aerodigestive tract: role in response to chemoprevention and cancer development. *Clin Cancer Res* 7, 3127–3134.
20. Emilion, G., Langdon, J.D., Speight, P., and Partridge, M. (1996) Frequent gene deletions in potentially malignant oral lesions. *Br J Cancer* 73, 809–813.
21. Roz, L., Wu, C.L., Porter, S., Scully, C., Speight, P., Read, A., et al. (1996) Allelic imbalance on chromosome 3p in oral dysplastic lesions: an early event in oral carcinogenesis. *Cancer Res* 56, 1228–1231.
22. Miracca, E.C., Kowalski, L.P., and Nagai, M.A. (1999) High prevalence of p16 genetic alterations in head and neck tumours. *Br J Cancer* 81, 677–683.
23. Esteller, M., Corn, P.G., Baylin, S.B., and Herman, J.G. (2001) A gene hypermethylation profile of human cancer. *Cancer Res* 61, 3225–3229.
24. Rosas, S.L., Koch, W., da Costa Carvalho, M.G., Wu, L., Califano, J., Westra, W., et al. (2001) Promoter hypermethylation patterns of p16, O6-methylguanine-DNA-methyltransferase, and death-associated protein kinase in tumors and saliva of head and neck cancer patients. *Cancer Res* 61, 939–942.
25. Hasegawa, M., Nelson, H.H., Peters, E., Ringstrom, E., Posner, M., and Kelsey, K.T. (2002) Patterns of gene promoter methylation in squamous cell cancer of the head and neck. *Oncogene* 21, 4231–4236.
26. Viswanathan, M., Tsuchida, N., and Shanmugam, G. (2003) Promoter hypermethylation profile of tumor-associated genes p16, p15, hMLH1, MGMT and E-cadherin in oral squamous cell carcinoma. *Int J Cancer* 105, 41–46.
27. El-Naggar, A.K., Lai, S., Clayman, G., Lee, J.K., Luna, M.A., Goepfert, H., et al. (1997) Methylation, a major mechanism of p16/CDKN2 gene inactivation in head and neck squamous carcinoma. *Am J Pathol* 151, 1767–1774.
28. Sanchez-Cespedes, M., Esteller, M., Wu, L., Nawroz-Danish, H., Yoo, G.H., Koch, W.M., et al. (2000) Gene promoter hypermethylation in tumors and serum of head and neck cancer patients. *Cancer Res* 60, 892–895.

29. Chen, K., Sawhney, R., Khan, M., Benninger, M.S., Hou, Z., Sethi, S., et al. (2007) Methylation of multiple genes as diagnostic and therapeutic markers in primary head and neck squamous cell carcinoma. *Arch Otolaryngol Head Neck Surg* 133, 1131–1138.
30. Zou, C.P., Youssef, E.M., Zou, C.C., Carey, T.E., and Lotan, R. (2001) Differential effects of chromosome 3p deletion on the expression of the putative tumor suppressor RAR beta and on retinoid resistance in human squamous carcinoma cells. *Oncogene* 20, 6820–6827.
31. Xu, X.C., Ro, J.Y., Lee, J.S., Shin, D.M., Hong, W.K., and Lotan, R. (1994) Differential expression of nuclear retinoid receptors in normal, premalignant, and malignant head and neck tissues. *Cancer Res* 54, 3580–3587.
32. Pegg, A.E. (1990) Mammalian O6-alkylguanine-DNA alkyltransferase: regulation and importance in response to alkylating carcinogenic and therapeutic agents. *Cancer Res* 50, 6119-6129.
33. Hirohashi, S. (1998) Inactivation of the E-cadherin-mediated cell adhesion system in human cancers. *Am J Pathol* 153, 333–339.
34. Pollack, J.R., Perou, C.M., Alizadeh, A.A., Eisen, M.B., Pergamenschikov, A., Williams, C.F., et al. (1999) Genome-wide analysis of DNA copy-number changes using cDNA microarrays. *Nat Genet* 23, 41–46.
35. Khan, J., Saal, L.H., Bittner, M.L., Chen, Y., Trent, J.M., and Meltzer, P.S. (1999) Expression profiling in cancer using cDNA microarrays. *Electrophoresis* 20, 223–229.
36. Hanash, S.M., and Teichroew, D. (1998) Mining the human proteome: experience with the human lymphoid protein database. *Electrophoresis* 19, 2004–2009.
37. Soltys, S.G., Le, Q.T., Shi, G., Tibshirani, R., Giaccia, A.J., and Koong, A.C. (2004) The use of plasma surface-enhanced laser desorption/ionization time-of-flight mass spectrometry proteomic patterns for detection of head and neck squamous cell cancers. *Clin Cancer Res* 10, 4806–4812.
38. Smeets, S.J., Braakhuis, B.J., Abbas, S., Snijders, P.J., Ylstra, B., van de Wiel, M.A., et al. (2006) Genome-wide DNA copy number alterations in head and neck squamous cell carcinomas with or without oncogene-expressing human papillomavirus. *Oncogene* 25, 2558–2564.
39. Worsham, M.J., Pals, G., Schouten, J.P., Van Spaendonk, R.M., Concus, A., Carey, T.E., et al. (2003) Delineating genetic pathways of disease progression in head and neck squamous cell carcinoma. *Arch Otolaryngol Head Neck Surg* 129, 702–708.
40. Worsham, M.J., Chen, K.M., Tiwari, N., Pals, G., Schouten, J.P., Sethi, S., et al. (2006) Fine-mapping loss of gene architecture at the CDKN2B (p15INK4b), CDKN2A (p14ARF, p16INK4a), and MTAP genes in head and neck squamous cell carcinoma. *Arch Otolaryngol Head Neck Surg* 132, 409–415.
41. Shaw, R.J., Liloglou, T., Rogers, S.N., Brown, J.S., Vaughan, E.D., Lowe, D., et al. (2006) Promoter methylation of P16, RARbeta, E-cadherin, cyclin A1 and cytoglobin in oral cancer: quantitative evaluation using pyrosequencing. *Br J Cancer* 94, 561–568.
42. Sanchez-Cespedes, M., Okami, K., Cairns, P., and Sidransky, D. (2000) Molecular analysis of the candidate tumor suppressor gene ING1 in human head and neck tumors with 13q deletions. *Genes Chromosomes Cancer* 27, 319–322.
43. Shah, S.I., Yip, L., Greenberg, B., Califano, J.A., Chow, J., Eisenberger, C.F., et al. (2000) Two distinct regions of loss on chromosome arm 4q in primary head and neck squamous cell carcinoma. *Arch Otolaryngol Head Neck Surg* 126, 1073–1076.
44. Sidransky, D. (2000) Circulating DNA. What we know and what we need to learn. *Ann N Y Acad Sci* 906, 1–4.
45. Maruya, S., Issa, J.P., Weber, R.S., Rosenthal, D.I., Haviland, J.C., Lotan, R., et al. (2004) Differential methylation status of tumor-associated genes in head and neck squamous carcinoma: incidence and potential implications. *Clin Cancer Res* 10, 3825–3830.
46. Worsham, M.J., Chen, K.M., Meduri, V., Nygren, A.O., Errami, A., Schouten, J.P., et al. (2006) Epigenetic events of disease progression in head and neck squamous cell carcinoma. *Arch Otolaryngol Head Neck Surg* 132, 668–677.
47. Stephen, J.K., Vaught, L.E., Chen, K.M., Sethi, S., Shah, V., Benninger, M.S., et al. (2007) Epigenetic events underlie the pathogenesis of sinonasal papillomas. *Mod Pathol.*
48. Stephen, J.K., Vaught, L.E., Chen, K.M., Shah, V., Schweitzer, V.G., Gardner, G., et al. (2007) An epigenetically derived monoclonal origin for recurrent respiratory papillomatosis. *Arch Otolaryngol Head Neck Surg* 133, 684–692.
49. Herman, J.G., Graff, J.R., Myohanen, S., Nelkin, B.D., and Baylin, S.B. (1996) Methylation-specific PCR: a novel PCR assay for methylation status of CpG islands. *Proc Natl Acad Sci U S A* 93, 9821–9826.
50. Huang, T.H., Perry, M.R., and Laux, D.E. (1999) Methylation profiling of CpG islands in human breast cancer cells. *Hum Mol Genet* 8, 459–470.

51. Nygren, A.O., Ameziane, N., Duarte, H.M., Vijzelaar, R.N., Waisfisz, Q., Hess, C.J. et al. (2005) Methylation-specific MLPA (MS-MLPA): simultaneous detection of CpG methylation and copy number changes of up to 40 sequences. *Nucleic Acids Res* 33, e128.
52. Wan, H., Oridate, N., Lotan, D., Hong, W.K., and Lotan, R. (1999) Overexpression of retinoic acid receptor beta in head and neck squamous cell carcinoma cells increases their sensitivity to retinoid-induced suppression of squamous differentiation by retinoids. *Cancer Res* 59, 3518–3526.
53. Youssef, E.M., Lotan, D., Issa, J.P., Wakasa, K., Fan, Y.H., Mao, L., et al. (2004) Hypermethylation of the retinoic acid receptor-beta(2) gene in head and neck carcinogenesis. *Clin Cancer Res* 10, 1733–1742.
54. Toyota, M., Sasaki, Y., Satoh, A., Ogi, K., Kikuchi, T., Suzuki, H., et al. (2003) Epigenetic inactivation of CHFR in human tumors. *Proc Natl Acad Sci U S A* 100, 7818–7823.
55. Uesugi, H., Uzawa, K., Kawasaki, K., Shimada, K., Moriya, T., Tada, A., et al. (2005) Status of reduced expression and hypermethylation of the APC tumor suppressor gene in human oral squamous cell carcinoma. *Int J Mol Med* 15, 597–602.
56. Eads, C.A., Lord, R.V., Kurumboor, S.K., Wickramasinghe, K., Skinner, M.L., Long, T.I. et al. (2000) Fields of aberrant CpG island hypermethylation in Barrett's esophagus and associated adenocarcinoma. *Cancer Res* 60, 5021–5026.
57. Capper, J.W., Bailey, C.M., and Michaels, L. (1983) Squamous papillomas of the larynx in adults. A review of 63 cases. *Clin Otolaryngol Allied Sci* 8, 109–119.
58. Bauman, N.M.and Smith, R.J. (1996) Recurrent respiratory papillomatosis. *Pediatr Clin North Am* 43, 1385–1401.
59. Batsakis, J.G.and Suarez, P. (2001) Schneiderian papillomas and carcinomas: a review. *Adv Anat Pathol* 8, 53–64.
60. Doyle, D.J., Henderson, L.A., LeJeune, F.E., Jr., and Miller, R.H. (1994) Changes in human papillomavirus typing of recurrent respiratory papillomatosis progressing to malignant neoplasm. *Arch Otolaryngol Head Neck Surg* 120, 1273–1276.
61. Buchwald, C., Franzmann, M.B., Jacobsen, G.K., and Lindeberg, H. (1995) Human papillomavirus (HPV) in sinonasal papillomas: a study of 78 cases using in situ hybridization and polymerase chain reaction. *Laryngoscope* 105, 66–71.
62. Brandwein, M., Steinberg, B., Thung, S., Biller, H., Dilorenzo, T., and Galli, R. (1989) Human papillomavirus 6/11 and 16/18 in Schneiderian inverted papillomas. In situ hybridization with human papillomavirus RNA probes. *Cancer* 63, 1708–1713.
63. Mounts, P., Shah, K.V., and Kashima, H. (1982) Viral etiology of juvenile- and adult-onset squamous papilloma of the larynx. *Proc Natl Acad Sci U S A* 79, 5425–5429.
64. Gabbott, M., Cossart, Y.E., Kan, A., Konopka, M., Chan, R., and Rose, B.R. (1997) Human papillomavirus and host variables as predictors of clinical course in patients with juvenile-onset recurrent respiratory papillomatosis. *J Clin Microbiol* 35, 3098–3103.
65. Gissmann, L., Wolnik, L., Ikenberg, H., Koldovsky, U., Schnurch, H.G., and zur Hausen, H. (1983) Human papillomavirus types 6 and 11 DNA sequences in genital and laryngeal papillomas and in some cervical cancers. *Proc Natl Acad Sci U S A* 80, 560–563.
66. Syrjanen, K.J. (2003) HPV infections in benign and malignant sinonasal lesions. *J Clin Pathol* 56, 174–181.
67. Syrjanen, S., Happonen, R.P., Virolainen, E., Siivonen, L., and Syrjanen, K. (1987) Detection of human papillomavirus (HPV) structural antigens and DNA types in inverted papillomas and squamous cell carcinomas of the nasal cavities and paranasal sinuses. *Acta Otolaryngol* 104, 334–341.
68. Hartley, C., Hamilton, J., Birzgalis, A.R., and Farrington, W.T. (1994) Recurrent respiratory papillomatosis--the Manchester experience, 1974-1992. *J Laryngol Otol* 108, 226–229.
69. Lie, E.S., Karlsen, F., and Holm, R. (1996) Presence of human papillomavirus in squamous cell laryngeal carcinomas. A study of thirty-nine cases using polymerase chain reaction and in situ hybridization. *Acta Otolaryngol* 116, 900–905.
70. Katori, H., Nozawa, A., and Tsukuda, M. (2005) Markers of malignant transformation of sinonasal inverted papilloma. *Eur J Surg Oncol* 31, 905–911.
71. Lele, S.M., Pou, A.M., Ventura, K., Gatalica, Z., and Payne, D. (2002) Molecular events in the progression of recurrent respiratory papillomatosis to carcinoma. *Arch Pathol Lab Med* 126, 1184–1188.
72. Hyams, V.J. (1971) Papillomas of the nasal cavity and paranasal sinuses. A clinicopathological study of 315 cases. *Ann Otol Rhinol Laryngol* 80, 192–206.
73. Wormald, P.J., Ooi, E., van Hasselt, C.A., and Nair, S. (2003) Endoscopic removal of sinonasal inverted papilloma including endoscopic medial maxillectomy. *Laryngoscope* 113, 867–873.

74. Lawson, W., Kaufman, M.R., and Biller, H.F. (2003) Treatment outcomes in the management of inverted papilloma: an analysis of 160 cases. *Laryngoscope* 113, 1548–1556.

75. Califano, J., Koch, W., Sidransky, D., and Westra, W.H. (2000) Inverted sinonasal papilloma : a molecular genetic appraisal of its putative status as a Precursor to squamous cell carcinoma. *Am J Pathol* 156, 333–337.

76. Stephen, J.K., Vaught, L.E., Chen, K.M., Sethi, S., Shah, V., Benninger, M.S., et al. (2007) Epigenetic events underlie the pathogenesis of sinonasal papillomas. *Mod Pathol* 20, 1019–1027.

77. Yeh, K.T., Chang, J.G., Lin, T.H., Wang, Y.F., Tien, N., Chang, J.Y., et al. (2003) Epigenetic changes of tumor suppressor genes, P15, P16, VHL and P53 in oral cancer. *Oncol Rep* 10, 659–663.

78. Shintani, S., Nakahara, Y., Mihara, M., Ueyama, Y., and Matsumura, T. (2001) Inactivation of the p14(ARF), p15(INK4B) and p16(INK4A) genes is a frequent event in human oral squamous cell carcinomas. *Oral Oncol* 37, 498–504.

79. Kaghad, M., Bonnet, H., Yang, A., Creancier, L., Biscan, J.C., Valent, A., et al. (1997) Monoallelically expressed gene related to p53 at 1p36, a region frequently deleted in neuroblastoma and other human cancers. *Cell* 90, 809–819.

80. Garcia, M., Derocq, D., Freiss, G., and Rochefort, H. (1992) Activation of estrogen receptor transfected into a receptor-negative breast cancer cell line decreases the metastatic and invasive potential of the cells. *Proc Natl Acad Sci U S A* 89, 11538–11542.

81. Issa, J.P., Ottaviano, Y.L., Celano, P., Hamilton, S.R., Davidson, N.E., and Baylin, S.B. (1994) Methylation of the oestrogen receptor CpG island links ageing and neoplasia in human colon. *Nat Genet* 7, 536–540.

82. Duggan, M.A., Lim, M., Gill, M.J., and Inoue, M. (1990) HPV DNA typing of adult-onset respiratory papillomatosis. *Laryngoscope* 100, 639–642.

83. Herman, J.G., Latif, F., Weng, Y., Lerman, M.I., Zbar, B., Liu, S., et al. (1994) Silencing of the VHL tumor-suppressor gene by DNA methylation in renal carcinoma. *Proc Natl Acad Sci U S A* 91, 9700–9704.

Chapter 12

Epigenome and DNA Methylation in Oral Squamous Cell Carcinoma

Mario Pérez-Sayáns García and Abel García-García

Abstract

Epigenetics studies and defines inherited changes in gene expression that are not encoded in the DNA sequence. The most studied epigenetic change in mammalian DNA is cytosine methylation in CpG dinucleotide areas. The other main group in epigenetic changes includes the posttranslational modifications of histones, mainly phosphorylation, deacetylation changes, and in the ubiquitinylation status. Oral squamous cell carcinoma is the most common malignancy of the oral cavity, and epigenetic changes are very common, as described in this chapter. Alterations in the DNA methylation status resulting from exposure to environmental stress agents have been documented even before birth. Although many epigenetic markers are potentially reversible, the mechanism still remains unclear and many epigenetic changes persist across cell lines and the life of the organism.

Key words: Epigenetics, Oral squamous cell carcinoma, Histones, Deacetylation, Hypermethylation

1. Introduction

Epigenetics studies and defines inherited changes in gene expression that are not encoded in the DNA sequence (1, 2). The most studied epigenetic change in mammalian DNA is cytosine methylation in CpG dinucleotide areas (cytosine residues in nucleotides). The other main group in epigenetic changes includes the posttranslational modifications of histones, mainly phosphorylation, deacetylation changes, and in the ubiquitinylation status (3, 4). Mechanisms frequently act together modifying the structure and function of chromatin. DNA methylation is a covalent biochemical modification of the mammalian genome, occurring predominantly in cytosine bases located in position 5′ to guanosine(5). Methylation turns off gene expression preventing the binding of transcription factors,

Ramona G. Dumitrescu and Mukesh Verma (eds.), *Cancer Epigenetics: Methods and Protocols*, Methods in Molecular Biology, vol. 863, DOI 10.1007/978-1-61779-612-8_12, © Springer Science+Business Media, LLC 2012

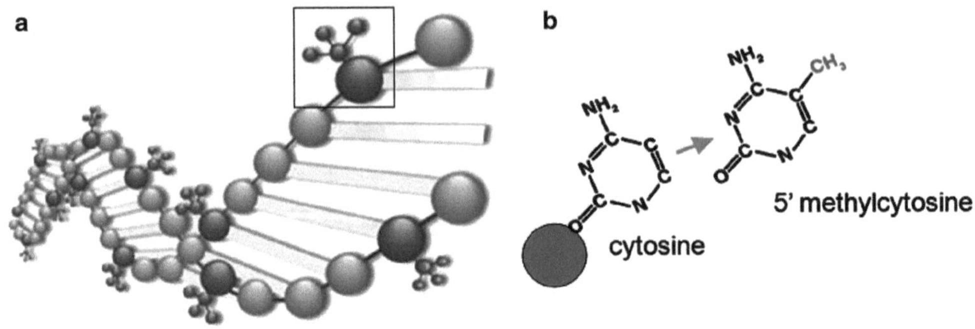

Fig. 1. (**a**) DNA methylation occurs on cytisine residue when it appears in the form of CG dinucleotide. (**b**) CpG island methylation consists of the addition of a methyl group to the 5′ of the cytosine in the region of promoter genes preventing DNA transcription.

even in normal cells (Fig. 1). While genetic aberrations change the expression altering the sequences of base pairs of adenine (A)-thymine (T) and cytosine (C)-guanine (G), epigenetic modifications do not affect the underlying base pair sequence (6).

CpGs are underrepresented regions in the genome; there are approximately 45,000 islands. Moreover, the regions rich in CpGs are not casually distributed throughout the genome but appear more frequently in the promoter regions and in the first exons of specific genes (7, 8).

The enzymes involved in DNA methylation include DNA methyltransferases (DNMTs) that establish and maintain the pattern of DNA methylation using S-adenosyl methionine (SAM) as a methyl group donor (9). When DNA is methylated, these methyl groups protrude from the cytosine nucleotide into the major groove of DNA, displacing the transcription factors that normally would be attached to DNA (10). Exhibited methylated sites attract methyl-binding proteins, the domain of methyl-CpG-binding proteins (MBD) involved in reading and recognition of methylated sites, affecting chromatin condensation by recruiting the deacetylase of histones that covalently modify the tails of histone proteins (4, 9). Histone deacetylation (HDAC) may lead to proteins with a positive charge that interacts with the DNA producing a negative close in structure to repress gene transcription and silencing (6, 11, 12) (Fig. 2).

Besides deacetylation, lysine methylation of histones is also involved in gene regulation. The combination of histone modification and acetylation is known as the "histone code" (13, 14).

The modification of histones results in gene silencing and chromatin compaction (12, 15). If chromatin is condensed, closely united, the factors involved in gene expression cannot access DNA. On the contrary, if chromatin is chemically modified and remains loose, with a more open pattern, the genes are turned on (4, 8).

It has always been believed that both alleles of tumor suppressor genes must be altered by mutations or deletions to be inactivated.

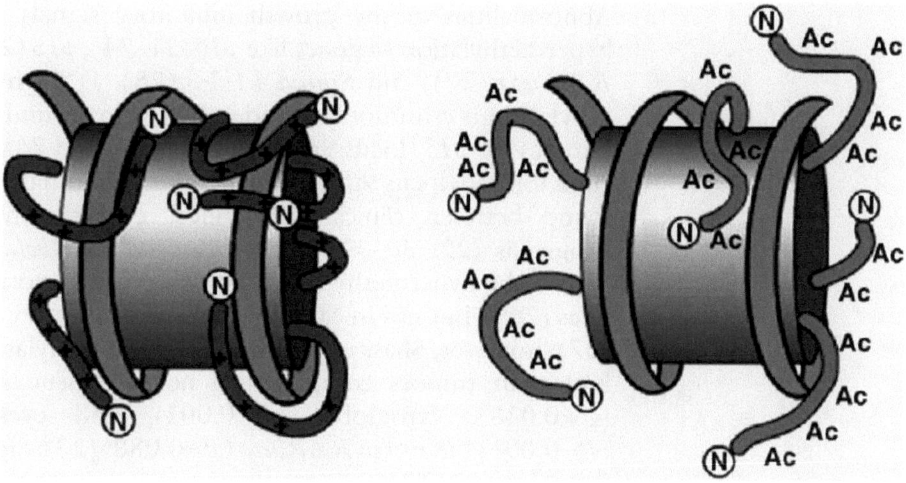

Fig. 2. Deacetylated nucleosome with tight structure (*left*) and acetylated nucleosome with loose structure (*right*) (62).

Gene silencing is possible in the absence of genetic changes, which suggests a new model of inactivation involving hypermethylation (16). This type of epigenetic change is called gene imprinting where the modification occurs only in one of the alleles of a gene and is traditionally associated with the X chromosome, aiming to regulate the gene dosage in men and women (9). Loss of imprinting (LOI) is associated with malignancy predisposition of genes associated with tumors, such as insulin-like growth factor 2 in gastric cancer, *PEG10* in hepatocellular carcinomas, or *p57KIP2* in head and neck squamous cell carcinoma (17). Such modifications appear to be associated with oropharyngeal cancers in young nonsmokers and nondrinkers; this has traditionally been called "bad genes." It is very important to take this into account for possible oral squamous cell carcinoma (OSCC) preventive strategies (18).

2. DNA Hypermethylation in Head and Neck Squamous Cell Carcinoma

Hanahan and Weinberg described six distinctive features that repeat themselves in all tumors, which they called "hallmarks of cancer." These were later modified by Choi et al. (19, 20):

(a) *Abnormalities in growth inhibitory signals*: retinoblastoma gene (*Rb*), *p53*, *p21*^{WAF1}, *p16*^{INK4a}, and *p15*

(b) *Acquisition of stimulating signals for self-sufficient growth*: for example, *ras* oncogene (especially *RASSF1A*)

(c) *Avoidance of apoptosis*: *p14*

(d) *Angiogenesis*: von Hippel-Lindau suppressor gene (*VHL* gene) and *p73*

(e) *Invasion and metastasis*: *ABO gene*

(a) Abnormalities in the growth inhibitory signals include hypermethylation of genes like *p16* (21–24), *p15* (25, 26), *RARbeta* (27), and *Sigma 14-3-3* (28). DNA hypermethylation is commonly found in OSCC in around 30% of samples for *p15* (locus 9p21) (29) and around 76% of the cases for *p16* (locus 9p21) (22), but no relationship has been found between clinical-pathological characteristics and prognosis (22, 30–32). In the case of *RARbeta* (locus 3p24), the hypermethylation appears linked to normal cell lines (26%) but not in cases of dysplasia or primary tumors (27); however, Shaw et al. found that the methylation was higher in tumors compared to normal tissue for *p16* ($P=0.048$), cytoglobin ($P=0.002$), and cyclin A1 ($P=0.001$) but not in *RARbeta* ($P=0.088$) (23). Sigma14-3-3 (locus 22q12) modifies the signals of glucocorticoids, and it has been discovered that its inactivation occurs by epigenetic hypermethylation rather than genetic mutations. Their alterations are a rare event and not always associated with *p53* mutations although with a reduced expression of the gene encoding cyclin D1 (33).

(b) Epigenetic alterations leading to the acquisition of self-sufficient growth stimulation signals in HNSCC (head and neck squamous cell carcinoma) include hypermethylation of ras oncogene, specifically *RASSF1A* (locus 3p21) (34, 35). Tran et al. found 93% hypermethylation in OSCC (36). Recently, hypermethylation of *RASSF2* has been observed in OSCC (35, 37).

(c) Alterations in genes involved in apoptosis, including *p14* gene (locus 9p21) whose hypermethylation has been associated with tumor pathogenesis in malignant tumors of the salivary glands, showing gene silencing in 31% of samples (38). In another study, surprisingly, *p14* methylation was associated with good tumor prognosis (26). *DAP-kinase* gene located at 19q34 locus, encodes a protein that has a p53-dependent proapoptotic effect. Several studies have found a hypermethylated pattern in HNSCC (39), in some cases reaching 68.3% (40).

(d) During angiogenesis, methylation of *VHL* and *p73* genes was observed in oral tumors. *VHL*, located at locus 3p26–25, is an angiogenesis suppressor gene, which has been found hypermethylated in OSCC with a relatively low frequency (4%) (41). The *p73* protein is related to apoptosis and angiogenesis inhibition; its gene methylation rarely appears in oral tumors (2%) (27).

(e) Tissue invasion, a process always inherent in OSCC and distant metastasis, includes epigenetic modifications in genes that encode E-cadherin (locus 16q22), the *ABO* blood group gene (9q34 locus), *IKKalpha* (I kappa B kinase-alpha, locus 10q24–q25), and *Syk* (spleen tyrosine kinase, locus 9q22). E-cadherin is closely linked to intercellular adhesion, and its loss of expression is linked to tumor invasiveness. Hypermethylation of *E-cadherin* gene has been demonstrated with a frequency of 46%, and this methylation has been associated with adverse histologic grades and poor survival (42–46). The ABO group is associated with mobility-related glycosylation of tumor cells through loss of expression of AB antigen, the AB allele, or allele O (47). IKKalpha shows an expression in the nucleus of the basal cells of normal oral mucosa, while the methylated form is marginally expressed or absent in 32.8% of OSCC (48). *Syk* is silenced in 62% of OSCC cases, by an epigenetic mechanism facilitating tumor metastatic ability (49).

In regard to markers associated with genomic instability in OSCC, we found hypermethylated patterns in the genes *DCC* (deleted in colorectal cancer, locus 18q21), *hMLH1* (MutL homolog 1, colon cancer, nonpolyposis type 2, locus 3p21), *MGMT* (O6-methylguanine-DNA-methyltransferase, locus 10q26), *HMT* (histone lysine methyltransferases) and *p53* (locus 17p13). The *DCC* gene product is intimately involved in the process of cell-cell adhesion and has been associated with OSCC with bone invasion in gingival tumors, with aggressive invasion in tongue tumors and survival reduction (26). *hMLH1* is involved in the DNA mismatch repair process, showing 8% of hypermethylation (50, 51). *MGMT* encodes a protein responsible for DNA repair for alkylated guanine (39), and it has been found methylated in 23%, according to Rose et al. (52), and by 18.1%, according to Zuo et al. (53); this hypermethylation has been associated with loss of protein expression, favoring the carcinogenic and mutagenic effects in DNA. Regarding the *HMT* gene, Aniello et al. studied four HMT types and found that levels of *SETB1*, *Eu-HMTase*, and *SET08* were higher in tumor tissue of pleomorphic adenoma of the salivary glands (54). The *p53* gene, which appears mutated in most tumors throughout the body, has also been found epigenetically modified in OSCC in 42% of the samples (55).

2.1. Epigenetic Changes in Other Genes Involved in HNSCCs

There are other epigenetically altered genes in HNSCCs, among which, we must mention *ATM* (ataxia telangiectasia mutated gene, locus 11q22), *GSTP1* (glutathione S-transferase 1, locus 11q13), *MINT* CpG islands (Msx2 interacting nuclear target), *PMCA* (plasma membrane Ca(2+) ATPase), *CKMT1* (ubiquitous mitochondrial creatine kinase, locus 15q15), *LRP1B* (low-density lipoprotein receptor-related protein 1B, 2q21), *PRTFDC1* (phosphoribosyl transferase domain containing 1, locus 10p12), *MTNR1A* (melatonin receptor 1A, locus 4q35), *PTEN* (phosphatase and tensin homolog, locus 10q23), *SFRP* (secreted frizzled-related proteins), *RUNX3* (runt-related transcription factor 3, locus 1p36), *TGM3* (transglutaminase 3, locus 20q11), *MALT1* (mucosa-associated lymphoid tissue lymphoma translocation gene 1, locus 18q21), *SERPINE 1* (serpin peptidase inhibitor, clade E—nexin, plasminogen activator inhibitor type 1, member 1, locus 7q21–q22), and *CSMD 1* (CUB and sushi multiple domains 1, locus 8p23).

ATM is directly involved in responding to genotoxic stress and radiotherapy, and its methylation occurs in 25% of OSCCs, correlating with its prognosis (56). *GSTP1*, involved in detoxification processes, appears hypermethylated in steroid-related neoplasia; however, it has not been found in OSCC (57, 58). This enzyme is responsible for detoxification of xenobiotic products such as carboplatin (chemotherapy), and its overexpression results in therapeutic resistance (59–61). CpG islands of the *MINT* family have been associated with several types of tumors and appear to be corepressors, probably involved in the regulation of different pathways such as the Notch pathway, blocking the differentiation of B cell precursors in marginal zone B cells. The methylation frequencies are the following: *MINT 1* (23%), *MINT 2* (8%), *MINT 27* (16%), and *MINT 31* (15%) (62, 63). *PMCA* gene has been linked to oral cancer and it appears epigenetically inactivated in OSCC (43%) and oral premalignant lesions (40%) but not mutated (64). *CKMT1* appears hypermethylated in OSCC leading to a reduction in the amount of protein expressed by 37% with no observable genetic mutations. This epigenetic reduction is related to tumor differentiation (65). *LRP1B* appears silenced by methylation in 47.1% of the tumors and can be clearly related to oral tumorigenesis (66). *PRTFDC1* appears methylated in 17% of the OSCC, reducing the activity of this potential tumor suppressor gene (67). *MTNR1A* is not expressed in 89% of the OSCCs because of the hypermethylation of the promoter region (68). *PTEN* is a tumor suppressor gene, and its epigenetic alterations appear to be related to the subexpression of its protein, although further studies are required (69). *SFRP1* (locus 8p11) appeared methylated in 41% of samples, *SFRP2* (locus 4q31) in 94% of OSCC cases, and *SFRP5* (locus 10q24) in 82% of the patients. Loss of function of these proteins contributes to the activation of the Wnt signal, leading to cell proliferation during oral carcinogenesis (70). *RUNX3* is an important functional component in the signaling pathway of transforming growth factor beta (TGF-beta) and appears underexpressed by promoter hypermethylation in OSCC (71). *TGM3* expression undergoes a reduction caused by hypermethylation of CpG islands, and there is a correlation of this methylation with histological differentiation of OSCCs (72). *MALT1* is located in a genomic region that encodes an unknown tumor suppressor gene that activates the nuclear factor-kappaB in lymphoid lines. However, its expression in the pathology of malignant epithelial tumors is unknown. Chiba et al. have found lack of *MALT1* expression in 45% of OSCCs through epigenetic modification (73). Elevated levels of plasminogen activator inhibitor-1 (*PAI-1*) or *SERPINE 1* have been associated with poor prognosis in human tumors, including OSCC. According to Gao et al., methylation levels in tumors and normal adjacent tissue are higher than those of healthy volunteers, although the CpG methylation is not the main determinant of the expression levels of *SERPINE 1* (74). *CSMD 1* appears to be a tumor suppressor gene, presenting normal DNA structure in one in 20 tumors, but the rest of the samples show methylation around the first exon of *CSMD 1*; aberrant splicing and epigenetic silencing are responsible for their reduction in OSCC (75).

3. Histone Modifications

Methylation of specific lysine residues in histone tails has been established as an epigenetic marker that directly affects chromatin structure (12). The levels of H3K4me1, me2, and me3 were analyzed by Mancuso et al. who found that levels of H3K4me2 and me3 were significantly different in OSCC; compared to normal tissues, the levels of H3K4me2 were higher while those of H3K4me3 decreased, and also no differences in H3K4me1 levels were observed (14).

All these genes and molecules can be analyzed, not only in the tissues themselves by means of a biopsy, but they can also be measured through the evaluation of free DNA in plasma/serum (76–78) and saliva/mouth wash (79).

Most of these epigenetic alterations can be used as a therapeutic target, based on the reversal of DNA methylation or inhibition of histone deacetylation. Some of these agents are 5-azacytidine (5AC) which is under research in head and neck malignant tumor clinical trials (80). Unfortunately, DNA methyltransferase inhibitors (MTI) are not specific to particular genes such as *p15* or *p16*, thus there may be problems with toxicity (81, 82). A similar case is that of HDAC inhibitors; some of which have had clinical efficacy in solid tumors (83–87).

4. Epigenetic Changes Inducing or Preceding Genetic Changes

Epigenetics can be seen as an important turning point in regard to the central dogma of molecular biology, recognizing that there is an epigenetic inheritance through systems independent of DNA sequences that can be transmitted in cell tissues and organism lineages (88). Thus, current epigenetics provides new insight not only to gene regulation and inheritance but also to evolution, genetics, and development. Environmental factors (ranging from stress to infections) can influence gene expression (89, 90). Moreover, these possible epigenetic modifications can occur throughout the life of the organism, i.e., from in utero life to more advanced stages of development, being accumulated in the tissues and modifying cellular gene expression patterns over time (89, 90).

The epigenome consists of the chromatin and its modifications and functions as an interface between the inherited genome and environmental dynamism (90). In this interaction with the environment, epigenetic modifications are promoted being specific patterns of DNA methylation, which result in relative stability or homeostasis of gene expression profiles (91). Chromatin modifications, including methylation of CpG, can sculpt the epigenome during development, modified by individual environmental exposures, providing a unique and absolute identity, even in monozygotic twins (90, 92).

Epigenetic changes are very important during embryonic development given that they dictate differentiation pathways, even in human adult cells (93). Epigenetic changes affect different genes involved in growth, especially tumor suppressor genes that are active in normal cells and silenced in cancer (9, 94). However, aging, autoimmune diseases, and cancer are diseases mediated by the gradual accumulation of epigenetic alterations, in which the main genes involved are tumor suppressor genes, genes related to DNA repair, genes related to hormone receptors, and angiogenesis inhibitor genes (95).

Methylation of promoter regions rich in GpGs is a mechanism used by mammals to prevent transcriptional initiation and to promote gene silencing in inactive X chromosome, imprinted genes, and parasitic DNAs (96). Such methylation can regulate gene expression in specific tissues and may be influenced by exogenous factors such as toxins or age, potentially increasing or decreasing transcription levels, depending on whether methylation inactivates places with positive or negative regulatory elements (36, 97). In normal cells, DNA methylation occurs predominantly in repetitive genomic regions, including satellite DNA and parasitic elements, such as long interspersed transposable elements (LINES), short interspersed transposable elements (SINES), and endogenous retroviruses, stabilizing the changes in gene expression (98, 99). Changes in the methylation status may also regulate the expression of microRNA (miRNA), which in turn modulates posttranslational gene expression and plays an important role in essential processes such as differentiation, growth, or cell death (100, 101).

The different profiles of DNA methylation and the histone acetylation patterns that arise among different tissues during the lifetime of monozygotic twins may contribute to the explanation of some of their phenotypic discordances and highlight the differences between the frequency/initiation of some of the most common diseases, based on the cumulative history of exogenous exposures (environment, nutritional factors, toxins, and infections) that reprogram the individual's epigenetic status (90, 93, 102).

The discovery that tumor suppressor genes often fail in their expression in the absence of detectable genetic abnormalities has raised interest in epigenetics and the time when these changes happen (13).

Alterations in the DNA methylation status resulting from exposure to environmental stress agents have been documented even before birth (103). Although many epigenetic markers are potentially reversible, the mechanism still remains unclear and many epigenetic changes persist across cell lines and the life of the organism, thus confirming Barker's hypothesis. This hypothesis argues that intrauterine exposures may result in fetal programming that persists into adulthood and may contribute to the risk of suffering diseases like cancer, through the acquisition of specific mutations, deletions, or other genetic alterations (104).

References

1. S. Gao, J. Worm, P. Guldberg, H. Eiberg, A. Krogdahl, C. J. Liu, J. Reibel, and E. Dabelsteen, (2004) Genetic and epigenetic alterations of the blood group ABO gene in oral squamous cell carcinoma. *Int J Cancer* 109, 230–237.
2. M. Perez-Sayans, J. M. Somoza-Martin, F. Barros-Angueira, M. D. Reboiras-Lopez, J. M. Gandara Rey, and A. Garcia-Garcia (2009) Genetic and molecular alterations associated with oral squamous cell cancer (review). *Oncol Rep* 22, 1277–1282.
3. A. Bird, (2002) DNA methylation patterns and epigenetic memory. *Genes Dev* 16, 6-21.
4. T. Vaissiere, C. Sawan, and Z. Herceg (2008) Epigenetic interplay between histone modifications and DNA methylation in gene silencing. *Mutat Res* 659, 40–48.
5. J. Murakami, J. Asaumi, Y. Maki, *et al* (2004) Influence of CpG island methylation status in O6-methylguanine-DNA methyltransferase expression of oral cancer cell lines. *Oncol Rep* 12, 339–345.
6. C. J. Piyathilake, W. C. Bell, J. Jones, O. L. Henao, D. C. Heimburger, A. Niveleau, and W. E. Grizzle (2005) Patterns of global DNA and histone methylation appear to be similar in normal, dysplastic and neoplastic oral epithelium of humans. *Dis Markers* 21, 147–151.
7. F. Larsen, G. Gundersen, R. Lopez, and H. Prydz (1992) CpG islands as gene markers in the human genome. *Genomics* 13, 1095–1107.
8. P. K. Ha and J. A. Califano (2006) Promoter methylation and inactivation of tumour-suppressor genes in oral squamous-cell carcinoma. *Lancet Oncol* 7, 77–82.
9. K. Gronbaek, C. Hother, and P. A. Jones (2007) Epigenetic changes in cancer. *APMIS* 115, 1039–1059.
10. A. T. Hark, C. J. Schoenherr, D. J. Katz, R. S. Ingram, J. M. Levorse, and S. M. Tilghman (2000) CTCF mediates methylation-sensitive enhancer-blocking activity at the H19/Igf2 locus. *Nature* 405, 486–489.
11. J. Murakami, J. Asaumi, N. Kawai, *et al* (2005) Effects of histone deacetylase inhibitor FR901228 on the expression level of telomerase reverse transcriptase in oral cancer, *Cancer Chemother Pharmacol* 56, 22–28.
12. A. P. Bird and A. P. Wolffe (1999) Methylation-induced repression--belts, braces, and chromatin. *Cell* 99, 451–454.
13. A. P. Feinberg (2001) Cancer epigenetics takes center stage. *Proc Natl Acad Sci USA* 98, 392–394.
14. M. Mancuso, D. S. Matassa, M. Conte, G. Colella, G. Rana, L. Fucci, and M. Piscopo (2009) H3K4 histone methylation in oral squamous cell carcinoma. *Acta Biochim Pol* 56, 405–410.
15. E. A. Vucic, C. J. Brown, and W. L. Lam (2008) Epigenetics of cancer progression. *Pharmacogenomics* 9, 215–234.
16. R. L. Momparler and V. Bovenzi (2000) DNA methylation and cancer. *J Cell Physiol* 183, 145–154.

17. M. Cruz-Correa, H. Cui, F. M. Giardiello, *et al* (2004) Loss of imprinting of insulin growth factor II gene: A potential heritable biomarker for colon neoplasia predisposition. *Gastroenterology* 126, 964–970.
18. X. Wu, H. Zhao, R. Suk, and D. C. Christiani (2004) Genetic susceptibility to tobacco-related cancer. *Oncogene* 23, 6500-6523.
19. D. Hanahan and R. A. Weinberg (2000) The hallmarks of cancer. *Cell* 100, 57–70.
20. S. Choi and J. N. Myers (2008) Molecular pathogenesis of oral squamous cell carcinoma: Implications for therapy. *J Dent Res* 87, 14–32.
21. A. K. El-Naggar, S. Lai, G. Clayman, J. K. Lee, M. A. Luna, H. Goepfert, and J. G. (1997) Batsakis, Methylation, a major mechanism of p16/CDKN2 gene inactivation in head and neck squamous carcinoma. *Am J Pathol* 151, 1767–1774.
22. R. Sailasree, A. Abhilash, K. M. Sathyan, K. R. Nalinakumari, S. Thomas, and S. Kannan. (2008) Differential roles of p16INK4A and p14ARF genes in prognosis of oral carcinoma. *Cancer Epidemiol Biomarkers Prev* 17, 414–420.
23. R. J. Shaw, T. Liloglou, S. N. Rogers, J. S. Brown, E. D. Vaughan, D. Lowe, J. K. Field, and J. M. Risk (2006) Promoter methylation of P16, RARbeta, E-cadherin, cyclin A1 and cytoglobin in oral cancer: Quantitative evaluation using pyrosequencing, *Br J Cancer* 94. 561–568.
24. C. Motsch, A. Giers, C. Boltze, M. Evert, B. Freigang, A. Roessner, and R. Schneider-Stock (2004) Biallelic inactivation of the p16-gen in a metachronous triple carcinoma in the oropharyngeal region. *Laryngorhinootologie* 83, 55–60.
25. S. Shintani, Y. Nakahara, M. Mihara, Y. Ueyama, and T. Matsumura (2001) Inactivation of the p14(ARF), p15(INK4B) and p16(INK4A) genes is a frequent event in human oral squamous cell carcinomas. *Oral Oncol* 37, 498–504.
26. K. Ogi, M. Toyota, M. Ohe-Toyota, N. Tanaka, M. Noguchi, T. Sonoda, G. Kohama, and T. Tokino (2002) Aberrant methylation of multiple genes and clinicopathological features in oral squamous cell carcinoma. *Clin Cancer Res* 8, 3164–3171.
27. S. Maruya, J. P. Issa, R. S. Weber, D. I. Rosenthal, J. C. Haviland, R. Lotan, and A. K. El-Naggar (2004) Differential methylation status of tumor-associated genes in head and neck squamous carcinoma: Incidence and potential implications. *Clin Cancer Res* 10, 3825–3830.
28. M. Gasco, A. K. Bell, V. Heath, *et al* (2002) Epigenetic inactivation of 14-3-3 sigma in oral carcinoma: Association with p16(INK4a) silencing and human papillomavirus negativity. *Cancer Res* 62, 2072–2076.
29. T. Daa, K. Kashima, Y. Kondo, N. Yada, M. Suzuki, and S. Yokoyama (2008) Aberrant methylation in promoter regions of cyclin-dependent kinase inhibitor genes in adenoid cystic carcinoma of the salivary gland. *APMIS* 116, 21–26.
30. M. J. Huang, K. T. Yeh, H. C. Shih, Y. F. Wang, T. H. Lin, J. Y. Chang, M. C. Shih, and J. G. Chang (2002) The correlation between CpG methylation and protein expression of P16 in oral squamous cell carcinomas. *Int J Mol Med* 10, 551–554.
31. S. Ohta, H. Uemura, Y. Matsui, *et al* (2009) Alterations of p16 and p14ARF genes and their 9p21 locus in oral squamous cell carcinoma. *Oral Surg Oral Med Oral Pathol Oral Radiol Endod* 107, 81–91.
32. M. A. Gonzalez-Moles, J. A. Gil-Montoya, I. Ruiz-Avila, F. Esteban, M. Delgado-Rodriguez, and A. Bascones-Martinez (2007) Prognostic significance of p21WAF1/CIP1, p16INK4a and CD44s in tongue cancer. *Oncol Rep* 18, 389–396.
33. U. K. Bhawal, K. Tsukinoki, T. Sasahira, F. Sato, Y. Mori, N. Muto, M. Sugiyama, and H. Kuniyasu (2007) Methylation and intratumoural heterogeneity of 14-3-3 sigma in oral cancer. *Oncol Rep* 18, 817–824.
34. S. M. Dong, D. I. Sun, N. E. Benoit, I. Kuzmin, M. I. Lerman, and D. Sidransky, (2003). Epigenetic inactivation of RASSF1A in head and neck cancer, *Clin Cancer Res* 9, 3635–3640.
35. K. H. Huang, S. F. Huang, I. H. Chen, C. T. Liao, H. M. Wang, and L. L. Hsieh (2009) Methylation of RASSF1A, RASSF2A, and HIN-1 is associated with poor outcome after radiotherapy, but not surgery, in oral squamous cell carcinoma. *Clin Cancer Res* 15, 4174–4180.
36. T. N. Tran, Y. Liu, M. Takagi, A. Yamaguchi, and H. Fujii (2005) Frequent promoter hypermethylation of RASSF1A and p16INK4a and infrequent allelic loss other than 9p21 in betel-associated oral carcinoma in a vietnamese non-smoking/non-drinking female population. *J Oral Pathol Med* 34, 150–156.
37. T. Imai, M. Toyota, H. Suzuki, *et al* (2008) Epigenetic inactivation of RASSF2 in oral squamous cell carcinoma. *Cancer Sci* 99, 958–966.
38. M. Nishimine, M. Nakamura, M. Kishi, M. Okamoto, K. Shimada, E. Ishida, T. Kirita,

and N. Konishi (2003) Alterations of p14ARF and p16INK4a genes in salivary gland carcinomas. *Oncol Rep* 10, 555–560.

39. C. A. Righini, F. de Fraipont, E. Reyt, and M. C. Favrot (2007) Aberrant methylation of tumor suppressor genes in head and neck squamous cell carcinoma: Is it clinically relevant? *Bull Cancer* 94, 191–197.
40. V. Kulkarni and D. Saranath (2004) Concurrent hypermethylation of multiple regulatory genes in chewing tobacco associated oral squamous cell carcinomas and adjacent normal tissues. Oral Oncol 40, 145–153.
41. K. T. Yeh, J. G. Chang, T. H. Lin, Y. F. Wang, N. Tien, J. Y. Chang, J. C. Chen, and M. C. Shih (2003) Epigenetic changes of tumor suppressor genes, P15, P16, VHL and P53 in oral cancer. *Oncol Rep* 10, 659–663.
42. S. Nakayama, A. Sasaki, H. Mese, R. E. Alcalde, T. Tsuji, and T. Matsumura (2001) The E-cadherin gene is silenced by CpG methylation in human oral squamous cell carcinomas. *Int J Cancer* 93, 667–673.
43. Y. Saito, H. Takazawa, K. Uzawa, H. Tanzawa, and K. Sato (1998) Reduced expression of E-cadherin in oral squamous cell carcinoma: Relationship with DNA methylation of 5′ CpG island. *Int J Oncol* 12, 293–298.
44. H. W. Chang, V. Chow, K. Y. Lam, W. I. Wei, and A. Yuen (2002) Loss of E-cadherin expression resulting from promoter hypermethylation in oral tongue carcinoma and its prognostic significance. *Cancer* 94, 386–392.
45. G. Maeda, T. Chiba, T. Aoba, and K. Imai (2007) Epigenetic inactivation of E-cadherin by promoter hypermethylation in oral carcinoma cells. *Odontology* 95, 24–29.
46. R. V. de Moraes, D. T. Oliveira, G. Landman, F. de Carvalho, O. Caballero, S. Nonogaki, I. Nishimoto, and L. P. Kowalski (2008) E-cadherin abnormalities resulting from CPG methylation promoter in metastatic and non-metastatic oral cancer. *Head Neck* 30, 85–92.
47. S. Gao, E. P. Bennett, J. Reibel, X. Chen, M. E. Christensen, A. Krogdahl, and E. Dabelsteen (2004) Histo-blood group ABO antigen in oral potentially malignant lesions and squamous cell carcinoma--genotypic and phenotypic characterization. *APMIS* 112, 11–20.
48. G. Maeda, T. Chiba, S. Kawashiri, T. Satoh, and K. Imai (2007) Epigenetic inactivation of IkappaB kinase-alpha in oral carcinomas and tumor progression. *Clin Cancer Res* 13, 5041–5047.
49. S. Ogane, T. Onda, N. Takano, T. Yajima, T. Uchiyama, and T. Shibahara (2009) Spleen tyrosine kinase as a novel candidate tumor suppressor gene for human oral squamous cell carcinoma. *Int J Cancer* 124, 2651–2657.
50. K. Liu, H. Huang, P. Mukunyadzi, J. Y. Suen, E. Hanna, and C. Y. Fan (2002) Promoter hypermethylation: An important epigenetic mechanism for hMLH1 gene inactivation in head and neck squamous cell carcinoma. *Otolaryngol Head Neck Surg* 126, 548–553.
51. M. Viswanathan, N. Tsuchida, and G. Shanmugam (2003) Promoter hypermethylation profile of tumor-associated genes p16, p15, hMLH1, MGMT and E-cadherin in oral squamous cell carcinoma. *Int J Cancer* 105, 41–46.
52. S. L. Rosas, W. Koch, M. G. da Costa Carvalho, L. Wu, J. Califano, W. Westra, J. Jen, and D. Sidransky (2001) Promoter hypermethylation patterns of p16, O6-methylguanine-DNA-methyltransferase, and death-associated protein kinase in tumors and saliva of head and neck cancer patients. *Cancer Res* 61, 939–942.
53. C. Zuo, L. Ai, P. Ratliff, J. Y. Suen, E. Hanna, T. P. Brent, and C. Y. Fan (2004) O6-methylguanine-DNA methyltransferase gene: Epigenetic silencing and prognostic value in head and neck squamous cell carcinoma. *Cancer Epidemiol Biomarkers Prev* 13, 967–975.
54. F. Aniello, G. Colella, G. Muscariello, A. Lanza, D. Ferrara, M. Branno, and S. Minucci (2006) Expression of four histone lysine-methyltransferases in parotid gland tumors. *Anticancer Res* 26, 2063–2067.
55. S. Mitra, S. Banerjee, C. Misra, R. K. Singh, A. Roy, A. Sengupta, C. K. Panda, and S. Roychoudhury (2007) Interplay between human papilloma virus infection and p53 gene alterations in head and neck squamous cell carcinoma of an Indian patient population. *J Clin Pathol* 60, 1040–1047.
56. L. Ai, Q. N. Vo, C. Zuo, L. Li, W. Ling, J. Y. Suen, E. Hanna, K. D. Brown, and C. Y. Fan (2004) Ataxia-telangiectasia-mutated (ATM) gene in head and neck squamous cell carcinoma: Promoter hypermethylation with clinical correlation in 100 cases. *Cancer Epidemiol Biomarkers Prev* 13, 150–156.
57. M. Esteller, P. G. Corn, S. B. Baylin, and J. G. Herman (2001) A gene hypermethylation profile of human cancer. *Cancer Res* 61, 3225–3229.
58. M. Sanchez-Cespedes, M. Esteller, L. Wu, H. Nawroz-Danish, G. H. Yoo, W. M. Koch, J. Jen, J. G. Herman, and D. Sidransky (2000) Gene promoter hypermethylation in tumors and serum of head and neck cancer patients. *Cancer Res* 60, 892–895.

59. J. B. Engel, A. V. Schally, G. Halmos, B. Baker, A. Nagy, and G. Keller (2005) Targeted therapy with a cytotoxic somatostatin analog, AN-238, inhibits growth of human experimental endometrial carcinomas expressing multidrug resistance protein MDR-1. *Cancer* 104, 1312–1321.
60. M. Koshiyama, H. Fujii, M. Kinezaki, Y. Morita, H. Nanno, and M. Yoshida (2001) Immunohistochemical expression of topoisomerase IIalpha (topo IIalpha) and multidrug resistance-associated protein (MRP), plus chemosensitivity testing, as chemotherapeutic indices of ovarian and endometrial carcinomas. *Anticancer Res* 21, 2925–2932.
61. M. Perez-Sayans, J. M. Somoza-Martin, F. Barros-Angueira, P. G. Diz, J. M. Rey, and A. Garcia-Garcia (2010) Multidrug resistance in oral squamous cell carcinoma: The role of vacuolar ATPases. *Cancer Lett* 295, 135–43
62. R. Shaw (2006) The epigenetics of oral cancer. *Int J Oral Maxillofac Surg* 35, 101-108.
63. M. Toyota, C. Ho, N. Ahuja, K. W. Jair, Q. Li, M. Ohe-Toyota, S. B. Baylin, and J. P. Issa (1999) Identification of differentially methylated sequences in colorectal cancer by methylated CpG island amplification. *Cancer Res* 59, 2307–2312.
64. K. Saito, K. Uzawa, Y. Endo, Y. Kato, D. Nakashima, K. Ogawara, M. Shiba, H. Bukawa, H. Yokoe, and H. Tanzawa (2006) Plasma membrane Ca2+ ATPase isoform 1 down-regulated in human oral cancer. *Oncol Rep* 15, 49–55.
65. T. Onda, K. Uzawa, Y. Endo, H. Bukawa, H. Yokoe, T. Shibahara, and H. Tanzawa (2006) Ubiquitous mitochondrial creatine kinase downregulated in oral squamous cell carcinoma. *Br J Cancer* 94, 698–709.
66. T. Nakagawa, A. Pimkhaokham, E. Suzuki, K. Omura, J. Inazawa, and I. Imoto (2006) Genetic or epigenetic silencing of low density lipoprotein receptor-related protein 1B expression in oral squamous cell carcinoma. *Cancer Sci* 97, 1070–1074.
67. E. Suzuki, I. Imoto, A. Pimkhaokham, T. Nakagawa, N. Kamata, K. I. Kozaki, T. Amagasa, and J. Inazawa (2007) PRTFDC1, a possible tumor-suppressor gene, is frequently silenced in oral squamous-cell carcinomas by aberrant promoter hypermethylation. *Oncogene* 26, 7921–7932.
68. E. Nakamura, K. Kozaki, H. Tsuda, *et al* (2008) Frequent silencing of a putative tumor suppressor gene melatonin receptor 1 A (MTNR1A) in oral squamous-cell carcinoma. *Cancer Sci* 99, 1390–1400.
69. Y. Kurasawa, M. Shiiba, M. Nakamura, K. Fushimi, T. Ishigami, H. Bukawa, H. Yokoe, K. Uzawa, and H. Tanzawa (2008) PTEN expression and methylation status in oral squamous cell carcinoma. *Oncol Rep* 19, 1429–1434.
70. Y. Sogabe, H. Suzuki, M. Toyota, K. Ogi, T. Imai, M. Nojima, Y. Sasaki, H. Hiratsuka, and T. Tokino (2008) Epigenetic inactivation of SFRP genes in oral squamous cell carcinoma. *Int J Oncol* 32, 1253–1261.
71. F. Gao, C. Huang, M. Lin, Z. Wang, J. Shen, H. Zhang, L. Jiang, and Q. Chen (2009) Frequent inactivation of RUNX3 by promoter hypermethylation and protein mislocalization in oral squamous cell carcinomas. *J Cancer Res Clin Oncol* 135, 739–747.
72. A. Negishi, M. Masuda, M. Ono, *et al* (2009) Quantitative proteomics using formalin-fixed paraffin-embedded tissues of oral squamous cell carcinoma. *Cancer Sci* 100, 1605–1611.
73. T. Chiba, G. Maeda, S. Kawashiri, K. Kato, and K. Imai (2009) Epigenetic loss of mucosa-associated lymphoid tissue 1 expression in patients with oral carcinomas. *Cancer Res* 69, 7216–7223.
74. S. Gao, B. S. Nielsen, A. Krogdahl, J. A. Sorensen, J. Tagesen, S. Dabelsteen, E. Dabelsteen, and P. A. Andreasen (2010) Epigenetic alterations of the SERPINE1 gene in oral squamous cell carcinomas and normal oral mucosa. *Genes Chromosomes Cancer* 49, 526–538.
75. T. M. Richter, B. D. Tong, and S. B. Scholnick (2005) Epigenetic inactivation and aberrant transcription of CSMD1 in squamous cell carcinoma cell lines. *Cancer Cell Int* 5, 29.
76. S. A. Leon, G. E. Ehrlich, B. Shapiro, and V. A. Labbate (1977) Free DNA in the serum of rheumatoid arthritis patients. *J Rheumatol* 4, 139–143.
77. B. Shapiro, M. Chakrabarty, E. M. Cohn, and S. A. Leon (1983) Determination of circulating DNA levels in patients with benign or malignant gastrointestinal disease. *Cancer* 51, 2116–2120.
78. A. Ziegler, U. Zangemeister-Wittke, and R. A. Stahel (2002) Circulating DNA: A new diagnostic gold mine? *Cancer Treat Rev* 28, 255–271.
79. M. Lopez, J. M. Aguirre, N. Cuevas, M. Anzola, J. Videgain, J. Aguirregaviria, and M. Martinez de Pancorbo (2003) Gene promoter hypermethylation in oral rinses of leukoplakia patients--a diagnostic and/or prognostic tool? *Eur J Cancer* 39, 2306–2309.
80. M. M. Coombes, K. L. Briggs, J. R. Bone, G. L. Clayman, A. K. El-Naggar, and S. Y. Dent (2003) Resetting the histone code at CDKN2A in HNSCC by inhibition of DNA methylation, *Oncogene* 22, 8902–8911.

81. M. Daskalakis, T. T. Nguyen, C. Nguyen, P. Guldberg, G. Kohler, P. Wijermans, P. A. Jones, and M. Lubbert (2002) Demethylation of a hypermethylated P15/INK4B gene in patients with myelodysplastic syndrome by 5-aza-2′-deoxycytidine (decitabine) treatment. *Blood* 100, 2957–2964.
82. J. Gilbert, S. D. Gore, J. G. Herman, and M. A. Carducci (2004) The clinical application of targeting cancer through histone acetylation and hypomethylation. *Clin Cancer Res* 10, 4589–4596.
83. J. L. Marshall, N. Rizvi, J. Kauh, *et al* (2002) A phase I trial of depsipeptide (FR901228) in patients with advanced cancer. *J Exp Ther Oncol* 2, 325–332.
84. V. Sandor, S. Bakke, R. W. Robey, *et al* (2002) Phase I trial of the histone deacetylase inhibitor, depsipeptide (FR901228, NSC 630176), in patients with refractory neoplasms. *Clin Cancer Res* 8, 718–728.
85. A. D. Donald, V. L. Clark, S. Patel, *et al* (2010) Design and synthesis of novel pyrimidine hydroxamic acid inhibitors of histone deacetylases. *Bioorg Med Chem Lett* 20, 6657–6660.
86. H. C. Yoon, E. Choi, J. E. Park, *et al* (2010) Property based optimization of delta-lactam HDAC inhibitors for metabolic stability. *Bioorg Med Chem Lett* 20, 6808–6811.
87. J. Kim, J. Guan, I. Chang, X. Chen, D. Han, and C. Y. Wang (2010) PS-341 and histone deacetylase inhibitor synergistically induce apoptosis in head and neck squamous cell carcinoma cells. *Mol Cancer Ther* 9, 1977–1984.
88. M. Nishimine, N. Konishi, K. Yamamoto, H. Nagai, M. Emi, T. Kirita, and M. Sugimura (2000) Epigenetic alterations in methylation in oral squamous cell carcinoma cell lines detected by two-dimensional gel electrophoresis. *Int J Oncol* 17, 743–747.
89. D. J. Smiraglia, L. T. Smith, J. C. Lang, L. J. Rush, Z. Dai, D. E. Schuller, and C. Plass (2003). Differential targets of CpG island hypermethylation in primary and metastatic head and neck squamous cell carcinoma (HNSCC). *J Med Genet* 40, 25–33.
90. S. Choudhuri, Y. Cui, and C. D. Klaassen (2010) Molecular targets of epigenetic regulation and effectors of environmental influences. *Toxicol Appl Pharmacol* 245, 378–393.
91. A. P. Feinberg (2008) Epigenetics at the epicenter of modern medicine. *JAMA* 299, 1345–1350.
92. M. F. Fraga, E. Ballestar, A. Villar-Garea, *et al* (2005) Loss of acetylation at Lys16 and trimethylation at Lys20 of histone H4 is a common hallmark of human cancer. *Nat Genet* 37, 391–400.
93. T. Ryba, I. Hiratani, J. Lu, M. Itoh, M. Kulik, J. Zhang, T. C. Schulz, A. J. Robins, S. Dalton, and D. M. Gilbert (2010) Evolutionarily conserved replication timing profiles predict long-range chromatin interactions and distinguish closely related cell types. *Genome Res* 20, 761–770.
94. N. M. Boyd and P. C. Reade (1988) Differences between preneoplastic cells, neoplastic cells and their normal counterparts. *J Oral Pathol* 17, 257–265.
95. B. C. Richardson (2002) Role of DNA methylation in the regulation of cell function: Autoimmunity, aging and cancer. *J Nutr* 132, 2401S–2405S.
96. K. Gronbaek, M. Treppendahl, F. Asmar, and P. Guldberg (2008) Epigenetic changes in cancer as potential targets for prophylaxis and maintenance therapy. *Basic Clin Pharmacol Toxicol* 103, 389–396.
97. D. C. Dolinoy, D. Huang, and R. L. Jirtle (2007) Maternal nutrient supplementation counteracts bisphenol A-induced DNA hypomethylation in early development. *Proc Natl Acad Sci USA* 104, 13056–13061.
98. J. A. Yoder, C. P. Walsh, and T. H. Bestor (1997) Cytosine methylation and the ecology of intragenomic parasites. *Trends Genet* 13, 335–340.
99. S. P. Barros and S. Offenbacher (2009) Epigenetics: Connecting environment and genotype to phenotype and disease. *J Dent Res* 88, 400–408.
100. E. A. Miska (2005) How microRNAs control cell division, differentiation and death. *Curr Opin Genet Dev* 15, 563–568.
101. P. D. Zamore and B. Haley (2005) Ribo-gnome: The big world of small RNAs, *Science* 309, 1519–1524.
102. K. T. Yeh, J. G. Chang, T. H. Lin, Y. F. Wang, J. Y. Chang, M. C. Shih, and C. C. Lin (2003) Correlation between protein expression and epigenetic and mutation changes of wnt pathway-related genes in oral cancer. *Int J Oncol* 23, 1001–1007.
103. W. S. Post, P. J. Goldschmidt-Clermont, C. C. Wilhide, A. W. Heldman, M. S. Sussman, P. Ouyang, E. E. Milliken, and J. P. Issa (1999) Methylation of the estrogen receptor gene is associated with aging and atherosclerosis in the cardiovascular system. *Cardiovasc Res* 43, 985–991.
104. D. J. Barker, J. G. Eriksson, T. Forsen, and C. Osmond (2002) Fetal origins of adult disease: Strength of effects and biological basis. *Int J Epidemiol* 31, 1235–1239.

Chapter 13

Clinical Implications of Epigenetic Alterations in Human Thoracic Malignancies: Epigenetic Alterations in Lung Cancer

Keiko Shinjo and Yutaka Kondo

Abstract

Besides known genetic aberrations, epigenetic alterations have emerged as common hallmarks of many cancer types, including lung cancer. Epigenetics is a process involved in gene regulation, mediated via DNA methylation, histone modification, chromatin remodeling, and functional noncoding RNAs, which influences the accessibility of the underlying DNA to transcriptional regulatory factors that activate or repress expression. Studies have shown that epigenetic dysregulation is associated with multiple steps during carcinogenesis. Since epigenetic therapy is now in clinical use in hematopoietic diseases and undergoing trials for lung cancer, a better understanding of epigenetic abnormalities is desired. Recent technologies for high-throughput genome-wide analyses for epigenetic modifications are promising and potent tools for understanding the global dysregulation of cancer epigenetics. In this chapter, studies of epigenetic abnormality and its clinical implication in lung cancers are discussed.

Key words: Lung cancer, Non-small cell lung cancer, Small cell lung cancer, Epithelial growth factor receptor, DNA methylation, CpG island methylator phenotype, Demethylating agent, Histone deacetylase, High-throughput methylation analysis

1. Introduction

Despite recent advances in targeted therapy, lung cancer is the leading cause of human cancer death worldwide (1, 2). Histologically and clinically, lung cancers can be divided into two major groups: small cell lung cancer (SCLC) and non-small cell lung cancer (NSCLC); the latter is further divided into adenocarcinoma, squamous cell carcinoma, and large cell carcinoma.

Recent targeted therapies have dramatically improved the survival of patients with certain types of lung cancer. Patients with epidermal growth factor receptor (EGFR) mutation-positive

Ramona G. Dumitrescu and Mukesh Verma (eds.), *Cancer Epigenetics: Methods and Protocols*, Methods in Molecular Biology, vol. 863, DOI 10.1007/978-1-61779-612-8_13, © Springer Science+Business Media, LLC 2012

NSCLC display particular benefit from EGFR tyrosine kinase inhibitors (TKIs) (3, 4), whereas EML4-ALK mutation-positive NSCLCs are highly sensitive to ALK inhibitors (5). Although these emergent treatments for NSCLC have shown some success, many patients with lung cancer still suffer from recurrence or relapse of disease. Therefore, elucidating the underlying mechanisms leading to the development of lung cancer is key to facilitating new advances in the treatment of this disease.

Studies have shown that in addition to copy number alterations, gene mutations, and genetic rearrangements, accumulation of epigenetic alterations play an important role in the tumorigenesis of lung cancers (6). Epigenetic mechanisms include DNA methylation, histone modification, chromatin remodeling, and functional noncoding RNA, which dynamically affect chromatin structure and are closely associated with gene regulation. Aberrant epigenetic mechanisms have been observed in many human malignancies (7, 8). Simultaneous dysregulation of multiple genes related to cell cycle, cell growth, cell death, or cell adhesion by epigenetic mechanisms may be a strong driving force to transformation and is sometimes correlated with potentiated aggressiveness of tumors (Fig. 1).

In addition to the pathogenic implications, DNA methylation profiles represent a source of molecular diagnostic information. DNA methylation in particular genes has been known to be associated

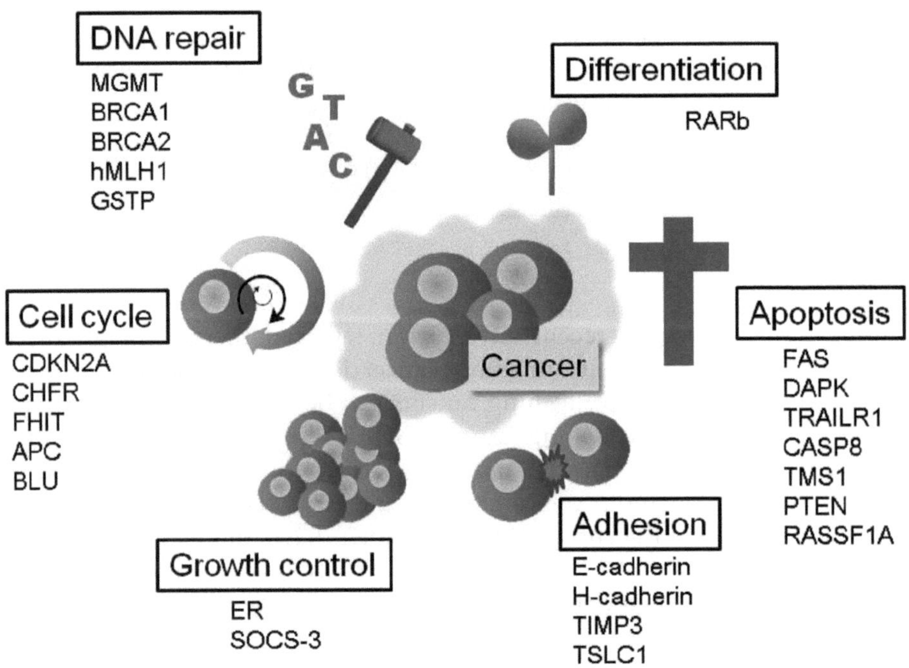

Fig. 1. Targets of DNA methylation during lung carcinogenesis involved in key cellular processes. These cellular processes are simultaneously dysregulated by aberrant epigenetic mechanisms in human neoplasia.

with patient outcome (9–11). Moreover, aberrant DNA methylation of certain genes can be detected in samples from the aerodigestive tract epithelium of cancer-free heavy smokers (12). Therefore, detection of aberrant DNA methylation in clinical specimens could be a potent biomarker for malignancies. Recent advances in technologies for high-throughput genome-wide DNA methylation analyses have facilitated epigenetic profiling of human malignancies (13). In the context of personalized therapy, epigenetic profiling of cancers may provide new molecular diagnostic tools for disease stratification, which may be of great benefit for cancer treatments.

2. Genetic Abnormalities in Lung Cancer

Studies in relation to genetic alterations and associated functional dysregulation have been broadly documented in the case of lung cancer. We will briefly overview some of the most common genetic abnormalities in lung cancer.

Partial deletion of chromosome 3p has been reported as a frequent event in lung cancer (14, 15). Several tumor suppressor genes are located in this region, including *FHIT*, *RASSF1A*, *SEMA3B*, *SEMA3F*, *MLH1*, and *RARB* (16).

TP53, a major tumor suppressor gene on chromosome 17p, is also a frequent target of genetic alterations (around 50% of NSCLCs and 90% of SCLCs) (17–19). Mutation of *TP53* appears to be associated with smoking history and aggressiveness of tumors (17, 20).

EGFR, encoding an important tyrosine kinase receptor, is frequently mutated in NSCLCs. *EGFR* mutations are present in about 10% of NSCLC cases in North America and Western Europe, while 30–50% of NSCLC cases with East Asian ethnicity exhibit this mutation. Incidence of EGFR mutations is associated with adenocarcinoma histology, a history of nonsmoking, and female gender (21, 22). Mutation of this gene causes constitutive activation leading to uncontrolled activation of downstream signaling pathways, such as the RAS/MAPK and PIK3CA/AKT pathways (23).

KRAS mutations are often found in adenocarcinoma (approximately 20%), but are less frequent in squamous cell carcinoma (approximately 5%). This mutation is associated with smoking history, resistance to TKI treatments, and poor prognosis of NSCLC patients (24–26). Interestingly, *KRAS* and *EGFR* mutations appear to be mutually exclusive genetic events, indicating that mutation of either *KRAS* or *EGFR* may activate an overlapping set of oncogenic pathways, which results in neoplastic transformation (21, 22).

Recently, *EML4-ALK*, a fusion-type protein tyrosine kinase, generated as a result of a small inversion within chromosome 2p, was identified in NSCLCs. This fusion was found in about 5% of

NSCLC patients, in which a high incidence was associated with adenocarcinoma histology, younger onset, and a history of non-smoking (27). Importantly, *EML4-ALK* mutations are mutually exclusive with *EGFR* mutations, suggesting that *EML4-ALK* mutations may be a particular new therapeutic target in NSCLC patients who are not sensitive to EGFR TKIs. Indeed, ALK inhibitors have demonstrated efficacy in *EML4-ALK* mutation-positive patients (5).

In addition to the above-mentioned genetic alterations, recent large-scale gene sequencing studies of adenocarcinomas identified 26 genes, including *TP53*, *KRAS*, *EGFR*, *STK11*, *CDKN2A*, which are frequently mutated in lung cancers (28). Strikingly, 132 out of 188 tumors displayed at least one mutation in the MAPK pathway, suggestive of an important role during lung carcinogenesis.

3. Epigenetics Abnormalities in Lung Cancer

Dysregulation of epigenetic transcriptional control is a fundamental feature of human malignancies; in particular, aberrant promoter DNA methylation and histone modifications are well documented in human neoplasia (29). Accumulating evidence has shown that inappropriate activation and inactivation of gene function by abnormal epigenetic mechanisms contribute to lung cancer development and progression (6).

3.1. DNA Methylation in Lung Cancer

Cancer cells generally demonstrate simultaneous global hypomethylation and regional hypermethylation. Methylation in promoter CpG islands (short stretches, up to 2 kb, of CpG-rich regions generally found in the promoters of approximately 60% of the genes) is closely linked to alterations of chromatin structure and is associated with gene silencing.

Multiple pathways and processes silenced by DNA methylation have been implicated in the transformation of normal lung epithelial cells to tumor cells (Fig. 1). CDKN2A is an inhibitor of cyclin-dependent kinase 4/6 and functions in control of the G1/S phase transition. Methylation of the *CDKN2A* gene in sputum DNA has been detected 3 years before the diagnosis of squamous cell carcinoma (12). Analysis of epithelial cells obtained through bronchoscopy from cancer-free smokers suggested that methylation of *CDKN2A* is probably one of the earliest epigenetic changes in lung cancer (30). Thus, methylation of the *CDKN2A* gene appears to be a very early step during lung cancer tumorigenesis. Cadherins are calcium-dependent cell-cell adhesion proteins. In NSCLCs, the *E-cadherin* (*CDH1*) and *H-cadherin* (*CDH13*) genes are frequently inactivated through DNA methylation (Table 1), which might have an association with prognosis in lung cancer (9).

Table 1
Frequently methylated target genes in lung cancer (%)

Pathway	Gene	Analysis method[a]	NSCLC	AD[a]	SQ[a]	SCLC	Reference
Cell cycle							
	CDKN2A	MSP	21–45	13–26	37–48	9–56	(37, 73–75, 83, 86)
		MethyLight	26–45	12	46		(76, 77)
		Pyrosequencing	21				(78)
	PAX5α	MSP		64	52		(79)
	PAX5β	MSP		74	61		(79)
	CHFR	MSP	19	5	30		(80, 81)
	FHIT	MSP	21–37				(73, 82)
	APC	MSP	41	42–53	16–24	12	(37, 74, 83)
		MethyLight	30–37	49	17		(76, 77)
	BLU	MSP	40–65	51	35		(35, 84)
		COBRA, MSP	19			14	(85)
DNA repair							
	MGMT	MSP	15–19	17–27	11–19	16	(83, 86)
		MethyLight	4	0	10		(77)
		Pyrosequencing	11				(78)
	BRCA1	MSP	4–30				(87, 88)
	BRCA2	MSP	0–42				(87, 88)
	hMLH1	MSP	12	5	10		(35, 74)
	GSTP	MSP	7–12	2–10	0–16	16	(73, 74, 83, 86)
Apoptosis							
	FAS	MSP	0			40	(89)
	DAPK	MSP	18	16–23	21–35		(74, 86)
		MethyLight	6–43	4	13		(76, 77)
		Pyrosequencing	18				(78)
	TRAILR1	MSP	0			40	(89)
	CASP8	MSP	0			35–52	(89, 90)
	TMS1	MSP	40			41	(91)
		MethyLight	8	14	5		(77)
	PTEN	MSP	26	24	30		(92)
		Pyrosequencing	49				(78)
	RUNX	MSP		28	7		(74)
		MethyLight	21	31	3		(77)
	RASSF1A	BS				79	(93)
		MSP	37–40	32–52	31–41	84–94	(37, 74, 75, 83, 84)
		MethyLight	30–45	31	18		(76, 77)
		Pyrosequencing	37				(78)
Growth control							
	ER	MSP	54	55	52		(94)
	SOCS3	BS, MSP	81				(95)
		MethyLight	5				(76)

(continued)

Table 1 (continued)

Pathway	Gene	Analysis method[a]	NSCLC	AD[a]	SQ[a]	SCLC	Reference
Adhesion							
	E-cadherin	MSP	8–34	16–34	19–34	56	(74, 83, 86)
		MethyLight	6–12	6	5		(76, 77)
		Pyrosequencing	26				(78)
	H-cadherin	MSP	40–42	29–52	16	16	(37, 73, 83)
		MethyLight	11–28	12	10		(76, 77)
	TIMP3	MSP	26	24	23		(86)
		COBRA	13				(96)
	TSLC1	BS	44	43	54		(97)
		BS, MSP	37	32	46	0	(98)
Differentiation							
	RARB	MSP	30–40	30–49	29–35	47	(37, 73, 83, 86)
		MethyLight	31	31	31		(77)

[a] *AD* adenocarcinoma, *BS* bisulfite sequencing, *MSP* methylation-specific PCR, *SQ* squamous cell carcinoma

Numerous examples of promoter hypermethylation have been described and are summarized in Fig. 1 and Table 1. Silencing these genes by epigenetic mechanisms may affect multiple oncogenic pathways in a gradual or stepwise manner.

3.2. Significance of CpG Island Methylator Phenotype in Lung Cancer

A remarkable study in colorectal cancers indicated that a subset of cases exhibit a high frequency of aberrant promoter hypermethylation, the so-called CpG island methylator phenotype (CIMP) (31). CIMP tumors in the context of colorectal cancer show distinct genetic and clinical features, such as high rates of *BRAF* and *KRAS* mutations, low frequency of *TP53* mutation, specific histology (mucinous, poorly differentiated), proximal location, and characteristic clinical outcome, suggesting that CIMP-related carcinogenesis may proceed through an unique pathway in which DNA methylation changes are the driving force for neoplastic transformation (32, 33).

In lung cancer, a few studies have demonstrated a distinct subgroup showing this characteristic high rate of aberrant DNA methylation (Table 2). Suzuki et al. first described the CIMP in NSCLCs that were methylation-positive in either the *CDH13* or *CRBP1* genes (34). These CIMP-positive cases appeared to be associated with poorer prognosis than non-CIMP cases. Liu et al. examined the methylation status of eight candidate genes in chromosome 3p and found that patients with CIMP-positive tumors had worse prognosis (35). Recently, using genome-wide analysis, Goto et al. demonstrated the existence of extensively methylated tumors in patients with adenocarcinomas, again suggestive of CIMP in lung

Table 2
CIMP in lung cancer

Marker	Method[a]	Criteria	Frequency of CIMP	Character of CIMP	Reference
CDH13, CRBP1	MSP	≥1	26/79 (33%)	CIMP(+) adenocarcinomas showed poorer prognosis than CIMP(−) tumors	(34)
APC, DAPK, GSTP1, LAMC2, RARB, RASSF1, SFRP1, SFRP2, SFRP4, SFRP5, PYCARD, CDH1, CDH13, CDKN2A, hMLH1, MGMT	MSP				(99)
Reprimo, p16, SPARC, DRM/gremlin, IL-12Rb2, RUNX3, SFRP1, SFRP2, SFRP5, Wif-1, Dkk3, APC	MSP	≥5	99/229 (43%)	CIMP(−) NSCLCs with COPD had worse prognosis	(100)
hOGG1, VHL, RARB, hMLH1, SEMM3B, RASSF1A, BLU, FHIT	MSP	≥4	34/60 (57%)	CIMP(+) NSCLCs had shorter survival	(35)

[a] *MSP* methylation-specific PCR

cancer (36). Given the evidence that frequent DNA methylation of certain candidate genes has been found in patients with smoking history or *EGFR* wild-type tumors (37), CIMP tumors may have a distinct molecular etiology from non-CIMP tumors, leading to different clinical phenotypes. However, in comparison to the considerable research activity on colorectal cancers in the context of CIMP markers, relatively little study has been performed in this area in respect to lung cancer. It is still not clear which marker or panel of markers will be most accurate for identifying CIMP in lung cancer. Thus, it is important to first define the relevant markers for CIMP tumors in this context. Establishing further accurate and practical classifications of methylation-dependent tumors might provide new therapeutic strategies in lung cancer (see below).

3.3. High-Throughput DNA Methylation Analysis in Lung Cancer

Early studies were focused on methylation status of single genes; however, recent development of high-throughput approaches has provided us a huge amount of information which will help to understand how epigenetic changes contribute to lung tumorigenesis. The methods utilized for DNA methylation analysis are summarized in Fig. 2. The first genome-wide methylation analysis in lung cancers

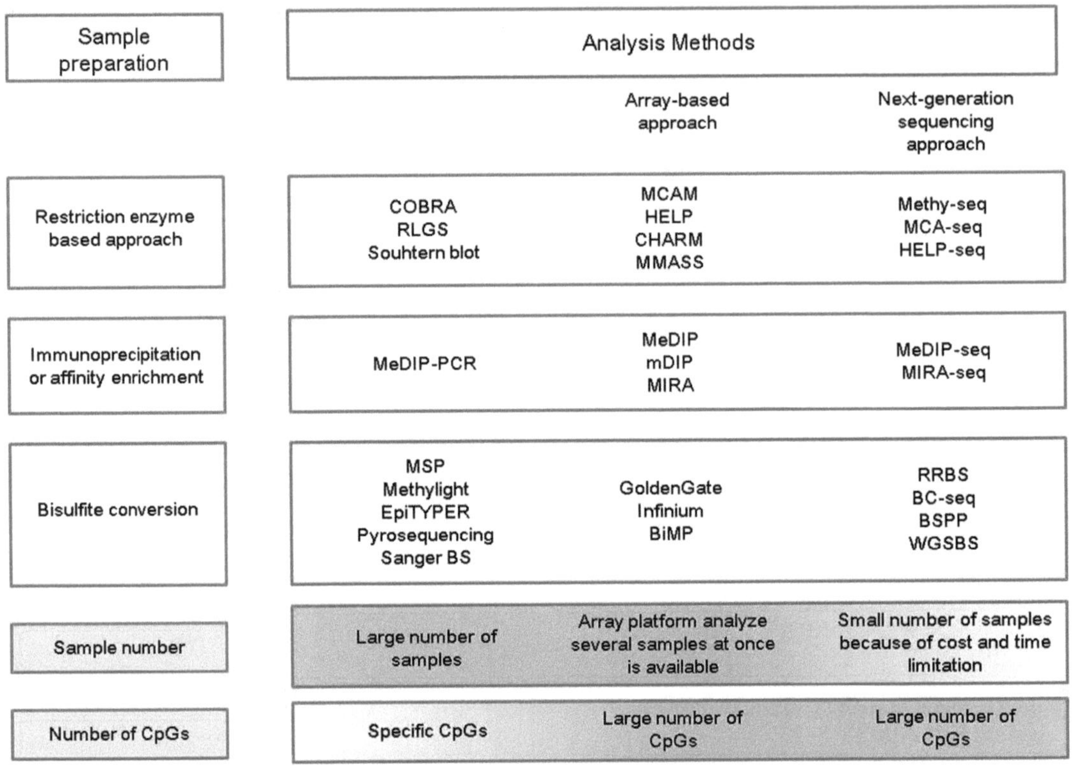

Fig. 2. DNA methylation analysis. *COBRA* combined bisulfite restriction analysis, *BC-seq* bisulfite conversion followed by capture and sequencing, *BiMP* bisulfite methylation profiling, *BS* bisulfite sequencing, *BSPP* bisulfite padlock probes, *CHARM* comprehensive high-throughput arrays for relative methylation, *HELP Hpa*II tiny fragment enrichment by ligation-mediated PCR, *MCA* methylated CpG island amplification, *MCAM* MCA with microarray hybridization, *MeDIP* methylated DNA immunoprecipitation, *MIRA* methylated CpG island recovery assay, *MMASS* microarray-based methylation assessment of single samples, *MSP* methylation-specific PCR, *RLGS* restriction landmark genomics scanning, *-seq* followed by sequencing, *RRBS* reduced representation bisulfite sequencing, and *WGSBS* whole-genome shotgun bisulfite sequencing (13).

was performed by restriction landmark genomics scanning (RLGS). Dai et al. analyzed 1,184 CpG islands in 16 primary NSCLCs, finding 11 genes, including *bone morphogenetic protein 3B* (*BMP3B*, also known as the *growth differentiation factor 10*, *GDF10* gene), a member of the TGF-β superfamily, that were differently methylated compared to matched normal lung tissue (38). Brena et al. investigated 40 NSCLCs using the RLGS technique and identified 47 DNA methylation targets that were differently methylated between adenocarcinomas and squamous cell carcinomas. Among the 47 genes, they further identified *oligodendrocyte transcription factor 1* (*OLIG1*) as being significantly correlated in expression terms with survival of NSCLC patients (39).

Epigenetic changes are reversible with DNA methyltransferase (DNMT) inhibitors and histone deacetylase (HDAC) inhibitors. In addition, DNMT inhibitors and HDAC inhibitors synergistically activate the expression of silenced genes (40). Indirect approaches which compare the gene expression patterns of cells treated with DNMT inhibitors and/or HDAC inhibitors by expression microarrays can be used to identify epigenetically repressed genes. Using this functional screening approach, Shames et al. examined seven NSCLC cell lines and found that 132 genes were effectively reactivated by 5-aza-2′-deoxycytidine treatment (41). Among the 132 genes, 31 genes were bona fide targets of DNA methylation in primary NSCLCs, with *ALDH1A3*, *BNC1*, *CCNA1*, *CTSZ*, *LOX*, *MSX1*, and *NRCAM* being particularly frequent targets. Zhong et al. compared the expression pattern before and after treatment with DNMT and HDAC inhibitors. Among 226 upregulated genes, *MT3*, *CST6*, and *NNAT* were frequently methylated in NSCLC cell lines, as well as primary tumors (42).

Combination of bisulfite conversion of DNA and BeadArray technology appears to be a powerful and widely used approach to interrogate DNA methylation in the genome, although reduction in sequence complexity after bisulfite conversion may sometimes be a problem, which results in some potential bias for the examined loci. Bibikova et al. analyzed 1,536 CpG sites in 371 cancer-related genes in primary lung adenocarcinoma and normal lung tissues (43). They identified 55 methylation markers, including *ASCL2*, *CDH13*, *HOXA5*, *HOXA11*, *NPY*, *RUNX3*, *TERT*, and *TP73*, which could distinguish adenocarcinoma from normal tissues. Christensen et al. used the same technique to compare the methylation profile of lung adenocarcinoma and malignant pleural mesothelioma and showed that DNA methylation status of 1,266 CpG loci was different between the two malignancies (44).

Enzyme-based and affinity enrichment-based DNA methylation analysis techniques, combined with microarray technology, are alternative ways of genome-wide study of epigenetic phenomena. These techniques have benefited by being easy to adapt to hybridization arrays, although enzyme-based assays have lower resolution coverage than other technologies in this arena due its intrinsic limitation on enzymatic recognition sites. Rauch et al. used tiling arrays in combination with the methylated CpG island recovery assay (MIRA), the latter approach being based on the high affinity of a complex of MBD2b and MBD3L1 protein for CpG-methylated DNA (45, 46). In the case of stage I squamous cell carcinoma samples, an average 537 out of 27,800 CpG islands were methylated (46). These investigators further identified the *OTX1*, *PAX6*, *IRX2*, *OC2*, *TFAP2A*, and *EVX2* genes as showing tumor-specific methylation and proposed that these genes might be useful for diagnostic applications. Fukasawa et al. used an enzyme-based (*Hpa*II and *Msp*I) approach to examine the methylation status of six NSCLC cell lines. They showed that about 11% of 288 cancer-related genes were methylated in cancer cell lines, among which the *ASC*, *PAX3*, and *RIPK3* genes were frequently methylated in primary lung cancers (47). Goto et al. analyzed 6,157 CpG islands using another set of restriction enzymes, namely,

*Xma*I and *Sma*I, in malignant pleural mesothelioma and lung adenocarcinoma (36). They revealed that these two malignancies were classified into distinct groups, as determined by DNA methylation patterns, with the frequency of tumor-specific DNA methylation being found to be higher in adenocarcinomas than in mesotheliomas.

Next-generation DNA sequencing provides more abundant information in relation to genome-wide epigenetic changes, with less input DNA, than microarray analysis (48, 49). Once sequencing costs come down and convenient bioinformatic analyses become more easily available, this will become an ideal method to analyze the whole genome in relation to epigenetic phenomena. In the near future, DNA methylation profiles from these high-throughput analyses will help us to understand lung cancer tumorigenesis in epigenetic terms, which may in turn improve prognosis of lung cancer patient.

3.4. DNA Methylation as a Diagnostic and Prognostic Marker

DNA methylation has been recognized as a powerful biomarker for early detection and monitoring of lung cancer (6). As described above, hundreds of aberrantly methylated genes have been identified in the context of this disease. Progressing from normal lung to atypical adenomatous hyperplasia to adenocarcinoma, stepwise accumulation of DNA hypermethylation within sets of genes has been observed, events which are positively associated with advanced histology (50). In relation to diagnostic detection of aberrant DNA methylation in lung cancer patients, sputum, blood, bronchoalveolar lavage (BAL), and bronchial brushings are useful samples obtained from minimally invasive procedures.

CDKN2A may be a good candidate gene for early detection of lung cancer. In a high-risk cohort with smoking history, methylation of three or more genes from a set of six, including *CDKN2A*, was shown to be closely associated with an increased risk for lung cancer (51). DNA methylation status has been also associated with prognosis in lung cancers. Stage I NSCLC patients who had recurrence after surgery showed a higher frequency of DNA methylation in the *CDKN2A* and *CDH13* genes than patients without recurrences (9). A study with combinatory use of methylation markers, *APC*, *CDKN2A*, and *RASSF1A*, in bronchial aspirates showed 63 and 44% of methylation-positive cases in central and peripheral lung cancers, respectively (52). Use of blood samples to examine the potential utility of DNA methylation as a diagnostic marker is more challenging than other tissue samples since identification of markers for tumor type-specific DNA methylation is required (53, 54). Analysis of DNA methylation in pleural effusions is sometimes useful for differential diagnosis of lung cancers and the other thoracic malignancies, such as malignant pleural mesotheliomas. Several genes, *CDKN2A*, *APC*, *ESR1*, *RASSF1A*, *DAPK*, and *RARB*, have been reported as candidate targets that are differentially methylated in lung cancers and malignant pleural mesotheliomas (55–57). Goto et al. reported specific methylation markers (*TMEM30B*, *KAZALD1*, and *MAPK13*) for malignant pleural mesotheliomas (36). The delineation of regional DNA methylation status, as well as broader DNA methylation profiles using high-throughput analyses, may provide important implications for understanding how aberrant DNA methylation contributes to lung tumorigenesis, which may potentially link in with the identification of effective diagnostic and prognostic markers for lung cancer.

4. Epigenetic Abnormalities as Therapeutic Targets in Lung Cancer

Epigenetic drugs targeting DNA methylation, such as 5-aza-2′-deoxycytidine (decitabine, DAC) and 5-azacytidine (azacitidine, AZA), have demonstrated clinical effectiveness in cancer treatment (58). Both drugs are now approved by the US Food and Drug Administration for the treatment of patients with myelodysplastic syndromes (59, 60). A phase I trial using DAC in patients with thoracic malignancies has been conducted, in which DAC modulated the expression of several genes repressed or upregulated in the primary tumor (61). Another study showed that a stage IV NSCLC patient could survive 81 months after treatment of five cycles of DAC (62). Such studies suggest that at least some patients have a clinical benefit from DAC treatment. A key challenge remains to identify and develop effective markers that can select those patients that are sensitive to demethylating agents (Fig. 3) (63), thereby carrying the promise of more effective epigenetic treatment strategies for lung cancer.

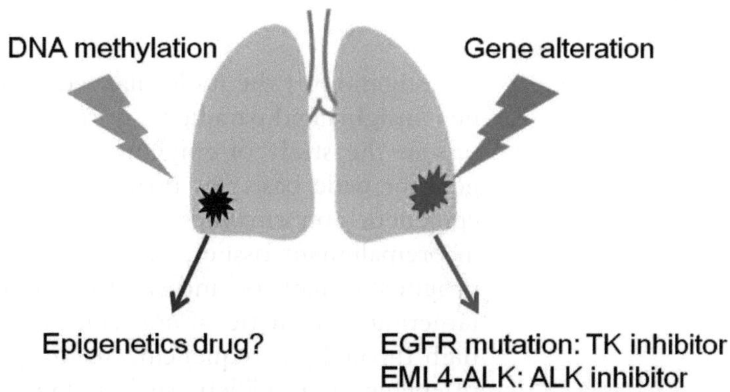

Fig. 3. Possible targeted therapy for lung cancers. In addition to TKIs and ALK inhibitors, epigenetic therapy might be useful approaches, especially for those individuals with high rate of aberrant epigenetic alterations.

In addition to single-agent use of DAC, combination therapy with other chemotherapies has also been investigated. Combination therapy of DAC and carboplatin in patients with solid tumors induced demethylation of *MAGE1A* in tumor cells (64). DAC may also have a role in increasing sensitivity to agents like carboplatin in drug-resistant ovarian and colon tumor xenografts (65).

There is an abundance of reports regarding the incidence of DNA methylation in lung cancer; however, relatively little is known about histone modifications in this disease. In patients with prostate cancer, high expression of EZH2, a histone H3 lysine 27 methyltransferase, is associated with aggressiveness and poor prognosis (66). In NSCLCs, tumors with high expression of EZH2 have been correlated with poorly differentiated adenocarcinoma, advanced stage, and poor prognosis (67). Global analysis of histone modification of NSCLCs revealed seven distinct groups of tumors based on different histone modifications, each showing different prognosis (68). These observations provide a rational basis for combination therapy incorporating standard chemotherapy with a histone modification drug, such as HDAC inhibitors. A recent study showed that a lung cancer cell line, once showed resistance to TKI treatment, recovered drug tolerance when treated with HDAC inhibitor (69). As mentioned previously, DNA methylation and HDAC inhibitors synergistically induce re-expression of epigenetically silenced genes (40). In a phase II trial of AZA and the HDAC inhibitor, entinostat, in relapsed NSCLC patients, some patients had benefit from the treatment (70). Thus, epigenetic therapy might be a useful approach, especially for those individuals who have been diagnosed with aberrant epigenetic alterations (e.g., exhibiting CIMP) but have not yet achieved clinical responses by other standard chemotherapies.

5. Conclusions

Investigation of the molecular pathology of lung cancer provides new insights and paradigms in respect to treatment. Recent progress in the study of epigenetic abnormalities in lung cancer on genome-wide basis has provided (1) information on the role of epigenetic abnormalities as early events in tumor formation, even in premalignant tissues, (2) identification of new diagnostic and prognostic markers, and (3) the establishment of a new strategy targeting epigenetic abnormalities. In addition, new powerful high-throughput sequencing techniques have revealed mutations of epigenetic modifiers, such as DNA methyltranseferase 3A and EZH2 in human malignancies (71, 72). Since it is important to elucidate the exact role of the key factors involved in the generation of epigenetic patterns, these findings may provide insight into answering the long-term question of how genetic mutation leads to epigenetic abnormalities in cancers. A more complete understanding of the basis of epigenetic abnormalities in lung cancer may provide better clinical capability for diagnosis and therapy.

References

1. Jemal, A., Siegel, R., Xu, J., and Ward, E. (2010) Cancer statistics, 2010, *CA Cancer J Clin* 60, 277–300.
2. Ferlay, J., Parkin, D. M., and Steliarova-Foucher, E. (2010) Estimates of cancer incidence and mortality in Europe in 2008, *Eur J Cancer* 46, 765–781.
3. Mok, T. S., Wu, Y. L., Thongprasert, S., Yang, C. H., Chu, D. T., Saijo, N., Sunpaweravong, P., Han, B., Margono, B., Ichinose, Y., Nishiwaki, Y., Ohe, Y., Yang, J. J., Chewaskulyong, B., Jiang, H., Duffield, E. L., Watkins, C. L., Armour, A. A., and Fukuoka, M. (2009) Gefitinib or carboplatin-paclitaxel in pulmonary adenocarcinoma, *N Engl J Med* 361, 947–957.
4. Mitsudomi, T., Morita, S., Yatabe, Y., Negoro, S., Okamoto, I., Tsurutani, J., Seto, T., Satouchi, M., Tada, H., Hirashima, T., Asami, K., Katakami, N., Takada, M., Yoshioka, H., Shibata, K., Kudoh, S., Shimizu, E., Saito, H., Toyooka, S., Nakagawa, K., and Fukuoka, M. (2010) Gefitinib versus cisplatin plus docetaxel in patients with non-small-cell lung cancer harbouring mutations of the epidermal growth factor receptor (WJTOG3405): an open label, randomised phase 3 trial, *Lancet Oncol* 11, 121–128.
5. Choi, Y. L., Soda, M., Yamashita, Y., Ueno, T., Takashima, J., Nakajima, T., Yatabe, Y., Takeuchi, K., Hamada, T., Haruta, H., Ishikawa, Y., Kimura, H., Mitsudomi, T., Tanio, Y., and Mano, H. (2010) EML4-ALK mutations in lung cancer that confer resistance to ALK inhibitors, *N Engl J Med* 363, 1734–1739.
6. Belinsky, S. A. (2004) Gene-promoter hypermethylation as a biomarker in lung cancer, *Nat Rev Cancer* 4, 707–717.
7. Jones, P. A., and Laird, P. W. (1999) Cancer epigenetics comes of age, *Nat Genet* 21, 163–167.
8. Jones, P. A., and Baylin, S. B. (2007) The epigenomics of cancer, *Cell* 128, 683–692.
9. Brock, M. V., Hooker, C. M., Ota-Machida, E., Han, Y., Guo, M., Ames, S., Glockner, S., Piantadosi, S., Gabrielson, E., Pridham, G., Pelosky, K., Belinsky, S. A., Yang, S. C., Baylin, S. B., and Herman, J. G. (2008) DNA methylation markers and early recurrence in stage I lung cancer, *N Engl J Med* 358, 1118–1128.
10. Shen, L., Catalano, P. J., Benson, A. B., 3rd, O'Dwyer, P., Hamilton, S. R., and Issa, J. P. (2007) Association between DNA methylation and shortened survival in patients with advanced colorectal cancer treated with 5-fluorouracil based chemotherapy, *Clin Cancer Res* 13, 6093–6098.
11. Noushmehr, H., Weisenberger, D. J., Diefes, K., Phillips, H. S., Pujara, K., Berman, B. P., Pan, F., Pelloski, C. E., Sulman, E. P., Bhat, K. P., Verhaak, R. G., Hoadley, K. A., Hayes, D. N., Perou, C. M., Schmidt, H. K., Ding, L., Wilson, R. K., Van Den Berg, D., Shen, H., Bengtsson, H., Neuvial, P., Cope, L. M., Buckley, J., Herman, J. G., Baylin, S. B., Laird, P. W., and Aldape, K. (2010) Identification of a CpG Island Methylator Phenotype that Defines a Distinct Subgroup of Glioma, *Cancer Cell* 17, 510–522.
12. Palmisano, W. A., Divine, K. K., Saccomanno, G., Gilliland, F. D., Baylin, S. B., Herman, J. G., and Belinsky, S. A. (2000) Predicting lung cancer by detecting aberrant promoter methylation in sputum, *Cancer Res* 60, 5954–5958.
13. Laird, P. W. (2010) Principles and challenges of genome-wide DNA methylation analysis, *Nat Rev Genet* 11, 191–203.
14. Brauch, H., Johnson, B., Hovis, J., Yano, T., Gazdar, A., Pettengill, O. S., Graziano, S., Sorenson, G. D., Poiesz, B. J., Minna, J. (1987) Molecular analysis of the short arm of chromosome 3 in small-cell and non-small-cell carcinoma of the lung, *N Engl J Med* 317, 1109–1113.
15. Hibi, K., Takahashi, T., Yamakawa, K., Ueda, R., Sekido, Y., Ariyoshi, Y., Suyama, M., Takagi, H., and Nakamura, Y. (1992) Three distinct regions involved in 3p deletion in human lung cancer, *Oncogene* 7, 445–449.
16. Zabarovsky, E. R., Lerman, M. I., and Minna, J. D. (2002) Tumor suppressor genes on chromosome 3p involved in the pathogenesis of lung and other cancers, *Oncogene* 21, 6915–6935.
17. Takahashi, T., Nau, M. M., Chiba, I., Birrer, M. J., Rosenberg, R. K., Vinocour, M., Levitt,

M., Pass, H., Gazdar, A. F., and Minna, J. D. (1989) p53: a frequent target for genetic abnormalities in lung cancer, *Science* 246, 491–494.

18. Forbes, S. A., Tang, G., Bindal, N., Bamford, S., Dawson, E., Cole, C., Kok, C. Y., Jia, M., Ewing, R., Menzies, A., Teague, J. W., Stratton, M. R., and Futreal, P. A. (2010) COSMIC (the Catalogue of Somatic Mutations in Cancer): a resource to investigate acquired mutations in human cancer, *Nucleic Acids Res* 38, D652–657.
19. Wistuba, II, Gazdar, A. F., and Minna, J. D. (2001) Molecular genetics of small cell lung carcinoma, *Semin Oncol* 28, 3–13.
20. Mounawar, M., Mukeria, A., Le Calvez, F., Hung, R. J., Renard, H., Cortot, A., Bollart, C., Zaridze, D., Brennan, P., Boffetta, P., Brambilla, E., and Hainaut, P. (2007) Patterns of EGFR, HER2, TP53, and KRAS mutations of p14arf expression in non-small cell lung cancers in relation to smoking history, *Cancer Res* 67, 5667–5672.
21. Kosaka, T., Yatabe, Y., Endoh, H., Kuwano, H., Takahashi, T., and Mitsudomi, T. (2004) Mutations of the epidermal growth factor receptor gene in lung cancer: biological and clinical implications, *Cancer Res* 64, 8919–8923.
22. Shigematsu, H., Lin, L., Takahashi, T., Nomura, M., Suzuki, M., Wistuba, II, Fong, K. M., Lee, H., Toyooka, S., Shimizu, N., Fujisawa, T., Feng, Z., Roth, J. A., Herz, J., Minna, J. D., and Gazdar, A. F. (2005) Clinical and biological features associated with epidermal growth factor receptor gene mutations in lung cancers, *J Natl Cancer Inst* 97, 339–346.
23. Sharma, S. V., Bell, D. W., Settleman, J., and Haber, D. A. (2007) Epidermal growth factor receptor mutations in lung cancer, *Nat Rev Cancer* 7, 169–181.
24. Le Calvez, F., Mukeria, A., Hunt, J. D., Kelm, O., Hung, R. J., Taniere, P., Brennan, P., Boffetta, P., Zaridze, D. G., and Hainaut, P. (2005) TP53 and KRAS mutation load and types in lung cancers in relation to tobacco smoke: distinct patterns in never, former, and current smokers, *Cancer Res* 65, 5076–5083.
25. Mascaux, C., Iannino, N., Martin, B., Paesmans, M., Berghmans, T., Dusart, M., Haller, A., Lothaire, P., Meert, A. P., Noel, S., Lafitte, J. J., and Sculier, J. P. (2005) The role of RAS oncogene in survival of patients with lung cancer: a systematic review of the literature with meta-analysis, *Br J Cancer* 92, 131–139.
26. Linardou, H., Dahabreh, I. J., Kanaloupiti, D., Siannis, F., Bafaloukos, D., Kosmidis, P., Papadimitriou, C. A., and Murray, S. (2008) Assessment of somatic k-RAS mutations as a mechanism associated with resistance to EGFR-targeted agents: a systematic review and meta-analysis of studies in advanced non-small-cell lung cancer and metastatic colorectal cancer, *Lancet Oncol* 9, 962–972.
27. Wong, D. W., Leung, E. L., So, K. K., Tam, I. Y., Sihoe, A. D., Cheng, L. C., Ho, K. K., Au, J. S., Chung, L. P., and Pik Wong, M. (2009) The EML4-ALK fusion gene is involved in various histologic types of lung cancers from nonsmokers with wild-type EGFR and KRAS, *Cancer* 115, 1723–1733.
28. Ding, L., Getz, G., Wheeler, D. A., Mardis, E. R., McLellan, M. D., Cibulskis, K., Sougnez, C., Greulich, H., Muzny, D. M., Morgan, M. B., Fulton, L., Fulton, R. S., Zhang, Q., Wendl, M. C., Lawrence, M. S., Larson, D. E., Chen, K., Dooling, D. J., Sabo, A., Hawes, A. C., Shen, H., Jhangiani, S. N., Lewis, L. R., Hall, O., Zhu, Y., Mathew, T., Ren, Y., Yao, J., Scherer, S. E., Clerc, K., Metcalf, G. A., Ng, B., Milosavljevic, A., Gonzalez-Garay, M. L., Osborne, J. R., Meyer, R., Shi, X., Tang, Y., Koboldt, D. C., Lin, L., Abbott, R., Miner, T. L., Pohl, C., Fewell, G., Haipek, C., Schmidt, H., Dunford-Shore, B. H., Kraja, A., Crosby, S. D., Sawyer, C. S., Vickery, T., Sander, S., Robinson, J., Winckler, W., Baldwin, J., Chirieac, L. R., Dutt, A., Fennell, T., Hanna, M., Johnson, B. E., Onofrio, R. C., Thomas, R. K., Tonon, G., Weir, B. A., Zhao, X., Ziaugra, L., Zody, M. C., Giordano, T., Orringer, M. B., Roth, J. A., Spitz, M. R., Wistuba, II, Ozenberger, B., Good, P. J., Chang, A. C., Beer, D. G., Watson, M. A., Ladanyi, M., Broderick, S., Yoshizawa, A., Travis, W. D., Pao, W., Province, M. A., Weinstock, G. M., Varmus, H. E., Gabriel, S. B., Lander, E. S., Gibbs, R. A., Meyerson, M., and Wilson, R. K. (2008) Somatic mutations affect key pathways in lung adenocarcinoma, *Nature* 455, 1069–1075.
29. Jones, P. A., and Baylin, S. B. (2002) The fundamental role of epigenetic events in cancer, *Nat Rev Genet* 3, 415–428.
30. Belinsky, S. A., Palmisano, W. A., Gilliland, F. D., Crooks, L. A., Divine, K. K., Winters, S. A., Grimes, M. J., Harms, H. J., Tellez, C. S., Smith, T. M., Moots, P. P., Lechner, J. F., Stidley, C. A., and Crowell, R. E. (2002) Aberrant promoter methylation in bronchial epithelium and sputum from current and former smokers, *Cancer Res* 62, 2370–2377.
31. Toyota, M., Ahuja, N., Ohe-Toyota, M., Herman, J. G., Baylin, S. B., and Issa, J. P. (1999) CpG island methylator phenotype in colorectal cancer, *Proc Natl Acad Sci U S A* 96, 8681–8686.

32. Issa, J. P. (2004) CpG island methylator phenotype in cancer, *Nat Rev Cancer* 4, 988–993.
33. Grady, W. M. (2007) CIMP and colon cancer gets more complicated, *Gut* 56, 1498–1500.
34. Suzuki, M., Shigematsu, H., Iizasa, T., Hiroshima, K., Nakatani, Y., Minna, J. D., Gazdar, A. F., and Fujisawa, T. (2006) Exclusive mutation in epidermal growth factor receptor gene, HER-2, and KRAS, and synchronous methylation of nonsmall cell lung cancer, *Cancer* 106, 2200–2207.
35. Liu, Z., Zhao, J., Chen, X. F., Li, W., Liu, R., Lei, Z., Liu, X., Peng, X., Xu, K., Chen, J., Liu, H., Zhou, Q. H., and Zhang, H. T. (2008) CpG island methylator phenotype involving tumor suppressor genes located on chromosome 3p in non-small cell lung cancer, *Lung cancer* 62, 15–22.
36. Goto, Y., Shinjo, K., Kondo, Y., Shen, L., Toyota, M., Suzuki, H., Gao, W., An, B., Fujii, M., Murakami, H., Osada, H., Taniguchi, T., Usami, N., Kondo, M., Hasegawa, Y., Shimokata, K., Matsuo, K., Hida, T., Fujimoto, N., Kishimoto, T., Issa, J. P., and Sekido, Y. (2009) Epigenetic profiles distinguish malignant pleural mesothelioma from lung adenocarcinoma, *Cancer Res* 69, 9073–9082.
37. Toyooka, S., Tokumo, M., Shigematsu, H., Matsuo, K., Asano, H., Tomii, K., Ichihara, S., Suzuki, M., Aoe, M., Date, H., Gazdar, A. F., and Shimizu, N. (2006) Mutational and epigenetic evidence for independent pathways for lung adenocarcinomas arising in smokers and never smokers, *Cancer Res* 66, 1371–1375.
38. Dai, Z., Lakshmanan, R. R., Zhu, W. G., Smiraglia, D. J., Rush, L. J., Fruhwald, M. C., Brena, R. M., Li, B., Wright, F. A., Ross, P., Otterson, G. A., and Plass, C. (2001) Global methylation profiling of lung cancer identifies novel methylated genes, *Neoplasia* 3, 314–323.
39. Brena, R. M., Morrison, C., Liyanarachchi, S., Jarjoura, D., Davuluri, R. V., Otterson, G. A., Reisman, D., Glaros, S., Rush, L. J., and Plass, C. (2007) Aberrant DNA methylation of OLIG1, a novel prognostic factor in non-small cell lung cancer, *PLoS medicine* 4, e108.
40. Cameron, E. E., Bachman, K. E., Myohanen, S., Herman, J. G., and Baylin, S. B. (1999) Synergy of demethylation and histone deacetylase inhibition in the re-expression of genes silenced in cancer, *Nat Genet* 21, 103–107.
41. Shames, D. S., Girard, L., Gao, B., Sato, M., Lewis, C. M., Shivapurkar, N., Jiang, A., Perou, C. M., Kim, Y. H., Pollack, J. R., Fong, K. M., Lam, C. L., Wong, M., Shyr, Y., Nanda, R., Olopade, O. I., Gerald, W., Euhus, D. M., Shay, J. W., Gazdar, A. F., and Minna, J. D. (2006) A genome-wide screen for promoter methylation in lung cancer identifies novel methylation markers for multiple malignancies, *PLoS medicine* 3, e486.
42. Zhong, S., Fields, C. R., Su, N., Pan, Y. X., and Robertson, K. D. (2007) Pharmacologic inhibition of epigenetic modifications, coupled with gene expression profiling, reveals novel targets of aberrant DNA methylation and histone deacetylation in lung cancer, *Oncogene* 26, 2621–2634.
43. Bibikova, M., Lin, Z., Zhou, L., Chudin, E., Garcia, E. W., Wu, B., Doucet, D., Thomas, N. J., Wang, Y., Vollmer, E., Goldmann, T., Seifart, C., Jiang, W., Barker, D. L., Chee, M. S., Floros, J., and Fan, J. B. (2006) High-throughput DNA methylation profiling using universal bead arrays, *Genome Res* 16, 383–393.
44. Christensen, B. C., Marsit, C. J., Houseman, E. A., Godleski, J. J., Longacker, J. L., Zheng, S., Yeh, R. F., Wrensch, M. R., Wiemels, J. L., Karagas, M. R., Bueno, R., Sugarbaker, D. J., Nelson, H. H., Wiencke, J. K., and Kelsey, K. T. (2009) Differentiation of lung adenocarcinoma, pleural mesothelioma, and nonmalignant pulmonary tissues using DNA methylation profiles, *Cancer Res* 69, 6315–6321.
45. Rauch, T., Wang, Z., Zhang, X., Zhong, X., Wu, X., Lau, S. K., Kernstine, K. H., Riggs, A. D., and Pfeifer, G. P. (2007) Homeobox gene methylation in lung cancer studied by genome-wide analysis with a microarray-based methylated CpG island recovery assay, *Proc Natl Acad Sci U S A* 104, 5527–5532.
46. Rauch, T. A., Zhong, X., Wu, X., Wang, M., Kernstine, K. H., Wang, Z., Riggs, A. D., and Pfeifer, G. P. (2008) High-resolution mapping of DNA hypermethylation and hypomethylation in lung cancer, *Proc Natl Acad Sci U S A* 105, 252–257.
47. Fukasawa, M., Kimura, M., Morita, S., Matsubara, K., Yamanaka, S., Endo, C., Sakurada, A., Sato, M., Kondo, T., Horii, A., Sasaki, H., and Hatada, I. (2006) Microarray analysis of promoter methylation in lung cancers, J *Hum Genet* 51, 368–374.
48. Meissner, A., Mikkelsen, T. S., Gu, H., Wernig, M., Hanna, J., Sivachenko, A., Zhang, X., Bernstein, B. E., Nusbaum, C., Jaffe, D. B., Gnirke, A., Jaenisch, R., and Lander, E. S. (2008) Genome-scale DNA methylation maps of pluripotent and differentiated cells, *Nature* 454, 766–770.

49. Lister, R., Pelizzola, M., Dowen, R. H., Hawkins, R. D., Hon, G., Tonti-Filippini, J., Nery, J. R., Lee, L., Ye, Z., Ngo, Q. M., Edsall, L., Antosiewicz-Bourget, J., Stewart, R., Ruotti, V., Millar, A. H., Thomson, J. A., Ren, B., and Ecker, J. R. (2009) Human DNA methylomes at base resolution show widespread epigenomic differences, *Nature* 462, 315–322.
50. Licchesi, J. D., Westra, W. H., Hooker, C. M., and Herman, J. G. (2008) Promoter hypermethylation of hallmark cancer genes in atypical adenomatous hyperplasia of the lung, *Clin Cancer Res* 14, 2570–2578.
51. Belinsky, S. A., Liechty, K. C., Gentry, F. D., Wolf, H. J., Rogers, J., Vu, K., Haney, J., Kennedy, T. C., Hirsch, F. R., Miller, Y., Franklin, W. A., Herman, J. G., Baylin, S. B., Bunn, P. A., and Byers, T. (2006) Promoter hypermethylation of multiple genes in sputum precedes lung cancer incidence in a high-risk cohort, *Cancer Res* 66, 3338–3344.
52. Schmiemann, V., Bocking, A., Kazimirek, M., Onofre, A. S., Gabbert, H. E., Kappes, R., Gerharz, C. D., and Grote, H. J. (2005) Methylation assay for the diagnosis of lung cancer on bronchial aspirates: a cohort study, *Clin Cancer Res* 11, 7728–7734.
53. Belinsky, S. A., Klinge, D. M., Dekker, J. D., Smith, M. W., Bocklage, T. J., Gilliland, F. D., Crowell, R. E., Karp, D. D., Stidley, C. A., and Picchi, M. A. (2005) Gene promoter methylation in plasma and sputum increases with lung cancer risk, *Clin Cancer Res* 11, 6505–6511.
54. Fujiwara, K., Fujimoto, N., Tabata, M., Nishii, K., Matsuo, K., Hotta, K., Kozuki, T., Aoe, M., Kiura, K., Ueoka, H., and Tanimoto, M. (2005) Identification of epigenetic aberrant promoter methylation in serum DNA is useful for early detection of lung cancer, *Clin Cancer Res* 11, 1219–1225.
55. Tsou, J. A., Galler, J. S., Wali, A., Ye, W., Siegmund, K. D., Groshen, S., Laird, P. W., Turla, S., Koss, M. N., Pass, H. I., and Laird-Offringa, I. A. (2007) DNA methylation profile of 28 potential marker loci in malignant mesothelioma, *Lung cancer* 58, 220–230.
56. Toyooka, S., Pass, H. I., Shivapurkar, N., Fukuyama, Y., Maruyama, R., Toyooka, K. O., Gilcrease, M., Farinas, A., Minna, J. D., and Gazdar, A. F. (2001) Aberrant methylation and simian virus 40 tag sequences in malignant mesothelioma, *Cancer Res* 61, 5727–5730.
57. Fischer, J. R., Ohnmacht, U., Rieger, N., Zemaitis, M., Stoffregen, C., Kostrzewa, M., Buchholz, E., Manegold, C., and Lahm, H. (2006) Promoter methylation of RASSF1A, RARbeta and DAPK predict poor prognosis of patients with malignant mesothelioma, *Lung cancer* 54, 109–116.
58. Issa, J. P., and Kantarjian, H. M. (2009) Targeting DNA methylation, *Clin Cancer Res* 15, 3938–3946.
59. Silverman, L. R., Demakos, E. P., Peterson, B. L., Kornblith, A. B., Holland, J. C., Odchimar-Reissig, R., Stone, R. M., Nelson, D., Powell, B. L., DeCastro, C. M., Ellerton, J., Larson, R. A., Schiffer, C. A., and Holland, J. F. (2002) Randomized controlled trial of azacitidine in patients with the myelodysplastic syndrome: a study of the cancer and leukemia group B, *J Clin Oncol* 20, 2429–2440.
60. Kantarjian, H., Issa, J. P., Rosenfeld, C. S., Bennett, J. M., Albitar, M., DiPersio, J., Klimek, V., Slack, J., de Castro, C., Ravandi, F., Helmer, R., 3rd, Shen, L., Nimer, S. D., Leavitt, R., Raza, A., and Saba, H. (2006) Decitabine improves patient outcomes in myelodysplastic syndromes: results of a phase III randomized study, *Cancer* 106, 1794–1803.
61. Schrump, D. S., Fischette, M. R., Nguyen, D. M., Zhao, M., Li, X., Kunst, T. F., Hancox, A., Hong, J. A., Chen, G. A., Pishchik, V., Figg, W. D., Murgo, A. J., and Steinberg, S. M. (2006) Phase I study of decitabine-mediated gene expression in patients with cancers involving the lungs, esophagus, or pleura, *Clin Cancer Res* 12, 5777–5785.
62. Momparler, R. L., and Ayoub, J. (2001) Potential of 5-aza-2′-deoxycytidine (Decitabine) a potent inhibitor of DNA methylation for therapy of advanced non-small cell lung cancer, *Lung cancer* 34 Suppl 4, S111–115.
63. Shen, L., Kantarjian, H., Guo, Y., Lin, E., Shan, J., Huang, X., Berry, D., Ahmed, S., Zhu, W., Pierce, S., Kondo, Y., Oki, Y., Jelinek, J., Saba, H., Estey, E., and Issa, J. P. (2010) DNA methylation predicts survival and response to therapy in patients with myelodysplastic syndromes, *J Clin Oncol* 28, 605–613.
64. Appleton, K., Mackay, H. J., Judson, I., Plumb, J. A., McCormick, C., Strathdee, G., Lee, C., Barrett, S., Reade, S., Jadayel, D., Tang, A., Bellenger, K., Mackay, L., Setanoians, A., Schatzlein, A., Twelves, C., Kaye, S. B., and Brown, R. (2007) Phase I and pharmacodynamic trial of the DNA methyltransferase inhibitor decitabine and carboplatin in solid tumors, *J Clin Oncol* 25, 4603–4609.
65. Plumb, J. A., Strathdee, G., Sludden, J., Kaye, S. B., and Brown, R. (2000) Reversal of drug

resistance in human tumor xenografts by 2′-deoxy-5-azacytidine-induced demethylation of the hMLH1 gene promoter, *Cancer Res* 60, 6039–6044.

66. Varambally, S., Dhanasekaran, S. M., Zhou, M., Barrette, T. R., Kumar-Sinha, C., Sanda, M. G., Ghosh, D., Pienta, K. J., Sewalt, R. G., Otte, A. P., Rubin, M. A., and Chinnaiyan, A. M. (2002) The polycomb group protein EZH2 is involved in progression of prostate cancer, *Nature* 419, 624–629.
67. Kikuchi, J., Kinoshita, I., Shimizu, Y., Kikuchi, E., Konishi, J., Oizumi, S., Kaga, K., Matsuno, Y., Nishimura, M., and Dosaka-Akita, H. (2010) Distinctive expression of the polycomb group proteins Bmi1 polycomb ring finger oncogene and enhancer of zeste homolog 2 in nonsmall cell lung cancers and their clinical and clinicopathologic significance, *Cancer* 116, 3015–3024.
68. Barlesi, F., Giaccone, G., Gallegos-Ruiz, M. I., Loundou, A., Span, S. W., Lefesvre, P., Kruyt, F. A., and Rodriguez, J. A. (2007) Global histone modifications predict prognosis of resected non small-cell lung cancer, *J Clin Oncol* 25, 4358–4364.
69. Sharma, S. V., Lee, D. Y., Li, B., Quinlan, M. P., Takahashi, F., Maheswaran, S., McDermott, U., Azizian, N., Zou, L., Fischbach, M. A., Wong, K. K., Brandstetter, K., Wittner, B., Ramaswamy, S., Classon, M., and Settleman, J. (2010) A chromatin-mediated reversible drug-tolerant state in cancer cell subpopulations, *Cell* 141, 69–80.
70. Juergens R. A., Vendetti F., Coleman B., Sebree R. S., Rudek M. A., Belinsky S., Brock M., Herman J., Baylin S., Rudin C. M. (2009) Interim analysis of a phase II trial of 5-azacitidine (5AC) and entinostat (SNDX-275) in relapsed advanced lung cancer (NSCLC), J Clin Oncol 27:15s, abstr 8055.
71. Ley, T. J., Ding, L., Walter, M. J., McLellan, M. D., Lamprecht, T., Larson, D. E., Kandoth, C., Payton, J. E., Baty, J., Welch, J., Harris, C. C., Lichti, C. F., Townsend, R. R., Fulton, R. S., Dooling, D. J., Koboldt, D. C., Schmidt, H., Zhang, Q., Osborne, J. R., Lin, L., O'Laughlin, M., McMichael, J. F., Delehaunty, K. D., McGrath, S. D., Fulton, L. A., Magrini, V. J., Vickery, T. L., Hundal, J., Cook, L. L., Conyers, J. J., Swift, G. W., Reed, J. P., Alldredge, P. A., Wylie, T., Walker, J., Kalicki, J., Watson, M. A., Heath, S., Shannon, W. D., Varghese, N., Nagarajan, R., Westervelt, P., Tomasson, M. H., Link, D. C., Graubert, T. A., DiPersio, J. F., Mardis, E. R., and Wilson, R. K. (2010) DNMT3A mutations in acute myeloid leukemia, *N Engl J Med* 363, 2424–2433.
72. Morin, R. D., Johnson, N. A., Severson, T. M., Mungall, A. J., An, J., Goya, R., Paul, J. E., Boyle, M., Woolcock, B. W., Kuchenbauer, F., Yap, D., Humphries, R. K., Griffith, O. L., Shah, S., Zhu, H., Kimbara, M., Shashkin, P., Charlot, J. F., Tcherpakov, M., Corbett, R., Tam, A., Varhol, R., Smailus, D., Moksa, M., Zhao, Y., Delaney, A., Qian, H., Birol, I., Schein, J., Moore, R., Holt, R., Horsman, D. E., Connors, J. M., Jones, S., Aparicio, S., Hirst, M., Gascoyne, R. D., and Marra, M. A. (2010) Somatic mutations altering EZH2 (Tyr641) in follicular and diffuse large B-cell lymphomas of germinal-center origin, *Nat Genet* 42, 181–185.
73. Kim, J. S., Kim, J. W., Han, J., Shim, Y. M., Park, J., and Kim, D. H. (2006) Cohypermethylation of p16 and FHIT promoters as a prognostic factor of recurrence in surgically resected stage I non-small cell lung cancer, *Cancer Res* 66, 4049–4054.
74. Yanagawa, N., Tamura, G., Oizumi, H., Takahashi, N., Shimazaki, Y., and Motoyama, T. (2003) Promoter hypermethylation of tumor suppressor and tumor-related genes in non-small cell lung cancers, *Cancer Sci* 94, 589–592.
75. Helmbold, P., Lahtz, C., Herpel, E., Schnabel, P. A., and Dammann, R. H. (2009) Frequent hypermethylation of RASSF1A tumour suppressor gene promoter and presence of Merkel cell polyomavirus in small cell lung cancer, *Eur J Cancer* 45, 2207–2211.
76. Shivapurkar, N., Stastny, V., Suzuki, M., Wistuba, II, Li, L., Zheng, Y., Feng, Z., Hol, B., Prinsen, C., Thunnissen, F. B., and Gazdar, A. F. (2007) Application of a methylation gene panel by quantitative PCR for lung cancers, *Cancer Lett* 247, 56–71.
77. Hawes, S. E., Stern, J. E., Feng, Q., Wiens, L. W., Rasey, J. S., Lu, H., Kiviat, N. B., and Vesselle, H. (2010) DNA hypermethylation of tumors from non-small cell lung cancer (NSCLC) patients is associated with gender and histologic type, *Lung cancer* 69, 172–179.
78. Buckingham, L., Penfield Faber, L., Kim, A., Liptay, M., Barger, C., Basu, S., Fidler, M., Walters, K., Bonomi, P., and Coon, J. (2010) PTEN, RASSF1 and DAPK site-specific hypermethylation and outcome in surgically treated stage I and II nonsmall cell lung cancer patients, *Int J Cancer* 126, 1630–1639.
79. Palmisano, W. A., Crume, K. P., Grimes, M. J., Winters, S. A., Toyota, M., Esteller, M., Joste, N., Baylin, S. B., and Belinsky, S. A. (2003) Aberrant promoter methylation of the transcription factor genes PAX5 alpha and

beta in human cancers, *Cancer Res* 63, 4620–4625.

80. Koga, T., Takeshita, M., Yano, T., Maehara, Y., and Sueishi, K. (2010) CHFR hypermethylation and EGFR mutation are mutually exclusive and exhibit contrastive clinical backgrounds and outcomes in non-small cell lung cancer, *Int J Cancer* 128, 1009–1017.
81. Mizuno, K., Osada, H., Konishi, H., Tatematsu, Y., Yatabe, Y., Mitsudomi, T., Fujii, Y., and Takahashi, T. (2002) Aberrant hypermethylation of the CHFR prophase checkpoint gene in human lung cancers, *Oncogene* 21, 2328–2333.
82. Zochbauer-Muller, S., Fong, K. M., Maitra, A., Lam, S., Geradts, J., Ashfaq, R., Virmani, A. K., Milchgrub, S., Gazdar, A. F., and Minna, J. D. (2001) 5 CpG island methylation of the FHIT gene is correlated with loss of gene expression in lung and breast cancer, *Cancer Res* 61, 3581–3585.
83. Toyooka, S., Toyooka, K. O., Maruyama, R., Virmani, A. K., Girard, L., Miyajima, K., Harada, K., Ariyoshi, Y., Takahashi, T., Sugio, K., Brambilla, E., Gilcrease, M., Minna, J. D., and Gazdar, A. F. (2001) DNA methylation profiles of lung tumors, *Mol Cancer Ther* 1, 61–67.
84. Marsit, C. J., Kim, D. H., Liu, M., Hinds, P. W., Wiencke, J. K., Nelson, H. H., and Kelsey, K. T. (2005) Hypermethylation of RASSF1A and BLU tumor suppressor genes in non-small cell lung cancer: implications for tobacco smoking during adolescence, *Int J Cancer* 114, 219–223.
85. Agathanggelou, A., Dallol, A., Zochbauer-Muller, S., Morrissey, C., Honorio, S., Hesson, L., Martinsson, T., Fong, K. M., Kuo, M. J., Yuen, P. W., Maher, E. R., Minna, J. D., and Latif, F. (2003) Epigenetic inactivation of the candidate 3p21.3 suppressor gene BLU in human cancers, *Oncogene* 22, 1580–1588.
86. Zochbauer-Muller, S., Fong, K. M., Virmani, A. K., Geradts, J., Gazdar, A. F., and Minna, J. D. (2001) Aberrant promoter methylation of multiple genes in non-small cell lung cancers, *Cancer Res* 61, 249–255.
87. Marsit, C. J., Liu, M., Nelson, H. H., Posner, M., Suzuki, M., and Kelsey, K. T. (2004) Inactivation of the Fanconi anemia/BRCA pathway in lung and oral cancers: implications for treatment and survival, *Oncogene* 23, 1000–1004.
88. Lee, M. N., Tseng, R. C., Hsu, H. S., Chen, J. Y., Tzao, C., Ho, W. L., and Wang, Y. C. (2007) Epigenetic inactivation of the chromosomal stability control genes BRCA1, BRCA2, and XRCC5 in non-small cell lung cancer, *Clin Cancer Res* 13, 832–838.
89. Hopkins-Donaldson, S., Ziegler, A., Kurtz, S., Bigosch, C., Kandioler, D., Ludwig, C., Zangemeister-Wittke, U., and Stahel, R. (2003) Silencing of death receptor and caspase-8 expression in small cell lung carcinoma cell lines and tumors by DNA methylation, *Cell death and differentiation* 10, 356–364.
90. Shivapurkar, N., Toyooka, S., Eby, M. T., Huang, C. X., Sathyanarayana, U. G., Cunningham, H. T., Reddy, J. L., Brambilla, E., Takahashi, T., Minna, J. D., Chaudhary, P. M., and Gazdar, A. F. (2002) Differential inactivation of caspase-8 in lung cancers, *Cancer Biol Ther* 1, 65–69.
91. Virmani, A., Rathi, A., Sugio, K., Sathyanarayana, U. G., Toyooka, S., Kischel, F. C., Tonk, V., Padar, A., Takahashi, T., Roth, J. A., Euhus, D. M., Minna, J. D., and Gazdar, A. F. (2003) Aberrant methylation of TMS1 in small cell, non small cell lung cancer and breast cancer, *Int J Cancer* 106, 198–204.
92. Marsit, C. J., Zheng, S., Aldape, K., Hinds, P. W., Nelson, H. H., Wiencke, J. K., and Kelsey, K. T. (2005) PTEN expression in non-small-cell lung cancer: evaluating its relation to tumor characteristics, allelic loss, and epigenetic alteration, *Human pathology* 36, 768–776.
93. Dammann, R., Takahashi, T., and Pfeifer, G. P. (2001) The CpG island of the novel tumor suppressor gene RASSF1A is intensely methylated in primary small cell lung carcinomas, *Oncogene* 20, 3563–3567.
94. Lai, J. C., Cheng, Y. W., Chiou, H. L., Wu, M. F., Chen, C. Y., and Lee, H. (2005) Gender difference in estrogen receptor alpha promoter hypermethylation and its prognostic value in non-small cell lung cancer, *Int J Cancer* 117, 974–980.
95. He, B., You, L., Uematsu, K., Zang, K., Xu, Z., Lee, A. Y., Costello, J. F., McCormick, F., and Jablons, D. M. (2003) SOCS-3 is frequently silenced by hypermethylation and suppresses cell growth in human lung cancer, *Proc Natl Acad Sci U S A* 100, 14133–14138.
96. Dammann, R., Strunnikova, M., Schagdarsurengin, U., Rastetter, M., Papritz, M., Hattenhorst, U. E., Hofmann, H. S., Silber, R. E., Burdach, S., and Hansen, G. (2005) CpG island methylation and expression of tumour-associated genes in lung carcinoma, *Eur J Cancer* 41, 1223–1236.
97. Kikuchi, S., Yamada, D., Fukami, T., Maruyama, T., Ito, A., Asamura, H., Matsuno,

Y., Onizuka, M., and Murakami, Y. (2006) Hypermethylation of the TSLC1/IGSF4 promoter is associated with tobacco smoking and a poor prognosis in primary nonsmall cell lung carcinoma, *Cancer* 106, 1751–1758.

98. Heller, G., Fong, K. M., Girard, L., Seidl, S., End-Pfutzenreuter, A., Lang, G., Gazdar, A. F., Minna, J. D., Zielinski, C. C., and Zochbauer-Muller, S. (2006) Expression and methylation pattern of TSLC1 cascade genes in lung carcinomas, *Oncogene* 25, 959–968.

99. Marsit, C. J., Houseman, E. A., Christensen, B. C., Eddy, K., Bueno, R., Sugarbaker, D. J., Nelson, H. H., Karagas, M. R., and Kelsey, K. T. (2006) Examination of a CpG island methylator phenotype and implications of methylation profiles in solid tumors, *Cancer Res* 66, 10621–10629.

100. Suzuki, M., Wada, H., Yoshino, M., Tian, L., Shigematsu, H., Suzuki, H., Alaa, M., Tamura, H., Fujiwara, T., Nagato, K., Motohashi, S., Moriya, Y., Hoshino, H., Yoshida, S., Shibuya, K., Hiroshima, K., Nakatani, Y., and Yoshino, I. (2010) Molecular characterization of chronic obstructive pulmonary disease-related non-small cell lung cancer through aberrant methylation and alterations of EGFR signaling, *Ann Surg Oncol* 17, 878–888.

Chapter 14

The Role of MicroRNAs in the Management of Liver Cancer

Krishna K. Banaudha and Mukesh Verma

Abstract

Four major components of epigenetic regulation are promoter methylation, histone modification, chromatin conformation changes, and altered expression of noncoding RNAs, especially microRNAs (miRNAs). MiRNAs are noncoding RNAs of single-stranded RNA molecules consisting of ~22 nucleotides that regulate gene expression at the posttranscriptional level. MiRNAs are endogenous and potentially can regulate every aspect of cellular activity, including development and proliferation, differentiation, metabolism, viral infection, epigenetic modulation, apoptotic cell death, and tumor genesis. Recent studies provide evidence that miRNAs are abundant in the liver and affect a diverse spectrum of liver functions. MiRNA expression and deregulation of miRNAs may be a major pathogenetic factor in many liver diseases. Although global downregulation is a common trait in human malignancies, including viral hepatitis, hepatocellular carcinoma, and polycystic liver diseases, specific miRNAs are upregulated in cancer and offer new diagnostic and therapeutic strategies to manage liver diseases. Here, the current status of the role of miRNAs in liver cancer is discussed along with areas for future research.

Key words: Biogenesis, Biomarkers, Epidemiology, Epigenetics, Hepatitis, Liver cancer, MiRNA, Treatment

Abbreviations

AFP	Alpha-fetoprotein
HCC	Hepatocellular carcinoma
HCV	Hepatitis C virus
IFN α/β	Interferon alpha/beta
MiRNAs	MicroRNAs
pri-miRNA	Primary microRNA
RISC	RNA-induced silencing complex
RNAi	RNA interference

Ramona G. Dumitrescu and Mukesh Verma (eds.), *Cancer Epigenetics: Methods and Protocols*, Methods in Molecular Biology, vol. 863, DOI 10.1007/978-1-61779-612-8_14,

1. Introduction: miRNAs Are an Integral Part of the Epigenetic Mechanism

During the past few years, emphasis has been placed on exploring gene structure and function. The role of genes and proteins was explained. In seeking to explain the initiation and development of cancer, the mechanisms that underlie some pathways could not be explained by the involvement of proteins alone. As a result, the idea of noncoding RNAs and their regulatory function in multiple genes, either as tumor suppressor genes or oncogenes, emerged (1–5). Among a number of noncoding RNAs, the role of microRNAs (miRNAs) has been established in cancer initiation, development, maintenance, and proliferation (6). MiRNAs are 19–24 nucleotide long, transcribed as a precursor, and interfere in posttranscriptional processes. Due to their sequence specificity and complementary sequence to mRNAs, miRNAs can be made target specific and used for therapeutic purposes. In recent years, several cancer-specific miRNAs have been identified (6, 7). A few miRNAs, such as miR-18a, miR-21, miR-101, miR-141, and miR-146a, have been reported in liver cancer (8–12). Recent studies have strong evidence that miRNA-mediated RNA-silencing pathway is involved in virus–host interactions (13). There are more than 500 miRNAs expressed in mammals. These are processed from noncoding regions of the genome by an enzymatic cascade that results in formation of an RNA-induced silencing complex (RISC) (14, 15). The RNA interference (RNAi) mechanisms have been reported to control viral infection in plants and invertebrates; later, it was shown that the IFN system superseded the requirement for an RNAi mechanism to control viral infection (16, 17). Padersen et al. have reported that IFNα/β upregulates several miRNAs that are capable of inhibi-ting hepatitis C virus (HCV) replication and infection. The downregulation of miR-122 in response to IFN-β contributes to the antiviral effect of interferons. These studies provide evidence of rapid modulation of cellular miRNAs as a component of the mammalian innate immune response.

Hepatocellular carcinoma (HCC) is a fatal disease that occurs worldwide and develops mainly in patients with chronic liver disease. Despite routine screening of individuals at high risk, most of the patients are diagnosed at late stages of HCC. In addition, the recurrence rate after surgical resection of small tumors is high. Liver cancer and the role of miRNAs in its development are discussed below.

2. Biogenesis of miRNAs

miRNAs are transcribed as a much larger molecule than their final size (9, 18). The miRNA genes are monocistronic as well as polycistronic clusters. Furthermore, miRNA genes are transcribed as nonprotein coding RNAs. They can be processed either from the sense or antisense strand of the gene that codes them. MiRNAs processing occurs in two different cell compartments: in the nucleus and in the cytoplasm. In the nucleus, miRNA genes are transcribed by RNA polymerase II as 70–100 nucleotide-long primary transcripts (pri-miRNA) that have a hairpin-like structure with a 5′-cap and a poly A tail (19). These primary transcripts are further processed in the nucleus to acquire the stem-loop structure of about 70 nucleotides. This processing is accomplished by a microprocessor protein complex consisting of a double-stranded RNA (dsRNA)-specific ribonuclease called Drosha and a double-stranded RNA-binding protein called Pasha (Fig. 1).

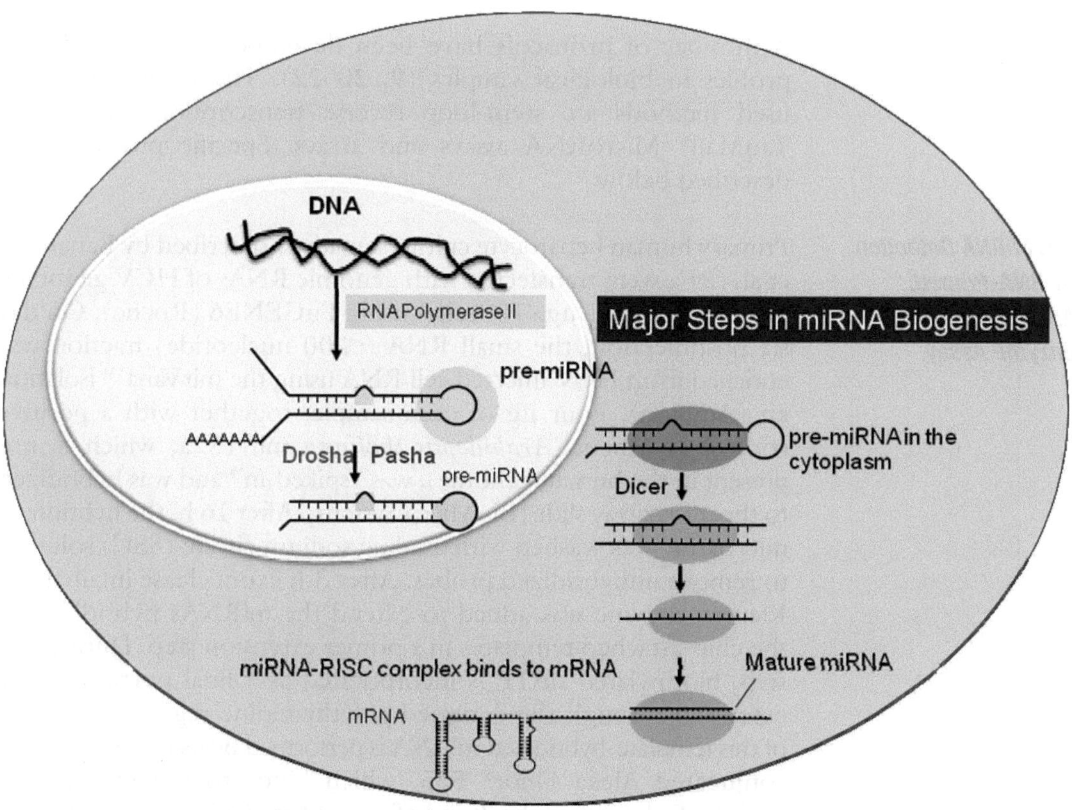

Fig. 1. miRNA biogenesis. The major steps and components of miRNA biogenesis are shown.

Efficient processing of pri-miRNA by Drosha requires the presence of extended single-stranded RNA on both the 3′- and 5′-ends of the hairpin molecule. These pre-miRNAs then are transported from the nucleus to the cytoplasm. The transport of pre-miRNAs is mediated by exportin-5 (a conserved nuclear export protein). These pre-miRNAs then are processed into mature miRNAs by interacting with a second RNAse III-like enzyme called Dicer, which generates 19–23 nucleotide-long miRNA that is bound by a complex similar to the RISC. RISC is responsible for miRNA-mediated gene silencing and RNAi. Upon cleaving of the pre-miRNA with Dicer, two complementary short RNA molecules are generated; however, only one of them is integrated into RISC. This strand is known as the "guide strand" and is selected by the argonaute protein, the catalytically active RNAse in RISC. The remaining strand, known as the "anti-guide" or "passenger strand" is degraded as a RISC substrate. After integration into the active RISC, miRNAs bind with their complementary mRNA molecules and induce mRNA degradation by the argonaute protein.

3. Protocols to Assay miRNA

A number of protocols have been developed to assay miRNA profiles in biological samples (9, 20–22). The most commonly used methods are stem-loop reverse transcription (RT)-based TaqMan® MicroRNA assays and arrays. Specific protocols are described below.

3.1. MiRNA Detection by RNA-Primed, Array-Based Klenow Enzyme Assay

Primary human hepatocyte cultures, made as described by Banaudha et al. (21), were transfected with genomic RNAs of HCV genotype 1a, 1b, and 2a (1 μg/10^6 cells) using FuGENE6 (Roche). On day six postinfection, the small RNA (≤200 nucleotide) fraction was enriched from HCV-infected cell RNA using the mirVana™ isolation kit (Ambion). Four μg of each sample, together with a positive control (synthetic *Arabidopsis thaliana* mir-157a, which is not present in the human genome), was "spiked-in" and was hybridized to the microarray slide (BioMicro System). After 16 h, the hybridized microarray was washed with a saline sodium citrate (SSC) solution to remove unhybridized probes. After 3-h exonuclease incubation, Klenow enzyme was added to extend the miRNAs hybridized to the chip-attached templates in a primer extension step. During this step, biotinylated dATP is incorporated as a final portion of the extension through the designed polythymidine region. Detection of this template-hybridized miRNA is performed by using streptavidin-conjugated Alexa Fluor® 555, which binds to the biotinylated stretch of adenines at the 3-end of the captured miRNA. Fluorescent data sets were collected using a GenePix 4000B scanner (Axon) as described by Yeung et al. (23).

3.2. Luciferase Reporter Assay

Primary human hepatocyte culture was cotransfected with a luciferase reporter containing DLC-1 3′-UTR (50 ng/10^6 cells), miR-141 (50 nM/10^6 cells, antagomir), or miR-141 (50 nM/10^6 cells, mimic) using Lipofectamine 2000 (Invitrogen). Luciferase assays (Promega, according to the manufacturer's instructions) were performed on the third day after the transfection (20–22).

4. miRNAs in the Management of Liver Cancer

The use of miRNAs as biomarkers has received increased attention in recent years (1, 24). Their role in regulating a great variety of targets and, as a consequence, multiple pathways allows their use as a diagnostic tool for early cancer detection, risk assessment, and prognosis, and for the design of innovative therapeutic strategies. HCC is an aggressive cancer with a poor prognosis, mainly due to metastasis. In addition to being aggressive, HCC has a tendency to recur after surgery. A number of biomarkers (histochemical, genetic, proteomic, and epigenetic) and risk factors, such as alcohol, infection, and family history, contribute to the development of liver cancer (25–29). A diagrammatic sketch of biomarkers and risk factors for liver cancer is presented in Fig. 2. Among all risk factors, chronic infection by the hepatitis B virus (HBV) and HCV appears to be the most significant causes of HCC (30, 31). Further characterization of infection mediated liver carcinogenesis demonstrated that aberrant promoter methylation is deeply involved in cancer including in HCC (32, 33). Varnholt et al. (31) have determined the miRNA gene expression profile of HCC patients who tested positive for HCV.

Serum fibrosis is a disease progression marker in hepatitis-positive patients who have not been informative in making a decision about hepatectomy (26). Three markers, alpha-fetoprotein (AFP), lens culinaris agglutinin A-reactive fraction of AFP (AFP-L3), and des-gamma-carboxy prothrombin (DCP), have been reported as effective in detecting and predicting the recurrence of liver cancer (28). This study also demonstrated that the biomarkers that are used effectively to detect liver cancer are not the same biomarkers that are effective in detecting the recurrence of liver cancer. AFP-L3 was found to be the best among all recurrence markers. Proteomic biomarkers have been identified from serum using matrix-assisted laser desorption ionization time of flight mass spectrometry (MALDI-TOF MS) (27). Among genetic markers for the early detection of liver cancer are mutations in *HSP70, CAP2,* and *GPC3* (34). These investigators have suggested that their liver cancer model should be considered an excellent model for understanding carcinogenesis because different steps in this multistage cancer can be followed by determining the expression of different markers at different stages of the disease.

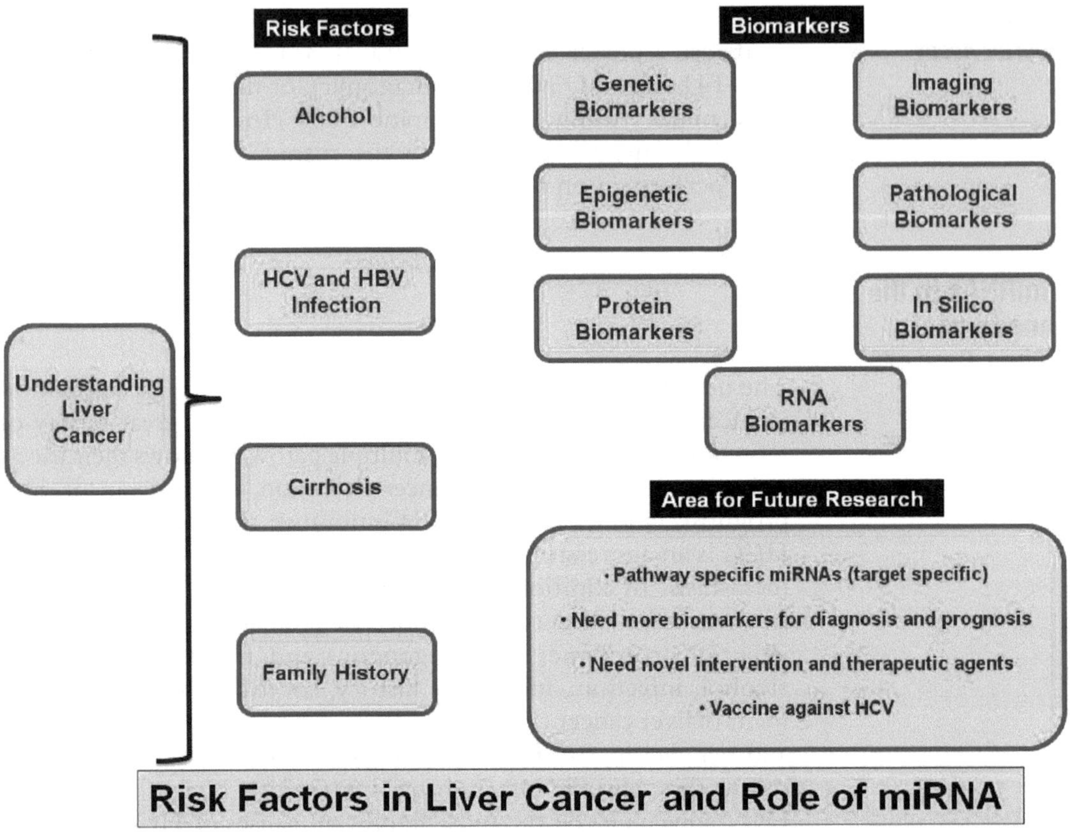

Fig. 2. Risk factors of liver cancer and involvement of miRNA. Few risk factors contributing to liver cancer are shown. At different steps of the disease development (initiation, progression, metastasis), different biomarkers are used. This information helps in better detection, diagnosis, prognosis, and follow-up of survival in cancer patients.

Because miRNAs are involved in multiple cancer-related pathways and regulate multiple genes, their role in coordinating cancer metastasis has been proposed in different scientific discussions and meetings (4, 19, 35). MiRNAs originate from highly structured pri-miRNA transcripts, which are processed in the nucleus and exported to the cytoplasm (19). The resulting miRNA duplexes are incorporated into RISC where one of the miRNA strands is degraded, while the strand that is complementary to the target mRNA serves in target selection and silencing, either by degradation (in the case of perfect base complementarity) or by inhibition of translation (in the case of imperfect sequence complementarity) (36). Thus, the expression of miRNAs in cell type-specific fashion shapes mRNA profiles. MiR-18a, miR-21, miR-141, and miR-146a are associated with HCV infection in liver cells (8–12, 20, 21). Currently, there is a big gap in the field of viral-induced HCC study model which is important for the development of drug. Long-term human hepatocyte culture developed by Banaudha et al. has a great advantage to study the HCV genotypes replication and chronic infection of HCV-induced in vitro system (21). The investigators have reported that efficient HCV replication requires miR-141-mediated suppression of DLC-1. An increase in miR-141 correlated with the inhibition of DLC-1 protein in HCV-infected cells. Furthermore, depletion of miR-141 with oligonucleotides complementary to the miRNAs inhibited virus replication, whereas artificially increased levels of miR-141 enhanced HCV replication (20, 21).

Regarding the management of liver cancer, intervention and therapeutic agents have been discovered and are targeted for components of pathways or viral genes and their products (19). For example, 4H-pyrazolo(1,5-a)pyrimidin-7-one was developed to inhibit HCV polymerase (32), and nonnucleoside inhibitors were developed by Beaulieu et al. using combinatorial library approaches (37). Protease inhibitors also show promise in inhibiting viral replication (38). A different class of therapeutics, called locked nucleic acid-modified oligonucleotides, has been used by Stenvang et al. (39). These oligonucleotides comprise a class of bicyclic conformational analogs of RNA, that exhibit a high affinity to complementary RNA molecules and are highly stable in blood and tissues. Additional classes of promising inhibitors and different treatment approaches are being developed by other investigators (19, 40–42).

5. Future Directions and Concluding Remarks

Because miRNAs are involved in cancer pathogenesis, their role in differentiation, self-renewal, and proliferation is critical. Moreover, a clearer understanding of miRNA regulation and identification of tissue-specific miRNA targets can be explored by employing transgenic/knockout animal models. Modulation in oligonucleotides may improve the understanding of liver physiology and pathology. Reliable models need to be developed to enhance the understanding of the biology of HCV-mediated carcinogenesis. A key breakthrough thus far has been the development of primary hepatocyte cells infected by HCV in which the role of miRNAs can be studied. Progress also has been made in developing computational tools to follow posttranscription regulation. Kinetic models of posttranscriptional regulation by miRNA also are needed to advance the understanding of liver carcinogenesis.

A number of biomarkers have been identified that can be useful in diagnosing liver cancer. To reduce false-positive results and improve the sensitivity and specificity of disease detection, however, multiple biomarkers should be used. A combination of biomarkers should be validated clinically before being applied in disease stratification among patients.

Patients with hepatitis are particularly susceptible to developing HCC, although the disease mechanisms are poorly understood. Attempts should be made to use metabolomics, an emerging field that provides new information on biological perturbations based on changes in multiple small-molecule metabolites. This is because new advances made in nuclear magnetic resonance (NMR) spectroscopy and mass spectrometry (MS) and their combination with multivariate statistical methods provide a promising approach for early disease diagnosis and for monitoring therapy. Presently, no highly reliable metabolite biomarkers have been identified for the early detection of HCC. Key metabolic signatures should be identified that may be diagnostic of the early onset of the disease, thus creating the possibility for earlier therapy and reduced overall mortality rates. Detecting liver cancer using metabolomics will be based on establishing key small molecular weight metabolite signatures in serum and tissue from human patients, as well as in serum samples from patients with nonmalignant liver disease and in healthy controls, using advanced NMR/MS techniques. Correlation of signals from tumor tissue and serum will help identify additional key metabolic signatures in serum that may be used to detect early liver cancer noninvasively. Validation of a statistical model based on these metabolic markers should be performed on a set of blinded samples. These advances may provide medical oncologists with new tools and knowledge to more efficiently care for liver cancer patients. This project will lay the foundation for clinical application of the metabolomics of early liver cancer diagnosis in a large number of patients and will advance scientific knowledge on disease mechanisms through basic research and finally to the clinical setting. Padersen and colleagues have certainly presented a novel mechanism for the actions of IFN against mammalian viruses. The development of miRNA-based therapeutics and delivery of 18–22 nucleotide bases miRNA molecules, it is possible that novel RNAi therapeutics strategies will help to fight HCV and other viral infections (20, 21, 43, 44).

Apart from potential benefits to liver cancer subtyping and clinical prognosis, long-term research can be directed to specific miRNAs and their target genes as interactive networks, with a focus on molecular targets amenable to novel and effective interventions. Through systematic analyses of miRNA expression profiles and genetic variations within miRNA coding sequences and predicted miRNA target sites, findings from this work may form the basis for further pathway-oriented research to either elucidate mechanisms of liver carcinogenesis or identify specific molecular pathways suitable for early screening and effective intervention.

Acknowledgement

We are thankful to Dr. Sita D. Gupta (Uniform Health Sciences University of Health) for the suggestions to improve the manuscript. We are also thankful to Christine Kaefer and Joanne Brodsky for reading the manuscript and providing their comments.

References

1. Bala, S., Marcos, M., and Szabo, G. (2009) Emerging role of microRNAs in liver diseases. *World J Gastroenterol* 15, 5633–5640.
2. Duncavage, E., Goodgame, B., Sezhiyan, A., Govindan, R., and Pfeifer, J. (2010) Use of microRNA expression levels to predict outcomes in resected stage I non-small cell lung cancer. *J Thorac Oncol* 5, 1755–1763.
3. Nana-Sinkam, S. P., Fabbri, M., and Croce, C. M. (2010) MicroRNAs in cancer: personalizing diagnosis and therapy. *Ann N Y Acad Sc* 1210, 25–33.
4. Ji, J. and Wang, X. W. (2009) New kids on the block: diagnostic and prognostic microRNAs in hepatocellular carcinoma. *Cancer Biol Ther* 8, 1686–1693.
5. Zhang, B., Pan, X., Cobb, G. P., Anderson, and T.A. (2007) microRNAs as oncogenes and tumor suppressors. *Dev Biol* 302, 1–12.
6. Neal, C. S., Michael, M. Z., Rawlings, L. H., Van der Hoek, M. B., and Gleadle, J. M. (2010) The VHL-dependent regulation of microRNAs in renal cancer. *BMC Med* 8, 64–65.
7. Zhang, H., Cai, X., Wang, Y., Tang, H., Tong, D., and Ji, F. (2010) microRNA-143, down-regulated in osteosarcoma, promotes apoptosis and suppresses tumorigenicity by targeting Bcl-2. *Oncol Rep* 24, 1363–1369.
8. Liu, W. H., Yeh, S. H., Lu, C. C., Yu, S. L., Chen, H. Y., Lin, C.Y., Chen, D.S., and Chen, P. J. (2009) MicroRNA-18a prevents estrogen receptor-alpha expression, promoting proliferation of hepatocellular carcinoma cells. *Gastroenterology* 136, 683–693.
9. Gramantieri, L., Fornari, F., Callegari, E., Sabbioni, S., Lanza, G., Croce, C. M., Bolondi, L., and Negrini, M. (2008) MicroRNA involvement in hepatocellular carcinoma. *J Cell Mol Med* 12, 2189–2204.
10. Su, H., Yang, J. R., Xu, T., Huang, J., Xu, L., Yuan, Y., and Zhuang, S. M. (2009) MicroRNA-101, down-regulated in hepatocellular carcinoma, promotes apoptosis and suppresses tumorigenicity. *Cancer Res* 69, 1135–1142.
11. Vinciguerra, M., Sgroi, A., Veyrat-Durebex, C., Rubbia-Brandt, L., Buhler, L. H., and Foti, M. (2009) Unsaturated fatty acids inhibit the expression of tumor suppressor phosphatase and tensin homolog (PTEN) via microRNA-21 up-regulation in hepatocytes. *Hepatology* 49, 1176–1184.
12. Xu, T., Zhu, Y., Wei, Q. K., Yuan, Y., Zhou, F., Ge, Y. Y., Yang, J. R., Su, H., and Zhuang, S. M. (2008) A functional polymorphism in the miR-146a gene is associated with the risk for hepatocellular carcinoma. *Carcinogenesis* 29, 2126–1131.
13. Houzet, L., Yaung, M. L., de Lame, V., Desai, D., Smith, S. M., and Jeang, K. T. (2008) MicroRNA profile changes in human immunodeficiency virus type 1 (HIV-1) seropositive individuals. *Rerovirology* 5, 118–119.
14. Cullen, B. R. (2006) Is RNA interference involved in intrinsic antiviral immunity in mammals? *Nat Immunol* 7, 563–567.
15. Berkhout, B. and Jeang, K. T. (2007) RISCy business MicroRNAs, pathogenesis, and viruses. *J Biol Chem* 282, 26641–26645.
16. Padersen, I. M., Cheng, G., Wieland, S., Volinia, S., Croce, C. M., Chisasi, F. V., and David, M. (2008) Control of HCV Replication: When Size Does Not Matter. *Hepatology* 47, 1092–1094.
17. Padersen, I. M., Cheng, G., Wieland, S., Volinia, S., Croce, C. M., Chisasi, F. V., and David, M. (2007) Interferon modulation of cellular microRNAs as an antiviral mechanism. *Nature* 18, 910–923.
18. Winter, J. and Diederichs, S. (2011) MicroRNA biogenesis and cancer. *Methods Mol Biol* 676, 6713–6722.
19. Rossi, J. J. (2009) New hope for a microRNA therapy for liver cancer. *Cell* 137, 990-992.
20. Banaudha, K., Kaliszewski, M., Korolnek, T., Florea, L., Yeung, M. L., Kuan, K. T., and Kumar, A. (2011a) MicroRNA silencing of tumor suppressor DLC-1 promotes efficient hepatitis C virus replication in primary human hepatocytes. *Hepatology* 53 (1) 53–61.

21. Banaudha, K., Orenstein, J. M., Korolnek, T. St Laurent, G. C. 3rd, Wakita, T., and Kumar A. (2010b) Primary hepatocyte culture supports hepatitis C virus replication: a model for infection-associated hepatocarcinogenesis. *Hepatology* 51, 1922–1932.
22. Chen, C., Tan, R., Wong, L., Fekete, R., and Halsey, J. (2011) Quantitation of microRNAs by real-time RT-qPCR. *Methods Mol Biol* 687, 113–134.
23. Yeung, M. L., Bennasser, Y., Myers, T. G., Jiang, G., Benkirane, M., and Jeang, K. T. (2005) Changes in microRNA expression profiles in HIV-1-transfected human cells. *Retrovirology* 28, 2, 81.
24. Xiong, Y., Fang, J. H., Yun, J. P., Yang, J., Zhang, Y., Jia, W. H., and Zhuang, S. M. (2010) Effects of microRNA-29 on apoptosis, tumorigenicity, and prognosis of hepatocellular carcinoma. *Hepatology* 51, 836–845.
25. Fontana, R. J., Dienstag, J. L., Bonkovsky, H. L., Sterling, R. K., Naishadham, D., Goodman, Z. D., Lok, A. S., Wright, E. C., Su, G. L., and HALT-C Trial Group. (2010) Serum fibrosis markers are associated with liver disease progression in non-responder patients with chronic hepatitis C. *Gut* 59, 1401–1409.
26. Kaibori, M., Ishizaki, M., Matsui, K., and Kwon, A. H. (2010) Predictors of microvascular invasion before hepatectomy for hepatocellular carcinoma. *J Surg Onco.* 102, 462–468.
27. Liu, C., Shen, J., Pan, C., Yang, L., Mou, S., Wang, H., and Liang, Y. (2010) MALDI-TOF MS combined with magnetic beads for detecting serum protein biomarkers and establishment of boosting decision tree model for diagnosis of hepatocellular carcinoma. *Am J Clin Pathol* 134, 235–241.
28. Beppu, T., Sugimoto, K., Shiraki, K., Tameda, M., Kusagawa, S., Nojiri, K., Tanaka, J., Yamamoto, N., Takei, Y., Takaki, H., Uraki, J., Nakatsuka, A., Yamakado, K., and Takeda, K. (2010) Clinical significance of tumor markers in detection of recurrent hepatocellular carcinoma after radiofrequency ablation. *J Mol Med* 26, 425–433.
29. Suriawinata, A. and Thung, S. N. (2010) Molecular signature of early hepatocellular carcinoma. *Oncology* 78, 36–39.
30. Deng, L., Adachi, T., Kitayama, K., Bungyoku, Y., Kitazawa, S., Ishido, S., Shoji, I., and Hotta, H. (2008) Hepatitis C virus infection induces apoptosis through a Bax-triggered, mitochondrion-mediated, caspase 3-dependent pathway. *J Virol* 82, 10375–10385.
31. Varnholt, H., Drebber, U., Schulze, F., Wedemeyer, I., Schirmacher, P., Dienes, H. P., and Odenthal, M. (2008) MicroRNA gene expression profile of hepatitis C virus-associated hepatocellular carcinoma. *Hepatology* 47, 1223–1232.
32. Deng, Y., Shipps, G. W. Jr., Wang, T., Popovici-Muller, J., Rosner, K. E., Siddiqui, M. A., Duca, J., Cooper, A. B., and Cable, M. (2009) Discovery of 4H-pyrazolo[1,5-a]pyrimidin-7-ones as potent inhibitors of hepatitis C virus polymerase. *Bioorg Med Chem Lett* 19, 5363–5367.
33. Deng, Y. B., Nagae, G., Midorikawa, Y., Yagi, K., Tsutsumi, S., Yamamoto, S., Hasegawa, K., Kokudo, N., Aburatani, H., and Kaneda, A. (2010) Identification of genes preferentially methylated in hepatitis C virus-related hepatocellular carcinoma. *Cancer Sci* 101, 1501–1510.
34. Sakamoto, M., Effendi, K., and Masugi, Y. (2010) Molecular diagnosis of multistage hepatocarcinogenesis. *Jpn J Clin Oncol* 40, 891–896.
35. Ji, J., Zhao, L., Budhu, A., Forgues, M., Jia, H. L., Qin, L. X., Ye, Q. H., Yu, J., Shi, X., Tang, Z. Y., and Wang, X. W. (2010) Let-7g targets collagen type I alpha2 and inhibits cell migration in hepatocellular carcinoma. *J Hepatol.* 52, 690–697.
36. Kumar, A. and Jeang, K. T. (2008) Insights into cellular microRNAs and human immunodeficiency virus type 1 (HIV-1). *J Cell Physiol* 216, 327–331.
37. Beaulieu, P. L., Bös, M., Bousquet, Y., Fazal, G., Gauthier, J., Gillard, J., Goulet, S., LaPlante, S., Poupart, M. A., Lefebvre, S., McKercher, G., Pellerin, C., Austel, V., and Kukolj, G. (2004) Non-nucleoside inhibitors of the hepatitis C virus NS5B polymerase: discovery and preliminary SAR of benzimidazole derivatives. *Bioorg Med Chem Let.* 14, 119–124.
38. Gal-Tanamy, M., Zemel, R., Bachmatov, L., Jangra, R. K., Shapira, A., Villanueva, R. A., Yi, M., Lemon, S. M., Benhar, I., and Tur-Kaspa, R. (2010) Inhibition of protease-inhibitor-resistant hepatitis C virus replicons and infectious virus by intracellular intrabodies. *Antiviral Res* 88, 95–106.
39. Stenvang, J., Lindow, M., and Kauppinen, S. (2008) Targeting of microRNAs for therapeutics. *Biochem Soc Trans* 36, 1197–1200.
40. Priet, S., Zlatev, I., Barvik, I., Geerts, K., Leyssen, P., Neyts, J., Dutartre, H., Canard, B., Vasseur, J. J., Morvan, F., and Alvarez, K. (2010) 3′-Deoxy phosphoramidate dinucleosides as improved inhibitors of hepatitis C virus subgenomic replicon and NS5B polymerase activity. *J Med Chem* 53, 6608–6617.

41. Arbuthnot, P. and Thompson, L. J. (2008) Harnessing the RNA interference pathway to advance treatment and prevention of hepatocellular carcinoma. *World J Gastroenterol* 14, 1670–1681.
42. Suzuki, T., Sakurai, F., Nakamura, S., Kouyama, E., Kawabata, K., Kondoh, M., Yagi, K., and Mizuguchi, H. (2008) miR-122a-regulated expression of a suicide gene prevents hepatotoxicity without altering antitumor effects in suicide gene therapy. *Mol Ther* 16, 1719–1726.
43. Gantier, M. P., Sadler, A. J., and Williams, B. R. (2007) Fine-tuning of the innate immune response by micrRNAs. *Immunol Cell Biol* 85, 458–462.
44. Kim, D. H. and Rossi, J. J. (2007) Strategies for silencing human disease using RNA interference. *Nat Rev Genes* 8, 173–184.

Chapter 15

Epigenetics in Ovarian Cancer

L.M.S. Seeber and P.J. van Diest

Abstract

Ovarian cancer is the most lethal gynecological cancer. Due to few early symptoms and a lack of early detection strategies, most patients are diagnosed with advanced-stage disease. Most of these patients, although initially responsive, eventually develop drug resistance. In this chapter, epigenetic changes in ovarian cancer are described. Various epigenetic changes including CpG island methylation and histone modification have been identified in ovarian cancer. These aberrations are associated with distinct disease subtypes and present in circulating serum of ovarian cancer patients. Several epigenetic changes have shown promise for their diagnostic, prognostic, and predictive capacity but still need further validation.

In contrast to DNA mutations and deletions, epigenetic modifications are potentially reversible by epigenetic therapies. Promising preclinical studies show epigenetic drugs to enhance gene re-expression and drug sensitivity in ovarian cancer cell lines and animal models.

Key words: Ovarian cancer, Methylation, Histone modification, MicroRNA, Epigenetic biomarkers, Epigenetic therapies

1. Introduction

1.1. Ovarian Cancer

Epithelial ovarian cancer is the fifth leading cause of cancer death in women and has the highest mortality rate of cancers of the reproductive organs (1). Due to few early symptoms and a lack of early detection strategies, most (>70%) patients are diagnosed with advanced-stage disease. Five-year survival rates are less than 20% for these advanced-stage patients, with only modestly improved survival over the past 40 years despite advances in chemotherapy (1, 2). Epithelial ovarian tumors account for ~60% of all ovarian neoplasms and 80–90% of malignant ovarian tumors. It is a clinically and pathologically heterogeneous disease comprised of serous, mucinous, clear cell, and endometrioid subtypes. Serous tumors are the most common subtype. Surgery and chemotherapy is the mainstay for treatment of ovarian cancer. Although the majority of patients are initially

Ramona G. Dumitrescu and Mukesh Verma (eds.), *Cancer Epigenetics: Methods and Protocols*, Methods in Molecular Biology, vol. 863, DOI 10.1007/978-1-61779-612-8_15, © Springer Science+Business Media, LLC 2012

responsive to chemotherapy, most of them eventually develop drug-resistant disease. Both genetic and epigenetic changes contribute to malignant transformation and progression. Only epigenetic modifications will be considered in this chapter.

2. Epigenetic Aberrations in Ovarian Cancer

2.1. Hypermethylated Genes

CpG island hypermethylation is a common phenomenon in ovarian cancer (3–19). However, the reported frequency of methylation in hypermethylated genes often varies widely between independent studies. Besides classical tumor suppressors that may be hypermethylated in ovarian cancer such as *BRCA1* (3), *p16* (4), and *MLH1* (5), examples of other genes hypermethylated in ovarian cancer include the putative tumor suppressors *OPCML* and *RASSF1A* (6, 7); the imprinted genes *ARHI* (*ARLTS1*), *PEG3* (8), *DLEC1* (9), *ARL11* (10), and *TCEAL7* (11); the proapoptotic genes *LOT1*, *DAPK*, *TMS1/ASC*, and *PAR-4* (12–14), the cell adhesion–associated genes *ICAM-1*, *CDH1* (15, 16), the cell signaling gene *HSulf-1* (17, 18), and the genome stability gene *PALB2* (19) (Table 1). Recently discovered candidate tumor suppressor genes hypermethylated in ovarian cancer are *SPARC* (20), *ANGPTL2* (21), and *CTGF* (22). In many cases, the functional effects of gene silencing on ovarian cancer pathogenesis are however not known.

One of the most studied genes in ovarian cancer is *BRCA1* due to its role in both inherited and sporadic forms of this disease (23). Studies investigating *BRCA1* hypermethylation report methylation in 5–24% of epithelial ovarian cancers (6, 23–29). A recent study investigating the different methylation profiles of sporadic and hereditary ovarian cancer showed *BRCA1* to be methylated in 14% of sporadic tumors, but never in hereditary ovarian cancer (30). In earlier studies, hypermethylation of the *BRCA1* promoter was reported to range from 5 to 40% in sporadic ovarian cancers. *BRCA1* methylation is strongly associated with loss of *BRCA1* RNA and protein (3) and significantly correlated with poor outcome in sporadic disease (31). No correlation of *BRCA1* methylation with histological subtypes or grade or stage has been found (32). *BRCA2* promoter methylation is rarely found in sporadic non hereditary ovarian cancers (31, 33).

Interestingly, gene methylation patterns are often associated with molecular, clinical, and pathological features of ovarian carcinomas. Comparing methylation status of *SFRP1*, *2*, *4*, 5, *SOX1*, *PAX1*, and *LMX1A* between patients with benign, borderline, and malignant ovarian tumors showed that methylation rates were highest in ovarian cancer patients and decreased progressively in patients with a borderline malignancy and nonmalignant ovarian tissue (34). Methylation of the embryonic developmentally regulated genes

Table 1
Overview of epigenetically altered genes in ovarian cancer

Regulator	Modification	Target
DNA methylation	Hypermethylation	*BRCA1*
		P16
		MLH1
		RASSF1A
		OPCML
		RASSF1A
		ARH1
		PEG3
		DLEC1
		ARL11
		TCEAL7
		LOT1
		DAPK
		TMS1/ASC
		PAR-4
		ICAM-1
		CDH1
		HSulf-1
		PALB2
		SPARC
		ANGPTL2
		CTGF
		HOXA10, HOXA11
		SFRP1,2,4,5
		SOX1
		PAX1
		LMX1A
		FBXO32
		IGFBP-3
		P14
		APC
		TIMP3
		CDH13
		PPP1R13B
		HSPA2
		HSD17B4
		ESR1
		GSTP1
		CYP1B1
		MYOD1
		SOCS1
		TITF1
		GSTM3
	Hypomethylation	*MCJ*
		SNCG
		TRAG-3
		BORIS
		IGF2
		Claudin-4

(continued)

Table 1 (continued)

Regulator	Modification	Target
miRNAs	Upregulation	miR-200a
		miR-141
		miR200c
		miR-200b
		miR-21
		miR-203
		miR-205
	Downregulation	miR-199a
		miR140
		miR-145
		miR-125b1
		Let-7i
Histone modifications	Upregulation	*HDAC1-3*
		Rb
		CDKN1
	Downregulation	*Class III β-tubulin*
		Survivin
		PACE4
		Claudin-3
		GATA4
		GATA6

HOXA10 and *HOXA11* was found to be highly discriminative between normal and malignant ovarian tissue (35).

Next to candidate gene studies also methylation microarrays have been used to examine global DNA hypermethylation in ovarian cancer (36). It has been demonstrated that ovarian tumors contain a large number of hypermethylated loci and that the degree of aberrant methylation is correlated with ovarian tumor progression. In a study of Wei et al. (36) 956 loci of the 7776 CpG islands studied were hypermethylated in the tumor compared to the normal control tissue.

DNA methylation profiles of the ovarian tumors also indicate clear differences between histological subtypes (37). For example, aberrant methylation of the promoters of *14-3-3 sigma*, *TMS1,* and *WT1* is a more frequent event in clear cell ovarian tumors than in other histological types (14, 29, 38–41). In a study by Houshdaran et al. (37), serous and endometrioid ovarian tumors were shown to be distinguishable by 70 of 90 CpG sites studied (corresponding with 52 genes), of which 49 CpG sites (36 genes) were on average more methylated in endometrioid tumors. Nineteen CpG sites (18 genes) and 12 CpG sites (10 genes) differed significantly in mean methylation between clear cell and serous tumors, or between clear cell and endometrioid tumors, respectively. Nearly all of the 26 CpG (23 genes) with differential methylation between clear cell tumors and serous or endometrioid tumors (or both) were on average more highly methylated in clear cell tumors.

2.2. Hypomethylated Genes

Not only is the well-studied hypermethylation of CpG islands in promoter regions associated with carcinogenesis, but also hypomethylation of certain other parts of the genome is a common cancer-associated phenomenon (42–44). There are, however, limited examples of specific gene activation by hypomethylation in ovarian cancer. Genes overexpressed in ovarian cancer association with promoter hypomethylation include *MCJ* (methylation-controlled DNAJ gene) (45), *SNCG* (synuclein-γ) (46, 47), *TRAG-3* (48), and *BORIS* (brother of the regulator of imprinted sites) (49). Other ovarian cancer hypomethylated genes are *IGF2* (50), and *claudin-4* (51).

Retrotransposons, a major class of middle repetitive sequences, have been identified as potential targets of hypomethylation (52, 53). Retrotransposons are classified into three subtypes: long interspersed elements (LINEs), short interspersed elements (SINEs), and long terminal repeat retrotransposons (*LTRs*) (54). The LINE-1 methylation pattern was hypomethylated in epithelial ovarian cancer specimens in 95% of cases (55). The methylation levels were lower compared with representative control tissue (55, 56). A decrease in the level of LINE-1 methylation was correlated with histological subtypes; mucinous tumors possessed higher methylation levels than endometrioid. Hypomethylation often involves satellite 2 (Sat2) DNA in the juxtacentromeric region of chromosome 1 and 16 in ovarian cancers (57). Hypomethylation of both chromosome 1 satellite 2 and chromosome 1 satellite α increased significantly from nonneoplastic toward ovarian cancer tissue. Serous and endometrioid tumors showed higher hypomethylation levels than mucinous tumors (58). Furthermore, extensive hypomethylation was more prevalent in tumors of advanced stage or high grade (58).

2.3. Histone Modifications

In addition to redistributions of DNA methylation patterns, another epigenetic aberration in ovarian cancer is atypical modifications of histones and dysregulated expression of histone-modifying enzymes. Many covalent posttranslational modifications of the histone tails have been documented, of which acetylation, methylation, and phosphorylation are most well characterized (59, 60). Histone modifications contribute to normal ovarian functions, including estrogen synthesis, folliculogenesis, and luteal phase activity (61). Ovarian cancer cells, however, significantly alter their expression of chromatin-modifying proteins (62). Like DNA methylation, histone modifications can play a role in silencing of tumor suppressor genes. Aberrant expression of class III β-tubulin protein (63), silencing of survivin (64), reduction of PACE4 expression (65), and lack of Claudin-3 expression (66) are linked to histone modifications in ovarian carcinogenesis. Similarly, altered histone modification of the promoter loci was found responsible for the silencing of the *GATA4* and *GATA6* transcription factors in ovarian cancer cell lines (67). This was associated with subsequent loss of a target gene, the tumor suppressor *Disabled-2* (67).

Histone acetylation is typically associated with increased transcription and is regulated by two opposing classes of enzymes: histone acetyltransferases and histone deacetylases (HDACs). HDACs1–3 have been shown to be overexpressed in ovarian cancer tissue and are thought to play a role in ovarian carcinogenesis (68). Two genes upregulated by histone acetylation include the tumor suppressor *Rb* and the cyclin-dependent kinase inhibitor *CDKN1* (69).

2.4. MicroRNA

The most recently discovered epigenetic phenomenon is posttranscriptional gene downregulation by small (21–23 nucleotides in length), non-protein-coding RNA molecules known as microRNAs (miRNAs) (70, 71). Tissue-specific miRNAs have been reported. Overexpression of miR-200a, miR-200b, miR-200c, and miR-141 has been described in ovarian cancer (72). On the other hand, miR-199a, miR-140, miR-145, and miR-125b1 were among the most downregulated ones (72, 73). miRNA signatures of ovarian cancer could be helpful to distinguish the tumors based on their histological subtype; miR200b and miR-141 were upregulated in endometrioid and serous subtypes (72). Moreover, the endometrioid histotypes seem to show the upregulation of three additional miRNAs: miR-21, miR-203, and miR-205. Nineteen miRNAs were downregulated in all the three histotypes in comparison with normal tissue, whereas miR-145 was downregulated in both serous and clear cell carcinomas and miR-222 in both endometrioid and clear cell carcinomas (72). Significant downregulation of miR-34c, miR-422b, miR-143, and miR-145, as well as increased expression of miR-29a and miR-29b, was seen in patients with BRCA1/2 abnormalities (74, 75).

Interestingly, the levels of miR-21, miR-203, and miR-205 that are upregulated in ovarian carcinomas compared to normal tissue were significantly increased after demethylating treatment, suggesting that the hypomethylation could be the mechanism responsible for their overexpression (72).

3. Epigenetics in Ovarian Cancer Management

As mentioned above, ovarian cancer is characterized by a number of epigenetic aberrations. Consequently, these specific hypomethylated sequences and individual or panels of hypermethylated genes represent potential biomarkers for diagnosis, staging, prognosis, and monitoring or predicting response to therapy.

3.1. Early Diagnosis Markers

Late presentation of symptoms and lack of screening modalities, making the timely detection of ovarian cancer difficult, contribute to high mortality rates. Early diagnosis is thus critical for the successful treatment of ovarian cancer. The detection of cancer at early stages by noninvasive methods may be aided by the identification of cancer-specific biomarkers detectable in body fluids. Despite little blood-borne spread, specific methylated DNA markers can be detected in the serum, plasma, and peritoneal fluid of ovarian cancer patients (6, 76). Although methylation assessment of single genes lacks sufficient specificity for ovarian cancer diagnostics, a panel of multiple methylation biomarkers may achieve the accuracy required for widespread population screening (77). Tumor-specific methylation of at least one of a panel of six tumor suppressor genes—*BRCA1*, *RASSF1A*, *APC*, *p14*^{arf}, *p16*^{ink4a}, and *DAPK* could be detected in serum of ovarian cancer patients with 100% specificity and 82% sensitivity (6). Hypermethylation was observed across histological cell types, grades, and stages. In contrast, no methylation was observed in nonneoplastic tissue, peritoneal fluid, or serum from 40 control women.

DAPK methylation in whole peripheral blood DNA of ovarian cancer patients has also been independently examined (78). In 20 (67%) of the tumor samples tested methylation of *DAPK* was observed. Comparison of the paired samples from these patients showed that 14 (54%) had also methylation in their peripheral blood. There were ten patients with unmethylated tumor DNA and unmethylated peripheral blood. There was no evidence of *DAPK* methylation in the blood DNA of healthy individuals.

Although several limitations still exist, including the sensitivity of methylation assays, detection of specific epigenetic markers in the blood circulation of patients appears a promising approach to early ovarian cancer detection.

3.2. Prognostic Markers

Tumor stage, residual disease after initial surgery, histological type, and tumor grade are the most important clinical-pathological factors related to ovarian cancer treatment outcome. To supplement these traditional prognostic factors, several epigenetically regulated genes have been assessed for their prognostic potential in ovarian cancer.

Individual methylated genes with possible prognostic value in ovarian cancer include *HOXA11*, linked with postsurgical residual tumor and overall poor prognosis (35), *FBXO32*, associated with a shorter progression-free survival (79), and *IGFBP*-3 associated with disease progression and death in ovarian cancer, particularly in patients with early-stage disease (80). Similarly, hypermethylation of 18S and 28S rDNA is associated with prolonged progression-free survival of ovarian cancer patients (81).

Although some of these methylated markers hold potential as prognostic indicators individually, it is likely that panels of genes will be more informative. The methylation status of *SFRP1*, *SFRP2*,

SOX1, and *LMX1A* correlated with recurrence and overall survival (34). Combining the data for *SFRP1*, *SFRP2*, and *SOX1* gave a relative risk for recurrence of 3.19 in patients with at least one gene methylated. The rate of cancer-related death was elevated by two times in patients with a single gene methylated and by six times in those with multiple genes methylated (34). Wei et al. (36) could stratify late-stage ovarian tumors into two distinct groups with significantly different outcome on the basis of methylation profiling of 956 CpG-island-containing loci. Further, a microarray analysis resulted in the identification of 112 highly discriminatory loci possessing a progression-free survival prediction accuracy of 95% in ovarian cancer patients (82). A higher degree of CpG island methylation was also associated with early disease recurrence after chemotherapy (36).

An examination of peritoneal fluid from 57 ovarian cancer patients revealed that methylation levels of a 15-gene panel (*TIMP3*, *CDH1*, *CDH13*, *APC*, *PPP1R13B*, *HSPA2*, *HSD17B4*, *ESR1*, *GSTP1*, *CYP1B1*, *BRCA1*, *MYOD1*, *SOCS1*, *TITF1*, and *GSTM3*) likewise could distinguish short vs. long overall survival (83).

Hypomethylation of certain chromosomal regions also appears to have prognostic value; patients with little or no hypomethylation of chromosome 1 satellite 2 or chromosome 1 Satellite α had a significantly longer disease free survival compared with patients with strong hypomethylation of these regions (58). Patients with greater hypomethylation of LINE-1 had poorer mean overall survival and a lower mean progression-free interval (55).

In terms of miRNAs, a lower ratio of miR-221 to miR-222 was also significantly correlated with worse overall survival in predominantly high-grade, advanced-stage sporadic ovarian carcinomas. This relationship remained significant after accounting for optimal vs. suboptimal surgical cytoreduction in a multivariate model (84). Additionally, low miR-200 family (formed by five microRNAs; miR-141, miR-200a, miR-200b, miR-200c, and miR-429) expression had a trend toward poor progression-free survival. Also after multivariate analysis adjusting for relevant clinicopathological variables (debulking status, tumor stage, and histological grade), a tendency was observed for the association of miR-429 expression with recurrence-free survival (85). In high-grade serous ovarian carcinomas with *BRCA1/2* abnormalities, lower levels of miR-422b and miR-34c were both associated with decreased disease-specific survival (74).

With regard to histone modifications, trimethylation of lysine 27 on histone (H3K27me3) showed significant prognostic impact in ovarian cancers. Patients with low expression of H3K27me3 had significantly shorter overall survival times compared to those with high H3K27me3 (86). High expression of class I HDACs is associated with a poor prognosis in endometrioid ovarian carcinomas, the absence of or only partial expression of class I HDACs indicating a very good prognosis (93% 10-year disease-specific survival) (87).

3.3. Predictive Markers

Variations in methylation patterns can occur within the same tumor type, and in addition to providing prognostic information, these patterns could be associated with response to therapy. A major impediment for improving survival of ovarian cancer patients is the development of chemoresistance. Several genes in ovarian cancer, including genes involved in apoptotic pathways related to chemotherapeutic action, are downregulated by epigenetic mechanisms. One well-documented example is the *MLH1* gene. Silencing of *MLH1* by methylation has been linked with platinum resistance in ovarian cancer cell lines (88–90). In a recent study by Hofstetter et al. (91), demethylation agent cytidine analog 5-azacytidine (azacitidine, 5-aza-CR; Vidaza, Celgene Corp., Summit, NJ, USA) has been shown to successfully demethylate *MLH1* (91). Interestingly, a recent report showed that the azacitidine may enhance the response to platinum in patients with platinum-resistant ovarian cancer (92). Methylation of the *TUBB3* gene has been linked to taxane resistance in ovarian cancer cell lines (63), and methylation of *MCJ* has been associated with chemoresistance (45). Furthermore, epigenetic silencing of *SFRP5* (a member of the secreted frizzled-related protein family) seems to lead to oncogenic activation of the Wnt pathway and contribute to ovarian cancer progression and chemoresistance (93).

Moreover, elevated expression due to hypomethylation can also induce drug resistance. For example, MAL (myelin and lymphocyte protein) overexpression due to decreased methylation of the MAL promoter region was associated with a poor prognosis in ovarian cancer. MAL transcription levels were also higher in the platinum-resistant ovarian cell lines. Consequently, it has potential as a marker of platinum sensitivity (94).

Methylation-induced *FANCF* inactivation is observed in ovarian cancer cells with a defective *BRCA2* pathway and is associated with increased sensitivity to cisplatin. Its relevance to clinical outcome following chemotherapy has however yet to be established (95).

With regard to miRNAs, a recent study has reported a significant link between the expression of 27 miRNAs and chemotherapy response (96). Furthermore, miRNA Let-7i has recently been found to be a tumor suppressor significantly downregulated in platinum-resistant ovarian tumors, and Let-7i gain of function was able to restore drug sensitivity of chemoresistant ovarian cancer cells (97). Further, miR-214 has been shown to target the tumor suppressor *PTEN* and correlate with platinum resistance (73).

4. Epigenetic Therapies

Complex epigenetic patterns involving DNA methylation, histone modifications, and miRNA abnormality contribute to ovarian cancer progression and drug resistance. Whereas genetic mutation, deletions, or allelic losses are fixed and irreversible, epigenetic abnormalities can potentially be corrected (98, 99). Consequently, reversing epigenetic events could be a promising treatment modality. In this regard, inhibitors of DNA methyltransferases (DNMT) or HDAC activity are now being studied.

4.1. DNA Methylation Inhibitors

Several drugs that inhibit DNMT activity have been discovered. In preclinical studies, various DNMT inhibitors, such as azacitidine, were found to cause DNA hypomethylation and reverse chemoresistance of platinum-resistant ovarian cancer cells (100–102). This effect seems to be due to re-expression of tumor suppressor genes by promoter demethylation. In cisplatin-resistant ovarian cancer cells, the methylation inhibitors decitabine and zebularine mediated resensitization to platinum by demethylation of *RASSF1A* and *MLH1* (102). In another study, treatment with decitabine induced re-expression of *MLH1* in platinum-resistant ovarian cancer cells (89). Xenograft tumors derived from these cells were sensitized by decitabine to cisplatin, carboplatin, temozolomide, and epirubicin (89). A recent clinical study showed that the combination of the demethylating agent azacitidine with carboplatin had clinical activity in patients with platinum-resistant ovarian cancer, indicating that a hypomethylating agent may partially reverse platinum resistance in patients with ovarian cancer (92). The predominant toxicities were fatigue and myelosuppression.

4.2. Histone Deacetylase Inhibitors

In ovarian cancer cells and xenografts, the HDAC inhibitor vorinostat has demonstrated potent antigrowth activity and minimal toxicity (103). A phase II trial for advanced ovarian cancer also showed however only minimal tumor response (104). Another HDAC inhibitor, PXD101 (belinostat; CuraGen Corp., Branford, CT), has also shown potent activity against human ovarian cancer xenografts that are generally refractory to chemotherapy (105). In a recent completed phase I trial, belinostat combined with carboplatin or paclitaxel in solid tumors including ovarian carcinomas was well tolerated, with no evidence of pharmacokinetic interaction. Further evaluation of antitumor activity is however needed. Another novel HDAC inhibitor, R306465, inhibited tumor growth of ovarian cancer cell xenografts (106). The HDAC inhibitor scriptaid showed to be highly antiproliferative in ovarian cancer cell lines (107).

While HDAC and DNMT inhibitors have demonstrated therapeutic activity as single agents, it is believed that combinations of these two inhibitors will be most effective in addition to conventional therapies (98). Microarray evaluation of ovarian cancer cell treatment with methylation (5-aza-2′-deoxycytidine) and/or deacetylation (trichostatin A) inhibitors showed that combined treatment resulted in synergistic reactivation of more genes (108). Consequently, a preclinical study showed that a combination of decitabine with belinostat elicited greater platinum resensitization of resistant ovarian cancer xenografts than decitabine alone (109).

5. Conclusion

It is increasingly evident that epigenetics plays a prominent role in ovarian carcinogenesis. Such modifications represent highly promising biomarkers for early detection, and predicting therapy response and prognosis. In addition, the fact that tumor-derived cell-free DNA is detectable in body fluids such as blood and serum means that noninvasive methods can be used to make such assessments. The more epigenetic markers are being identified, the more specific and accurate algorithms could be developed for the detection of ovarian cancer. Further, epigenetically silenced genes offer new targets for therapeutic approaches based on re-expression of tumor suppressor genes via demethylating and deacetylating drugs.

References

1. Jemal, A., Siegel, R., Ward, E., Hao, Y., Xu, J., Thun, M.J. (2009) Cancer statistics, 2009. *CA Cancer J Clin* 59, 225–249.
2. Barnholtz-Sloan, J.S., Schwartz, A.G., Qureshi, F., Jacques, S., Malone, J., Munkarah, A.R. (2003) Ovarian cancer: changes in patterns at diagnosis and relative survival over the last three decades. *Am J Obstet Gynecol* 189, 1120–1127.
3. Press, J.Z., De Luca, A., Boyd, N., Young, S., Troussard, A., Ridge, Y., Kaurah, P., Kalloger, S.E., Blood, K.A., Smith, M., Spellman, P.T., Wang, Y., Miller, D.M., Horsman, D., Faham, M., Gilks, C.B., Gray, J., Huntsman, D.G. (2008) Ovarian carcinomas with genetic and epigenetic BRCA1 loss have distinct molecular abnormalities. *BMC Cancer* 8, 17.
4. Milde-Langosch, K., Ocon, E., Becker, G., Loning, T. (1998) p16/MTS1 inactivation in ovarian carcinomas: high frequency of reduced protein expression associated with hypermethylation or mutation in endometrioid and mucinous tumors. *Int J Cancer* 79, 61–65.
5. Balch, C., Huang, T.H., Brown, R., Nephew, K.P. (2004) The epigenetics of ovarian cancer drug resistance and resensitization. *Am J Obstet Gynecol* 191, 1552–1572.
6. Ibanez de Caceres, I., Battagli, C., Esteller, M., Herman, J.G., Dulaimi, E., Edelson, M.I., Bergman, C., Ehya, H., Eisenberg, B.L., Cairns, P.(2004) Tumor cell-specific BRCA1 and RASSF1A hypermethylation in serum, plasma, and peritoneal fluid from ovarian cancer patients. *Cancer Res* 64, 6476–6481.
7. Sellar, G.C., Watt, K.P., Rabiasz, G.J., Stronach, E.A., Li, L., Miller, E.P., Massie, C.E., Miller, J., Contreras-Moreira, B., Scott, D., Brown, I., Williams, A.R., Bates, P.A., Smyth, J.F., Gabra, H. (2003) OPCML at 11q25 is epigenetically inactivated and has tumor-suppressor function in epithelial ovarian cancer. *Nat Genet* 34, 337–343.
8. Feng, W., Marquez, R.T., Lu, Z., Liu, J., Lu, K.H., Issa, J.P., Fishman, D.M., Yu, Y., Bast, R.C. Jr. (2008) Imprinted tumor suppressor genes ARHI and PEG3 are the most frequently

down-regulated in human ovarian cancers by loss of heterozygosity and promoter methylation. *Cancer* 112, 1489–1502.

9. Kwong, J., Lee, J.Y., Wong, K.K., Zhou, X., Wong, D.T., Lo, K.W., Welch, W.R., Berkowitz, R.S., Mok, S.C. (2006) Candidate tumor-suppressor gene DLEC1 is frequently downregulated by promoter hypermethylation and histone hypoacetylation in human epithelial ovarian cancer. *Neoplasia* 8, 268–278.
10. Petrocca, F., Iliopoulos, D., Qin, H.R., Nicoloso, M.S., Yendamuri, S., Wojcik, S.E., Shimizu, M., Di Leva, G., Vecchione, A., Trapasso, F., Godwin, A.K., Negrini, M., Calin, G.A., Croce, C.M. (2006) Alterations of the tumor suppressor gene ARLTS1 in ovarian cancer. *Cancer Res* 66, 10287–10291.
11. Chien, J., Staub, J., Avula, R., Zhang, H., Liu, W., Hartmann, L.C., Kaufmann, S.H., Smith, D.I., Shridhar, V. (2004) Epigenetic silencing of TCEAL7 (Bex4) in ovarian cancer. *Oncogene* 24, 5089–5100.
12. Cvetkovic, D., Pisarcik, D., Lee, C., Hamilton, T.C., Abdollahi, A. (2004) Altered expression and loss of heterozygosity of the LOT1 gene in ovarian cancer. *Gynecol Oncol* 95, 449–455.
13. Pruitt, K., Ulku, A.S., Frantz, K., Rojas, R.J., Muniz-Medina, V.M., Rangnekar, V.M., Der, C.J., Shields, J.M. (2005) Ras-mediated loss of the pro-apoptotic response protein Par-4 is mediated by DNA hypermethylation through Raf-independent and Raf-dependent signaling cascades in epithelial cells. *J Biol Chem* 280, 23363–23370.
14. Terasawa, K., Sagae, S., Toyota, M., Tsukada, K., Ogi, K., Satoh, A., Mita, H., Imai, K., Tokino, T., Kudo, R. (2004) Epigenetic inactivation of TMS1/ASC in ovarian cancer. Clin *Cancer Res* 10, 2000–2006.
15. Arnold, J.M., Cummings, M., Purdie, D., Chenevix-Trench, G. (2001) Reduced expression of intercellular adhesion molecule-1 in ovarian adenocarcinomas. *Br J Cancer* 85, 1351–1358.
16. Yuecheng, Y., Hongmei, L., Xiaoyan, X. (2006) Clinical evaluation of E-cadherin expression and its regulation mechanism in epithelial ovarian cancer. *Clin Exp Metastasis*; 23, 65–74.
17. Backen, A.C., Cole, C.L., Lau, S.C., Clamp, A.R., McVey, R., Gallagher, J.T., Jayson, G.C. (2007) Heparan sulphate synthetic and editing enzymes in ovarian cancer. *Br J Cancer* 96, 1544–1548.
18. Staub, J., Chien, J., Pan, Y., Qian, X., Narita, K., Aletti, G., Scheerer, M., Roberts, L.R., Molina, J., Shridhar, V. (2007) Epigenetic silencing of HSulf-1 in ovarian cancer:implications in chemoresistance. *Oncogene* 26, 4969–4978.
19. Potapova, A., Hoffman, A.M., Godwin, A.K., Al-Saleem, T., Cairns, P. (2008) Promoter hypermethylation of the PALB2 susceptibility gene in inherited and sporadic breast and ovarian cancer. *Cancer Res* 68, 998–1002.
20. Socha, M.J., Said, N., Dai, Y., Kwong, J., Ramalingam, P., Trieu, V., Desai, N., Mok, S.C., Motamed, K. (2009) Aberrant promoter methylation of SPARC in ovarian cancer. *Neoplasia* 11, 126–135.
21. Kikuchi, R., Tsuda, H., Kozaki, K., Kanai, Y., Kasamatsu, T., Sengoku, K., Hirohashi, S., Inazawa, J., Imoto, I. (2008) Frequent inactivation of a putative tumor suppressor, angiopoietin-like protein 2, in ovarian cancer. *Cancer Res* 68, 5067–5075.
22. Kikuchi, R., Tsuda, H., Kanai, Y., Kasamatsu, T., Sengoku, K., Hirohashi, S., Inazawa, J., Imoto, I. (2007) Promoter hypermethylation contributes to frequent inactivation of a putative conditional tumor suppressor gene connective tissue growth factor in ovarian cancer. *Cancer Res* 67, 7095–7105.
23. Baldwin, R.L., Nemeth, E., Tran, H., Shvartsman, H., Cass, I., Narod, S., Karlan, B.Y. (2000) BRCA1 promoter region hypermethylation in ovarian carcinoma: a population-based study. *Cancer Res* 60, 5329–5333.
24. Strathdee, G., Appleton, K., Illand, M., Millan, D.W., Sargent, J., Paul, J., Brown, R. (2001) Primary ovarian carcinomas display multiple methylator phenotypes involving known tumor suppressor genes. *Am J Pathol* 158, 1121–1127.
25. Catteau, A., Harris, W.H., Xu, C.F., Solomon, E. (1999) Methylation of the BRCA1 promoter region in sporadic breast and ovarian cancer: correlation with disease characteristics. *Oncogene* 18, 1957–1965.
26. Geisler, J.P., Hatterman-Zogg, M.A., Rathe, J.A., Buller, R.E. (2002) Frequency of BRCA1 dysfunction in ovarian cancer. *J Natl Cancer Inst* 94, 61–67.
27. Buller, R.E., Shahin, M.S., Geisler, J.P., Zogg, M., De Young, B.R., Davis, C.S. (2002) Failure of BRCA1 dysfunction to alter ovarian cancer survival. *Clin Cancer Res* 8, 1196–1202.
28. Rathi, A., Virmani, A.K., Schorge, J.O., Elias, K.J., Maruyama, R., Minna, J.D., Mok, S.C., Girard, L., Fishman, D.A., Gazdar, A.F. (2002) Methylation profiles of sporadic ovarian tumors and nonmalignant ovaries from high-risk women. *Clin Cancer Res* 8, 3324–3331.

29. Teodoridis, J.M., Hall, J., Marsh, S., Kannall, H.D., Smyth, C., Curto, J., Siddiqui, N., Gabra, H., McLeod, H.L., Strathdee, G., Brown, R. (2005) CpG island methylation of DNA damage response genes in advanced ovarian cancer. *Cancer Res* 65, 8961–8967.
30. Bol, G.M., Suijkerbuijk, K.P., Bart, J., Vooijs, M., van der Wall, E., van Diest, P.J. (2010) Methylation profiles of hereditary and sporadic ovarian cancer. *Histopathology* 57, 363–370.
31. Hilton, J.L., Geisler, J.P., Rathe, J.A., Hattermann-Zogg, M.A., DeYoung, B., Buller, R.E. (2002) Inactivation of BRCA1 and BRCA2 in ovarian cancer. *J Natl Cancer Inst* 94, 1396–1406.
32. Wilcox, C.B, Baysal, B.E., Gallion, H.H., Strange, M.A., DeLoia, J.A. (2005) High-resolution methylation analysis of the BRCA1 promoter in ovarian tumors. *Cancer Genet Cytogenet* 159, 114–122.
33. Gras, E., Cortes, J., Diez, O., Alonso, C., Matias-Guiu, X., Baiget, M., Prat, J. (2001) Loss of heterozygosity on chromosome 13q12-q14, BRCA-2 mutations and lack of BRCA-2 promoter hypermethylation in sporadic epithelial ovarian tumors. *Cancer* 92, 787–795.
34. Su, H.Y., Lai, H.C., Lin, Y.W., Chou, Y.C., Liu, C.Y., Yu, M.H. (2009) An epigenetic marker panel for screening and prognostic prediction of ovarian cancer. *Int J Cancer* 124, 387–393.
35. Fiegl, H., Windbichler, G., Mueller-Holzner, E., Goebel, G., Lechner, M., Jacobs, I.J., Widschwendter, M. (2008) HOXA11 DNA methylation--a novel prognostic biomarker in ovarian cancer. *Int J Cancer* 123, 725–729.
36. Wei, S.H., Chen, C.M., Strathdee, G., Harnsomburana, J., Shyu, C.R., Rahmatpanah, F., Shi, H., Ng, S.W., Yan, P.S., Nephew, K.P., Brown, R., Huang, T.H. (2002) Methylation microarray analysis of late-stage ovarian carcinomas distinguishes progression-free survival in patients and identifies candidate epigenetic markers. *Clin Cancer Res* 8, 2246–2252.
37. Houshdaran, S., Hawley, S., Palmer, C., Campan, M., Olsen, M.N., Ventura, A.P., Knudsen, B.S., Drescher, C.W., Urban, N.D., Brown, P.O., Laird, P.W. (2010) DNA methylation profiles of ovarian epithelial carcinoma tumors and cell lines. *PLoS One* 5, e9359.
38. Akahira, J., Sugihashi, Y., Suzuki, T., Ito, K., Niikura, H., Moriya, T., Nitta, M., Okamura, H., Inoue, S., Sasano, H., Okamura, K., Yaegashi, N. (2004) Decreased expression of 14-3-3 sigma is associated with advanced disease in human epithelial ovarian cancer: its correlation with aberrant DNA methylation. *Clin Cancer Res* 10, 2687–2693.
39. Akahira, J., Sugihashi, Y., Ito, K., Niikura, H., Okamura, K., Yaegashi, N. (2004) Promoter methylation status and expression of TMS1 gene in human epithelial ovarian cancer. *Cancer Sci* 95, 40–43.
40. Kaneuchi, M., Sasaki, M., Tanaka, Y., Shiina, H., Yamada, H., Yamamoto, R., Sakuragi, N., Enokida, H., Verma, M., Dahiya, R.. (2005) WT1 and WT1-AS genes are inactivated by promoter methylation in ovarian clear cell adenocarcinoma. *Cancer* 104, 1924–1930.
41. Kaneuchi, M., Sasaki, M., Tanaka, Y., Shiina, H., Verma, M., Ebina, Y., Nomura, E., Yamamoto, R., Sakuragi, N., Dahiya, R. (2004) Expression and methylation status of 14-3-3 sigma gene can characterize the different histological features of ovarian cancer. *Biochem Biophys Res Commun* 316, 1156–1162.
42. Ehrlich, M. (2006) Cancer-linked DNA hypomethylation and its relationship to hypermethylation. *Curr Top Microbiol Immunol* 310, 251–274.
43. Feinberg, A.P., Vogelstein, B. (1983) Hypomethylation distinguishes genes of some human cancers from their normal counterparts. *Nature* 301(5895):89–92.
44. Gama-Sosa, M.A., Midgett, R.M., Slagel, V.A., Githens, S., Kuo, K.C., Gehrke, C.W., Ehrlich, M. (1983) Tissue-specific differences in DNA methylation in various mammals. *Biochim Biophys Acta* 740, 212–219.
45. Strathdee, G., Vass, J.K., Oien, K.A., Siddiqui, N., Curto-Garcia, J., Brown, R. (2005) Demethylation of the MCJ gene in stage III/IV epithelial ovarian cancer and response to chemotherapy. *Gynecol Oncol* 97, 898–903.
46. Czekierdowski, A., Czekierdowska, S., Wielgos, M., Smolen, A., Kaminski, P., Kotarski, J. (2006) The role of CpG islands hypomethylation and abnormal expression of neuronal protein synuclein-gamma (SNCG) in ovarian cancer. *Neuro Endocrinol Lett* 27, 381–386.
47. Gupta, A., Godwin, A.K., Vanderveer, L., Lu, A., Liu, J. (2003) Hypomethylation of the synuclein gamma gene CpG island promotes its aberrant expression in breast carcinoma and ovarian carcinoma. *Cancer Res* 63, 664–673.
48. Yao, X., Hu, J.F., Li, T., Yang, Y., Sun, Z., Ulaner, G.A., Vu, T.H., Hoffman, A.R. (2004) Epigenetic regulation of the taxol resistance-associated gene TRAG-3 in human tumors. *Cancer Genet Cytogenet* 151, 1–13.

49. Woloszynska-Read, A., James, S.R., Link, P.A., Yu, J., Odunsi, K., Karpf, AR. (2007) DNA methylation-dependent regulation of BORIS/CTCFL expression in ovarian cancer. *Cancer Immun* 7, 21.

50. Murphy, S.K., Huang, Z., Wen, Y., Spillman, M.A., Whitaker, R.S., Simel, L.R., Nichols, T.D., Marks, J.R., Berchuck, A. (2006) Frequent IGF2/H19 domain epigenetic alterations and elevated IGF2 expression in epithelial ovarian cancer. *Mol Cancer Res* 4, 283–292.

51. Litkouhi, B., Kwong, J., Lo, C.M., Smedley, J.G., III, McClane, B.A., Aponte, M., Gao, Z., Sarno, J.L., Hinners, J., Welch, W.R., Berkowitz, R.S., Mok, S.C., Garner, E.I. (2007) Claudin-4 overexpression in epithelial ovarian cancer is associated with hypomethylation and is a potential target for modulation of tight junction barrier function using a C-terminal fragment of Clostridium perfringens enterotoxin. *Neoplasia* 9, 304–314.

52. Florl, A.R., Lower, R., Schmitz-Drager, B.J., Schulz, W.A. (1999) DNA methylation and expression of LINE-1 and HERV-K provirus sequences in urothelial and renal cell carcinomas. *Br J Cancer* 80, 1312–1321.

53. Lorincz, M.C., Schubeler, D., Groudine, M. (2001) Methylation-mediated proviral silencing is associated with MeCP2 recruitment and localized histone H3 deacetylation. *Mol Cell Biol* 21, 7913–7922.

54. Lander, E.S., Linton, L.M., Birren, B., Nusbaum, C., Zody, M.C., Baldwin, J., et al. (2001) Initial sequencing and analysis of the human genome. *Nature* 409, 860–921.

55. Pattamadilok, J., Huapai, N., Rattanatanyong, P., Vasurattana, A., Triratanachat, S., Tresukosol, D., Mutirangura, A. (2008) LINE-1 hypomethylation level as a potential prognostic factor for epithelial ovarian cancer. *Int J Gynecol Cancer* 18, 711–717.

56. Menendez, L., Benigno, B.B., McDonald, J.F. (2004) L1 and HERV-W retrotransposons are hypomethylated in human ovarian carcinomas. *Mol Cancer* 3, 12.

57. Qu, G., Dubeau, L., Narayan, A., Yu, M.C., Ehrlich, M. (1999) Satellite DNA hypomethylation vs. overall genomic hypomethylation in ovarian epithelial tumors of different malignant potential. *Mutat Res* 423, 91–101.

58. Widschwendter, M., Jiang, G., Woods, C., Muller, H.M., Fiegl, H., Goebel, G., Marth, C., Muller-Holzner, E., Zeimet, A.G., Laird, P.W., Ehrlich, M. (2004) DNA hypomethylation and ovarian cancer biology. *Cancer Res* 64, 4472–4480.

59. Zhang, K., Dent, S.Y. (2005) Histone modifying enzymes and cancer: going beyond histones. *J Cell Biochem* 96, 1137–1148.

60. Santos-Rosa, H., Caldas, C. (2005) Chromatin modifier enzymes, the histone code and cancer. *Eur J Cancer* 41, 2381–2402.

61. LaVoie, H.A. (2005) Epigenetic control of ovarian function: the emerging role of histone modifications. *Mol Cell Endocrinol* 243, 12–18.

62. Ozdag, H., Teschendorff, A.E., Ahmed, A.A., Hyland, S.J., Blenkiron, C., Bobrow, L., Veerakumarasivam, A., Burtt, G., Subkhankulova, T., Arends, M.J., Collins, V.P., Bowtell, D., Kouzarides, T., Brenton, J.D., Caldas, C. Differential expression of selected histone modifier genes in human solid cancers. *BMC Genomics* 7, 90.

63. Izutsu, N., Maesawa, C., Shibazaki, M., Oikawa, H., Shoji, T., Sugiyama, T., Masuda, T. (2008) Epigenetic modification is involved in aberrant expression of class III beta-tubulin, TUBB3, in ovarian cancer cells. *Int J Oncol* 32, 1227–1235.

64. Mirza, A., McGuirk, M., Hockenberry, T.N., Wu, Q., Ashar, H., Black, S., Wen, S.F., Wang, L., Kirschmeier, P., Bishop, W.R., Nielsen, L.L., Pickett, C.B., Liu, S. (2002) Human survivin is negatively regulated by wild-type p53 and participates in p53-dependent apoptotic pathway. *Oncogene* 21, 2613–2622.

65. Fu, Y., Campbell, E.J., Shepherd, T.G., Nachtigal, M.W. (2003) Epigenetic regulation of proprotein convertase PACE4 gene expression in human ovarian cancer cells. Mol *Cancer Res* 1, 569–576.

66. Honda, H., Pazin, M.J., Ji, H., Wernyj, R.P., Morin, P.J. (2006) Crucial roles of Sp1 and epigenetic modifications in the regulation of the CLDN4 promoter in ovarian cancer cells. *J Biol Chem* 281, 21433–21444.

67. Caslini, C., Capo-chichi, C.D., Roland, I.H., Nicolas, E., Yeung, A.T., Xu. X.X. (2006) Histone modifications silence the GATA transcription factor genes in ovarian cancer. *Oncogene* 25, 5446–5461.

68. Jin, K.L., Pak. J.H., Park, J.Y., Choi, W.H., Lee, J.Y., Kim, J.H., Nam, J.H. (2008) Expression profile of histone deacetylases 1, 2 and 3 in ovarian cancer tissues. *J Gynecol Oncol* 19, 185–190.

69. Strait, K.A., Dabbas, B., Hammond, E.H., Warnick, C.T., Iistrup, S.J., Ford, C.D. (2002) Cell cycle blockade and differentiation of ovarian cancer cells by the histone deacetylase inhibitor trichostatin A are associated with changes in p21, Rb, and Id proteins. Mol *Cancer Ther* 1, 1181–1190.

70. Lopez, J., Percharde, M., Coley, H.M., Webb, A., Crook, T. (2009) The context and potential of epigenetics in oncology. *Br J Cancer* 100, 571–577.
71. Schickel, R., Boyerinas, B., Park, S.M., Peter, M.E. (2008) MicroRNAs: key players in the immune system, differentiation, tumorigenesis and cell death. *Oncogene* 27, 5959–5974.
72. Iorio, M.V., Visone, R., Di, L.G., Donati, V., Petrocca, F., Casalini, P., Taccioli, C., Volinia, S., Liu, C.G., Alder, H., Calin, G.A., Menard, S., Croce, C.M. (2007) MicroRNA signatures in human ovarian cancer. *Cancer Res* 67, 8699–8707.
73. Yang, H., Kong, W., He, L., Zhao, J.J., O'Donnell, J.D., Wang, J., Wenham, R.M., Coppola, D., Kruk, P.A., Nicosia, S.V., Cheng, J.Q. (2008) MicroRNA expression profiling in human ovarian cancer: miR-214 induces cell survival and cisplatin resistance by targeting PTEN. *Cancer Res* 68, 425–433.
74. Lee, C.H., Subramanian, S., Beck, A.H., Espinosa, I., Senz, J., Zhu, S.X., Huntsman, D., van de Rijn, M., Gilks, CB. (2009) MicroRNA profiling of BRCA1/2 mutation-carrying and non-mutation-carrying high-grade serous carcinomas of ovary. *PLoS One* 4, e7314.
75. Corney, D.C., Hwang, C.I., Matoso, A., Vogt, M., Flesken-Nikitin, A., Godwin, A.K., Kamat, A.A., Sood, A.K., Ellenson, L.H., Hermeking, H., Nikitin, A.Y. (2010) Frequent downregulation of miR-34 family in human ovarian cancers. *Clin Cancer Res* 16, 1119–1128.
76. Teschendorff, A.E., Menon, U., Gentry-Maharaj, A., Ramus, S.J., Gayther, S.A., Apostolidou, S., Jones, A., Lechner, M., Beck, S., Jacobs, I.J., Widschwendter, M. (2009) An epigenetic signature in peripheral blood predicts active ovarian cancer. *PLoS One* 4, e8274.
77. Laird PW. (2003) The power and the promise of DNA methylation markers. *Nat Rev Cancer* 3, 253–266.
78. Collins, Y., Dicioccio, R., Keitz, B., Lele, S., Odunsi, K. (2006) Methylation of death-associated protein kinase in ovarian carcinomas. *Int J Gynecol Cancer* 16 Suppl 1, 195–199.
79. Chou, J.L., Su, H.Y., Chen, L.Y., Liao, Y.P., Hartman-Frey, C., Lai, Y.H., Yang, H.W., Deatherage, D.E., Kuo, C.T., Huang, Y.W., Yan, P.S., Hsiao, S.H., Tai, C.K., Lin, H.J., Davuluri, R.V., Chao, T.K., Nephew, K.P., Huang, T.H., Lai, H.C., Chan, M.W. (2010) Promoter hypermethylation of FBXO32, a novel TGF-beta/SMAD4 target gene and tumor suppressor, is associated with poor prognosis in human ovarian cancer. *Lab Invest* 90, 414–425.
80. Wiley, A., Katsaros, D., Chen, H., Rigault de la Longrais, I.A., Beeghly, A., Puopolo, M., Singal, R., Zhang, Y., Amoako, A., Zelterman, D., Yu, H. (2006) Aberrant promoter methylation of multiple genes in malignant ovarian tumors and in ovarian tumors with low malignant potential. *Cancer* 107, 299–308.
81. Chan, M.W., Wei, S.H., Wen, P., Wang, Z., Matei, D.E., Liu, J.C., Liyanarachchi, S., Brown, R., Nephew, K.P., Yan, P.S., Huang, T.H. (2005) Hypermethylation of 18S and 28S ribosomal DNAs predicts progression-free survival in patients with ovarian cancer. *Clin Cancer Res* 11, 7376–7383.
82. Wei, S.H., Balch, C., Paik, H.H., Kim, Y.S., Baldwin, R.L., Liyanarachchi, S., Li, L., Wang, Z., Wan, J.C., Davuluri, R.V., Karlan, B.Y., Gifford, G., Brown, R., Kim, S., Huang, T.H., Nephew, K.P. (2006) Prognostic DNA methylation biomarkers in ovarian cancer. *Clin Cancer Res* 12, 2788–2794.
83. Muller, H.M., Millinger, S., Fiegl, H., Goebel, G., Ivarsson, L., Widschwendter, A., Muller-Holzner, E., Marth, C., Widschwendter, M. (2004) Analysis of methylated genes in peritoneal fluids of ovarian cancer patients: a new prognostic tool. *Clin Chem* 50, 2171–2173.
84. Wurz, K., Garcia, R.L., Goff, B.A., Mitchell, P.S., Lee, J.H., Tewari, M., Swisher, E.M. (2010) MiR-221 and MiR-222 alterations in sporadic ovarian carcinoma: Relationship to CDKN1B, CDKNIC and overall survival. *Genes Chromosomes Cancer* 49, 577–584.
85. Leskela, S., Leandro-Garcia, L.J., Mendiola, M., Barriuso, J., Inglada-Perez, L., Munoz, I., Martinez-Delgado, B., Redondo, A., de Santiago, J., Robledo, M., Hardisson, D., Rodriguez Antona, C. (2010) miR-200 family controls {beta}-tubulin III expression and is associated with paclitaxel-based treatment response and progression-free survival in ovarian cancer patients. *Endocr Relat Cancer.*
86. Wei, Y., Xia, W., Zhang, Z., Liu, J., Wang, H., Adsay, N.V., Albarracin, C., Yu, D., Abbruzzese, J.L., Mills, G.B., Bast, R.C. Jr, Hortobagyi, G.N., Hung, MC. (2008) Loss of trimethylation at lysine 27 of histone H3 is a predictor of poor outcome in breast, ovarian, and pancreatic cancers. *Mol Carcinog* 47, 701–706.
87. Weichert, W., Denkert, C., Noske, A., rb-Esfahani, S., Dietel, M., Kalloger, S.E., Huntsman, D.G., Kobel, M. (2008) Expression of class I histone deacetylases indicates poor prognosis in endometrioid subtypes of ovarian

and endometrial carcinomas. *Neoplasia* 10, 1021–1027.

88. Strathdee, G., MacKean, M.J., Illand, M., Brown, R. (1999) A role for methylation of the hMLH1 promoter in loss of hMLH1 expression and drug resistance in ovarian cancer. *Oncogene* 18, 2335–2341.
89. Plumb, J.A., Strathdee, G., Sludden, J., Kaye, S.B., Brown, R. (2000) Reversal of drug resistance in human tumor xenografts by 2 -deoxy-5-azacytidine-induced demethylation of the hMLH1 gene promoter. *Cancer Res* 60, 6039–6044.
90. Brown, R., Hirst, G.L., Gallagher, W.M., McIlwrath, A.J., Margison, G.P., van der Zee, A.G., Anthoney, D.A. (1997) hMLH1 expression and cellular responses of ovarian tumour cells to treatment with cytotoxic anticancer agents. *Oncogene* 15, 45–52.
91. Hofstetter, B., Niemierko, A., Forrer, C., Benhattar, J., Albertini, V., Pruschy, M., Bosman, F.T., Catapano, C.V., Ciernik, I.F. (2010) Impact of genomic methylation on radiation sensitivity of colorectal carcinoma. *Int J Radiat Oncol Biol Phys* 76, 1512–1519.
92. Fu, S., Hu, W., Iyer, R., Kavanagh, J.J., Coleman, R.L., Levenback, C.F., Sood, A.K., Wolf, J.K., Gershenson, D.M., Markman, M., Hennessy, B.T., Kurzrock, R., Bast, R.C. Jr. (2010) Phase 1b-2a study to reverse platinum resistance through use of a hypomethylating agent, azacitidine, in patients with platinum-resistant or platinum-refractory epithelial ovarian cancer. *Cancer.*
93. Su, H.Y., Lai, H.C., Lin, Y.W., Liu, C.Y., Chen CK, Chou YC, Lin SP, Lin WC, Lee HY, Yu MH. (2010) Epigenetic silencing of SFRP5 is related to malignant phenotype and chemoresistance of ovarian cancer through Wnt signaling pathway. *Int J Cancer* 127, 555–567.
94. Lee, P.S., Teaberry, V.S., Bland, A.E., Huang, Z., Whitaker, R.S., Baba, T., Fujii, S., Secord, A.A., Berchuck, A., Murphy, S.K. (2010) Elevated MAL expression is accompanied by promoter hypomethylation and platinum resistance in epithelial ovarian cancer. *Int J Cancer* 126, 1378–1389.
95. Taniguchi, T., Tischkowitz, M., Ameziane, N., Hodgson, S.V., Mathew, C.G., Joenje, H., Mok, S.C., D'Andrea, A.D. (2003) Disruption of the Fanconi anemia-BRCA pathway in cisplatin-sensitive ovarian tumors. *Nat Med* 9, 568–574.
96. Boren, T., Xiong, Y., Hakam, A., Wenham, R., Apte, S., Chan, G., Kamath, S.G., Chen, D.T., Dressman, H., Lancaster, JM. (2009) MicroRNAs and their target messenger RNAs associated with ovarian cancer response to chemotherapy. *Gynecol Oncol* 113, 249–255.
97. Yang, N., Kaur, S., Volinia, S., Greshock, J., Lassus, H., Hasegawa, K., Liang, S., Leminen, A., Deng, S., Smith, L., Johnstone, C.N., Chen, X.M., Liu, C.G., Huang, Q., Katsaros, D., Calin, G.A., Weber, B.L., Butzow, R., Croce, C.M., Coukos, G., Zhang, L. (2008) MicroRNA microarray identifies Let-7i as a novel biomarker and therapeutic target in human epithelial ovarian cancer. *Cancer Res* 68, 10307–10314.
98. Jones, P.A., Baylin, SB. (2007) The epigenomics of cancer. *Cell* 128, 683–692.
99. Esteller, M. (2008) Epigenetics in cancer. *N Engl J Med* 358, 1148–1159.
100. Li, Y., Hu, W., Shen, D.Y., Kavanagh, J.J., Fu, S. (2009) Azacitidine enhances sensitivity of platinum-resistant ovarian cancer cells to carboplatin through induction of apoptosis. *Am J Obstet Gynecol* 200, 177–179.
101. Lenzi, R., Frost, P., Abbruzzese, J.L. (1994) Modulation of cisplatin resistance by 2′-deoxy-5-azacytidine in human ovarian tumor cell lines. *Anticancer Res* 14, 247–251.
102. Balch, C., Yan, P., Craft, T., Young, S., Skalnik, D.G., Huang, T.H., Nephew, K.P. (2007) Antimitogenic and chemosensitizing effects of the methylation inhibitor zebularine in ovarian cancer. *Mol Cancer Ther* 4, 1505–1514.
103. Takai, N., Narahara. H. (2007) Human endometrial and ovarian cancer cells: histone deacetylase inhibitors exhibit antiproliferative activity, potently induce cell cycle arrest, and stimulate apoptosis. *Curr Med Chem* 14, 2548–2553.
104. Modesitt, S.C., Sill, M., Hoffman, J.S., Bender, D.P. (2008) A phase II study of vorinostat in the treatment of persistent or recurrent epithelial ovarian or primary peritoneal carcinoma: a Gynecologic Oncology Group study. *Gynecol Oncol* 109, 182–186.
105. Plumb, J.A., Finn, P.W., Williams, R.J., Bandara, M.J., Romero, M.R., Watkins, C.J,, La Thangue, N.B., Brown, R. (2003) Pharmacodynamic response and inhibition of growth of human tumor xenografts by the novel histone deacetylase inhibitor PXD101. *Mol Cancer Ther* 2, 721–728.
106. Arts, J., Angibaud, P., Marien, A., Floren, W., Janssens, B., King, P., van Dun, J., Janssen, L., Geerts, T., Tuman, R.W., Johnson, D.L., Andries, L., Jung, M., Janicot, M., van Emelen, K. (2007) R306465 is a novel potent inhibitor of class I histone deacetylases with broad-spectrum antitumoral activity against solid and haematological malignancies. *Br J Cancer* 97, 1344–1353.

107. Takai, N., Ueda, T., Nishida, M., Nasu, K., Narahara, H. (2006) A novel histone deacetylase inhibitor, Scriptaid, induces growth inhibition, cell cycle arrest and apoptosis in human endometrial cancer and ovarian cancer cells. *Int J Mol Med* 17, 323–329.
108. Shi, H., Wei, S.H., Leu, Y.W., Rahmatpanah, F., Liu, J.C., Yan, P.S., Nephew, K.P., Huang, T.H. (2003) Triple analysis of the cancer epigenome: an integrated microarray system for assessing gene expression, DNA methylation, and histone acetylation. *Cancer Res* 63, 2164–2171.
109. Steele, N., Finn, P., Brown, R., Plumb, J.A. (2009) Combined inhibition of DNA methylation and histone acetylation enhances gene re-expression and drug sensitivity in vivo. *Br J Cancer*, 100, 758-763.

Part III

Methods and Technologies used for Epigenetic Changes' Detection

Chapter 16

DNA Methylation in Pancreatic Cancer: Protocols for the Isolation of DNA and Bisulfite Modification

Katja Biewusch*, Marie Heyne*, Robert Grützmann, and Christian Pilarsky

Abstract

Pancreatic ductal adenocarcinoma (PDAC) is an aggressive tumor and still remains a challenge for its lack of effective therapeutic strategies, which is due to the late diagnosis of this disease. Methylation markers might improve early detection and surveillance of PDAC. Furthermore, analysis of hypermethylation in the tumor tissue might help to identify new targets for therapeutic intervention and improve the understanding of the pathophysiological changes occurring in pancreatic cancer. Methylation specific PCR is the method of choice if a small number of genes will be tested in a larger set of patient samples. After DNA isolation by standard procedure, the DNA is then modified using sodium bisulfite. This DNA can then be used in qualitative and quantitative PCR assays.

Key words: Pancreatic cancer, Methylation, Bisulfide, Plasma tissue, Polymerase chain reaction

1. Introduction

Pancreatic cancer is still one of the most malignant and aggressive types of cancer in humans with a very poor prognosis. With 40,000 new cases diagnosed in the United States each year, it is the fourth male and the fifth female leading cause of cancer-related death in the western world (1). The most abundant form of exocrine pancreatic cancer is ductal adenocarcinoma (PDAC) (2). In the last decades, only small therapeutic improvements could be made, which is mainly due to the delayed appearance of symptoms causing a late diagnosis. The vast majority of the patients show an organ overlapping growth of the tumor when the disease is discovered and only the remaining approximately 15% of patients have an opportunity of curative surgical treatment. Therefore, the actual 5-year survival rate is about 5% for all patients (1).

*KB and MH contributed equally.

Ramona G. Dumitrescu and Mukesh Verma (eds.), *Cancer Epigenetics: Methods and Protocols*, Methods in Molecular Biology, vol. 863, DOI 10.1007/978-1-61779-612-8_16, © Springer Science+Business Media, LLC 2012

DNA hypermethylation of the coding areas of the human genome is a hallmark in cancer development and was identified in a series of landmark investigations in the late twentieth century (3, 4). Since then DNA hypermethylation has been investigated in nearly all cancers, and it has been shown that the detection of DNA hypermethylation might be a useful tumor marker (3). Methylation marker candidates might be identified in different ways, either direct by using large-scale analysis of the methyliome (5, 6) or by bioinformatics analysis of gene expression data, linking the observed under expression of genes with data from other sources.

In pancreatic cancer, several studies have investigated DNA hypermethylation in tumor tissue and body fluids revealing more than 100 possible marker genes available for testing in different settings (6–8). However, a major impediment is the low number of primary samples analyzed. Therefore, new studies are needed to investigate those markers in a large number of samples of PDAC and other form of pancreatic cancers and chronic pancreatitis to establish reliable methylation marker for early diagnosis, clinical monitoring, and prognosis.

2. Materials

For all the experiments routine lab ware is needed. The performance of enzymes, chemicals, plasticware, and equipment from high-quality providers is nearly identical. Performing a large number of PCR experiments requires high standard of cleanliness to reduce the risk of cross contaminants to bare minimum.

1. PDAC tissue can be used from different sources like fresh frozen or formalin fixed paraffin embedded (FFPE). However, due to the heterogeneity of PDAC it is of outmost importance that each tissue sample used should be evaluated by a trained pathologist.
2. Blood plasma can be obtained easily from patients during routine blood draws. It is critical that the plasma is free from white blood cells; therefore the plasma should be centrifuged twice.
3. QIAamp DNA Mini Kit (Qiagen, Hilden, Germany) for DNA isolation.
4. EZ DNA Methylation-Gold Kit (Zymo Research, Orange, CA, USA) for bisulfite modification.
5. PBS (Phosphate buffered saline, 1.06 mM KH_2PO_4, 115.17 mM NaCl, 2.97 mM Na_2HPO_4) pH 7.4.
6. Ethanol p.a.

7. Distilled Water. Beware of your source of water; sloppy prepared water is the number one cause of contaminants of reactions and therefore the number one reason why experiments fail.

For primer design several tools are available. However, we have had our best results with Methprimer (http://www.urogene.org/methprimer/index1.html). Another source is the usage of already described primer combinations. All primers should be tested on fully methylated DNA, which can be obtained from Millipore (Billerica, MA, USA).

3. Methods

3.1. DNA-Isolation from Plasma

1. Add 200 μL plasma to the microcentrifuge tube. If the sample volume is less than 200 μL add the appropriate volume of PBS (see Note 1).
2. Add 200 μL buffer AL to the sample. Mix thoroughly by pulse-vortexing for 15 s.
3. Incubate at 56°C for 10 min.
4. Add 200 μL ethanol (96–100%) to the sample, and mix again by pulse-vortexing for 15 s. After mixing, briefly centrifuge the 1.5-mL microcentrifuge tube to remove drops from the inside of the lid (see Note 2).
5. Carefully apply the mixture from step 4 to the QIAamp Mini spin column (in a 2-mL collection tube) without wetting the rim. Close the cap, and centrifuge at 6,000 × *g* for 1 min. Place the column in a clean 2-mL collection tube, and discard the tube containing the filtrate (see Note 3).
6. Open the column and add 500 μL buffer AW1 without wetting the rim. Close the cap and centrifuge at 6,000 × *g* for 1 min. Place the column in a clean 2-mL collection tube, and discard the collection tube containing the filtrate.
7. Carefully open the column and add 500 μL buffer AW2 without wetting the rim. Close the cap and centrifuge at 20,000 × *g* for 3 min.
8. Place the column in a new 2-mL collection tube (not provided) and discard the old collection tube with the filtrate. Centrifuge at 20,000 × *g* for 1 min.
9. Place the column in a clean 1.5-mL microcentrifuge tube and discard the collection tube containing the filtrate. Carefully open the column and add 200 μL buffer AE or distilled water. Incubate at room temperature (15–25°C) for 1 min, and then centrifuge at 6,000 × *g* for 1 min (see Note 4).

3.2. DNA-Isolation from Frozen or Formalin Fixed Paraffin Embedded Tissue

1. Excise the tissue sample or remove it from storage. Determine the amount of tissue. Do not use more than 25 mg (see Note 5).
2. If samples are large mechanically disrupt the tissue sample (see Note 6).
3. Add 20 μL proteinase K solution, mix by vortexing, and incubate at 56°C until the tissue is completely lysed. Vortex occasionally during incubation to disperse the sample, or place in a shaking water bath or on a rocking platform (see Note 7).
4. Briefly centrifuge the 1.5-mL microcentrifuge tube to remove drops from the inside of the lid.
5. Add 200 μL buffer AL to the sample, mix by pulse-vortexing for 15 s, and incubate at 70°C for 10 min. Briefly, centrifuge the 1.5-mL microcentrifuge tube to remove drops from inside the lid. It is essential that the sample and buffer AL are mixed thoroughly to yield a homogeneous solution.
6. Add 200 μL ethanol (96–100%) to the sample, and mix by pulse-vortexing for 15 s. After mixing, briefly centrifuge the 1.5-mL microcentrifuge tube to remove drops from inside the lid. Follow the protocol for Plasma DNA isolation from step 6.

3.3. Bisulfite Modification

1. Determine the concentration of the DNA you have prepared using a photometer. For the bisulfite modification samples containing 25 pg–100 pg/μl of DNA can be used.
2. Prepare the conversion reagent. Add 900 μL water, 300 μL of M-Dilution buffer, and 50 μL M-Dissolving buffer to a tube of CT conversion reagent.
3. Mix at room temperature with frequent vortexing or shaking for 10 min (see Note 8).
4. Preparation of M-Wash buffer: Add 24 mL of 100% ethanol to 6 mL M-Wash buffer before use.
5. Add 130 μL of the CT conversion reagent to 20 μL of your DNA sample in a PCR tube.
6. Place the sample tube in a thermal cycler and perform the following steps (see Note 9):

   98°C for 10 min.

   64°C for 2.5 h.

   4°C storage up to 20 h.
7. Add 600 μL of M-Binding buffer to a Zymo-Spin IC column and place the column into a provided collection tube.
8. Load the sample (from step 2) into the column containing the M- Binding buffer. Close the cap and mix by inverting the column several times.
9. Centrifuge at 20,000 × *g* for 30 s. Discard the flow-through.

10. Add 100 μL of M-Wash buffer to the column. Centrifuge at 20,000 × *g* for 30 s.
11. Add 200 μL of M-Desulphonation buffer to the column and let stand at room temperature (20–30°C) for 15–20 min. After incubation centrifuge at 20,000 × *g* for 30 s.
12. Add 200 μL of M-Wash buffer to the column. Centrifuge at 20,000 × *g* for 30 s. Add another 200 μL of M-Wash buffer and centrifuge at 20,000 × *g* for an additional 30 s.
13. Place the column into a 1.5-mL microcentrifuge tube. Add 10 μL of M-Elution buffer directly to the column matrix. Centrifuge for 30 s at 20,000 × *g* to elute the DNA (see Note 10).

4. Results

Using the protocols described above, we have isolated, modified, and amplified DNA from various sources including 15 year old FFPE tissue. We were also able to demonstrate changes in methylated genes between different types of pancreatic cancer like PDAC (n = 14) and tumors of the ampulla Vateri (AVT, n = 7). Those genes were selected from several publications describing methylation-specific PCR (MSP) in cancer (10–13). Analysis of the bisulfite modified DNA showed methylation differences in reelin (RELN, PDAC: 63%, AVT: 37%), ADAM metallopeptidase with thrombospondin type 1 motif, 8 (ADAMTS8, PDAC: 37%, AVT: 14%), BCL2/adenovirus E1B 19 kDa interacting protein 3 (BNIP3, PDAC: 85%, AVT: 50%), secreted frizzled-related protein 1 (SFRP1, PDAC: 84%, AVT: 100%) and inhibitor of DNA binding 4, dominant negative helix-loop-helix protein (ID4, PDAC: 93%, AVT: 62%). Interestingly, for tissue factor pathway inhibitor 2 (TFPI2) both tumors types showed nearly the same incidence of methylation events (PDAC: 86%, AVT: 87%). In conclusion, methylation analysis of human genes has become a common and easy adaptable technique. Therefore analysis of the methylation status in different tumors will become an integral part of translational oncology.

5. Notes

1. It is possible to add QIAGEN Protease (or proteinase K) to samples that have already been dispensed into microcentrifuge tubes. In this case, it is important to ensure proper mixing after adding the enzyme.

2. If the sample volume is larger than 200 μL, increase the amount of QIAGEN Protease (or proteinase K), buffer AL and Ethanol proportionally. Do not add QIAGEN Protease or proteinase K directly to buffer AL 4. Close each spin column to avoid aerosol formation during centrifugation.
3. Incubating the column loaded with buffer AE or water for 5 min at room temperature before centrifugation generally increases DNA yield. A second elution step with a further 200 μL buffer AE will increase yields by up to 15%. Volumes of more than 200 μL should not be eluted into a 1.5-mL microcentrifuge tube because the spin column will come into contact with the eluate. Elution with volumes of less than 200 μL increases the final DNA concentration in the eluate significantly, but slightly reduces the overall DNA yield.
4. For long-term storage of DNA, eluting in buffer AE and storing at −20°C is recommended, since DNA stored in water is subject to acid hydrolysis.
5. The QIAamp DNA Mini Kit can also be used to isolate DNA from fixed tissues. However, the length of DNA isolated from fixed tissues is usually <650 bp, depending on the type and age of the sample and the quality of the fixative used (9). Use of fixatives such as alcohol and formalin are recommended. Fixatives that cause cross-linking, such as osmium tetroxide, are not recommended as it can be difficult to obtain amplifiable DNA from tissue fixed with these agents. From FFPE tissue cut slices of 10 μm thickness and collect 1–10 of them in a 1.5-mL microcentrifuge tube and proceed with step 3. It is not necessary to remove the paraffin in advance since it will melt during the incubation at 56 C.
6. Some tissues require undiluted buffer ATL for complete lysis. In this case, grinding in liquid nitrogen is recommended. Samples cannot be homogenized directly in buffer ATL, which contains detergent.
7. Proteinase K must be used. Lysis time varies depending on the type of tissue processed. Lysis is usually complete in 1–3 h. In order to ensure efficient lysis, a shaking water bath or a rocking platform should be used. If not available, vortexing 2–3 times/h during incubation is recommended.
8. It is normal to see trace amounts of undissolved reagent in the CT conversion reagent. Each tube of CT conversion reagent is designed for 10 separate DNA treatments. Storage: The CT conversion reagent is light sensitive; so minimize its exposure to light. For best results, the CT conversion reagent should be used immediately following preparation. If not used immediately, the CT conversion reagent solution can be stored overnight at room temperature, 1 week at 4°C, or up to 1 month at −20°C.

Stored CT conversion reagent solution must be warmed to 37°C, then vortexed prior to use.

9. For DNA volumes >20 μL, an adjustment needs to be made during the preparation of the CT conversion reagent. The amount of water is decreased 100 μL for each 10 μL increase in DNA sample volume. For example, for a 40 μL DNA sample, 700 μL of water is added to make the CT conversion reagent. The maximum DNA sample volume to be used for each conversion reaction is 50 μL. Do not adjust the volumes of either the M-Dissolving buffer or M-Dilution buffer. The capacity of the collection tube with the column inserted is 800 μL. Empty the collection tube whenever necessary to prevent contamination of the column contents by the flow-through. Alternatively, water or TE (pH ≥ 6.0) can be used for elution if required for your experiments.
10. The DNA is ready for immediate analysis or can be stored at or below −20°C for later use. For long-term storage, store at or below −70°C. We recommend using 1–4 μL of eluted DNA for each PCR, however, up to 10 μL can be used if necessary. The elution volume can be >10 μL depending on the requirements of your experiments, but small elution volumes will yield more concentrated DNA.

Acknowledgements

I am grateful to Beatrix Jahnke for performing DNA isolation and bisulfite modification in our lab. Thanks also to Alfred E. Neumann for fruitful discussions.

References

1. Jemal, A., Siegel, R., Xu, J., and Ward, E. (2010) Cancer statistics, 2010. *CA Cancer J Clin* 60, 277–300.
2. Schneider, G., Siveke, J.T., Eckel, F., and Schmid, R.M. (2005) Pancreatic cancer: basic and clinical aspects. *Gastroenterology* 128, 1606–1625.
3. Kulis, M. and Esteller, M. (2010) DNA methylation and cancer. *Adv Genet* 70, 27–56.
4. Nakhasi, H.L., Lynch, K.R., Dolan, K.P., Unterman, R.D., and Feigelson P. (1981) Covalent modification and repressed transcription of a gene in hepatoma cells. *Proc Natl Acad Sci USA* 78, 834–837.
5. Lofton-Day, C., Model, F., Devos, T., Tetzner, R., Distler, J., Schuster, M. *et al* (2008) DNA methylation biomarkers for blood-based colorectal cancer screening. *Clin Chem* 54, 414–423.
6. Tan, A.C., Jimeno, A., Lin, S.H., Wheelhouse, J., Chan, F., Solomon, A. *et al* (2009) Characterizing DNA methylation patterns in pancreatic cancer genome. *Mol Oncol* 3, 425–438.
7. Wehrum, D., Grutzmann, R., Hennig, M., Saeger, H.D., and Pilarsky, C. (2008) Recent patents concerning diagnostic and therapeutic applications of aberrantly methylated sequences in pancreatic cancer. *Recent Pat DNA Gene Seq* 2, 97–106.
8. Kuroki, T., Tajima, Y., and Kanematsu, T. (2004) Role of hypermethylation on carcinogenesis in the pancreas. *Surg Today* 34, 981–986.

9. Wright, D.K. and Manos, M.M. (1990). Sample preparation from paraffin-embedded tissues. In: Innis M.A., Gelfont D.H., Sninsky J.J. and White T.J. (eds). *PCR Protocols: A guide to methods and applications*. Academic Press, San Diego. pp 153–158.
10. Hong, S.M., Kelly, D., Griffith, M., Omura, N., Li, A., Li, C.P. et al. (2008). Multiple genes are hypermethylated in intraductal papillary mucinous neoplasms of the pancreas. *Mod Pathol* 12, 1499–1507.
11. Noetzel, E., Veeck, J., Niederacher, D., Galm, O., Horn, F., Hartmann, A. et al. (2008) Promoter methylation-associated loss of ID4 expression is a marker of tumour recurrence in human breast cancer. *BMC Cancer* 8, 154.
12. Okami, J., Simeone, D.M., and Logsdon, C.D. (2004) Silencing of the hypoxia-inducible cell death protein BNIP3 in pancreatic cancer. *Cancer Res* 64, 5338–5346.
13. Dunn, J.R., Panutsopulos, D., Shaw, M.W. Heighway, J., Dormer, R., Salmo, E.N. et al. (2004) METH-2 silencing and promoter hypermethylation in NSCLC. *Br J Cancer* 91, 1149–1154.

Chapter 17

Detection and Analysis of DNA Methylation by Pyrosequencing

Hilary A.A. Colyer, Richard N. Armstrong, Daniel J. Sharpe, and Ken I. Mills

Abstract

Pyrosequencing is a "sequencing by synthesis" technique which can be used to quantify DNA methylation at specific CpG sites within the target region of interest. Biotin labelled polymerase chain reaction (PCR) products form the template for base-pair nucleotide incorporation causing a light emitting cascade reaction resulting in the formation of a pyrogram and the calculation of the percentage methylation for each site. Prior to pyrosequencing, it is essential to bisulphite-convert the DNA sample and then perform locus-specific PCR for the region of interest. One of the PCR primers needs to be biotinylated and a separate sequencing primer is required for the pyrosequencing itself.

Key words: Pyrosequencing, DNA, Methylation, Epigenetics, Bisulphite, Pyrogram, CpG

1. Introduction

Pyrosequencing, developed by Professor Pål Nyrén in 1996 (1), is a "sequencing by synthesis" technique which can be used in the quantification of DNA methylation at CpG sites within a defined region of interest. Biotin-labelled amplicons are created during polymerase chain reaction (PCR) amplification by the use of one standard and one biotinylated primer. The amplicons are denatured in the pyrosequencing preparation stage so that the ssDNA biotin labelled PCR amplicons can be utilized as a template to which a sequencing primer is bound. This allows base-pair extension of the complimentary strand to occur during the pyrosequencing reaction, (see Fig. 1) (2). During pyrosequencing single nucleotide aliquots are released. If incorporated into the sequence in a complimentary

Ramona G. Dumitrescu and Mukesh Verma (eds.), *Cancer Epigenetics: Methods and Protocols*, Methods in Molecular Biology, vol. 863, DOI 10.1007/978-1-61779-612-8_17,

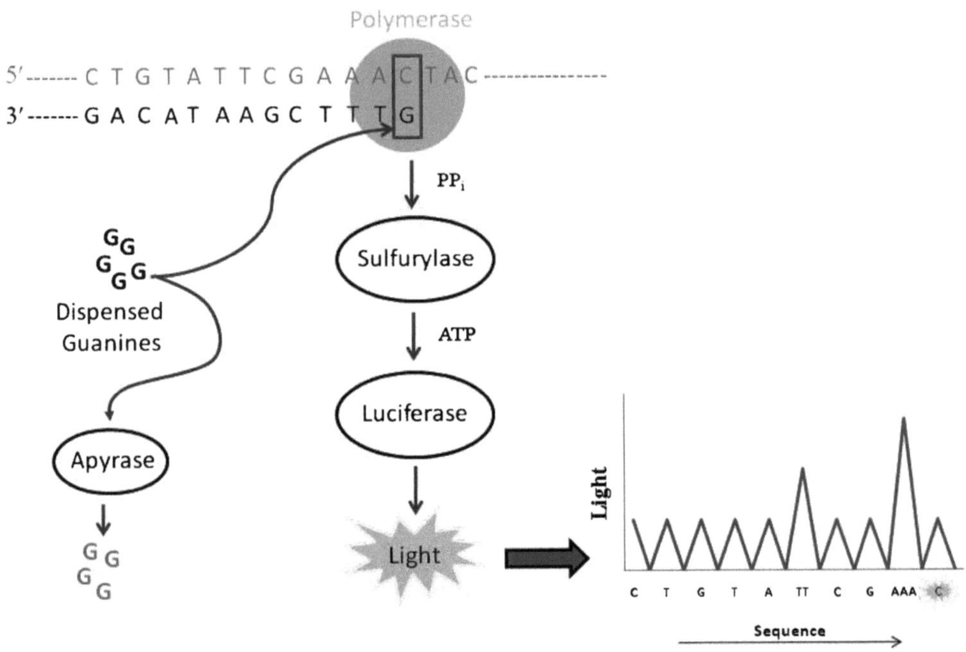

Fig. 1. The pyrosequencing cascade reaction. A nucleotide base aliquot is released and if complimentary to the template strand is incorporated by polymerase. The incorporation yields inorganic pyrophosphate (PP_i) which is converted by sulfurylase to adenosine triphosphate (ATP). Luciferase utilizes ATP as its substrate and the reaction produces light. The light captured by the charge-coupled device (CCD) camera is proportional to the number of incorporated bases in the sequence. Unincorporated nucleotides are degraded by apyrase before the next base is released to be incorporated.

base-pair wise manner, an inorganic pyrophosphate molecule (PPi) is released as a reaction by-product and a cascade reaction begins. The PPi, in the presence of adenosine 5′-phosphosulphate, is converted to adenosine triphosphate (ATP) by the enzyme ATP sulfurylase. The ATP drives luciferase to convert luciferin to oxyluciferin. This reaction generates visible light which is proportional to the amount of ATP, and therefore proportional to the number of bases of the dispensed and incorporated nucleotide (3). A charge coupled device (CCD) chip detects the visible light, which is recorded as a peak on the pyrogram (raw data output graph). Peak height is proportional to the number of nucleotide bases incorporated. Between each release of nucleotide aliquots apyrase efficiently hydrolyses unincorporated nucleoside triphosphates to nucleoside monophosphates, which prevents incorporation into the growing stand and thereby maintains specificity and sensitivity of the reaction. The next nucleotide base is then dispensed into the reaction for incorporation and the cascade begins again. One pyrosequencing assay is performed for each biological sample, and negative controls are included on the plate for both the pre-pyrosequencing PCR reaction and the pyrosequencing reaction itself to check for contamination of reagents.

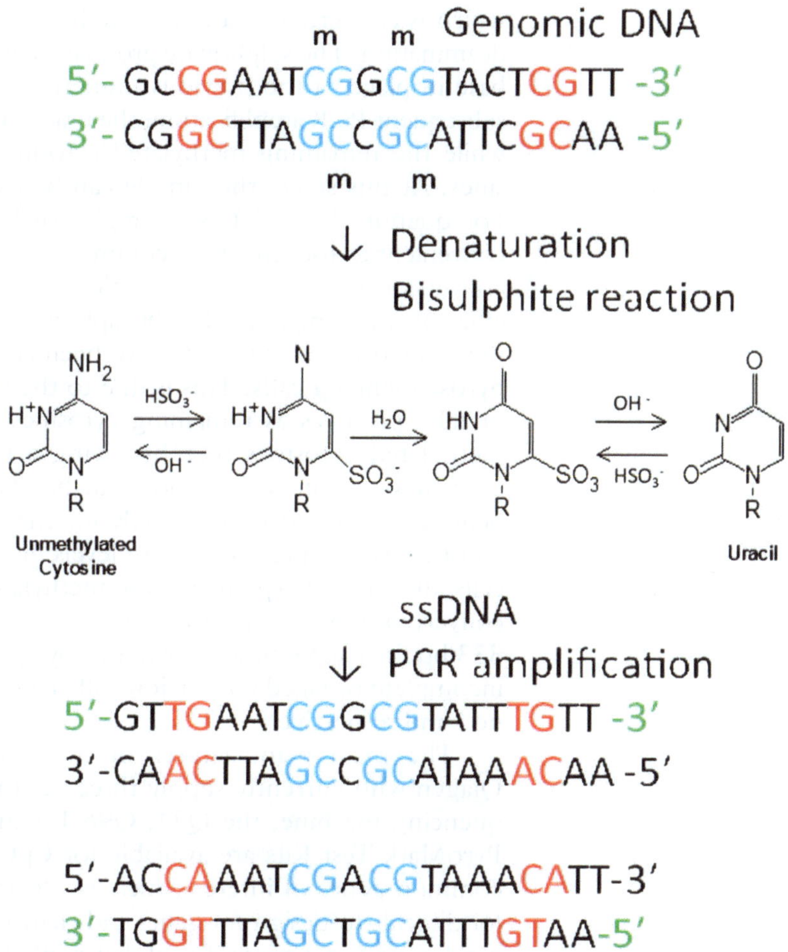

Fig. 2. Stages of bisulphite conversion. *Top*: genomic DNA is pictured with methylation indicating by "*m*". *Middle*: the bisulphite reaction deaminates unmethylated cytosines to uracil, resulting in single-stranded DNA. *Bottom*: during PCR amplification uracil becomes thymine allowing discrimination between the original unmethylated cytosines (now thymine) and methylated cytosine (remains as cytosine).

Before pyrosequencing for DNA methylation quantification can occur it is essential to bisulphite-convert the DNA sample. This allows the pyrosequencing reaction to detect methylation sites (see Note 1 and Fig. 2). This technique was first described by Frommer et al. (4) and has since become a standard method of discriminating between pre-conversion unmethylated cytosines and methylated cytosines in a sequence. The principle behind bisulphite conversion, which is specific to single-strand DNA (ssDNA), is that double-strand DNA (dsDNA) is denatured and unmethylated cytosines are rapidly deaminated in reaction with sodium bisulphite while methylated cytosines remain unchanged. The bisulphite reaction yields a cytosine-sulphonate derivative which is converted to a uracil-sulphonate derivative by hydrolytic deamination. The sulphonate group is then removed to yield a uracil base in place of the previous unmethylated cytosine (5). During subsequent PCR amplification, the uracils are amplified as thymines, while the remaining methylated cytosines are amplified as cytosines. At this stage, the sample can be used for pyrosequencing. For quantity limited DNA samples such as patient samples it is convenient to use any of the commercially available DNA bisulphite conversion kits which are capable of converting low yield DNA efficiently. Incomplete DNA bisulphite conversion, where not all of the unmethylated cytosines have been converted, can cause failed pyrosequencing calls. This is due to the internal bisulphite check or false positives as remaining cytosines are "read" as originally methylated cytosines thereby giving a false higher methylation percentage result. Conversion can be checked quickly and inexpensively by performing a PCR for the *Calponin* gene which is constitutively expressed at high levels in smooth- and non-muscle cells and in wild-type form is unmethylated (6). Fully bisulphite-converted DNA will, after conversion, yield a strong band of 333 bp for *Calponin* when run out by agarose gel electrophoresis, incomplete or failed conversion will yield a weak *Calponin* band or no band respectively.

The main manufacturer of pyrosequencing instruments is Qiagen who currently supply three versions of PyroMark pyrosequencing machine, the Q24, Q96 ID and Q96 MD. Associated PyroMark Test Kits are available for CpG methylation analysis of common genes of interest, such as *MGMT*, *MLH1*, and *P16* and for difficult-to-design-for genes and elements such as LINE1, which can be used as a proxy for global methylation analysis (7). These optimized kits contain forward, reverse and sequencing primers and PCR thermocycling conditions. Primers required for genes of interest other than those available in kit form can be designed using software, such as the PyroMark Assay Design Software (currently version 2.0), which is capable of designing PCR and sequencing primers taking into account the bisulphite-converted DNA sequence. The PCR reaction can be performed with standard PCR reagents; although a PyroMark PCR kit is available for use with both PyroMark Test Kits and self-designed primers.

2. Materials

2.1. Primer Design for Pyrosequencing

- PyroMark Assay Design Software.
- DNA region of interest in sequence format (e.g. FASTA).

2.2. Calponin PCR Control for Complete Bisulphite Conversion (see Note 2)

- 5′-GGAAGGTAGTTGAGGTTGTG-3′ (forward) and 5′-CC CAAACTCAAAACTCTAACCTAAC-3′ (reverse) primers for *Calponin* gene (8).
- Qiagen PCR buffer (10×, containing $MgCl_2$).
- $MgCl_2$ (25 mM).
- 200 μM each dNTP.
- 10 pmol each primer.
- 1 U HotStarTaq.
- 150 ng bisulphite-converted DNA (assume no conversion loss).
- Ultra-pure water.

2.3. Region-of-Interest Specific PCR

- PyroMark PCR kit or standard PCR reagents with self-designed primers (see Subheading 2.2).

2.4. Gel Electrophoresis of Specific Product

- Agarose crystals (electrophoresis grade).
- Buffer TAE (Tris-acetate and EDTA) (1%).
- Ethidium Bromide (10 μg/mL) (Caution: Carcinogen).
- DNA Loading buffer (if PyroMark PCR kit not used, which uses Coral-load buffer).
- DNA Ladder (100 bp).

2.5. Pyrosequencing

- Binding Buffer (Qiagen). Store at 4°C, equilibrate to room temperature before use.
- Streptavidin Sepharose High Performance Beads (GE Healthcare). Store at 4°C, equilibrate to room temperature before use.
- Ultra-pure water H_2O.
- PCR product for region of interest (see Subheading 2.3).
- Annealing Buffer (Qiagen). Store at 4°C, equilibrate to room temperature before use.
- Sequencing Primer (reconstituted in annealing buffer). Store at −20°C, thaw before use.
- 24-well 0.2 mL microtube plates (Abgene).
- Q-24 pyrosequencing plates (Qiagen).
- PyroMark reagents kit, contains enzyme and substrate (both light sensitive) which need reconstituting in ultra-pure water, incubate at room temperature for 5–10 min, do not shake; swirl to mix, store in aliquots at −20°C, thaw before use. Kits also contain dNTPs, including modified ATP (which is not a substrate for luciferase).

- Denaturation solution (Qiagen). Store at 4°C, equilibrate to room temperature before use. ~0.2 M NaOH solution; corrosive; risk of chemical burn.
- Wash buffer (Qiagen). Store stock at 4°C, dilute 2:20 and equilibrate to room temperature before use.

3. Methods

3.1. Primer Design for Pyrosequencing

1. Identify a region of interest of suitable length for investigating DNA methylation, e.g. the promoter region of a gene of interest (see Note 3).
2. Recommended: investigate the CpG enrichment of the DNA sequence analysis (see Note 4).
3. Open the PyroMark Assay Design 2.0 software. For a familiarization diagram of the software interface, please see Note 5 (Fig. 3).
4. Enter the sequence of interest for primer design into the original sequence editor tab. This can be done manually or by copy and pasting from other formats. This sequence will automatically be "bisulphite-converted" by the software and CpG sites will be recognized.
5. Highlight a region target containing CpG sites for methylation profiling, right click and select "Target region".
6. Click "Run Assay Design" to allow the software to automatically find suitable primer sets for this target. By default this

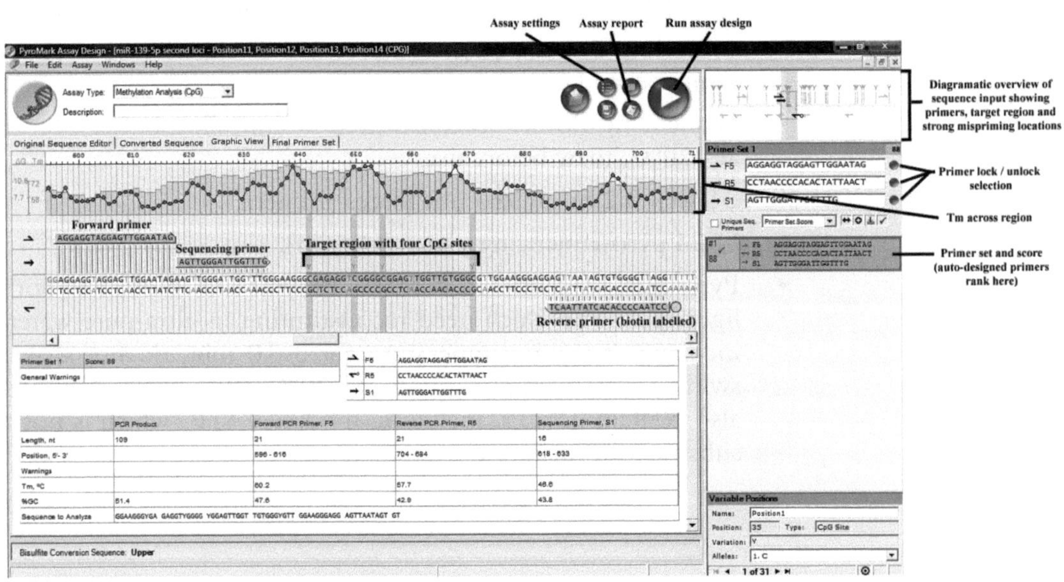

Fig. 3. Pyromark assay design 2.0 software interface.

process may be lengthy, we recommend following the set-up parameters described in Note 6. Ensure that the PCR product size is a suitable length (see Note 7). If the software returns no viable primer sets, please see Note 8 for help with manual primer design.

7. The software will rank primer sets for the target sequence. We consider a primer set score of >85 to be excellent, however, primer sets of >70 can work very well. Note 9 describes a technique for enriching the primers to increase primer set score. To understand what is penalizing the primer sets, one must look at the primer report. Here, we can identify problematic features of the primer sets such as primer dimerization, differential Tm and mispriming. In some instances, primer sets may work efficiently despite these penalties (see Note 10).

3.2. Calponin PCR Check of Complete Bisulphite Conversion (Optional)

1. The PCR is performed in a 25 μL volume containing:
   (a) 2.5 μL Qiagen PCR buffer (1× final concentration containing $MgCl_2$).
   (b) 1.5 μL $MgCl_2$ (25 mM).
   (c) 200 μM each dNTP.
   (d) 10 pmol each forward and reverse primer.
   (e) 1 U Qiagen HotStarTaq.
   (f) 150 ng bisulphite-converted DNA.
2. Thermocycling conditions are as follows:
   (a) 95°C for 5 min (for HotStarTaq activation) then 35 cycles of
      - Denaturation 95°C for 30 s.
      - Annealing 63°C for 30 s.
   (b) Extension 72°C for 30 s followed by a final hold at 72°C for 10 min.
3. If DNA bisulphite conversion is successful PCR products of 333 bp will form a strong band when separated on 1.5% agarose gel electrophoresis. No product or weak bands indicate incomplete bisulphite conversion.

3.3. Region-of-Interest Specific PCR

If using PyroMark PCR kit:
This kit contains PyroMark Mastermix, $MgCl_2$, Coral-load buffer, Q-solution and water. The kit follows a standard protocol which may require optimization for $MgCl_2$ and/or Q-solution but frequently does not require this. Cycling conditions have been optimized for this kit.

If using standard PCR reagents:
The PCR reaction may need optimization. Consider $MgCl_2$ concentration, primer concentration and annealing temperatures. PCR thermocycling conditions may require extra cycles, it is not uncommon for 50 cycles of the denaturation, annealing and extension steps to be needed.

3.4. Gel Electrophoresis of Specific Product

1. Check for PCR specificity and contamination by running products on 1.5% agarose electrophoresis gel. Heat the following until a clear solution:
   (a) 0.75 g agarose.
   (b) 50 mL buffer TAE.
2. Allow gel to cool slightly before adding
   (a) 1 μL Ethidium bromide.
3. Run 4 μL of PCR product with appropriate loading dye. Loading dye is not required if the PyroMark PCR kit is used.
4. Visualize bands under UV light. Strong bands indicating a strong PCR product is required (see Note 11).

3.5. Pyrosequencing

1. Allow binding buffer, denaturation solution, sepharose beads and annealing buffer to equilibrate to room temperature.
2. Assay plate layout for a pyrosequencing run is set up by the user using PyroMark software (see Note 12). This enables the user to assign wells for the appropriate sample assay. Include control wells for positive and/or negative PCR samples and a negative control for the pyrosequencing reagent mix. The assay design should be saved to a memory-stick to use in the PyroMark Q-24 pyrosequencer.
3. Pre-run information is calculated by the software for the volumes of enzyme and substrate mixes required as well as for each nucleotide. These are aliquoted into the cartridge as shown on the pre-run information. The enzyme and substrate are light-sensitive therefore insert the cartridge into the machine now.
4. Make a master-mix of (per sample) Binding Buffer (40 μL), Sepharose Beads (2 μL) and Ultra-pure water (18 μL).
5. Aliquot 60 μL of master-mix to each well of a 24-well 0.2-mL microtube plate and add 20 μL of appropriate PCR products according to layout of plate set-up.
6. Apply microtube caps or an adhesive film to the plate and agitate the microtube plate for 5–10 min at high speed in a H+P Labortechnik monoshaker or equivalent.
7. Fill the PyroMark Vacuum station troughs with ultra-pure water, 70% ethanol, denaturation solution, and wash-buffer.
8. Prepare the Q-24 well plate by aliquoting 25 μL of 0.3 μM sequencing primer in annealing buffer into the appropriate wells for the plate set-up.
9. Turn the vacuum tool on and immerse in water trough to clean. Wait until approximately 70 mL water has been flushed through the tool then hold tool vertically to drain.
10. Samples are attached to the filter probes of the vacuum tool by lowering the probes into the 24-well microtube plate once the

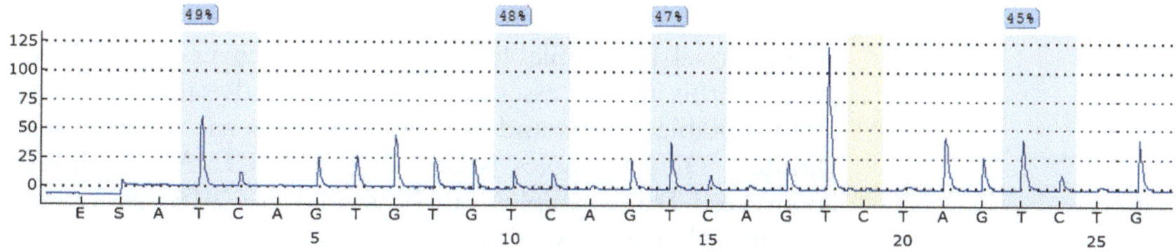

Fig. 4. The pyrosequencing pyrogram. *Y*-axis: (arbitrary units) peak height is determined by amount of light recorded by the charge-coupled device (CCD camera). Light is proportional to the number of that base incorporated in the sequence. *X*-axis: *E* enzyme mix released; *S* substrate mix released; *G, T, A, C* nucleotide bases. Peak height relates to the number of nucleotide base incorporated. *Blue* columns; location of CpG site within the sequence with the methylation shown as a percentage at the top of the column. *Yellow* column; internal bisulphite conversion check, a peak at this point would indicate the bisulphite conversion was not efficient.

adhesive cover is removed. The solution should be vacuumed-up within 15 s (see Note 13).

11. Immerse the probes into the 70% ethanol trough for 5 s, then denaturation solution for 5 s then Wash Buffer for 10 s. Hold the vacuum tool vertically to drain fluid from tool.
12. Lower the tool onto the Q-24 well plate containing sequencing primer (see Note 14). Agitate the tool gently to release the template from the vacuum filter probes.
13. Incubate the Q-24 plate at 80°C for 2 min then incubate at room temperature for 5 min to allow primers to anneal. Clean the vacuum tool by agitating in water with pump off then lowering into clean water with pump on until approximately 45 mL water has been vacuumed though the probes.
14. Place the Q-24 plate into the PyroMark Q24 and start the respective assay run. When the run is complete the memory-stick can be removed.
15. Open the results file on the memory stick within the Q-24 software. The resulting data is presented as a pyrogram which is analyzed using PyroMark Q24 software (see Fig. 4). Methylation is shown as a percentage for each CpG site assayed. Quality control information is given (see Note 11).
16. Clean the cartridge by washing through with ultra-pure water and leave to dry before re-use.

4. Notes

1. Necessity of bisulphite conversion.

   If using pyrosequencing for applications other than DNA methylation detection, such as SNP analysis, it is unnecessary to perform a DNA bisulphite conversion. There are several commercial kits available for bisulphite conversion of DNA. Kits for this are not essential, but they are advisable for consistent, reliable results and are convenient to use for precious/limited DNA samples such as patient DNA. Bisulphite-converted DNA samples can be stored at −20°C short term (<6 months) and −80°C long term.

2. PCR for the Calponin gene to check bisulphite conversion. DNA bisulphite conversion check by PCR for the *Calponin* gene is optional but recommended. Incomplete bisulphite conversion can cause unreliable results and it is cost-effective to ensure conversion is complete before pyrosequencing commences.

3. Selecting a input sequence of suitable length for pyrosequencing primer design.
   For methylation analysis, typically, it is reasonable to select sequence length that is ~350 bp upstream and downstream of a locus of interest such as a transcriptional start site. Choosing a sequence that is too long will increase the likelihood of erroneous pyrosequencing primer design reports due to misprimings. These penalties may be irrelevant when taking into account the severe fragmentation of DNA after bisulphite conversion and corresponding reduced potential for large PCR product amplification.

4. Identifying CpG enrichment within a sequence prior to pyrosequencing primer design.
   A commonly used tool for this is the EMBOSS CpG Plot/CpG report/Isochore tool (http://www.ebi.ac.uk/Tools/emboss/cpgplot/). This tool is useful for identifying CpG island regions and CpG enrichment within a sequence of interest and accepts sequences in GCG, FASTA, EMBL, GenBank, PIR, NBRF or Phylip format. From this information, one can better ascertain which CpG regions within the sequence may be worth investigating using pyrosequencing for DNA methylation investigations e.g. defined CpG islands.

5. An annotated picture of the PyroMark Assay Design 2.0 software interface

6. Increasing the efficiency of PyroMark Assay design software.
   By default, the PyroMark Assay design software will look for up to 100 primer sets for a given target, sequentially working from highest to lowest scored primer sets. In practice, this is a very inefficient set-up for assay design and it will take the software a long time to process this number of primer sets. It is therefore recommended that under Assay settings the "primer set #" is adjusted to five. The rationale for this is that only the top scoring primer sets should be taken forward for use.

7. Selecting an optimal PCR product length and target region for pyrosequencing.
   It is advised to limit PCR products size to 200 bp, but optimally around 100–150 bp. This is because bisulphite conversion of DNA will result in DNA fragmentation and as a result, large PCR products are difficult to produce. Additionally it is advisable to limit the dispensations during pyrosequencing to 45 to maintain pyrosequencing accuracy. Options for overcoming these restraints are designing multiple sets of primers for a region of interest to limit the PCR product size or designing multiple sequencing primers to reduce dispensation number.
8. Designing primer sets in PyroMark Assay design when the software returns no viable options.
   If the software returns no viable primer set options for a target sequence, it is recommended to create a manual sequencing primer or PCR primer. This primer can then be locked in to the assay set and the others can be automatically assigned. It is important to look at the Assay reports for each primer set to identify why individual primers are given a low score and make adjustments accordingly. Ensure to use single base alterations to primer sequences as slight changes can make a substantial difference to primer set scores. Additionally, always look to design primers which have stable T_m across binding site.
9. A technique for enriching for quality primer sets in PyroMark Assay Design.
   Whether presented with well or poorly scored primer sets, one can enrich for better primers by sequentially locking in any two primers (see Note 3) at a given time and clicking "Run Assay Design" to better design the third primer. For example, lock in the forward and reverse primer but let the software design a sequencing primer, then afterwards, lock in the sequencing primer and forward primer and allow the software to design a reverse primer. This method improved each primer at a time based on adjustments made to primers in the preceding cycles. We recommend repeating this technique until the primer set score no longer increases.
10. Knowing when to ignore mispriming warnings in PyroMark Assay Design.
    By default, the software will identify mispriming across the entire sequence inputted in to the software and these will have a detrimental effect on the primer set score. Only mispriming scores >20 in the Assay report should be considered as a moderate misprime. Any mispriming within the amplicon region should be considered detrimental but, in contrast, mispriming upstream or downstream of the target may not be problematic if no strong PCR product would result, regardless of the misprime score. Remember to factor in the likelihood of DNA

fragmentation during bisulphite conversion not allowing large PCR products (see Note 7).

11. Failed runs due to lack of analyzable sample.
    A common reason for poor assay runs are not a strong enough PCR product. Pyrosequencing requires 10–20 μL of PCR product. If after using the maximum volume the run is still failing, repeat the PCR with an increased bisulphite-converted DNA input, adjusting water in the reaction as necessary.
12. General notes about the PyroMark Q24 machine.
    This information is for use with the PyroMark Q24 machine using PyroMark software. Pyrosequencing is not limited to CpG methylation detection and has multiple applications including allele quantification and sequence analysis on the PyroMark Q24 which can be performed during one run. The PyroMark Assay design Software can be utilized for designing primers for all of these applications.
13. Attaching the sample to the filter probes.
    It is sometimes necessary to agitate the vacuum tool gently to allow suction of the sample due to surface tension of the liquid.
14. Applying the vacuum tool to the PyroMark Q-24 plate.
    The vacuum station should switch the tool off automatically but it is advised to ensure that the tool is switched off before lowering into the Q-24 plate containing the sequencing primer.

References

1. Nyren, P. (2007) The history of pyrosequencing, *Methods Mol Biol* 373, 1–14.
2. Tost, J., and Gut, I. G. (2007) DNA methylation analysis by pyrosequencing, *Nat Protoc* 2, 2265–2275.
3. Tost, J., and Gut, I. G. (2007) Analysis of gene-specific DNA methylation patterns by pyrosequencing technology, *Methods Mol Biol* 373, 89–102.
4. Frommer, M., McDonald, L. E., Millar, D. S., Collis, C. M., Watt, F., Grigg, G. W., Molloy, P. L., and Paul, C. L. (1992) A genomic sequencing protocol that yields a positive display of 5-methylcytosine residues in individual DNA strands, *Proc Natl Acad Sci USA* 89, 1827–1831.
5. Clark, S. J., Statham, A., Stirzaker, C., Molloy, P. L., and Frommer, M. (2006) DNA methylation: bisulphite modification and analysis, *Nat Protoc* 1, 2353–2364.
6. Gusev, N. B. (2001) Some properties of caldesmon and calponin and the participation of these proteins in regulation of smooth muscle contraction and cytoskeleton formation, *Biochemistry (Mosc)* 66, 1112–1121.
7. Hsiung, D. T., Marsit, C. J., Houseman, E. A., Eddy, K., Furniss, C. S., McClean, M. D., and Kelsey, K. T. (2007) Global DNA methylation level in whole blood as a biomarker in head and neck squamous cell carcinoma, *Cancer Epidemiol Biomarkers Prev* 16, 108–114.
8. Sriraksa, R., Chaopatchayakul, P., Jearanaikoon, P., Leelayuwat, C., and Limpaiboon, T. Verification of complete bisulfite modification using Calponin-specific primer sets, *Clin Biochem* 43, 528–530.

Chapter 18

Screening for miRNA Expression Changes Using Quantitative PCR (Q-PCR)

Richard N. Armstrong, Hilary A.A. Colyer, and Ken I. Mills

Abstract

In this section, we describe the use of Applied Biosystems TaqMan Array microRNA Card Set 3.0 to identify miRNA expression in a given RNA sample. This array set includes an array "A" and an array "B" which each have 384 wells that contain specific forward, reverse, and probe oligoinucleotides for measuring the expression of individual miRNAs during a Real-Time PCR (Q-PCR) reaction. Array "A" includes assays for profiling the comparatively higher expressed and better characterized miRNAs. Presently there are 1,048 mature miRNAs annotated in miRBase (release 16). The relatively small amount of miRNAs in comparison to protein-coding genes makes this format a viable option for measuring genome-wide miRNA expression changes. The Applied Biosystems TaqMan miRNA array set 3.0, which includes two separate arrays, can profile 754 miRNAs.

Key words: miRNAs, Applied biosystems, TaqMan, Array, Epigenetics, Real-time PCR, qPCR

1. Introduction

MicroRNAs (miRNAs) are small RNA molecules approximately ~21 nucleotides in length that can act as the transcriptional regulators of targeted messenger RNAs (mRNA). MiRNAs perform this regulation by blocking mRNA translation or cleaving mRNA transcripts (for partial and high miRNA-mRNA complementarity, respectfully). MiRNAs are important regulators of proliferation, apoptosis, differentiation, and invasion (1–4) and computational approaches suggest that miRNAs may negatively regulate one third of the genome (5). It is therefore no surprise that miRNAs have been implicated in many diseases and have become a focus of increasing interest from the research community in recent years. In 2003, Calin et al. showed that ~50% of miRNAs known at that time were located in cancer-associated genomic regions or fragile sites, suggesting their dysfunctional role in cancer phenotypes.

Ramona G. Dumitrescu and Mukesh Verma (eds.), *Cancer Epigenetics: Methods and Protocols*, Methods in Molecular Biology, vol. 863, DOI 10.1007/978-1-61779-612-8_18, © Springer Science+Business Media, LLC 2012

Subsequent studies have shown that miRNA expression profiles can classify disease subtypes (6) and in the case of oncology, help identify potential tumour suppressor and oncogenic miRNAs.

Alike to traditional protein-coding genes, some miRNAs have been shown to be epigenetically regulated via DNA methylation and associated histone modifications (7–9). Increasingly, DNA methylation of miRNA promoters is emerging as a common hallmark of cancer.

There are several options when considering an miRNA profiling platform, including hybridization, qPCR, and next–generation sequencing methods. When selecting a platform, it is important that it offers the best accuracy and reproducibility within budget constraints. In the future, next-generation is expected to be gold standard for profiling miRNA due to its quantitative ability, namely measuring direct copy number. However, at present it is a relatively undeveloped technique that is considerably more expensive than the other methods available.

An advantage of using miRNA qPCR arrays is that most molecular labs have experience with the technology, methodology, and data output. Additionally, the majority of labs will use qPCR as a means of validating microarray, thus in principle, it is more specific profiling method than microarray technology.

This chapter describes the methodology for using the TaqMan microRNA arrays for expression profiling. Unlike other PCR methods that employ the double-stranded DNA binding cyanine dye SYBR Green chemistry, the TaqMan array-based approach uses a reporter-quencher probe to measure miRNA expression. This method reduces the likelihood of false fluorescence signal during qPCR that arises from mispriming.

Although using the TaqMan array-based approach can involve the use of specific reverse-transcription (RT) primers, such specific primers are not always required, particularly when validating multiple miRNAs of interest. For the purpose of validating multiple miRNAs from a single RT, one may use a universal miRNA RT approach, such as the RT^2 miRNA qPCR method offered by SABiosciences, Qiagen. The RT step for this technique includes a polyadenylation of all mature miRNAs and subsequent cDNA generation from a universal poly-adenosine binding primer. This method also has the benefit of creating cDNA from miRNAs which have not been identified to date.

The TaqMan Array MicroRNA profiling method is a two-step approach to relative quantification of miRNA expression. First, a pool of stem loop primers are used in a multiplex reverse transcription PCR to yield miRNA specific complementary DNA (cDNA) from a total RNA sample (Fig. 1). Second, a cDNA real-time PCR mix is loaded into the array and subjected to a real-time PCR (qPCR) reaction. Each well within the array contains a specific forward primer, reverse primer, and a TaqMan probe for

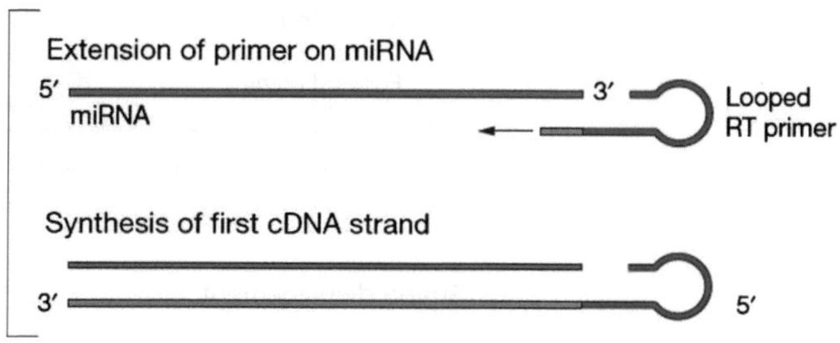

Fig. 1. The stem-loop is used to increase the T_m of the miRNA specific primer. During the PCR elongation step, cDNA templates are created from each miRNA copy. (Image courtesy of Applied Biosystems™).

an miRNA or endogenous small nucleolar RNA (snoRNA). When the cDNA mix is loaded, the primers and probe are hydrated to create 1 μL reaction volume. The real-time reaction is described in the Fig. 2.

During the qPCR reaction, the fluorescence emitted during DNA amplification is plotted against the PCR cycle number and presented as an XY plot. A threshold value is used to identify the exponential phase of the reaction and determine the cycle at which a gene is expressed. The cycle number at which this fluorescence threshold is met is referred to as the cycle threshold (C_T).

Figure 3 is an example of an amplification plot for two samples which show differential expression of a gene of interest (goi). The TaqMan miRNA arrays are used to find the miRNA expression fold difference between samples using the comparative C_T ($2^{-\Delta\Delta CT}$) method (where $\Delta\Delta C_T = \Delta C_{T\ \mathrm{sample}} - \Delta C_{T\ \mathrm{calibrator}}$ and ΔC_T is defined as a goi normalized to an endogenous control).

2. Materials

2.1. Megaplex™ Pool Reverse Transcription of RNA Samples

- Total RNA sample (250–1,000 ng within a 3-μL volume).
- Applied Biosystems reverse transcription kit.
- Megaplex™ RT primers (specific to array A or array B).

2.2. Preparing and Loading the TaqMan MicroRNA Array Card via Centrifugation

- TaqMan Universal Master Mix, No AmpErase, UNG, 2×.
- Custom Sorvall/Heraeus bucket and array holder.
- Sorvall/Heraeus EasySET™ or QuickSet centrifuge.

2.3. Sealing the TaqMan Array MicroRNA Card

- The Applied Biosystems array card sealer.

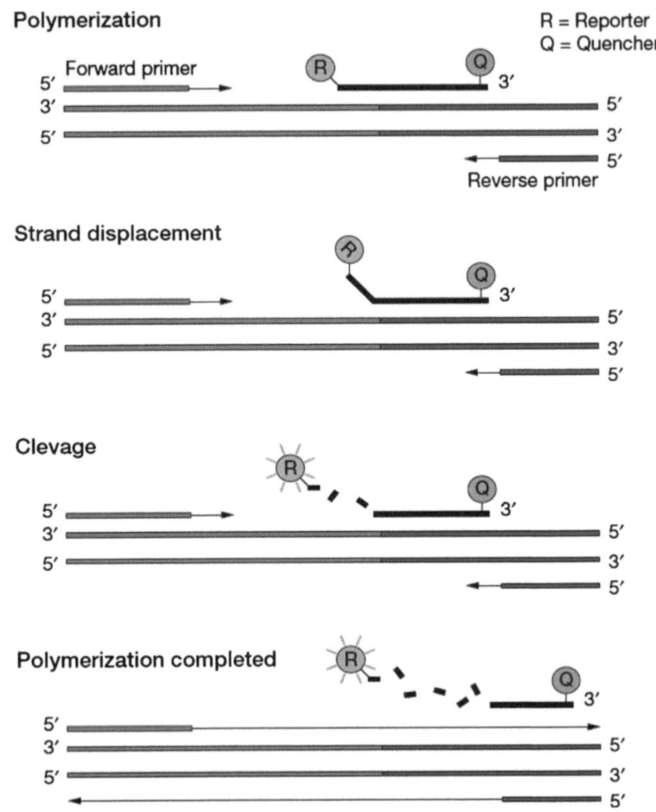

Fig. 2. *Polymerization*: during cooling from 95 to 60°C, the Taqman probe is first used to anneal with a sequence within the DNA oligonucleotide. The forward and reverse primers subsequently bind to the DNA. *Strand displacement*: during PCR primer elongation, the reporter end of the probe is displaced from the cDNA *Cleavage*: the AmpliTaq gold enzyme cleaves the reporter molecule from the probe via its 5′ nuclease activity. *Polymerization completed*: the probe is released from the DNA strand. With the reporter and quencher molecule separated, a fluorescence signal is emitted from the reporter. (Image courtesy of Applied Biosystems™).

2.4. Running the TaqMan Array MicroRNA Card on the ABI PRISM 7900HT Instrument

- The ABI PRISM 7900HT sequence detection system.
- Applied Biosystems SDS Enterprise software package.

3. Method (10, 11)

The method in this section profiles 350–1,000 ng total RNA within a 3 μL eluted volume (see Note 1). For lesser RNA quantities (1–350 ng/μL), Applied Biosystems miRNA reverse transcription kit provides a cDNA preamplification step not covered in this section.

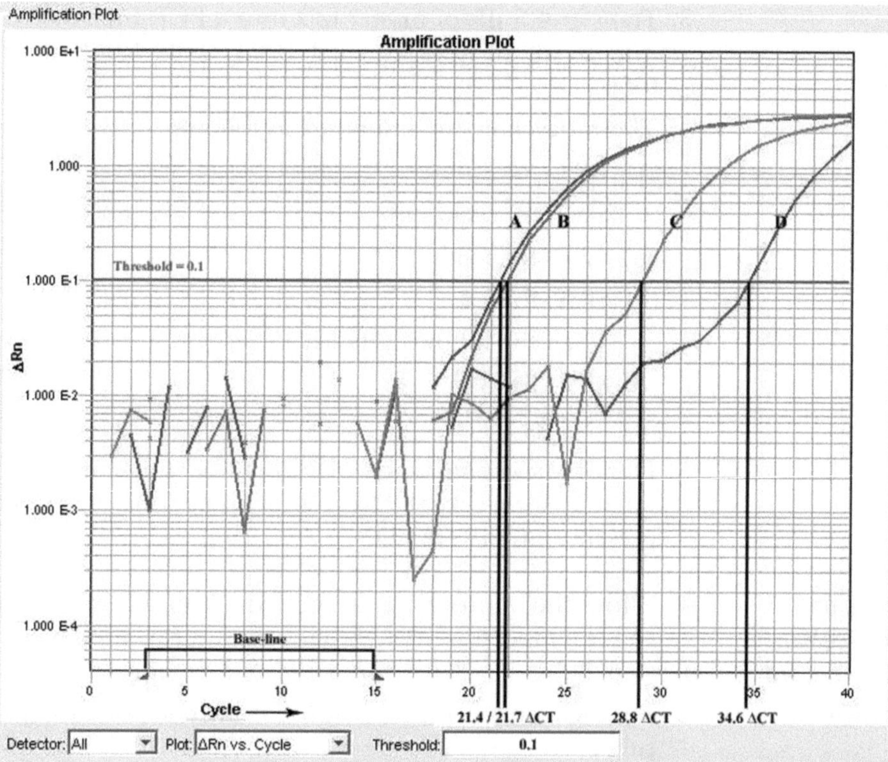

Fig. 3. An amplification plot of an endogenous gene and gene of interest (goi) from two different samples. For each gene, the threshold value must be set to cross the exponential phase of the sigmoidal curve to obtain accurate cycle threshold (C_T) values. The base-line must be set to nullify the early PCR background signal without affecting the signal created during the amplification. Sample 1 and 2 share a similar C_T for their endogenous control (labelled *A* and *B* respectfully). However, the goi from sample 1 (labelled *C*) has reached its C_T considerably earlier than in sample 2 (labelled *D*). The comparative C_T method will identify the relative goi fold difference between these samples ($2^{-\Delta\Delta CT}$).

3.1. Megaplex™ Pool Reverse Transcription of RNA Samples

1. Thaw on ice the components from the Applied Biosystems® miRNA reverse transcription kit and the Megaplex™ RT primers specific to array card A and/or B. Mix by inverting and spin briefly.
2. The following components are combined at the given volumes for each Megaplex™ pool RT reaction. For multiple samples we advise preparing a Megaplex™ RT master mix in a 1.5-mL tube. Additionally, adding 10% extra volume of each component will allow for loss of volume during pipetting.
   (a) 0.8 μL of RT buffer (10×).
   (b) 0.2 μL dNTPs with dTTP (100 mM).
   (c) 0.9 μL $MgCl_2$ (25 mM).
   (d) 0.1 μL RNase Inhibitor (20 U/μL).
   (e) 0.8 μL of array specific Megaplex™ pool RT primers (10×).
   (f) 1.5 μL MultiScribe™ Reverse Transcriptase (50 U/μL).
   (g) 0.2 μL Nuclease-free water.

3. Transfer 4.5 μL of master mix into a PCR tube or PCR plate. Add 3 μL of sample Total RNA (350–1,000 ng RNA in total).
4. Thermocycling conditions are as follows:
   (a) 16°C for 2 min.
   Then 40 cycles of
   (b) 42°C for 1 min.
   (c) 50°C for 1 s.
   Then the following holds
   (d) 85°C for 5 min.
   (e) 4°C for ∞.
5. Optional stopping point. cDNA can be stored at −15 to −25°C for at least a week. See Note 2 for an optional step to verify the presence of miRNA cDNA.

3.2. Preparing and Loading the TaqMan™ MicroRNA Array Card via Centrifugation

1. Allow the appropriate array card (A or B) to equilibrate at room temperature for 15 min (during this time proceed with step 2).
2. For each sample, prepare the following components in a 1.5-mL tube:
   (a) 450 μL TaqMan Universal Master Mix, No AmpErase, UNG, 2×.
   (b) 6 μL Megaplex™ RT cDNA product.
   (c) 444 μL Nuclease-free water.
3. Mix the tube by inverting several times, then centrifuging briefly. Do not vortex this solution (see Note 3).
4. Pipette 100 μL of the mix into each of the eight wells on the card. Ensure to pipette in the bigger "fill port" in each well (Fig. 4). Stop dispensing the volume at the first "pipette stop" to prevent injection of air in to the well.

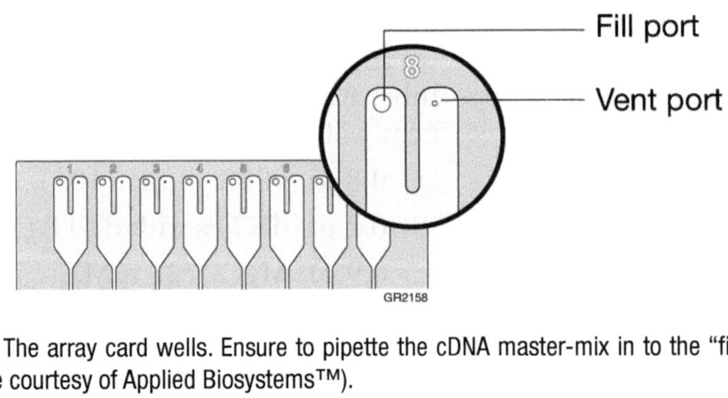

Fig. 4. The array card wells. Ensure to pipette the cDNA master-mix in to the "fill port". (Image courtesy of Applied Biosystems™).

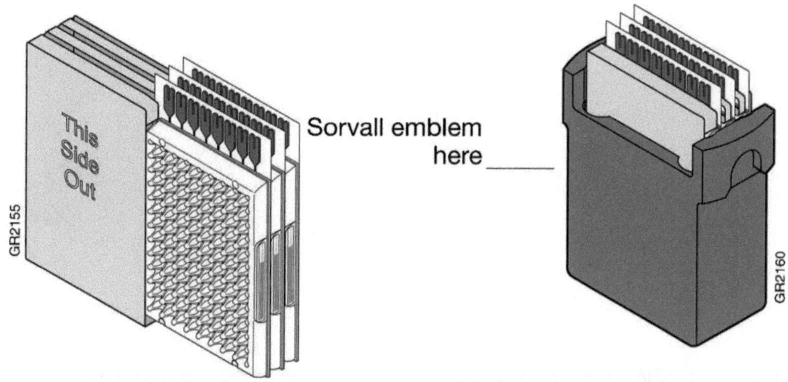

Fig. 5. The custom Sorvall/Heraeus bucket and array holder combo. Each combo can hold three arrays. Ensure the arrays are inserted in to the holder as shown above and that when loading the bucket in to the centrifuge, the array wells face outwards. (Image courtesy of Applied Biosystems™).

5. Place the custom Sorvall/Heraeus bucket containing an array holder on the bench. Insert up to three arrays per array holder/bucket combo ensuring that the reservoir wells protrude out from the top of the holder and that the reaction wells face the same direction as the "This side out label" (Fig. 5).
6. Place the bucket containing array in to a Sorvall/Heraeus centrifuge ensuring that the array wells face outwards.
7. Set the bucket type to 15679 on the centrifuge. For an EasySet touchpad centrifuge (For QuikSet knob-operated centrifuges see Note 4) set the following parameters:
   (a) Up Ramp rate = 9.
   (b) Down Ramp rate = 9.
   (c) Speed = 1,200 rpm (331 × *g*).
   (d) Duration = 1 min.
8. Repeat step 7 again after the centrifuge has stopped (see Note 5).
9. Remove the array from the bucket combo and inspect the array to ensure that the wells have drained (see Note 6).

3.3. Sealing the TaqMan Array MicroRNA Card

1. Ensure the sealer is on a sturdy surface with the start position closest to you and the end facing away. Move the carriage to the start position.
2. Insert the array into the sealer so that the wells are facing down. Ensure that the array is secured by the four spring clips.
3. Slowly and continually push the carriage upwards to seal the plate (Fig. 6).
4. With the carriage in the end position, remove the sealed array. Do not return the carriage to the start position until the array has been removed.

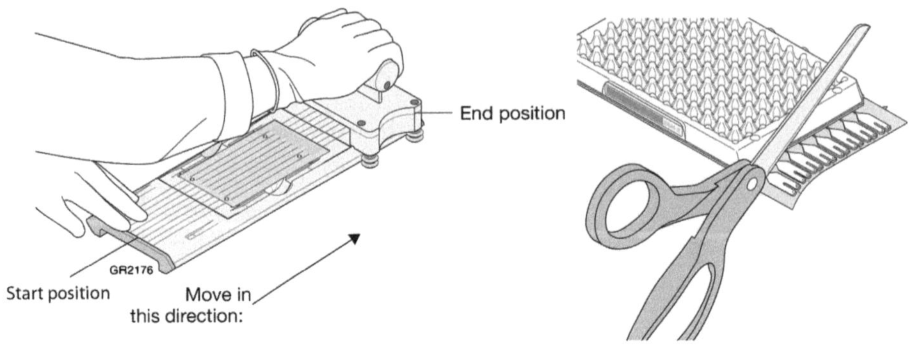

Fig. 6. The miRNA array is sealed by pushing the carriage across the restrained array from the start position towards the end position. After sealing, the array is the trimmed to remove the 8-well strip. (Image courtesy of Applied Biosystems™).

5. Inspect the sealing indentation, ensuring they match up with each well channel. Discard array if indentation not as intended.
6. Use scissors to remove the strip of wells.

3.4. Running the TaqMan Array MicroRNA Card on the ABI PRISM® 7900HT Instrument

1. This part of the protocol assumes a TaqMan array block and plate adapter is installed in the 7900HT. If this is not the case, ensure these are changed accordingly.
2. Open up the SDS software and select File > New.
3. Select the following options: assay type >$\Delta\Delta C_T$ (RQ) A.K.A. Relative Quantification, Container >384 TaqMan Low Density Array. One can optionally scan the array barcode at this stage.
4. Place the appropriate miRNA cd that came with each array type into the computer. Click File > Import. Now navigate to the cd and load the sds setup text file, e.g. "4400797_SDS_miRNA_Human_A.txt". This will label the appropriate wells with a corresponding miRNA ID/snoRNA ID.
5. Highlight the plate and enter a sample name in the designated box.
6. Save the run as a run document (.sds file).
7. Select the instrument tab and then the Real-Time tab. Click connect to instrument if necessary.
8. Select open to eject the plate holder.
9. Place the array on the holder so that well A1 is closest to the "A1" mark on the plate adapter.
10. Begin the qPCR reaction by clicking Run.
11. After the run, results are analysed by importing the finished run files in to the RQ manager software. This allows the user to import up to ten arrays into single study. Threshold and base-line settings must be selected for each gene and maintained across a study. The ΔC_T or C_T values for each gene can be exported from this program using the File > Export.

4. Notes

1. Suitability of RNA extraction methods for miRNA profiling.
This protocol assumes previous extraction of high-quality total RNA from samples. It is important that total RNA extraction methods are used such as phenol-chloroform based protocols. Many column-based extraction methods will remove small (<200 base long) oligonucleotides such as miRNAs and snoRNAs from samples.
2. Optional step to ensure the Megaplex™ RT has worked.
To ensure that the RT reaction has worked before using an array, we suggest assaying the expression of an endogenous gene profiled by the array using a TaqMan miRNA single assay. For this we alter the default single assay protocol to create the following qPCR reaction volume:
   (a) 10 μL Universal PCR Master mix, no AmpErase, UNG, 2×.
   (b) 9 μL Nuclease-free water.
   (c) 1 μL MegaPlex™ cDNA.
3. Do not vortex TaqMan master mix prior to loading the miRNA array.
Vortexing the Real-Time master mix will result in bubbles. This may prevent correct loading of the array during centrifugation.
4. Centrifuge settings for a QuickSet™knob-operated centrifuge.
If centrifuging the arrays with a QuickSet™ knob-operated centrifuge use the following parameters:
   (a) Up Ramp rate = 3.
   (b) Speed = 331 ×*g*.
   (c) Duration = 2 × 1 min.
5. Loading the miRNA arrays via centrifugation.
It is essential that the arrays are centrifuged for 2 × 1 min and *not* 2 min continuous. This allows the real-time master mix to settle during centrifugation, preventing the solution from pushing out of the wells.
6. A suggestion for arrays that fail to load correctly.
After centrifugation of the array(s), all wells with harbour residual master-mix. The outside wells will have master-mix along the outer walls sometimes making it appear as if there is greater volume left in these wells. If one or more wells have a moderate volume of master-mix, it is acceptable to repeat a 1 min spin as described in step 7. If this volume persists, a new array should be used.

References

1. Johnson, C. D., Esquela-Kerscher, A., Stefani, G., Byrom, M., Kelnar, K., Ovcharenko, D., Wilson, M., Wang, X., Shelton, J., Shingara, J., Chin, L., Brown, D., and Slack, F. J. (2007) The let-7 microRNA represses cell proliferation pathways in human cells, *Cancer Res* 67, 7713–7722.
2. Cimmino, A., Calin, G. A., Fabbri, M., Iorio, M. V., Ferracin, M., Shimizu, M., Wojcik, S. E., Aqeilan, R. I., Zupo, S., Dono, M., Rassenti, L., Alder, H., Volinia, S., Liu, C. G., Kipps, T. J., Negrini, M., and Croce, C. M. (2005) miR-15 and miR-16 induce apoptosis by targeting BCL2, *Proc Natl Acad Sci USA* 102, 13944–13949.
3. Esau, C., Kang, X., Peralta, E., Hanson, E., Marcusson, E. G., Ravichandran, L. V., Sun, Y., Koo, S., Perera, R. J., Jain, R., Dean, N. M., Freier, S. M., Bennett, C. F., Lollo, B., and Griffey, R. (2004) MicroRNA-143 regulates adipocyte differentiation, *J Biol Chem* 279, 52361–52365.
4. Ma, L., Teruya-Feldstein, J., and Weinberg, R. A. (2007) Tumour invasion and metastasis initiated by microRNA-10b in breast cancer, *Nature 449*, 682–688.
5. Griffiths-Jones, S., Saini, H. K., van Dongen, S., and Enright, A. J. (2008) miRBase: tools for microRNA genomics, *Nucleic Acids Res* 36, D154–158.
6. Calin, G. A. and Croce, C. M. (2006) MicroRNA signatures in human cancers, *Nat Rev Cancer* 6, 857–866.
7. Suzuki, H., Yamamoto, E., Nojima, M., Kai, M., Yamano, H. O., Yoshikawa, K., Kimura, T., Kudo, T., Harada, E., Sugai, T., Takamaru, H., Niinuma, T., Maruyama, R., Yamamoto, H., Tokino, T., Imai, K., Toyota, M., and Shinomura, Y. Methylation-associated silencing of microRNA-34b/c in gastric cancer and its involvement in an epigenetic field defect, *Carcinogenesis* 31, 2066–2073.
8. Lujambio, A., Calin, G. A., Villanueva, A., Ropero, S., Sanchez-Cespedes, M., Blanco, D., Montuenga, L. M., Rossi, S., Nicoloso, M. S., Faller, W. J., Gallagher, W. M., Eccles, S. A., Croce, C. M., and Esteller, M. (2008) A microRNA DNA methylation signature for human cancer metastasis, *Proc Natl Acad Sci USA* 105, 13556–13561.
9. Saito, Y., Suzuki, H., Tsugawa, H., Nakagawa, I., Matsuzaki, J., Kanai, Y., and Hibi, T. (2009) Chromatin remodeling at Alu repeats by epigenetic treatment activates silenced microRNA-512-5p with downregulation of Mcl-1 in human gastric cancer cells, *Oncogene* 28, 2738–2744.
10. Biosystems, A. Megaplex™ Pools For microRNA Expression Analysis Protocol (P/N: 4399721).
11. Biosystems, A. User Bulletin: Applied Biosystems Taqman Low Density Array.

Chapter 19

Genome-Wide Methylation Analysis

Alexander Unterberger, Adrian M. Dubuc, and Michael D. Taylor

Abstract

The disruption and alteration of genomic methylation patterns is a hallmark of cancer and other disease states. Understanding and characterizing genome-wide methylation will have a profound effect on our understanding of tumorigenesis and provide novel avenues for therapy. This chapter serves to describe techniques that examine genome-wide methylation patterns including luminometric methylation assay, restriction landmark genome scanning, and the cytosine extension assay, which utilize methylation-sensitive restriction enzymes. Additional techniques such as nucleotide separation assays (nearest neighbor analysis and high-performance capillary electrophoresis) and the infinium methylation assay are discussed. These techniques allow for the determination of changes in global methylation levels, as well as regional changes in methylation throughout the genome.

Key words: Global methylation levels, CG methylation, Luminometric methylation assay, Restriction landmark genome scanning, Cytosine extension assay, CpGlobal, Nearest neighbor analysis, Capillary electrophoresis, Infinium methylation assay

1. Introduction

While numerous techniques examine gene-specific DNA methylation, these methods are limited by their inability to assay total genomic DNA methylation. Consequentially, considerable information is lost, limiting our ability to fully understand consequences of epigenetic changes. Fortunately, novel techniques designed to analyze genome-wide DNA methylation have been developed. These methods include the use of methylation-sensitive restriction enzymes, regional sequencing of sodium bisulfite-converted DNA, as well as nucleotide separation and microarray analysis.

A commonly accepted hallmark of human cancer is the genome-wide hypomethylation with regional promoter hypermethylation (1–3). Examination of genomic DNA methylation changes has

Ramona G. Dumitrescu and Mukesh Verma (eds.), *Cancer Epigenetics: Methods and Protocols*, Methods in Molecular Biology, vol. 863, DOI 10.1007/978-1-61779-612-8_19, © Springer Science+Business Media, LLC 2012

allowed researchers to identify distinct cancer subtypes (4–7), permitting targeted therapy. Despite cytosine methylation having been discovered in the 1940s (8), its role in cancer was not explored in-depth until the advent of restriction enzyme-based methods of analysis in the 1970s (9). Since this point, genome-wide techniques of examining DNA methylation have been developed to start examining the role of epigenetics in cancer.

In this chapter, three different approaches for genome-wide methylation analysis have been discussed. The first examines the differences in DNA methylation profiles from restriction enzyme isoschizomers that are sensitive to DNA methylation. The techniques discussed are luminometric methylation assay (LUMA), restriction landmark genome scanning (RLGS), and the cytosine extension assay. The second approach visualizes separated methylated and unmethylated cytosines from genomic extracts. The techniques discussed are nearest neighbor analysis (NNA) and high-performance capillary electrophoresis (HPCE). The final approach discussed is a genome-wide genotyping of CG dinucleotides of sodium bisulfite-converted DNA. The technique discussed in this chapter is the infinium methylation assay (IMA).

1.1. Methylation-Sensitive Restriction Enzyme-Based Methods

1.1.1. Luminometric Methylation Assay

LUMA is a pyrosequencing-based method for detecting and quantifying DNA methylation. It uses the methylation-sensitive and -insensitive isoschizomer restriction enzymes *HpaII/MspI* and a luminometric polymerase reaction to quantify the levels of genomic methylation (10).

LUMA requires minimal amounts of DNA to fully assess the genomic methylation profile. 250–500 ng of genomic DNA is digested with the CG methylation-sensitive restriction enzyme *HpaII* and *EcoRI* or with the CG methylation-insensitive restriction enzyme *MspI* and *EcoRI*. *EcoRI* is included in each digestion to serve as a normalizing reference. *HpaII/MspI* leaves a 5′CG overhang, while *EcoRI* leaves a 5′ AATT overhang, which can be differentiated during the pyrosequencing reaction. Once the digestion is completed, the DNA overhangs are then filled in through a multistep polymerase extension using the pyrosequencing assay. dNTPs are incorporated into the overhangs in a stepwise process and a luminescent reaction is produced for each nucleotide. In the first step, dATP is incorporated into the *EcoRI* cut site, which serves as the normalization control. The second step incorporates both dCTP and dGTP into the HpaII/MspI overhang. This step serves as the signal for degree of methylation. The third step incorporates dTTP into the remaining overhand of the *EcoRI* cut site. The C+G (step 2) signal for each isoschizomer restriction enzyme is normalized to the A (step 1) signal. The normalized methylation digest (*HpaII*) is compared to the normalized non-methylation digest (*MspI*) and provides a quantification of the degree of methylation at all the *HpaII/MspI* cut sites of the genome. This assay can be adapted for other methylation-sensitive restriction enzymes that recognize other CG-containing consensus sequences.

Due to the rapid nature of analysis, LUMA has been used in clinical and nonclinical investigations. These include a study that examined the differences in genomic methylation in different human blood cell types (11). One study used LUMA to determine genome-wide methylation levels in human patients with acute myeloid leukemia and observed a positive correlation between increased genome-wide promoter-associated methylation and improved patient survival (12). This technique is advantageous for large-scale epidemiological studies due to the rapid nature of analysis, and high-throughput capabilities of the assay, which can be completed in less than 6 hour permitting hundreds of samples to be processed in a single day. Other benefits include the small amounts of genomic DNA requires, as well as being nonradioactive. Drawbacks include the access to a pyrosequencing machine, as well as being limited to profiling genomic methylation levels at *HpaII/MspI* cut sites.

1.1.2. Restriction Landmark Genome Scanning

RLGS is a sequence-independent method of evaluating CG methylation across the genome (13). Digestion of genomic DNA with a methylation-sensitive restriction enzyme and radiolabeling of cleaving sites is followed by a two-dimensional electrophoresis system designed to visualize and quantify the changes in methylation of two different samples.

Genomic DNA is digested with a methylation-sensitive restriction enzyme that has a CG in their recognition sequence. Popular restriction enzymes include *NotI* (GC\GGCCGC), *AscI* (GG\CGCGCC), *BssHII* (G\CGCGC), and *EagI* (C\GGCCG). The DNA is then radiolabeled at the cleavage sites. Due to the infrequent nature of these sequences, the sample is then digested with a second restriction enzyme, commonly *EcoRV*. The digested labeled DNA is separated through a tube-shaped non-denaturing polyacrylamide gel and digested with a third restriction enzyme to increase the number of fragments, typically *HinfI*. The gel is then unrolled and undergoes electrophoresis in a direction perpendicular to the first separation prior to drying and autoradiography, which generates a profile of genomic sites (RLGS fragments) on a two-dimensional space. When compared to control sample (normal tissue), differences of signal intensity for each fragment indicate changes in DNA methylation.

The identity of each fragment can be determined in a number of ways. Originally, a duplicate gel was run in parallel using digested DNA that was not radiolabeled. The RLGS fragments would then be excised from identical sites on the parallel gel, cloned, and sequenced. However, the identities of a large number (>800) of RLGS fragments from a *NotI-EcoRV-HinfI* digestion have been determined (14–16). This allows the identification of RLGS fragments from an experimental gel based on similar localization on a virtual RLGS (vRLGS). RLGS fragments that exhibit changes in DNA methylation that are not featured in a vRLGS can be excised and sequenced as previously mentioned or they can be predicted through *in silico* prediction of the RLGS fragments in two-dimensional model. To increase the resolution of this method, samples can be analyzed with different combinations of methylation-sensitive restriction enzymes, which increase the number of CG sites this technique can visualize and quantify.

Advantages of this technique include the resolution and ability to quantify and identify the sequence/location DNA methylation changes. Another advantage is that RLGS is PCR-independent, unlike promoter methylation arrays, and therefore does not introduce any amplifications biases. Disadvantages to this technique include radiolabeling and the restriction enzyme digests, limiting the resolution of RLGS to genomic regions containing restriction sites. Preparation of the samples also requires technical expertise as integrity of genomic DNA may affect the profile of RLGS fragments. A comprehensive protocol is detailed in a recent review (17).

1.1.3. Cytosine Extension Assay

The isotopic/nonisotopic cytosine extension assay (ICEA/NICEA) is a methylation-sensitive restriction enzyme-based system for examination of changes in global methylation levels. Differences in genomic cytosine methylation levels can be inferred by the number of methylation-sensitive restriction enzyme cut sites, detected through either radionucleotide incorporation (ICEA) (18, 19) or biotinylated-nucleotide incorporation (NICEA) (20).

The amount of genomic DNA used in this system varies between the ICEA and NICEA methods. ICEA requires 1 μg of genomic DNA while NICEA is much more sensitive and can be scaled down to as little as 100 ng. Genomic DNA is digested with a methylation-sensitive restriction enzyme (such as the commonly used *HpaII*), and cleaved (unmethylated) sites are then labeled through polymerase-dependent incorporation of labeled nucleotides, with either a [^{3}H] dCTP nucleotide (ICEA) or a biotin-14-dCTP (NICEA) (Fig. 1) as the donor. Quantitative detection of the number of cleaved sites is directly proportional to the number of unmethylated sites, as unmethylated sites are end-labeled. Methylated CGs remain uncut and unlabeled. A parallel reaction using *MspI*, the methylation-insensitive isoschizomer of *HpaII*, serves as a measurement for the total number of possible cut sites. With ICEA, the digested and radiolabeled DNA is then filtered and measured. With NICEA, the digested and biotinylated DNA is immobilized on a membrane and visualized with a streptavidin-alkaline phosphatase reaction.

A variation of the cytosine extension assay is the CpGlobal technique (21). Using genomic DNA aliquoted in a 96-well plate, this technique follows the same principle of digesting the DNA with *HpaII* or *MspI* and determining the degree of methylation through

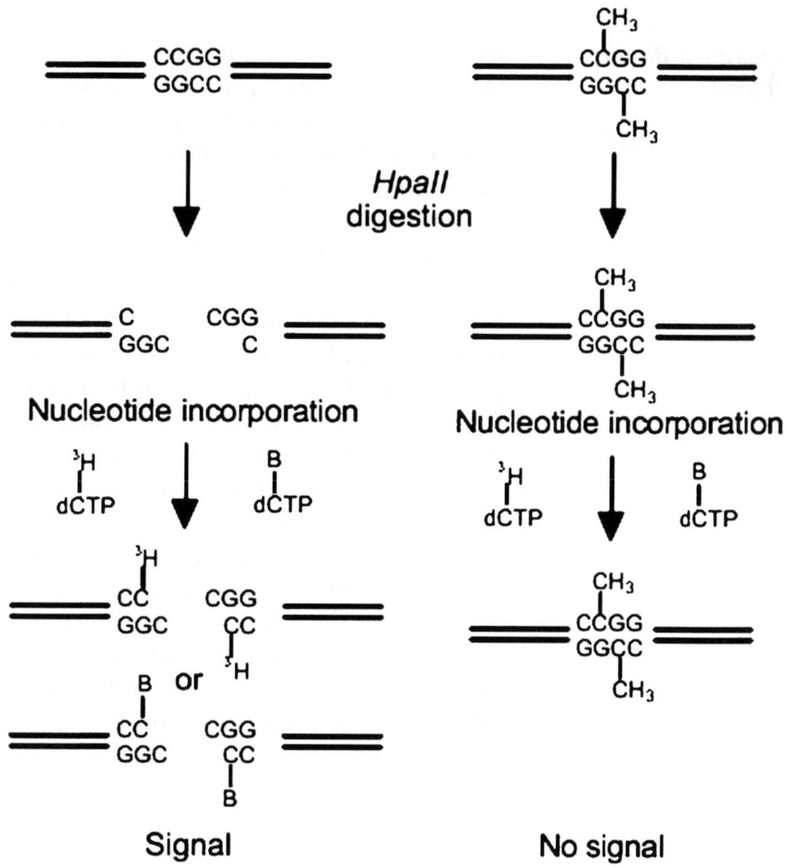

Fig. 1. Cytosine extension assay. Genomic DNA is digested with *HpaII* restriction enzyme. Recognition sites that are unmethylated are cleaved, while methylated recognition sites remain intact. [^{3}H] dCTP (ICEA) or biotinylated dCTP (NICEA) are incorporated into cleavage sites and measured. Signal strength is directly proportional to unmethylated CGs at *HpaII* cleavage sites. The degree of methylation can be inferred using this technique.

incorporation of biotinylated dCTP and dGTP oligonucleotides into the cleavage sites. Similarly to ICEA/NICEA, the degree of incorporated biotinylated nucleotides is directly proportional to the number of cleaved sites. The labeled cleavage sites are measured through the chemiluminescent HRP-Neutravidin detection of biotin. The degree of methylation for these techniques is calculated through the difference of the *HpaII* (unmethylated cytosine) and *MspI* (total cytosine) signals over the total signal ((*HpaII*-*MspI*)/*MspI*).

The cytosine extension assay is a rapid method for detection of global methylation changes using only a small amount of genomic DNA; however, it does have disadvantages. Being based on restriction enzymes, this assay biases itself for CGs located only in the target sequences of the restriction enzymes and does not examine all CGs in the genome. NICEA, in particular, requires the use of tritiated dCTP, with the appropriate facilities for correct handling.

1.2. Nucleotide Separation-Based Methods

1.2.1. Nearest Neighbor Analysis

NNA was originally developed as a method to determine the sequence identity of dinucleotide pairs in the genome (22, 23). As DNA methylation is primarily restricted to cytosine residues in the context of CG dinucleotides, this method was later adapted to quantify the amount of methylated and unmethylated cytosines in the genome (24, 25).

Briefly, DNA is digested with MboI (GATC), and all 3′ neighbors of the guanosine are labeled with [α-32P] dGTP. The labeled DNA is then separated from unincorporated [α-32P] dGTP through a size-exclusion column of Sephadex G50 beads. After purification, DNA is further digested using an exonuclease, spleen phosphodiesterase, and an endonuclease—micrococcal nuclease. The radiolabeled neighboring nucleotide will now appear as a mononucleotide residue with the incorporated [α-32P] serving as its 3′ phosphate group. The labeled mononucleotides are then separated by two-dimensional thin-layer chromatography (TLC), which allows for separation and quantification of adenosine, guanosine, thymidine, cytosine, and 5-methyl cytosine residues neighboring the MboI cut site, which are visualized through autoradiography (Fig. 2). This method is a modification of an earlier nick-labeling technique that utilizes random DNA nicking from DNaseI instead of a restriction enzyme (24). MboI was utilized to enrich for CG sites. Alternative restriction enzymes can be used for

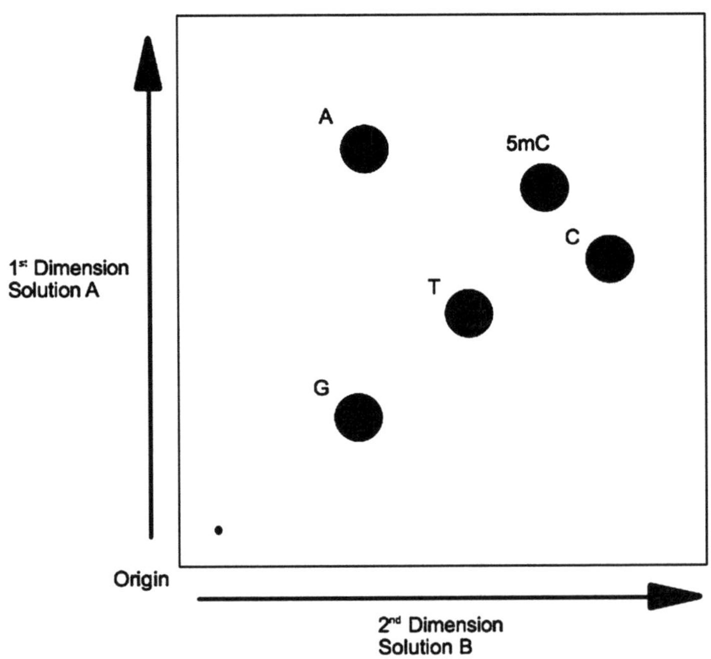

Fig. 2. Nearest neighbor nucleotide distribution. Expected positions of labeled mononucleotides after two-dimensional thin-layer chromatography.

CG enrichment. These include enzymes that cut 5′ of guanosine and have cytosine as a potential neighbor (Tsp45I), methylation-insensitive enzymes that digest at CG dinucleotide sites, which liberate the cytosine as the 3′ neighbor.

This technique is advantageous as it allows for the identification and quantification of all possible methylation modifications in the genome, as well as being cost-effective. The main drawback is that it is a radioactive technique and requires the appropriate facilities for handling radioactivity, as well as being selective for methylation levels at MboI cut sites.

1.2.2. High-Performance Capillary Electrophoresis

HPCE quantification of global DNA methylation is a technique that examines every methylated and unmethylated residue in the genome and quantifies their absolute level of methylation (26–28). As cytosine and 5-methyl cytosine have different separation constants, these nucleotides can be separated and quantified by UV/VIS spectrophotometry.

Genomic DNA is digested with Nuclease P1 and dephosphorylated with alkaline phosphatase, producing 2′-deoxymononucleosides. The nucleotides are then resolved through separation in an uncoated fused-silica capillary. An electric current is passed through a capillary tube at a length of 57 cm and the mononucleotides separate based on their respective migration rates. At the end of the capillary tube, a UV/VIS spectrophotometer measures the presence of each separated nucleotide as they pass through a detection window. Using this technique each nucleotide in the genome as well as any known modification can be effectively quantified.

HPCE has been widely used as an effective method for examining levels of methylated and unmethylated cytosine in clinical and experimental studies. HPCE was initially used to quantify differences in DNA methylation between species (28) and the effect of anti-cancer therapeutic treatments on the epigenome of different cancers was determined using this technique (29, 30). The primary advantage of this technique is that it examines global DNA methylation in an unbiased approach, independent of restriction enzymes, allowing for accurate determination of the methylation status of every cytosine nucleotide. Additionally the rapid time of analysis (~10 min/sample), low amounts of genomic DNA (1–2 μg), and the automated high-throughput nature of this method make it suitable for analysis of genomic methylation levels. Disadvantages with this technique include the high cost of the machinery involved, as well as a requirement for constant calibration with standardized nucleotides. While HPCE allows for the determination of global cytosine methylation levels, it does not provide any information about the localization of these levels. This technique would have to be paired with a method that can determine regional changes. This technique has also not been adapted for detection of the recently discovered 5-hydroxymethyl cytosine, as well as non-cytosine methylation.

1.3. Sodium Bisulfite-Based Method

1.3.1. Infinium Methylation Assay

A technique for examining genome-wide changes in DNA methylation, the illumina methylation assay or IMA, was recently developed. This system examines a large number of CG sites (>27,000) located in over 14,000 genes. Using immobilized beads and fluorescent staining, IMA examines individual CG sites for presence and absence of methylation, giving further significance to the perceived state of DNA methylation.

This method uses sodium bisulfite conversion to examine changes in DNA methylation. 1 μg genomic DNA is treated with sodium bisulfite, which converts cytosine to uracil (uracil is subsequently replaced by thymidine after DNA amplification), while methylated cytosines remain protected and unconverted (31). Therefore, a methylated CG site remains CG; however, an unmethylated CG dinucleotide is converted to TG. The DNA then undergoes whole genome amplification and fragmentation into 50 bp fragments, allowing for proper hybridization. The converted DNA fragments are then hybridized to an Illumina Methylation BeadChip. This chip contains beads that have a complimentary sequence for over 27,000 CG loci in the human genome, and each DNA fragment hybridizes to the bead with a corresponding complimentary sequence. For each locus, two beads are present. One bead corresponds to the unmethylated CG locus, with a CA dinucleotide sequence at the end allowing for complementarity with a converted unmethylated locus. The other bead corresponds to the methylated CG locus, with a CG dinucleotide sequence at the end allowing for complementarity with the methylated locus. After hybridization, each allele undergoes single nucleotide extension with a labeled nucleotide. T and A nucleotides are labeled with DNP, stained as red, while C and G nucleotides are labeled with a Biotin label, stained as green (Fig. 3). The overall methylation value for each locus is determined by the ratio of the intensity of the fluorescent signal of the methylated bead to the combined fluorescent signals of the locus.

Though recently developed, IMA has already been used in a number of studies. Groups have used IMA to determine subtype of breast cancer using differential DNA methylation profiles (32, 33), as well as determining an epigenetic basis of type 1 diabetes mellitus (34). The primary advantage of IMA is the large number of CG sites this technique can examine. The Illumina Methylation BeadChip was designed to examine CG sites located in a large set of gene promoters, CG islands, repetitive elements, miR promoters, as well as tumor or stem cell-specific CGs. While this method allows for a comprehensive genome-wide analysis of DNA methylation, it still does not feature complete coverage of every CG dinucleotide in the human genome, as well as only examining CG in 14,495 genes out of a reported 17,000 genes. Consequently, this method is not a complete determination of all CG methylation.

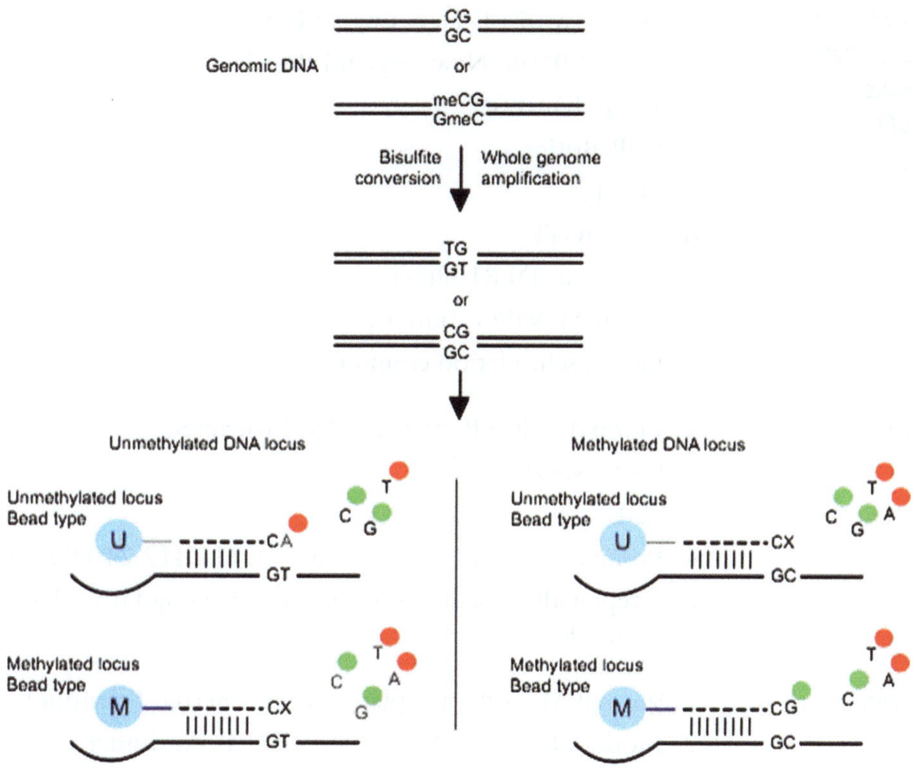

Fig. 3. Infinium methylation assay. Genomic DNA undergoes bisulfite conversion and whole genome amplification. Unmethylated cytosines (C) are converted into thymidine (T) while methylated cytosines (meC) remain as cytosines (C) after amplification. Bisulfite genomic DNA is hybridized to locus specific beads and undergoes single-base extension. Unmethylated CG locus is detected as red, while methylated CG locus is detected as green. DNA methylation values for each CG locus are calculated as a ratio of the methylated bead to the total fluorescence of the locus.

The presence of both a methylated and unmethylated bead for each locus allows the user to determine allelic-specific methylation, as well as strand specificity. Furthermore, 12 samples can be processed per chip, allowing for high-throughput processing. Despite this, a sample requires 2 weeks of processing to be fully analyzed. Moreover, the high cost of this technique is also prohibitive. A comprehensive protocol is detailed in a recent study (35).

2. Materials

2.1. Reagents and Materials for LUMA

1. *HpaII* (M0214. New England Biolabs).
2. *MspI* (R0106. New England Biolabs).
3. *EcoRI* (R0101. New England Biolabs).
4. Tango Buffer: 33 mM Tris-acetate pH 7.9, 10 mM Mg-acetate, 66 mM K-acetate, 0.1 mg/mL BSA.
5. Pyrosequencer.
6. PSQ 96 SNP reagents (40-0023. Biotage).

2.2. Reagents and Materials for Cytosine Extension Assays (ICEA/NICEA)

2.2.1. ICEA

1. *HpaII* (M0214. New England Biolabs).
2. *MspI* (R0106. New England Biolabs).
3. Taq polymerase.
4. PCR Buffer.
5. $MgCl_2$.
6. [^{3}H] dCTP.
7. Whatman DE81 filters.
8. 500 mM $NaPO_4$ buffer pH 7.0.
9. Liquid scintillation counter.

2.2.2. NICEA

1. Biotin-14-dCTP (19518-018. Invitrogen).
2. 0.4N NaOH.
3. TBE.
4. Positively charged nylon membrane (11 417 240 001. Roche).
5. Streptavidin Alkaline Phosphatase Imaging kit for biotinylated molecules.

2.2.3. CpGlobal

1. 96 well Microfluor 2 plate (7805. Thermo Scientific).
2. Biotin-11-dCTP (NEL538001EA. PerkinElmer).
3. Biotin-11-dGTP (NEL541001EA. PerkinElmer).
4. Sequenase (E70775Y. GE Healthcare).
5. 5× Sequenase Reaction Buffer: 200 mM Tris–HCl pH 7.5, 100 mM $MgCl_2$, 250 mM NaCl.
6. Reacti-Bind DNA Coating Solution (17250. Pierce).
7. TBS.
8. HRP Neutravidin (31001. Pierce).
9. Detector Block Solution (71-83-00. KPL).
10. Biotin Wash Solution (50-63-06. KPL).
11. LumiGlo chemiluminescence substrate (54-61-00. KPL).
12. PerkinElmer multilabel reader (PerkinElmer).

2.3. Reagents and Materials for Nearest Neighbor Analysis

1. MboI (R0147. New England Biolabs).
2. [α-32P] dGTP.
3. Klenow fragment (M0210. New England Biolabs).
4. Klenow labeling buffer.
5. Micrococcal nuclease (N3755. Sigma).
6. Calf spleen phosphodiesterase (Worthington Biochemical Corporation).
7. 2× Micrococcal nuclease/spleen phosphodiesterase digestion buffer: 15 mM $CaCl_2$, 100 mM Tris–HCl.

8. 0.2 M EDTA.
9. Sephadex G50 Spin Columns (Roche).
10. Solution A: 66 mL isobutyric acid, 18 mL water, 3 mL 30% ammonia solution.
11. Solution B: 80 mL saturated ammonium sulfate, 18 mL 1 M acetic acid, 2 mL isopropanol.
12. Glass backed 20 × 20 cm cellulose TLC plates (Whatman).
13. TLC developing tanks.

2.4. Reagents for High-Performance Capillary Electrophoresis

1. Nuclease P1. 200 U/mL in 30 mM Sodium Acetate (N8630. Sigma-Aldrich).
2. Alkaline Phosphatase. 50 U/mL in 2.5 M Ammonium Sulfate (Sigma-Aldrich).
3. 10 mM $ZnSO_4$.
4. 0.5 M Tris pH 8.3.
5. Nucleotide standards.
   (a) 2′-deoxyadenosine (Sigma-Aldrich).
   (b) 2′-deoxythymidine (Sigma-Aldrich).
   (c) 2′-deoxyguanosine (Sigma-Aldrich).
   (d) 2′-deoxycytidine (Sigma-Aldrich).
   (e) 5-methyl 2′-deoxycytidine (Sigma-Aldrich).
6. Running Buffer: 48 mM $NaCHO_3$ pH 9.6.
7. 0.25 m filtered water.
8. Uncoated fused-silica capillary, 60 cm × 75 m (Beckman Coulter).
9. Capillary Electrophoresis P/ACE (Beckman Coulter).

3. Methods

3.1. Methods for LUMA

1. Mix A: Digest 250–500 ng genomic DNA with 5 U *EcoRI*, 5 U *HpaII*, 2 μL Tango buffer in a total volume of 20 μL for 4 h at 37°C.
2. Mix B: Digest 250–500 ng genomic DNA with 5 U *EcoRI*, 5 U *MspI*, 2 μL Tango buffer in a total volume of 20 μL for 4 h at 37°C.
3. Add 20 μL Pyrosequencer Annealing Buffer to solutions. Transfer samples to 96-well pyrosequencing plates.
4. Run pyrosequencer machine in SNP mode and assay sequence as: AC/TCGA. Define nucleotide addition as ACTCGA.

(a) Mix 50 μL dATPαS with 50 μL H_2O and added to the "A" chamber of the pyrosequencing cartridge.

(b) Mix 50 μL dTTP with 50 μL H_2O and added to the "T" chamber of the pyrosequencing cartridge.

(c) Mix 50 μL dCTP with 50 μL dGTP and added to the "C" chamber of the pyrosequencing cartridge.

(d) Add 100 μL H_2O to the "G" chamber of the pyrosequencing cartridge.

(e) Start run.

5. Calculate the ratio of (peak "C")/(peak "A") for each sample. This represents the *HpaII/EcoRI* ratio for Mix A and the *MspI/EcoRI* ratio for Mix B, respectively. The HpaII/MspI ratio is calculated by comparing the (peak "C")/(peak "A") ratio for both digestions.

3.2. Methods for ICEA/NICEA

3.2.1. ICEA

1. Digest 1 μg of genomic DNA with 10 U *HpaII* or *MspI* in a volume of 10 μL for 8 h at 37°C.
2. Add 0.5 U Taq, 1× PCR Buffer, 1.0 mM $MgCl_2$, [^{3}H] dCTP (42.9 Ci/mmol) and digested DNA to a final volume of 25 μL. Label digested DNA for 1 h at 56°C.
3. Filter samples through Whatman DE81filters. Wash filters with 500 mM $NaPO_4$ Buffer.
4. Measure [^{3}H] dCTP by liquid scintillation counter.

3.2.2. NICEA

1. Digest 100 ng of genomic DNA with 1 U *HpaII* or *MspI* in a volume of 50 μL for 8 h at 37°C.
2. Add digested DNA to 1 U Taq, 1× PCR Buffer, 15 mM $MgCl_2$, 5 μL of 0.4 mM biotin-14-dCTP to a final volume of 100 μL. Label digested DNA for 1 h at 56°C.
3. Apply 2 μL of each sample to a defined area of a positively charged nylon membrane. The membrane is blocked with 0.4 M NaOH for 2 min and neutralized and washed with TBE. Dry membrane for 20 min at 80°C.
4. Visualize biotinylated dCTP with streptavidin alkaline phosphatase imaging kit.

3.2.3. CpGlobal

1. 100 ng of genomic DNA is digested with 5 U *HpaII* or *MspI* in a total volume of 30 μL in a 96-well microfluor 2 plate for 3 h at 37°C.
2. 20 μL of 0.1 μM of biotin-11-dCTP and biotin-11-dGTP each, 0.1 U sequenase and 1× sequenase buffer are added to each well. Label DNA for 30 min at 37°C.
3. Add 100 μL of Reacti-Bind DNA Coating Solution to each well to immobilize DNA. Wash wells four times with TBS.

4. Add 200 μL of Detector Block Solution to each well and incubate at 37°C for 30 min.
5. Aspirate solution. Add 150 μL of Detector Block Solution with 0.5 μg/mL of HRP Neutravidin to each well and incubate at room temperature for 30 min.
6. Wash wells five times with Biotin Wash Solution.
7. Add 150 μL of LumiGlo Chemiluminescence substrate to each well. Incubate at room temperature for 2 min. Quantify luminescence with plate reader.

3.3. Method for Nearest Neighbor Analysis

1. Digest 1 μg genomic DNA with 10 U of *MboI* at 37°C.
2. Heat-inactivate reaction at 70°C for 20 min.
3. Precipitate DNA in ethanol and resuspend in 10 μL of water.
4. Labeling reaction. Add 10–30 μCi [α-^{32}P] dGTP, 1.5 μL 10× Klenow labeling buffer, and 0.5 μL (2.5 U) Klenow. Incubate at 25°C for 20 min.
5. Add 2 μL 0.2 M EDTA to terminate the reaction.
6. Apply labeled DNA to Sephadex G50 column. Spin at 1,100 × *g* for 4 min, collecting the flow-through in a collection tube.
7. Digest 3 μL purified labeled DNA with 1 μL (0.2 U) micrococcal nuclease and 1 μL (2 μg) spleen phosphodiesterase in 5 μL digestion buffer for 4 h at 37°C.
8. Spot digestion reaction on 10 × 10 cm cellulose TLC plate 1 cm from the bottom left hand corner.
9. Run plate in first dimension with solution A in TLC developing tank.
10. Dry plate and rotate 90°.
11. Run plate in second dimension with solution B in TLC developing tank.
12. Dry plate.
13. Expose plate to autoradiogram.

3.4. Methods for High-Performance Capillary Electrophoresis

1. Digest 1.5 μg genomic DNA with 1.25 μL Nuclease P1 and 0.75 μL 10 mM $ZnSO_4$ in a total volume of 5 μL for 16 h at 37°C.
2. Dephosphorylate sample with 1.5 μL 0.5 M Tris and 0.75 μL Alkaline Phosphatase for 4 h at 37°C.
3. Run nucleotide standards at a concentration of 5 mM in a capillary of 57 cm length at a voltage of 298 V/cm at 20°C to determine correct separation and migration.
4. Run digested genomic samples.

5. Quantify methylation in samples as the percentage of mdC of total cytidines. mdC peak area/(mdC peak area + dC peak area) × 100.

In conclusion, the techniques outlined in this chapter examine changes in DNA methylation throughout the genome. Whether they determine the genome-wide methylation status of CG dinucleotides or the methylation status of specific regions of the genome, these techniques are useful and practical tools for determining epigenetic events in cancer.

References

1. Baylin, S. B., Esteller, M., Rountree, M. R., Bachman, K. E., Schuebel, K., and Herman, J. G. (2001) Aberrant patterns of DNA methylation, chromatin formation and gene expression in cancer, *Hum Mol Genet* 10, 687–692.
2. Ehrlich, M., Jiang, G., Fiala, E., Dome, J. S., Yu, M. C., Long, T. I., Youn, B., Sohn, O. S., Widschwendter, M., Tomlinson, G. E., Chintagumpala, M., Champagne, M., Parham, D., Liang, G., Malik, K., and Laird, P. W. (2002) Hypomethylation and hypermethylation of DNA in Wilms tumors, *Oncogene* 21, 6694–6702.
3. Ehrlich, M. (2002) DNA methylation in cancer: too much, but also too little, *Oncogene* 21, 5400–5413.
4. Lin, Z., Hegarty, J., Cappel, J., Yu, W., Chen, X., Faber, P., Wang, Y., Kelly, A., Poritz, L., Peterson, B., Schreiber, S., Fan, J. B., and Koltun, W. (2010) Identification of disease-associated DNA methylation in intestinal tissues from patients with inflammatory bowel disease, *Clin Genet.*
5. Houshdaran, S., Hawley, S., Palmer, C., Campan, M., Olsen, M. N., Ventura, A. P., Knudsen, B. S., Drescher, C. W., Urban, N. D., Brown, P. O., and Laird, P. W. (2010) DNA methylation profiles of ovarian epithelial carcinoma tumors and cell lines, *PLoS One* 5, e9359.
6. Vaissiere, T., Hung, R. J., Zaridze, D., Moukeria, A., Cuenin, C., Fasolo, V., Ferro, G., Paliwal, A., Hainaut, P., Brennan, P., Tost, J., Boffetta, P., and Herceg, Z. (2009) Quantitative analysis of DNA methylation profiles in lung cancer identifies aberrant DNA methylation of specific genes and its association with gender and cancer risk factors, *Cancer Res* 69, 243–252.
7. Zhu, J. and Yao, X. (2009) Use of DNA methylation for cancer detection: promises and challenges, *Int J Biochem Cell Biol* 41, 147– 154.
8. Hotchkiss, R. D. (1948) The quantitative separation of purines, pyrimidines, and nucleosides by paper chromatography, *J Biol Chem* 175, 315–332.
9. Razin, A. and Riggs, A. D. (1980) DNA methylation and gene function, *Science* 210, 604–610.
10. Karimi, M., Johansson, S., Stach, D., Corcoran, M., Grander, D., Schalling, M., Bakalkin, G., Lyko, F., Larsson, C., and Ekstrom, T. J. (2006) LUMA (LUminometric Methylation Assay)--a high throughput method to the analysis of genomic DNA methylation, *Exp Cell Res* 312, 1989–1995.
11. Wu, H. C., Delgado-Cruzata, L., Flom, J. D., Kappil, M., Ferris, J. S., Liao, Y., Santella, R. M., and Terry, M. B. (2011) Global methylation profiles in DNA from different blood cell types, *Epigenetics* 6.
12. Deneberg, S., Grovdal, M., Karimi, M., Jansson, M., Nahi, H., Corbacioglu, A., Gaidzik, V., Dohner, K., Paul, C., Ekstrom, T. J., Hellstrom-Lindberg, E., and Lehmann, S. (2010) Gene-specific and global methylation patterns predict outcome in patients with acute myeloid leukemia, *Leukemia* 24, 932–941.
13. Kawai, J., Hirose, K., Fushiki, S., Hirotsune, S., Ozawa, N., Hara, A., Hayashizaki, Y., and Watanabe, S. (1994) Comparison of DNA methylation patterns among mouse cell lines by restriction landmark genomic scanning, *Mol Cell Biol* 14, 7421–7427.
14. Matsuyama, T., Kimura, M. T., Koike, K., Abe, T., Nakano, T., Asami, T., Ebisuzaki, T., Held, W. A., Yoshida, S., and Nagase, H. (2003) Global methylation screening in the Arabidopsis thaliana and Mus musculus genome: applications of virtual image restriction landmark genomic scanning (Vi-RLGS), *Nucleic Acids Res* 31, 4490–4496.
15. Smiraglia, D. J., Kazhiyur-Mannar, R., Oakes, C. C., Wu, Y. Z., Liang, P., Ansari, T., Su, J., Rush, L. J., Smith, L. T., Yu, L., Liu, C., Dai, Z., Chen, S. S., Wang, S. H., Costello, J.,

Ioshikhes, I., Dawson, D. W., Hong, J. S., Teitell, M. A., Szafranek, A., Camoriano, M., Song, F., Elliott, R., Held, W., Trasler, J. M., Plass, C., and Wenger, R. (2007) Restriction landmark genomic scanning (RLGS) spot identification by second generation virtual RLGS in multiple genomes with multiple enzyme combinations, *BMC Genomics* 8, 446.

16. Zardo, G., Tiirikainen, M. I., Hong, C., Misra, A., Feuerstein, B. G., Volik, S., Collins, C. C., Lamborn, K. R., Bollen, A., Pinkel, D., Albertson, D. G., and Costello, J. F. (2002) Integrated genomic and epigenomic analyses pinpoint biallelic gene inactivation in tumors, *Nat Genet* 32, 453–458.
17. Costello, J. F., Hong, C., Plass, C., and Smiraglia, D. J. (2009) Restriction landmark genomic scanning: analysis of CpG islands in genomes by 2D gel electrophoresis, *Methods Mol Biol* 507, 131–148.
18. Boyko, A. and Kovalchuk, I. (2010) Detection of changes in global genome methylation using the cytosine-extension assay, *Methods Mol Biol* 631, 33–39.
19. Pogribny, I., Yi, P., and James, S. J. (1999) A sensitive new method for rapid detection of abnormal methylation patterns in global DNA and within CpG islands, *Biochem Biophys Res Commun* 262, 624–628.
20. Fujiwara, H., and Ito, M. (2002) Nonisotopic cytosine extension assay: a highly sensitive method to evaluate CpG island methylation in the whole genome, *Anal Biochem* 307, 386–389.
21. Anisowicz, A., Huang, H., Braunschweiger, K. I., Liu, Z., Giese, H., Wang, H., Mamaev, S., Olejnik, J., Massion, P. P., and Del Mastro, R. G. (2008) A high-throughput and sensitive method to measure global DNA methylation: application in lung cancer, *BMC Cancer* 8, 222.
22. Josse, J., Kaiser, A. D., and Kornberg, A. (1961) Enzymatic synthesis of deoxyribonucleic acid. VIII. Frequencies of nearest neighbor base sequences in deoxyribonucleic acid, *J Biol Chem* 236, 864–875.
23. Swartz, M. N., Trautner, T. A., and Kornberg, A. (1962) Enzymatic synthesis of deoxyribonucleic acid. XI. Further studies on nearest neighbor base sequences in deoxyribonucleic acids, *J Biol Chem* 237, 1961–1967.
24. Gruenbaum, Y., Stein, R., Cedar, H., and Razin, A. (1981) Methylation of CpG sequences in eukaryotic DNA, *FEBS Lett* 124, 67–71.
25. Unterberger, A., Szyf, M., Nathanielsz, P. W., and Cox, L. A. (2009) Organ and gestational age effects of maternal nutrient restriction on global methylation in fetal baboons, *J Med Primatol* 38, 219–227.
26. Fraga, M. F., Rodriguez, R., and Canal, M. J. (2000) Rapid quantification of DNA methylation by high performance capillary electrophoresis, *Electrophoresis* 21, 2990–2994.
27. Fraga, M. F., Rodriguez, R., and Canal, M. J. (2002) Genomic DNA methylation-demethylation during aging and reinvigoration of Pinus radiata, *Tree Physiol* 22, 813–816.
28. Fraga, M. F., Uriol, E., Borja Diego, L., Berdasco, M., Esteller, M., Canal, M. J., and Rodriguez, R. (2002) High-performance capillary electrophoretic method for the quantification of 5-methyl 2′-deoxycytidine in genomic DNA: application to plant, animal and human cancer tissues, *Electrophoresis* 23, 1677–1681.
29. Hellebrekers, D. M., Jair, K. W., Vire, E., Eguchi, S., Hoebers, N. T., Fraga, M. F., Esteller, M., Fuks, F., Baylin, S. B., van Engeland, M., and Griffioen, A. W. (2006) Angiostatic activity of DNA methyltransferase inhibitors, *Mol Cancer Ther* 5, 467–475.
30. Villar-Garea, A., Fraga, M. F., Espada, J., and Esteller, M. (2003) Procaine is a DNA-demethylating agent with growth-inhibitory effects in human cancer cells, *Cancer Res* 63, 4984–4989.
31. Clark, S. J., Harrison, J., Paul, C. L., and Frommer, M. (1994) High sensitivity mapping of methylated cytosines, *Nucleic Acids Res* 22, 2990–2997.
32. Li, L., Lee, K. M., Han, W., Choi, J. Y., Lee, J. Y., Kang, G. H., Park, S. K., Noh, D. Y., Yoo, K. Y., and Kang, D. (2010) Estrogen and progesterone receptor status affect genome-wide DNA methylation profile in breast cancer, *Hum Mol Genet* 19, 4273–4277.
33. Van der Auwera, I., Yu, W., Suo, L., Van Neste, L., van Dam, P., Van Marck, E. A., Pauwels, P., Vermeulen, P. B., Dirix, L. Y., and Van Laere, S. J. (2010) Array-based DNA methylation profiling for breast cancer subtype discrimination, *PLoS One* 5, e12616.
34. Bell, C. G., Teschendorff, A. E., Rakyan, V. K., Maxwell, A. P., Beck, S., and Savage, D. A. (2010) Genome-wide DNA methylation analysis for diabetic nephropathy in type 1 diabetes mellitus, *BMC Med Genomics* 3, 33.
35. Thirlwell, C., Eymard, M., Feber, A., Teschendorff, A., Pearce, K., Lechner, M., Widschwendter, M., and Beck, S. (2010) Genome-wide DNA methylation analysis of archival formalin-fixed paraffin-embedded tissue using the Illumina Infinium HumanMethylation27 BeadChip, *Methods* 52, 248–254.

Chapter 20

Microarray for Epigenetic Changes: Gene Expression Arrays

Hilary A.A. Colyer, Richard N. Armstrong, and Ken I. Mills

Abstract

Microarrays can be used to examine changes involving all aspects of the epigenetic interactions. As the relationship between DNA methylation, histone modifications, and gene expression is elucidated, an important aspect to investigate is how the epigenetic status regulates the cell through differential expression of genes. This can provide data from work including experimental drug investigations from cell line models, or more directly patient comparison data.

Key words: Microarray, Affymetrix, Expression, Screening, GeneChip

1. Introduction

Microarrays were developed by Fodor et al. in the late 1980s and presented a variety of potential applications and have since had an accelerating presence in research. Affymetrix, founded by Stephen Fodor, released the first commercially available array, the GeneChip® Hu6800, in 1998 (1). Microarrays, from various companies, have since been developed into single chip applications from the multiple chips first developed. The clinical application of some arrays has been shown as they have gained US Food and Drug Administration (FDA) approval as prognostic, diagnostic, or clinically relevant patient phenotype classification tools in some disease types (2–4).

The development of microarray technology has allowed for high-throughput investigation of biological materials such as DNA, RNA, and protein for analysis on a molecular level with regard to diseases such as cancer. The large amount of data yielded by microarrays requires careful analysis to gain insights into the material assayed which must then be validated using an alternative method before investigation can proceed.

Ramona G. Dumitrescu and Mukesh Verma (eds.), *Cancer Epigenetics: Methods and Protocols*, Methods in Molecular Biology, vol. 863, DOI 10.1007/978-1-61779-612-8_20, © Springer Science+Business Media, LLC 2012

Affymetrix GeneChip HG-U133 Plus 2.0 chips are gene expression arrays covering the human genome. The cartridges contain over 54,000 probe sets of 25 mer for ~47,000 transcripts and variants of 38,500 genes. There are 11 control sequences for hybridization control and constitutively expressed "housekeeping" genes in addition to 100 probe sets which are utilized in the normalization of the arrays (5). One Affymetrix GeneChip HG-U133 Plus 2.0 array cartridge is required per sample assayed.

The principle behind the Affymetrix GeneChip HG-U133 Plus 2.0 array preparation procedure is as follows: Total RNA, isolated from the sample to be assayed, is converted to complimentary DNA (cDNA) and purified. The cDNA is used as a template to convert to biotin-labeled complimentary RNA (cRNA) by an in vitro transcription reaction. The cRNA is then purified and fragmented, and controls are added. Hybridization occurs overnight; the sample is removed the next morning; the arrays are subjected to a series of washes and staining in an Affymetrix GeneChip fluidics station and are then scanned in an Affymetrix GeneChip Scanner. Scanning the arrays produces intensity-based CEL files for each array that can be exported for analysis.

2. Materials

2.1. cDNA Synthesis and Purification

- Total RNA, preferable at least 2 μg, but 1 μg can be used (see Note 1)
- Poly-A RNA Control Kit (see Note 2)
- One-Cycle cDNA Synthesis Kit
- Sample Cleanup Module

2.2. cRNA Conversion with Biotin Labeling and Purification

- IVT Labeling Kit
- Sample Cleanup Module

2.3. Sample Hybridization to Affymetrix GeneChip HG-U133 Plus 2.0 Arrays

- GeneChip Hybridization Wash and Stain Kit (Module 1)
- GeneChip Eukaryotic Hybridization Control Kit
- Control Oligo B2 (3 nM)
- Affymetrix hybridization oven

2.4. Washing and Staining the GeneChip Prior to Scanning

- GeneChip Hybridization Wash and Stain Kit (Box 1 and 2)
- Tough-Spots™ label dots (USA Scientific)
- Affymetrix wash station 450 (or 250)

2.5. Scanning Affymetrix GeneChip HG-U133 Plus 2.0 Arrays

- Affymetrix Scanner 3000

3. Methods (6, 7)

3.1. cDNA Synthesis and Purification

1. Make a serial dilution of the poly-A RNA control. For 2 μg of total RNA this means a 1:20 first dilution, 1:50 second dilution, and 1:25 third dilution. The resulting spike-in volume and all dilutions should be kept at 2 μL or above. For other starting amounts of RNA, see Note 3 for dilutions. Using the cDNA synthesis kit reagents, prepare the following in a 200 μL PCR tube:
   - Total RNA sample 2 μg (variable volume)
   - Poly-A RNA control dilution 2 μL
   - T7-Oligo(dT) primer (50 μM) 2 μL
   - RNase-free water to 12 μL (variable volume)
2. Flick to mix, then centrifuge briefly.
3. Incubate at 70°C for 10 min.
4. Cool at 4°C for 2 min, then centrifuge briefly.
5. Prepare the First Strand Master Mix per sample (prepare +10% for >2 samples):
   - 5× First Strand Reaction Mix 4 μL.
   - DTT (0.1 μM) 2 μL.
   - dNTP (10 mM) 1 μL

   Mix by gently flicking tube then centrifuge briefly.
6. Aliquot 7 μL of First Strand Master Mix to each sample tube, gently flick to mix, and centrifuge briefly.
7. Incubate at 42°C for 2 min.
8. Add 1 μL of SuperScript II to each sample tube (see Note 4), flick to mix, and centrifuge briefly.
9. Incubate at 42°C for 60 min, then incubate at 4°C for 2 min. Centrifuge briefly.
10. Prepare the Second Strand Master Mix as follows for each sample:
    - RNase-free water 91 μL.
    - 5× Second Strand Reaction Mix 30 μL.
    - dNTP (10 mM) 3 μL.
    - *E. coli* DNA ligase 1 μL.

- *E. coli* DNA polymerase I 4 μL.
- RNase H 1 μL

Mix well by flicking, then centrifuge briefly.

11. Aliquot 130 μL to each sample (total volume of Master Mix and sample is 150 μL).
12. Incubate at 16°C for 2 h.
13. Add 2 μL of T4 DNA polymerase and incubate at 16°C for a further 5 min.
14. Add 10 μL EDTA (0.5 M).
15. Cleaning of the samples is performed at room temperature using the Sample Cleanup Module (see Note 5), and it is advised to perform the cleanup uninterrupted. Transfer samples to 1.5 μL microcentrifuge tubes.
16. Add 600 μL cDNA binding buffer to each sample, and mix by quick vortexing (see Note 6).
17. Transfer 500 μL of sample to a cDNA cleanup spin column in a collection tube and centrifuge at ≥8,000 × *g* for 1 min. Discard flow through and repeat with remaining sample.
18. Transfer the spin column to a clean-labeled collection tube, add 750 μL cDNA wash buffer and centrifuge at ≥8,000 × *g* for 1 min and discard flow through.
19. Open the spin column and centrifuge at maximum speed for 5 min to dry the membrane.
20. Transfer the spin column to a clean 1.5-mL microcentrifuge tube and apply 14 μL of cDNA elution buffer to the spin column membrane.
21. Incubate at room temperature for 1 min, then centrifuge at maximum speed for 1 min.

3.2. cRNA Conversion with Biotin Labeling and Purification (see Note 7)

1. Working at room temperature, prepare template cDNA (see Note 8) and RNase-free water to 20 μL.
2. Make a master mix of the following:
   - 10× IVT Labeling buffer 4 μL
   - IVT Labeling NTP Mix 12 μL
   - IVT Labeling Enzyme Mix 4 μL
3. Add 20 μL of master mix to each sample (total sample volume is now 40 μL), mix by pipetting, then briefly centrifuge.
4. Incubate samples at 37°C for 16 h. (Recommended: use a thermocycler to prevent condensation.)
5. Labeled cRNA can now be frozen at −70°C if required.
6. The Sample Cleanup Module is again used to purify the biotin-labeled cRNA (see Note 9). Add 60 μL of RNase-free water to each sample and mix by quick vortex.

7. Add 350 μL of IVT cRNA binding buffer to each sample and mix by quick vortex.
8. Add 250 μL ethanol (96–100% v/v) and mix by pipetting.
9. Transfer sample to an IVT cRNA cleanup spin column in a collection tube and centrifuge at ≥8,000 × *g* for 15 s. Discard flow through and collection tube.
10. Transfer the spin column to a clean-labeled collection tube and add 500 μL IVT cRNA wash buffer. Centrifuge at ≥8,000 × *g* for 15 s. Discard flow through.
11. Add 500 μL ethanol (80% v/v). Centrifuge at ≥8,000 × *g* for 15 s. Discard flow through.
12. Centrifuge Spin Column at maximum speed for 5 min with lids open to dry the membrane.
13. Transfer the Spin Column to a labeled 1.5-mL microcentrifuge tube and add 11 μL RNase-free water directly to the membrane. Centrifuge at maximum speed for 1 min.
14. Add another 10 μL of RNase-free water and centrifuge at maximum speed for 1 min.
15. cRNA samples can now be stored at −20°C (short-term) or −70°C (long-term) if required.
16. Quantify cRNA using a spectrophotometer and Agilent Bioanalyzer (see Note 10).

3.3. Sample Fragmentation and Hybridization to Affymetrix GeneChip HG-U133 Plus 2.0 Arrays (Fig. 1)

1. Switch on heat-block to 94°C.
2. Prepare in a 1.5-mL microcentrifuge tube the following:
   - cRNA 15 μg
   - 5× fragmentation buffer 6 μL
   - RNase-free water to 30 μL
3. Incubate tubes at 94°C for 35 min, then incubate on ice for >2 min (see Note 11).
4. Equilibrate arrays to room temperature, heat hybridization oven to 45°C, and alter heat-block to 99°C if moving onto hybridization from step 3 in 3.3.
5. Prepare the hybridization cocktail for each sample in 1.5-mL microcentrifuge tubes:
   - Fragmented and labeled cRNA 10 μg
   - Control oligonucleotide B2 (3 nM) 3.3 μL
   - 20× Eukaryotic hybridization controls (*bioB*, *bioC*, *bioD*, *cre*) (see Note 11) 10 μL
   - 2× Hybridization Mix 100 μL
   - DMSO 20 μL
   - Nuclease-free water to final volume of 200 μL

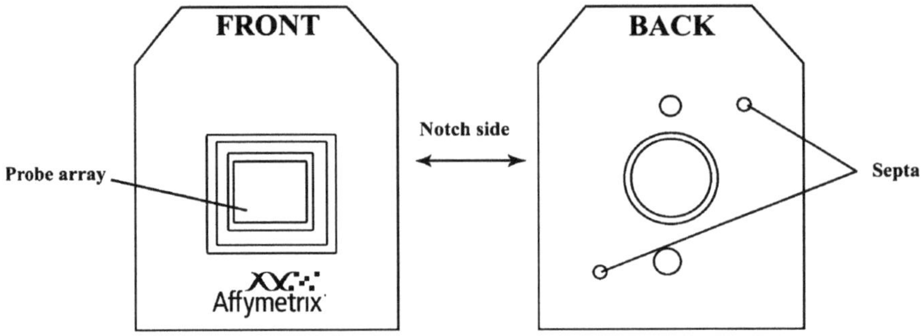

Fig. 1. A front and rear image of the GeneChip array cartridge window showing the probe array and septa ports, respectively.

6. Incubate hybridization cocktail at 99°C for 5 min.
7. Inject 130 μL of Pre-Hybridization Mix into the array and incubate rotating at 45°C for 10 min. See Note 12 for array injection procedure.
8. Incubate hybridization cocktail at 45°C for 5 min.
9. Centrifuge hybridization cocktail at maximum speed for 5 min.
10. Vent the array cartridge and remove the Pre-Hybridization Mix from the array (see Note 12) and inject in 130 μL of sample hybridization cocktail from the top of the microcentrifuge tube to avoid pelleted debris. Maintain sample temperature at 45°C if performing several array hybridizations.
11. Seal ports with Tough-Spots stickers to prevent evaporation and load array cartridges into the holding buckets and load into the hybridization oven in a balanced manner. Hybridize at 45°C and 60 RPM for 16 h.

3.4. Washing and Staining the GeneChip Prior to Scanning (see Note 13)

1. Prime the fluidics station (see Note 14). This should be done at start-up and shut down of the station as well as when wash solutions are changed.
2. After hybridization remove Tough-Spots stickers and vent the array using one septa port and a clean pipette tip and remove the hybridization cocktail through the other septum. The cocktail can be stored at −20°C and re-hybridized to another array if needed.
3. Pipette 160 μL of wash buffer A into the cartridge using the septum port (see Note 15).
4. For each array aliquot 600 μL of each stain cocktail (1 and 2) and 800 μL of array holding buffer into clean microcentrifuge tubes. Stain cocktail 1 should be protected from light. Avoid introducing bubbles into the solutions.
5. On the master station computer, select the appropriate fluidics protocol for each module used, and enter the sample information for each cartridge used (see Note 16).

6. Move the module lever down and insert the array into the assigned module and push the lever back up to engage. Instructions for positioning stain cocktails and array holding buffer vials will be shown on the LCD. Lift the needle lever, position vials, and move lever back down to move needles into place. Start run on the command console for each module used.

3.5. Scanning Affymetrix GeneChip HG-U133 Plus 2.0 Arrays

When the run is over, remove the array by releasing the lever, and inspect array window for bubbles. If bubbles are identified, return the array to the wash module and engage lever to drain and refill array (see Note 17). Continue with the shutdown protocol activated using the command console if all arrays are processed. Cover the septa ports with Tough-Spots and slot arrays into the Affymetrix GeneChip Scanner 3000 (see Note 18) and start the scan. Data is saved as .CEL files (Affymetrix Cell Intensity File) which can be exported for analysis (Materials courtesy of Affymetrix, Inc. All rights reserved).

4. Notes

1. *Isolation and qualitative/quantitative assessment of eukaryotic total RNA*
   It is recommended to use a kit such as QIAGEN RNeasy mini-kits to isolate RNA from cells, or TRIzol/QIAzol followed by a QIAGEN RNeasy mini-kit cleanup procedure for tissues. The quality and integrity of the RNA is important, and it is recommended to check this before starting the microarray protocol. An RNA Integrity Number (RIN) value can be obtained by running a sample of RNA on an Agilent 2100 Bioanalyser (8). RIN values are given 1 (fully degraded) to 10 (intact), and an RNA RIN value of 8 or more is advised where possible (Fig. 2). For a starting concentration of <1 μg, a modified procedure can be used which incorporates an additional cDNA synthesis cycle.
2. *Reagents used for Affymetrix GeneChip HG-U133 Plus 2.0 arrays*
   All reagents have been developed, optimized, and tested specifically for Affymetrix microarrays and are available from Affymetrix either as single reagents or kit form for 30 reactions.
3. *Poly-A RNA control reagent*
   For all total RNA concentrations between 1 and 10 μg, the first 2 dilutions needed are 1:20 and 1:50. The third dilution is altered depending on total RNA. For 1, 5, and 10 μg, the third dilution is 1:50, 1:10, and 1:5, respectively, with the volume of the third dilution used being 2 μL.

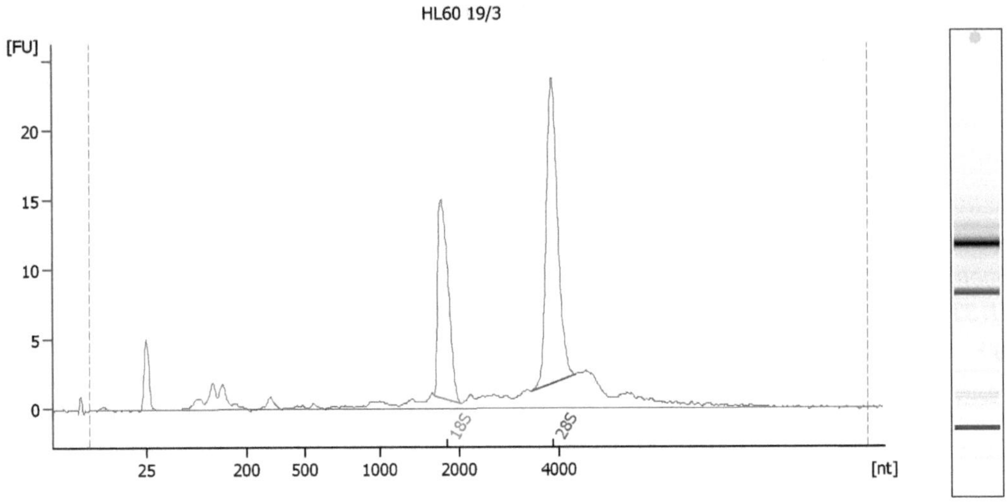

Overall Results for sample 8 : HL60 19/3

RNA Area:	122.6	RNA Integrity Number (RIN):	9.6 (B.02.07)
RNA Concentration:	169 ng/µl	Result Flagging Color:	
rRNA Ratio [28s / 18s]:	1.6	Result Flagging Label:	RIN: 9.60

Fragment table for sample 8 : HL60 19/3

Name	Start Size [nt]	End Size [nt]	Area	% of total Area
18S	1,689	2,043	24.8	20.3
28S	3,446	4,339	38.6	31.5

Fig. 2. Agilent Bioanalyzer 2100 Electropherogram (*top left*) and virtual gel (*top right*) for HL-60 total RNA. High-quality RNA is defined by strong 18 and 28S ribosomal RNA FU peaks. The ratio should approach 2:1 for the 28 and 18S bands, and the calculated RNA Integrity Number (RIN) should be approaching 10 (values given in the data summary).

4. *SuperScript II volumes for different RNA quantities*
   SuperScript II is added at different quantities depending on RNA quantity. For 1–8 µg of RNA, 1 µL is sufficient. For 8–15 µg of RNA, 2 µL of SuperScript II should be used. For <1 µg of mRNA and for every subsequent micrograms of mRNA, use 1 µL of SuperScript II.
5. *Preparation of the Sample Cleanup Module*
   Reagents in the module should be prepared as stated on the bottles by the addition of ethanol (96–100% v/v).
6. *cDNA binding buffer should remain yellow when added to sample*
   If the sample color is not yellow after the addition of cDNA binding buffer, 10 µL of sodium acetate (3M, pH 5.0) should be added. Mix by pipetting.
7. *GeneChip IVT labeling kit*
   The labeling kit should be stored in a −20°C non-frost-free freezer. Thaw reagents and centrifuge briefly before use. Use all of the cDNA sample if <8 µg total RNA or ≤0.5 µg mRNA was initially used, or 6 µL if >8 µg total RNA or >1 µg mRNA was initially used. Use 9 µL of cDNA sample if 0.6–1 µg mRNA was initially used.

8. *Purification of labeled cRNA samples*
This step is performed in order to remove unincorporated NTPs and should be done using the Cleanup Module to maintain yield. IVT cRNA binding buffer may require heating to 30°C to dissolve precipitants, but equilibrate to room temperature before using. Perform all steps uninterrupted at room temperature.

9. *Quantification of cRNA by spectrophotometer and Agilent Bioanalyzer*
An A_{260}/A_{280} ratio of between 1.9 and 2.1 is acceptable for a measurement of pure RNA. If total RNA was used at the beginning of this protocol, adjusted cRNA quantification must be obtained using the following equation:

$$\textit{adjusted cRNA quantification} = \textit{cRNA yeild} - (\textit{starting quantity of RNA})(\textit{fraction of cDNA used in IVT reaction})$$

A cRNA sample run on an Agilent 2100 Bioanalyzer should represent an average size of 1,580 nt.

10. *Fragmentation quality of sample and storage conditions*
An aliquot of the fragmented sample can be run on an Agilent Bioanalyzer to ensure fragmentation has occurred correctly. Samples should contain fragments of ~35 to 200 nucleotide bases. Samples at this stage can be frozen at −70°C.

11. *Preparation of 20× GeneChip eukaryotic hybridization controls*
This control mix requires heating to 65°C for 5 min to resuspend the solution fully.

12. *Sample injection into array via septa*
The GeneChip cartridge has two septa ports which seal the vacuum of the array surface. One port should be "pierced" with a clean 200-μL pipette tip to enable sample inject through the remaining port.

13. *Registering sample information*
A sample file with an ARR extension must be created in the Affymetrix GeneChip Command Console. This file will contain sample attribute information, such as experimental conditions and array information for arrays used with the sample. Information on this can be found in the AGGC user manual.

14. *Priming the fluidics station*
Fill the buffer reserve containers with the appropriate Wash Solutions (in GeneChip® Hybridization Wash and Stain Kit), deionized water. Place empty 1.5-mL microcentrifuge tubes in positions 1, 2, and 3. Lower the needles into the microcentrifuge tubes. Run the "Prime_450" protocol from the AGCC Fluidics Control program.

15. *Performing multiple arrays*
Array cartridges can be held at 4°C at this point until washing and scanning. This is useful when working with multiple array cartridges. Equilibrate to room temperature before continuing.
16. *Entering sample information for each module used*
The barcode from each cartridge should be scanned; each valid barcode will provide sample file names, array name, and probe array type automatically. The correct protocol should be selected for the array type.
17. *Dealing with bubbles on the surface of an array*
Bubbles are sometimes present when the array is removed from the wash module. These are usually removed by replacing the array in the wash module, allowing it to be drained and refilled. If this does not remove the bubbles, arrays can be drained and refilled with array holding buffer manually. Repeated attempts will reduce image quality. Arrays should then be stored in the dark at 4°C until scanned for a maximum of 24 h.
18. *The Affymetrix GeneChip Scanner 3000*
The scanner laser should be allowed to warm for a minimum of 10 min before scanning arrays. Arrays should be equilibrated to room temperature before scanning. Arrays fit in the scanner in one orientation only.

References

1. Fodor, S. P., Rava, R. P., Huang, X. C., Pease, A. C., Holmes, C. P., and Adams, C. L. (1993) Multiplexed biochemical assays with biological chips, *Nature* 364, 555–556.
2. Glas, A. M., Floore, A., Delahaye, L. J., Witteveen, A. T., Pover, R. C., Bakx, N., Lahti-Domenici, J. S., Bruinsma, T. J., Warmoes, M. O., Bernards, R., Wessels, L. F., and Van't Veer, L. J. (2006) Converting a breast cancer microarray signature into a high-throughput diagnostic test, *BMC Genomics* 7, 278.
3. Gutman, S. I. (2004) Evaluation of Automatic Class III Designation Roche AmpliChip CYP450 Test, (Administration, F. a. D., Ed.), pp 1–3, Department of Health and Human Services, Rockville MD.
4. Li, X., Quigg, R. J., Zhou, J., Gu, W., Nagesh Rao, P., and Reed, E. F. (2008) Clinical utility of microarrays: current status, existing challenges and future outlook, *Curr Genomics* 9, 466–474.
5. Affymetrix. (2004) Data Sheet GeneChip Human Genome Arrays, Santa Clara.
6. Affymetrix. (2002) GeneChip Expression Analysis: Technical Manual (P/N 701021 rev 1).
7. Affymetrix. (2009) GeneChip Expression Analysis: Technical Manual With Specific Protocols for Using the GeneChip Hybridization, Wash, and Stain Kit (P/N 702232 Rev. 3).
8. Schroeder, A., Mueller, O., Stocker, S., Salowsky, R., Leiber, M., Gassmann, M., Lightfoot, S., Menzel, W., Granzow, M., and Ragg, T. (2006) The RIN: an RNA integrity number for assigning integrity values to RNA measurements, *BMC Mol Biol* 7, 3.

Chapter 21

Detecting DNA Methylation Using the Methylated CpG Island Amplification and Microarray Technique

Hilary A.A. Colyer, Margaret Dellett, and Ken I. Mills

Abstract

Methylated CpG island amplification and microarray (MCAM) is a two-color array technique that quantifies DNA methylation by hybridizing equimolar amounts of treated vs. control cell-line DNA to an array platform. Sample preparation, hybridization, and scanning are performed over 1 week, but multiple samples can be prepared simultaneously, allowing for high-throughput processing and data acquisition. One microarray slide is required for each sample assayed, with a control sample hybridized with each test sample.

Key words: MCAM, Microarray, DNA, Methylation, Epigenetics, CpG

1. Introduction

Methylated CpG island amplification and microarray (MCAM) is a high-throughput method of analyzing DNA methylation. The method was developed and tested in both cancer cell lines and primary tumor tissues by Estécio et al. (1) from the original method described by Toyota et al. (2). It is a two-color array technique that allows the comparison of two samples, such as tumor vs. normal tissues or time course vs. control to identify genome-wide differential DNA methylation levels.

The principle behind this method is that genomic DNA is digested by two enzymes, a methylation-sensitive and methylation-insensitive enzyme, which results in only the methylated DNA fraction remaining in the sample after purification. This fraction is amplified by a polymerase chain reaction (PCR) step before the fluorochromes Cy3 and Cy5 are used to label the experimental and control sample amplicons, respectively. Equal quantities of the experimental and control sample are combined, condensed, and hybridized to the chosen microarray platform (Fig. 1).

Ramona G. Dumitrescu and Mukesh Verma (eds.), *Cancer Epigenetics: Methods and Protocols*, Methods in Molecular Biology, vol. 863, DOI 10.1007/978-1-61779-612-8_21, © Springer Science+Business Media, LLC 2012

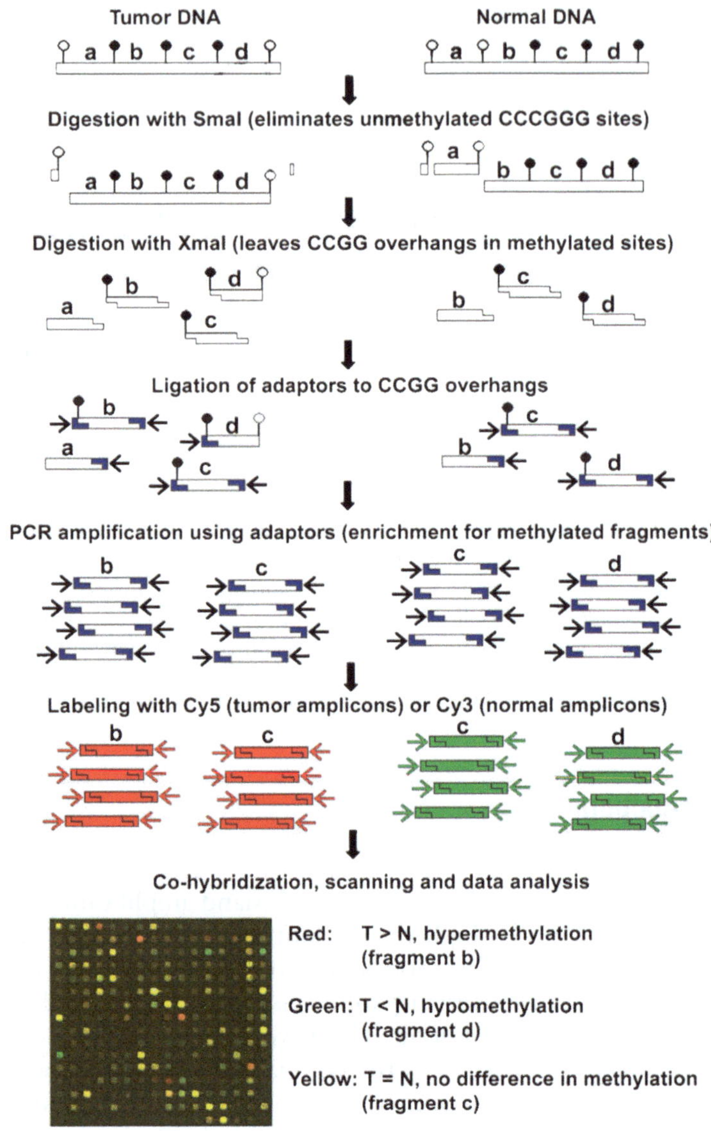

Fig. 1. A schematic diagram of the process involved in the technique of MCAM. Both experimental (tumor) and control (normal) global DNA samples are double digested with *SmaI* (methylation-sensitive) and *XmaI* (methylation-insensitive) enzymes. Adaptors are ligated to the resulting methylated fragments to allow PCR amplification of the samples. Amplicons are labeled with fluorochromes Cy5 (typically the experimental sample), and Cy3 (typically the control sample) is followed by co-hybridization to the chosen microarray platform. The scanned image fluorochrome intensities are analyzed to identify differential gene methylation levels. Hypermethylation of experimental samples appears red (Cy5), hypomethylation appears green (Cy3), and equally methylated experimental and control samples appear *yellow* (Image Copyright holder Cold Spring Harbor Laboratory Press).

The advantages of this technique are sensitivity, specificity, and reproducibility. During validation of the technique by bisulphite-PCR, sensitivity of hypermethylation detection was 93.8%, while specificity of hypomethylation detection was 94.1%. Reproducibility was assessed by duplicate MCAM experiments using cell lines, and correlation was statistically significant ($P < 0.0001$) with an average Pearson r value of 0.903 (1). Although false positives and false negatives have a low occurrence using the MCAM technique, they may be explained by the difficulty in amplifying and hybridizing certain sequences owing to differences in CG content (3).

The use of enzymes *SmaI* and *XmaI* reduces the complexity of the sample, and the ligated adapters allow methylated CpG islands to be amplified with greater specificity than techniques using other methylation-sensitive enzymes such as *HpaII/MspI* (3, 4). The limitation of using enzyme *SmaI* is that recognition sites need to be less than 2 kb apart for the generation of MCA amplicons. This however occurs in ~80% of promoter CpG islands in the human genome, so relatively good coverage is achieved (3).

2. Materials

This protocol is slightly modified from the protocol by Estécio et al. (3).

2.1. DNA Digestion

- Buffer 4 with BSA (New England Biolabs)
- *SmaI* (New England Biolabs)
- Sample and control DNA
- Ultrapure H_2O
- *XmaI* (New England Biolabs)

2.2. Purification of Digested DNA

- QIAquick PCR purification kit (QIAGEN)

2.3. Preparation of Adaptor Mix

- RMCA or RMXA primers (see Note 1)
- Ultrapure H_2O

2.4. Ligation of Adapters to Digested DNA

- Digested DNA (from step 1)
- Adaptor mix (from step 3)
- T4 DNA ligase buffer (10×)
- T4 DNA ligase (400 units)
- Ultrapure H_2O

2.5. MCA Reaction

- 10× PCR buffer (QIAGEN)
- dNTP mix (25 mM)
- HotStarTaq + (QIAGEN)
- Dimethyl sulfoxide (DMSO)

- Ultrapure water H_2O
- Ligation reaction product (step 4)
- RMCA24 primer

2.6. Agarose Gel to Check Amplicon Range

- 0.75-g agarose crystals
- 50 mL 1× TAE buffer
- Loading dye
- 100-bp ladder

2.7. Amplicon Labeling

- MCA PCR product (from step 5)
- Random primer (2.5×) (random Octomer 8 N) (Invitrogen)
- 10× React2 buffer
  - H_2O 890 μL
  - 1 M Tris–Cl (pH 8.0) 50 μL
  - 1 M $MgCl_2$ 10 μL
  - 1 M NaCl 50 μL
- 10× Low C dNTP mix
  - 0.5 M EDTA 1 μL
  - 1 M Tris–Cl (pH 7.5) 5 μL
  - 100 mM dATP 6 μL
  - 100 mM dTTP 6 μL
  - 100 mM dGTP 6 μL
  - 100 mM dCTP 1.5 μL
- Cy3 dCTP (GE Healthcare) (keep in dark)
- Cy5 dCTP (GE Healthcare) (keep in dark)
- Klenow fragments (40 U/mL. Bioprime DNA Labeling System (Invitrogen))

2.8. Sample Concentration

- Microcon YM-30 spin tubes (Millipore)
- Ultrapure H_2O

2.9. Sample Hybridization to Array Platform

- Human Cot1 (Invitrogen)
- 2X SDS hybridization solution (Genisphere)
- Microarray slide platform (see Note 2)
- Prehybridization solution:
  - 100% formamide 125 mL
  - 20× SSC (Ambion) 125 mL
  - 10% SDS (Ambion) 5 mL
  - 0.1% Bovine serum albumin (BSA) powder 50 mg
  - H_2O to 500 mL

- Ethanol (96–100%)
- Benchtop slide spinner
- Isopropanol
- KimWipes
- Compressed air (optional)
- Lifter slips (see Note 3)
- Wash 2 (see Subheading 2.10)

2.10. Washing the Arrays Prior to Scanning

- Wash 1
  - 20× SSC 25 mL
  - 10% SDS 5 mL
  - H_2O (distilled) 470 mL
- Wash 2
  - 20× SSC 5 mL
  - H_2O (distilled) 495 mL
- 1× SSC
  - 20× SSC 10 mL
  - H_2O (distilled) 190 mL
- 0.1× SSC
  - 20× SSC 1 mL
  - H_2O (distilled) 199 mL

2.11. Scanning

A microarray scanner appropriate for microarray platform used (see Note 2)

3. Methods

3.1. Preparing the Amplicons: DNA Digestion with SmaI

Digest 5 μg genomic DNA using 100 units *SmaI* with incubation at 25°C for 16 h (see Note 4).

- Buffer 4 (with BSA) 5 μL (10% of reaction volume)
- *SmaI* 5 μL (100 units)
- DNA 5 μg (variable volume)
- H_2O variable (to make up to 50 μL)

For convenience this reaction takes place overnight on day 1 to the morning of day 2

3.2. DNA Digestion with XmaI and Preparation of Adaptor Mix

Add 20 units (2 μL) of *XmaI* and incubate at 37°C for 6 h

This reaction lasts until the afternoon of day 2

Toward the end of this reaction make the adaptor mix

1. Dilute RMCA primers to 100 μM
2. Combine 50 μL RMCA24 with 50 μL RMCA12
3. Incubate at 65°C for 3 min, cool at room temperature for 1 h (can be stored at −20°C <6 months)

3.3. Purification of Digested DNA

An efficient way of purifying the digested DNA is using QIAquick PCR purification kits, following in-kit protocols, which is a column-based method.

After purification quantify the digested DNA using a spectrophotometer.

Samples can be stored at −20°C at this stage (see Note 5)

3.4. Ligation of Adaptors to Digested DNA

Combine the following reagents in a microcentrifuge tube and incubate at 16°C for 16 h:

- Digested DNA (500 ng) variable
- Adapter mix 10 μL
- 10× ligase buffer 3 μL
- T4 DNA ligase (400 units) 1 μL
- H_2O to 30 μL

For convenience this incubation is performed overnight from day 2 to the morning of day 3.

3.5. MCA Reaction (see Note 1)

a. Make a master mix by combining the following reagents, allowing four aliquots per sample into 200 μL PCR tubes (see Note 6)

   - QIAGEN 10× buffer 10 μL × 4
   - dNTP mix (25 mM) 1.2 μL × 4
   - HotStarTaq + 1 μL × 4
   - DMSO 5 μL × 4
   - H_2O 75.8 μL × 4

   Aliquot 93 μL per tube, then add 3 μL of ligation reaction (step 4) per tube and incubate at 82°C.

b. Combine the following, incubate at 95°C for 1 min, then add 4 μL to each PCR tube

   - RMCA24 primer 20 μL
   - H_2O 60 μL

c. Use the following conditions for the samples in a thermocycler machine:

- 95°C – 10 mins.
- 95°C – 1 min. } 30 cycles.
- 65°C – 90 secs } 30 cycles.
- 72°C – 2 mins } 30 cycles.
- 72°C – 10 mins.
- 4°C – hold

3.6. Agarose Gel Electrophoresis to Check Sample Quality (see Note 1)

Prepare 1.5% agarose gel and electrophorese 10 μL of each PCR sample to check quality. A relatively strong smear (300 bp to 1 kb) should be visible.

3.7. Purification of PCR Amplicons

The contents of the four tubes per sample should be combined and purified; it is suggested to use the QIAquick PCR purification kit, using manufacturer's instructions. After purification quantify the samples using a spectrophotometer.

3.8. Amplicon Labeling

1. Assemble each labeling reaction in a microcentrifuge tube:
   - MCA PCR product 5 μg (made up to 25 μL with H_2O).
   - Random primer (2.5×) 10 μl

   Incubate at 100°C for 5 min, transfer immediately to ice.

   Note: Where practical, work in the dark from this stage onwards (see Note 7).

   Add to each tube (total volume 50 μL):
   - 10× React2 buffer 5 μL.
   - 10× LowC dNTP mix 5 μL.
   - Cy3-dCTP *or* Cy5-dCTP 3 μL.
   - Klenow or exo-Klenow 2 μL.

   Incubate at 37°C for 2 h.

3.9. Purification of Labeled Samples

The labeled samples should be purified; it is suggested to use the QIAquick PCR purification kit, using manufacturer's instructions, and to elute in 50 μL of ultrapure H_2O. After purification quantify the samples using a spectrophotometer with a microarray setting, measuring each sample dye individually (see Note 7).

3.10. Preparing for Hybridization

Allow Cot1 and 2×SDS hybridization solutions to thaw. Chill ~30 mL of 100% ethanol in a 50 mL centrifuge tube at −20°C.

3.11. Combining Control and Experimental Samples and Reducing Overall Volume

1. Combine equal pmol amounts of each sample (control and experimental sample) (between 250 and 400 pmol each) and make up to 500 μL with H_2O.
2. Reduce volume using microcon YM-30 spin tubes according to the manufacturer's instructions. Bring sample volume to 15 μL with sterile H_2O, if necessary. Hold on ice.

3.12. Hybridization: Sample Preparation

To each sample add:

- Human CotI 10 μL.
- 2× SDS hybridization solution 25 μL.

Mix gently and heat at 95°C for 2 min to denature. Hold at 60°C until hybridization.

3.13. Hybridization: Slide Preparation (see Note 8)

1. Rinse slides at room temperature H_2O.
2. Place slides in boiling water for 1 min.
3. Place slides in chilled ethanol for 1 min.
4. Dry slides by spinning in benchtop slide spinner, and lay in hybridization chamber.
5. Add 50 μL wash 2 solution under each end of the slide.
6. Dip lifter slips in isopropanol, dry with KimWipe, and blow with compressed air.
7. Lay the lifter slips ridge-side-down on the microarray slide.
8. Pipette sample carefully at lifter slip edge, capillary action will draw the sample under.
9. Close chamber tightly, wrap loosely in foil, and incubate in water bath at 60°C for 16 h.

This hybridization incubation stage is carried out overnight from the third day to the morning of the fourth day.

3.14. Washing the Microarrays Prior to Scanning (see Note 9)

Remove lifter slips quickly and gently by dipping the slide in 1× SSC solution; slips should slide off. In rotating hybridization oven using 50 mL centrifuge tubes:

1. Three 15 min washes at 55°C (Wash 1 solution, use new tube for each wash stage).

   On a gyrating platform using staining jars:
2. Two 3 min washes at room temperature (1× SSC solution).
3. Two 3 min washes at room temperature (Wash 2 solution).
4. Two 3 min washes at room temperature (0.1× SSC solution).
5. One 3 min wash at room temperature (Ultrapure H_2O).

3.15. Drying the Microarrays Prior to Scanning (see Note 10)

Rinse by pouring ultrapure water on slide toward the label end of the slide (see Note 11), put slide label end first directly into a 50 mL centrifuge tube with a small amount of absorbent paper towel in the end, with one KimWipe on top to protect the slide from being scratched.

1. Centrifuge at $370 \times g$ for 7 min.
2. Spin in benchtop slide spinner to dry any remaining moisture spots.

3.16. Scanning the Microarrays

If there is a preview option, scan slides to check appearance, then start a full scan. Slides can be rewashed if necessary but often the appearance of the microarrays is not improved by re-washing. Slides can be stored 4°C for up to 24 h in the dark.

4. Notes

1. *RMCA or RXMA primers*

   RMCA primers: RMCA24: 5′-CCACCGCCATCCGAGCCT TTCTGC-3′.

   RMCA12: 5′-CCGGGCAGAAAG-3′.

   RXMA Primers: RXMA24: 5′-AGCACTCTCCAGCCTCTC ACCGAC-3′.

   RXMA12 : 5′-CCGGGTCGGTGA-3′.

   Either set of primers may be used but represent different CpG island subsets therefore consistent use of one primer set is recommended as results differ slightly although specificity and sensitivity are comparable (3).

   Optimization of the MCA PCR reaction (step 5) may be required. DMSO is not required in the PCR reaction if using RXMA primers. When running products by electrophoresis a smear of between 200 bp and 1 kb should be visible for RMCA primers and between 300 bp and 2 kb when using RXMA primers.

2. *Microarray platforms*

   This protocol is optimized for use with Human CpG island 12K Array (HCGI12K) from University Health Network (www.microarrays.ca). Suitable scanning equipment include GenePix scanners (e.g., GenePix 4400A scanner) and software such as GenePix Pro 7 software (MDS Analytical Technologies). Other microarray platforms such as oligonucleotide, tiling, or custom-made arrays also may be used.

3. *Lifter slips*
   Lifter slips (e.g., from Thermo Scientific) are slightly longer and heavier than cover slips and cover the entire UHN HCGI12K microarray surface area.
4. *DNA digestion with lower concentrations of genomic DNA*
   If 5 μg DNA >50 μL, use a 100 μL reaction with 10% buffer, 5 μL *SmaI* and variable water.
5. *Freezing samples at stages throughout the protocol*
   When working with many samples it may be convenient to store samples at certain stages throughout the protocol as factors such as the number of hybridization chambers may limit how many samples can be processed fully simultaneously. It is advisable to limit the number of stages that samples are frozen at and to keep the freezing stages consistent for groups of samples such as time courses.
6. *Performing 4 MCA reactions per sample*
   It is necessary to prepare 4 MCA PCR reactions per sample to have an adequate amount of amplicons to proceed with the labeling. It is sometimes enough to perform fewer PCR reactions but the amplicon yield may be too low to continue.
7. *Characteristics of fluorochromes Cy3 and Cy5*
   Cy3 and Cy5 (used for labeling control and experimental samples respectively) are sensitive to light and therefore it is recommended to work in the dark as much as possible in order to maintain standards. Cy3 is a pink reagent and is used to label control samples. Cy5 is a blue reagent and is used to label the experimental sample.

   When quantifying labeled sample using a spectrophotometer the following should be used:

   - Cy3: Absorbance maximum = 550 nm; emission maximum = 570 nm.
   - Cy5: Absorbance maximum = 649 nm; emission maximum = 670 nm.

8. *Preparation of microarray slide*
   The method of preparation may depend on the microarray platform used. See manufacturer's instructions.
9. *Washing the microarray slide prior to scanning*
   This stage is important for improving the quality of the scanned slide. A mix of washes of varying degrees of stringency helps to decrease background and remove un-hybridized sample.
10. *Drying the microarray slide prior to scanning*
   The slides must be dry before inserting into the microarray scanner. It is important that the slides dry uniformly and quickly to prevent moisture marks on the slide.

11. *Microarrays with labels*
Microarray slides with labels attached tend to absorb sample. It is advisable to rinse the slide with the water directed toward the label so that un-hybridized dyes are not streaked across the microarray surface on the final washes.

References

1. Estecio, M. R., Yan, P. S., Ibrahim, A. E., Tellez, C. S., Shen, L., Huang, T. H., and Issa, J. P. (2007) High-throughput methylation profiling by MCA coupled to CpG island microarray, *Genome Res* 17, 1529–1536.
2. Toyota, M., Ho, C., Ahuja, N., Jair, K. W., Li, Q., Ohe-Toyota, M., Baylin, S. B., and Issa, J. P. (1999) Identification of differentially methylated sequences in colorectal cancer by methylated CpG island amplification, *Cancer Res* 59, 2307–2312.
3. Estécio, M. R. H., Yan, P. S., Huang, T. H-M., Issa, J-P. J. (2008) Methylated CpG Island Amplification and Microarray (MCAM) for high-throughput analysis of DNA methylation, in *Cold Spring Harb. Protoc.*, Cold Spring Harbor Laboratory Press, Cold Spring Harbor.
4. Hatada, I., Fukasawa, M., Kimura, M., Morita, S., Yamada, K., Yoshikawa, T., Yamanaka, S., Endo, C., Sakurada, A., Sato, M., Kondo, T., Horii, A., Ushijima, T., and Sasaki, H. (2006) Genome-wide profiling of promoter methylation in human, *Oncogene* 25, 3059–3064.

Part IV

Factors that Influence the Epigenetic Changes in Cancer

Chapter 22

Nutrigenomics: Implications for Breast and Colon Cancer Prevention

Gabriela Riscuta and Ramona G. Dumitrescu

Abstract

Nutrigenomics refers to the interaction between one's diet and his/her genes. These interactions can markedly influence digestion, absorption, and the elimination of bioactive food components, as well as influence their site of actions/molecular targets. Nutrigenomics comprises nutrigenetics, epigenetics, and transcriptomics, coupled with other "omic," such as proteomics and metabolomics, that apparently account for the wide variability in cancer risk among individuals with similar dietary habits. Multiple food components including essential nutrients, phytochemical, zoochemicals, fungochemical, and bacterochemicals have been implicated in cancer risk and tumor behavior, admittedly with mixed results. Such findings suggest that not all individuals respond identically to a diet. This chapter highlights the influence of single-nucleotide polymorphism, copy number, epigenetic events, and transcriptomic homeostasis as factors influencing the response to food components and ultimately health, including cancer risk. Both breast and colorectal cancers are reviewed as examples about how nutrigenomics may influence the response to dietary intakes. As the concept that "one size fits all" comes to an end and personalized approaches surface, additional research data will be required to identify those who will benefit most from dietary change and any who might be placed at risk because of an adjustment.

Key words: Nutrigenomics, Nutrigenetics, Cancer prevention, Breast cancer, Colon cancer, Methylation

1. Introduction

Nutrigenomics is the scientific study by which specific genes and bioactive food components interact. It provides a fundamental foundation for understanding how the health consequences of eating behaviors may vary across individuals. The concept of nutrigenomics builds on the premise that:

- Diet and dietary components can alter the risk of disease by modulating multiple processes involved with the onset, incidence, progression, and/or severity

Ramona G. Dumitrescu and Mukesh Verma (eds.), *Cancer Epigenetics: Methods and Protocols*, Methods in Molecular Biology, vol. 863, DOI 10.1007/978-1-61779-612-8_22, © Springer Science+Business Media, LLC 2012

- Food components can act on the human genome, either directly or indirectly, to alter the expression of genes and gene products
- The health consequences of a diet are dependent on the balance of health and disease states and on an individual's genetic background (1)

In addition to a great diversity in the inherited genome between ethnic groups and individuals which influences nutrient bioavailability and metabolism, two central factors which underpin nutrigenomics are that people differ greatly in their food/nutrient availability and choices depending on cultural, economical, geographical, and taste perception differences, and that inappropriate nutrition (deficiency or excess) can affect genome stability leading to mutations or chromosomal instability which influences gene expression and may lead to phenotypic changes throughout life. Overall, the study of nutrigenomics and associated changes in proteomics and metabolomics will ultimately identify molecular targets for nutritional preemption. This information is essential to development of a personalized approach to nutrition, which will ultimately allow for the identification of positive responders, nonresponders, and negative responders to dietary intervention strategies. A personalized approach will require an assessment of not only the individual's genetic background but also his/her health and nutritional status, and nutritional needs based on age, body composition, work, and physical activities. The integration of data collected from genomic, proteomic, and metabolomic analyses will be a key in defining a "nutritional phenotype" and thus targeted intervention strategies (2).

Nutrients and nonnutritive dietary components are being examined for their effects on human metabolism and diseases, including coronary heart disease (CHD), hypertension, diabetes, and cancer. It is increasingly apparent that multiple dietary constituents are capable of modifying, either increasing or decreasing, cancer risk and tumor behavior. These bioactive food components may arise from plants (phytochemical), animal sources (zoochemicals), mushrooms (fungochemicals), or from the metabolism of food components by bacteria within the gastrointestinal tract (bacterochemicals) (3–5).

In the past 2 decades, increasing attention has been given to the importance of genetic variation, and gene–nutrient interactions for establishing the nutritional needs and for prevention/therapy strategies for reducing chronic diseases (6–8). Based on these studies genetic susceptibility has been identified for different types of cancers including breast, colon, prostate, and lung cancers, for lupus, age-related macular degeneration, diabetes, and Crohn's disease (9). Actually, it is increasingly difficult in finding a disease/condition that does not have a genetic link. Nutrigenetics is a term used to describe the impact that the genetic code has on the ability of a food component to influence growth, development, and disease resistance. Fluctuations caused by genetic polymorphism, variation in copy number, deletion, insertions, or translocations can influence the magnitude and sometime direction of the response to food components. Similar to pharmacogenetics, nutrigenetics seeks to optimize the health benefits of tailored interventions based on an individual's genetic background (10).

In 2007, the World Cancer Research Fund/American Institute for Cancer Research (WCRF/AICR) concluded that fruits and non-starchy vegetables probably protect against some types of cancers including the mouth, larynx, pharynx, esophagus, and stomach cancer and that allium vegetables and garlic probably protect against stomach cancer. Also, fruits show a protective effect against lung cancer (11). This chapter will review some of these findings and suggest that nutrigenomics likely accounts for the variation in findings across epidemiological and controlled intervention studies.

2. Multiple Cellular Processes Are Influenced by Genetics and Foods

All major signaling pathways are deregulated in cancer, including cell proliferation, apoptosis, DNA repair, carcinogen metabolism, inflammation, immunity, differentiation, and angiogenesis. Increasingly, evidence points to each of these as molecular targets for cancer prevention. Since several of these sites appear to be modified by multiple dietary components, it becomes challenging to tease apart nutrient–nutrient interactions and thus what constitutes an ideal diet for health promotion (12). For example, the apoptosis or programmed cell death, that is essential in the fight against cancer through two pathways either the intrinsic, mitochondrial-mediated pathway or the extrinsic, death receptor-mediated pathway could be a target for dietary bioactive agents including genistein, curcumin, resveratrol, luteolin, lupeol, indole 3-carbinol, etc. (13, 14). Dietary components can modulate apoptosis through effects at different levels all of which culminate in changes in gene expression. However, biological systems are very complex and exhibit properties that extend far beyond observations associated with one single cellular process. Therefore, it is critical to evaluate the multiple cancer-related processes simultaneously.

3. New Technologies

In the past decade, DNA microarray technology has been widely used for the studies of functional genomics, systems biology, and pharmacogenomics (15). DNA microarray technology is a powerful tool for the evaluation of gene expression in different tissues, especially in response to factors that can modify these expression profiles. In addition, this technology together with bioinformatics tools is used in nutrigenomics studies of the interaction between nutrients and/or other dietary bioactive compounds and the genome in order to understand how nutrients influence gene expression. The use of these technologies may provide information that can be used to improve one's diet and to discover new agents that may prevent or treat diseases including cancer (16). For example, caloric restriction is one of the most consistent approaches to reduce experimentally induced cancer. Recent gene expression microarray analysis of visceral white adipose tissue revealed 209 genes responsive to both caloric restriction and treadmill exercise, relative to a diet-induced obesity in female mice group. Interestingly, caloric restriction uniquely altered expression of an additional 496 genes (17). Of the genes distinctly responsive to caloric restriction, 17 were related to carbohydrate metabolism and glucose transport, including glucose transporter 4.

Soy intake has been reported in some cases to be linked to a reduction in breast cancer risk. Recently, Satih et al. identified 278 and 334 differentially expressed genes after treatment with two soy constituents, genistein or daidzein, respectively, in estrogen-positive (MCF-7) and estrogen-negative (MDA-MB-231, MCF-10a) cells (18). Hierarchical clustering of this data revealed significant shifts in the molecular pathways that relate to cell communication, biodegradation of xenobiotics, lipid metabolism, signal transduction, and cell growth/death. While these examples provide clues about molecular targets, it must be noted that the response is highly dependent on the amount of the bioactive component examined and the duration of the exposure to cells, animals or humans. Thus, these are windows and any interpretation must be done with caution.

The cytokinesis-block micronucleus cytome (CBMN cyt) assay is a new technique used to measure DNA damage, cytostasis, and cytotoxicity in different tissue types, including lymphocytes. The DNA damage events scored include micro-nuclei (MNi), a biomarker of chromosome loss and/or chromosome breakage; nucleoplasmic bridges (NPBs), a biomarker of DNA misrepair and/or telomere end-fusions; and nuclear buds (NBUDs), a biomarker of elimination of amplified DNA and/or DNA repair complexes. Cytostatic effects are measured via the proportion of mono-, bi-, and multinucleated cells and cytotoxicity via necrotic and/or apoptotic cell ratios.

The assay has been applied to the biomonitoring of in vivo exposure to genotoxins, in vitro genotoxicity testing, and in nutrigenomics and pharmacogenomics (19). Dose–response curves for the impact of many individual nutrients on DNA damage are beginning to be studied in more detail. While folate and selenium have been examined in more detail, other food components deserve the same attention (20). The micronuclei index differs with age and gender, but the impact of these variables on bioavailability and metabolism of specific nutrients, and genetic backgrounds has not been determined and is essential for the advancement of personalized nutrition.

Most of the studies done in nutrition research have focused on few genetic variants at a time and on the opportunity to modify the risk associated with these genetic variants by different nutritional interventions. Lately, much more it is known about genetic variation, especially after microarrays containing around 500,000 single nucleotide polymorphisms (SNPs) (500K arrays) became available. For example, the Cancer Genetic Markers of Susceptibility (CGEMS) project is currently using these chips to identify candidate loci for cancer. When disease-association studies will validate specific SNPs microarrays, further information could be obtained to fully understand the interaction between nutrition and these SNPs so that targeted interventions could be provided for prevention (21).

4. Epigenetics Changes

Epigenetics can also modify genetic expressions without a change in the DNA sequence. Site-specific hypomethylation is commonly found in cancer cells and is usually associated with increased oncogene expression. CpG region methylation may limit transcription factors' ability to bind a specific DNA sequence and consequently leads to gene silencing. DNA hypomethylation, for the same reason, may be associated with gene activation. As there are more than 500 genes implicated in cancer developing, needless to debate over the importance of these genes methylation status.

Bioactive food components may influence DNA methylation through several mechanisms including providing methyl groups for *S*-adenosylmethionine (SAM) synthesis, participating in DNA demethylation, and DNA methyltransferase activity. Cells' response to food components will be influenced by DNA methylation status. Moderate folate deficiency has been reported by Jacob et al. to reduce DNA methylation. Hypomethylation was reversed by increased plasma folate concentrations using food folate (22). Severe induced folate deficiency in rats leads to *p53* and global DNA hypomethylation in the liver (23), and also dietary selenium and zinc deficiency may induce DNA hypomethylation (24, 25). In utero, changes in epigenetics may be influenced by maternal diet and may cause relatively stable changes in gene expression in mice and predispose the offspring to multiple diseases (26, 27). In agouti mice feeding a methyl donor supplemented diet is accompanied by marked changes in methylation patterns and with a reduction in obesity and increased longevity (27).

Histone regulation is another important epigenetic regulator. Histones posttranslational modifications, relatively stable alterations may influence chromatin structure. Histone hyperacetylation of specific sites may be associated with active chromatin while histone deacetylation may associate with inactive chromatin and gene silencing. The global loss of monoacetylation and trimethylation of histone H4 is a common hallmark of human tumor cells (28). Several food items including butyrate, allyl sulfur, and sulforaphane have been found to modify histone deacetylase activity (29, 30).

5. Breast Cancer

Breast cancer is the second leading cause of cancer-related deaths among women in most Western countries (31). Among all breast cancer cases, only 5–10% cases are believed to be due to inherited susceptibility and thus environmental factors including one's eating habits are likely major contributors to risk.

Mutations in two genes *BRCA1* and *BRCA2* are associated with familial cases of early-onset breast cancer (32). Other germline mutations in *p53* gene, cell cycle-checkpoint kinase gene (*CHEK2*) as well as *PTEN* gene were associated with familial cases of breast cancer. Diet may be an important modifier even for those with increased susceptibility. A number of nutritional factors have been examined for their role in the etiology of breast cancer in vulnerable population. In a case–control study in a French–Canadian population, it was observed that consumption of fruits and vegetables in *BRCA* mutations carriers may be associated with reduced breast cancer risk with a case-odds ratio equal to 0.27 (33). Another study examined the influence of *BRCA1/BRCA2* expression in mammary cells following genistein exposure (34, 35). It was found that when genistein 50 μg daily is provided in the diet prepubertal leads to increased *BRCA1* expression in the mammary gland (36), lowering the risk of mammary gland malignant transformation. While intriguing, these findings need to be confirmed in humans.

Understanding the relationship between diet and breast cancer, especially among sporadic cancers, may provide information not only about breast cancer pathogenesis but also targets for the prevention strategies. Several studies of sporadic breast cancers have shown that fruits and vegetables (37), fish, monounsaturated and polyunsaturated fatty acids (38, 39), vitamin D, calcium, and phytoestrogens may reduce the risk of breast cancer, although there are inconsistencies in the literature (40). High intake of meat, poultry, total energy, and total fat and saturated fatty acids has been reported to be associated with increased risk for breast cancer (40), again with considerable variability in the literature. In the Women's Healthy Eating and Living (WHEL) randomized trial, it has been observed that high intake of vegetables, fruit, and fiber and low intake in fat did not reduce breast cancer recurrence or mortality among early-stage breast cancer survivors (41).

When the association between meat consumption and breast cancer was analyzed in a nested case–control study among postmenopausal women included in the "Diet, Cancer and Health" cohort study, it has been found that the association between meat consumption and breast cancer risk is limited to carriers of a genetic variant for the *N*-acetyl transferase 2 polymorphism (42), again pointing to the likelihood that not all may be equally susceptible to risk.

Folic acid is an essential nutrient and required for a host of biological reactions. Folate deficiency may impair de novo biosynthesis of purines and thymidylate and thereby disrupt DNA and RNA metabolism, homocysteine remethylation, methionine biosynthesis, and subsequent formation of SAM (the universal methyl donor) which in turn may lead to altered methylation reactions. This impaired folate-dependent intracellular metabolism can lead to several key pathologies including, for example, megaloblastic anemia, homocysteinemia, cardiovascular disease, embryonic defects, in particular neural tube defects (NTDs), congenital heart defects, and cancer. The association between folate intake and breast cancer has been reported to be modified by genetic variants of one-carbon metabolism genes, especially the folate-metabolizing enzyme methylenetetrahydrofolate reductase (MTHFR). Malmö Diet and Cancer cohort examined the association between dietary folate equivalents (DFE) and breast cancer among carriers of two genetic polymorphisms for *MTHFR* gene (*MTHFR* 677C/T and 1298A/C). A positive association between DFE and breast cancer among women carriers of *MTHFR* 677CT/TT-1298AA occurred while an inverse association was observed in 677CT-1298AC women (43). In a nested case–control study, Maruti et al. reported that postmenopausal women with two copies of variant T alleles (TT genotype) had increased risk of breast cancer. In addition, the intake of other B vitamins may influence the relationship between the MTHFR genetic variants and breast cancer risk. It has been found that the most pronounced MTHFR-breast cancer risk was observed among women with the lowest intakes of dietary folate and vitamin B6 (44).

Furthermore, the MTHFR C677T mutation was found to induce cell-specific changes in genomic DNA methylation and uracil misincorporation, suggesting the molecular basis for the breast cancer risk modification (45).

In a nested case–control study within the Singapore Chinese Health Study, it has been observed that there is an inverse relationship between breast cancer risk and low folate intake and weekly/daily green tea intake compared with reduced green tea intake. Also, women carrying the high-activity *MTHFR/TYMS* genotypes with 0–1 variant allele and weekly/daily green tea intake had a lower breast cancer risk, especially women who also had low folate intake. No association was observed among women carriers of two variant alleles. These findings suggest one of the mechanism through which green tea can provide protection against breast cancer is through folate regulation (10).

The anticancer effect of the EGCG (tea polyphenol (−)-epigallocatechin-3-gallate) may be mediated by the regulation of epigenetic processes. It was found that EGCG can lead to ERα reactivation in the ERα negative breast cancer cell lines by remodeling the chromatin structure of the ERα promoter by the alteration of the histone acetylation and methylation status (46). Further, it has been reported that EGCG inhibits the telomerase by decreasing the hTERT promoter methylation and ablating the histone H3 Lys9 acetylation in the MCF-7 cell lines (47).

Another study reported the inverse relationship between green tea intake and breast cancer risk among Asian-Americans (48) as a function of the catechol-*O*-methyltransferase (*COMT*) genotype. This enzyme is recognized to be involved in the metabolism of the tea polyphenols. More specifically, a reduced risk of breast cancer was observed only among tea (green and black) drinkers carriers of at least one low-activity *COMT* allele. These findings of reduced breast cancer risk with tea catechins, especially in women who had the low activity *COMT* alleles, suggest that these women were less efficient in eliminating tea catechins so therefore optimizing the benefits from the tea and its associated bioactive constituent (49).

The Shanghai Breast Cancer Study examined the relationship between breast cancer risk, *GSTP1* genetic variants, and other diet components, the cruciferous vegetables. The *GSTP1* Val/Val genotype was associated with increased breast cancer risk, especially in premenopausal women with low intake of cruciferous vegetables. Thus, cruciferous vegetable intake with high isothiocyanates may reduce breast cancer risk and modify the effect of the *GSTP1* genotype (50) and not necessarily be beneficial to all women. Finally, the response to marine *n*-3 fatty acids with breast cancer risk may depend on genetics. Women with genetic variants that encode lower or no enzymatic activity of GSTT1 have a 30% lower breast cancer risk from the marine-3 fatty acids, when compared with women with high activity genotypes. These data suggest that the peroxidation products of *n*-3 fatty acids may be involved in the protection against breast cancer (50). This is not that unusual since other food components have been reported to inhibit tumors by generating free radicals (51, 52). Watercress, a rich source of phenethyl isothiocyanates (PEITC), has been proposed to have anticancer activity. A crude watercress extract was reported to inhibit cancer cell growth and hypoxia-inducible factor (HIF) activity and reduced angiogenesis by decreasing the phosphorylation of the translation regulator 4E binding protein 1 (4E-BP1) (53).

In a breast case–control study that examined the association of the 5-lipoxygenase gene (*ALOX5*) and 5-lipoxygenase-activating protein gene (*ALOX5AP*) polymorphisms and dietary linoleic acid intake with breast cancer risk, it was found that women carriers of two variant alleles for the *ALOX5AP* 4900 A/G who had a diet rich in linoleic acid had a greater breast cancer risk compared with women carrying AG or GG genotypes. These results suggest that genetic predisposition related to *n*-6 polyunsaturated fatty acid metabolism should be taken into account when the relation between dietary fat and breast cancer risk is examined (54).

Moreover, dietary omega-3 polyunsaturated fatty acids downregulate the expression of the polycomb group (PcG) protein, enhancer of zeste homologue 2 (EZH2) in breast cancer cells. This study reported a decrease in histone 3 lysine 27 trimethylation (H3K27me3) activity of EZH2 and upregulation of E-cadherin and insulin-like growth factor-binding protein 3. The treatment with omega-3 PUFAs led to decrease in the invasion capacity of the breast cancer cells (55).

Additionally, a nested case–control study of postmenopausal women examined the interaction between oxidative stress-related genes including catalase (CAT) C262T, myeloperoxidase (*MPO*) G463A, endothelial nitric oxide synthase (*NOS3*) G894T, and heme oxygenase-1 (*HO-1*) GT (*n*) dinucleotide length polymorphism and level of vegetable and fruit intake on breast cancer risk. The study found that women with low intake of vegetables and fruits and the low-risk *CAT CC* genotypes appeared to be associated with increased breast cancer risk, especially those women with four or more low-risk alleles, suggestive of the role of endogenous and exogenous antioxidants in breast carcinogenesis (56).

Iwasaki et al. examined the effect of four SNPs in cytochrome P450c17alpha (*CYP17*), aromatase (*CYP19*), 17beta-hydroxysteroid dehydrogenase type I (*17beta-HSD1*), and sex hormone-binding globulin (*SHBG*) genes on the association between isoflavone intake and breast cancer risk. The study identified an inverse association between isoflavone intake and breast cancer risk among women with at least one variant allele for the *17beta-HSD1* polymorphism and among postmenopausal Japanese women with GG genotype for *SHBG* gene, indicating that genetic variants of the *17beta-HSD1* and *SHBG* genes may modify the relationship between isoflavone intake and breast cancer risk (57).

The association between isoflavones and breast cancer risk may be explained by the antiestrogenic effect of the isoflavones and the effect on the DNA methylation. It has been reported that the daily administration of isoflavones to healthy premenopausal women led to dose-specific changes in *RARbeta2* and *CCND2* gene promoter methylation, changes that correlated with genistein levels. Additionally, an inverse correlation between estrogenic marker complement C3 and genistein was observed suggesting an antiestrogenic effect (58).

Furthermore, genistein has been associated with specific epigenetic changes. For example, the long-term exposure to genistein of the MCF-7 breast cancer cell lines has been found to lead to reduced expression of the acetylated histone 3 (H3). Additionally, this exposure was associated with alteration in growth responses to mitogenic factors and histone deacetylase inhibitors (59).

Dietary berries have been proposed to influence breast cancer risk (AICR Report), although considerable variability in response is observed. Preclinical studies demonstrate that tumor formation is suppressed as a result of the levels of E(2)-metabolizing enzymes during the early phase of E(2) carcinogenesis (60).

Environmental exposures other than the diet may also influence breast cancer risk. Recently, a Western diet and associated exposure to heterocyclic amines such as 2-amino-1-methyl-6-phenylimidazo [4,5-b]pyridine (PhIP), a genotoxic carcinogen derived from cooked meat, has been proposed to be associated with increased breast cancer risk. While the mechanism is still being examined, it may be due to the estrogenic properties of PhIP that can also influence metastatic potential. The PhIP-induced invasive phenotype was associated with expression of cathepsin D, cyclooxygenase-2, and matrix metalloproteinase activity, suggesting the effect of this component from cooked meat on mammary gland-specific carcinogenesis (61).

6. Colorectal Cancer

Worldwide, over one million cases of colorectal cancer (CRC) were reported in 2002, with a 50% mortality rate, making CRC the second most common cancer in adults (62). Similar to other cancers, complex interaction between nutrients and genes occur. Several nutrients have been implicated in the risk of CRC including folate, vitamin D, butyrate, calcium, selenium, curcumin, etc.

Inadequate intake of folate has been found to be linked to an increase in CRC risk. However, not all individuals appear to have the same response to folate deficiency. Genetic polymorphism MTHFR at 677TT appears to determine beneficial effect at least in some individuals (62). Several studies, but not all, reveal the

TT genotype is associated with decreased risk, particularly in combination with high dietary folate (21). In addition, interactions between riboflavin availability may have a role in risk since it is required for the folate bioactivation. Many genes are involved with folate metabolism, so the number of polymorphisms is huge and makes the assessment of biological response difficult. It has been hypothesized that a temporal relationship between folic acid fortification of food in the 1980s and the increase in cancer of the colon in the 1990s may be related to the promoting effects of folate on tumor growth and is a concern that provision of folate could increase tumorigenesis among individuals with existing preneoplastic lesions of the colon and rectum (12).

Moreover, changes to folate intake appear to be capable of modulating DNA methylation levels in the human colonic mucosa and this may potentially alter CRC risk (63). Some other factors beside folate level/supplementation may play important roles as cancer risk modifiers. Folate supplementation, 5 mg/day in patients with resected colonic adenomas, was associated with a decreased degree of DNA methylation in patient with one single polyp and in patients with multiple lesions caloric and fat intake show a more determinant role (64). It seems that although DNA methylation status is an important factor in colon cancer risk, it is difficult to establish a clear relation between this type of cancer, its location on the right or on the left side, and folate status and DNA methylation (65).

Glutathione *S*-transferase (GSTs) is another enzyme that is likely involved with overall CRC risk. It is involved in phase II detoxification process of drugs and endogenous compounds. GSTM1 and GSTT1 null genotypes confer additional risk for CRC in Caucasian populations while the association in Chinese subjects was not significant (66). Could diet be a reason why GSTs surface in some but not all populations? Does the frequency of the mutation vary among these populations? In some cancers, like CRC, a polymorphism in the vitamin D receptor (VDR) may serve as a predictive marker for those who will benefit most from ensuring adequate intakes of dietary fat or calcium (67). Among those with either low calcium or low fat intake (below the median values in controls), the risk for CRC increased in a gene-dose-dependent manner such that individuals possessing the ff genotype displayed an approximately 2.5-fold increased risk that was statistically significant (67). The findings suggest that the effect was present only in deficient diet and disappeared once the inadequacy was corrected.

Further, there are in utero epigenetic events that may play a role in vitamin D feedback catabolism, maximizing active vitamin D bioavailability at the feto-maternal interface. No methylation of the *VDR* and *CYP27B1* genes was found in any placental tissues but *CYP24A1*, *CYP27B1*, and *VDR* genes were hypermethylated in choriocarcinoma cell lines (68).

The association of colorectal polyps with intake of calcium, magnesium, or both and Thr1482Ile polymorphism in the TRPM7 gene is modified by the Ca:Mg intake (69). This is a complex interrelationship, and it remains unclear as to what are the ideal absolute amounts and/or ratio need to maximize benefits. In the Tennessee Colorectal Polyp Study, an increased intake of magnesium was associated with decreased risk of colorectal adenoma. The risk of hyperplastic polyps is increased by Thr1482Ile polymorphism. The subject who carried one or more 1482Ile allele and who consumed diets with a high Ca:Mg intake were at a higher risk of adenoma and hyperplasic polyps than were the subjects who did not carry the polymorphism (69).

The increased risk of CRC to meat has been reported to vary with polymorphisms in several Cytochrome P450 genes (70). These data suggest a particularly vulnerable population exists and depending on number selected for epidemiological studies there might or might not be a relationship with meat intake. Clearly these types of gene–food interactions need to be examined as determinants of risk at several cancer sites.

An accepted risk factor for CRC in some population is high intake of red meat especially when cooked at high temperature and/or contains *N*-nitroso compounds. Base excision repair (BER) pathway, as a DNA repair mechanism may modify the risk for CRC in subjects consuming higher amounts of meat. Four BER genes were found statistically significant in population eating meat cooked at high temperature: *APEX1* Gln51His, Asp148Glu; *OGG1* Ser236Cys; *PARP* Val742Ala; *XRCC1* Arg194Trp, Arg280His, Arg399Gln (70). While fat intake increases the *APC* D1822V-adenoma association, further studies are warranted (71). Overall, it is likely that several genes may be involved in the increased risk of CRC and that all individuals are not equally susceptible to disease as a consequence of exaggerated intakes.

Curcumin, the active ingredient in curry powder, potentially modifies gene expression and may play a role in cancer prevention and treatment. A multitude of preclinical studies have demonstrated antioxidant and anti-inflammatory effects of curcumin through downregulating constitutive NfkB and Il-8 (72, 73). Interestingly, the evidence is strongest in CRC than other cancer sites but it is unclear why this is so unless it relates to exposures to the mucosa due to poor bioavailability. Recently, curcumin was found to inhibit the transcriptional regulation of miR-21 via AP-1; suppresses cell proliferation, tumor growth, invasion, and in vivo metastasis; and stabilizes expression of tumor suppressor Pdcd4 in CRC (74). The development of curcumin for clinical use as a regulator of epigenetic changes, however, needs further investigation to determine novel and effective chemopreventive strategies, either alone or in combination with other anticancer agents, for improving cancer treatment (75).

Other risk factors include obesity per se or hypercaloric diet. It is not clear if this effect is a direct stimulatory effect on the neoplasma or secondary to hormonal changes including changes in insulin. It should be noted the response to calories is mixed between a BMI of 25 and 30 but increases 20% or more above 30. These findings suggest that obesity per se may be insensitive to monitor risk and thus changes in bioenergetics may be better indicators. Available data about alcohol consumption also indicate a possible risk-increasing effect (76). Whether this relates to energetic or to improved solubility of potential carcinogens remains an active area of investigation—something about bioenergetics and maybe associated genetics is logical to induce. Overall, several food items are implicated in CRC risk. However, it is clear that not all individuals respond identically to these food items or components. A more comprehensive review about the relationship with diet is provided in the WCRF/AICR report (11).

7. Conclusions

Nutrigenomics will change the way scientists and healthcare providers understand the effect of diet as a cancer prevention tool and lead toward personalized diet as "one size fits all" is coming to an end. Yet, at this time we do not have all the knowledge needed to design an appropriate personalized diet.

Developments in nutrigenetics, epigenomics, transcriptomics, proteomics, and metabolomics will help with the understanding of a more comprehensive picture of key regulatory sites in normal and cancerous cells. This knowledge will help identify those individuals, who will benefit most or be placed at risk due to dietary change, important for the development of personalized diets with minimal adverse events.

References

1. Büchner, F.L., Bueno-de-Mesquita, H.B., Ros, M.M. et al. (2009) Consumption of vegetables and fruit and the risk of bladder cancer in the European Prospective Investigation into Cancer and Nutrition. *Int J Cancer* 125, 2643–2651.
2. Migianno, G.A. and De Sanctis, R. (2006) Nutritional Genomics :toward a personalized diet. *Clin Ter* 157, 355–361.
3. Milner, J.A. (2004) Molecular targets for bioactive food components. *J Nutr* 134, 2492S–2498S.
4. Tan, A.C., Konczak, I, Sze, D.M., et al. (2011) Molecular pathways for cancer chemoprevention by dietary phytochemicals. *Nutr Cancer* 63, 495–505.
5. Newman, D.J. and Cragg, G.M. (2009) Microbial antitumor drugs: natural products of microbial origin as anticancer agents. *Curr Opin Investig Drugs* 10, 1280–1296.
6. Fenech, M., El-Sohemy, A., Cahill, L., et al. (2011) Nutrigenetics and Nutrigenomics: Viewpoints on the Current Status and Applications in Nutrition Research and Practice. *J Nutrigenet Nutrigenomics* 28, 69–89.
7. Ross, S.A. (2010) Evidence for the relationship between diet and cancer. *Exp Oncol* 32, 137–142.

8. Trujillo, E., Davis, C., and Milner, J. (2010) Nutrigenomics, proteomics, metabolomics, and the practice of dietetics. *J Am Diet Assoc* 106, 403–443.
9. Simopoulos, A.P. (2010) Genetic variants in the metabolism of omega-6 and omega-3 fatty acids: their role in the determination of nutritional requirements and chronic disease risk. *Exp Biol Med* 235,785–795.
10. Inoue, M., Robien, K., Wang, R., et al. (2008) Green tea intake, MTHFR/TYMS genotype and breast cancer risk: the Singapore Chinese Health Study. *Carcinogenesis* 1967–1972.
11. World Cancer Research Fund/American Institute for Cancer Research. *Food, Nutrition, Physical Activity, and the Prevention of Cancer: A Global Perspective.* 2007. American Institute for Cancer Research, Washington, DC. Retrieved February 20, 2009, from: http://www.dietandcancerreport.org.
12. Milner, J.A., Romagnolo, D.F., et al. (2010) *Bioactive compounds and Cancer* 45–46, 393, 469–496, 580.
13. Martin, K.R. (2007) Using nutrigenomics to evaluate apoptosis as a preemptive target in cancer prevention. *Curr Cancer Drug Targets* 7, 438–446.
14. Davis, C.D., Emenaker, N.J., and Milner, J.A. (2010) Cellular proliferation, apoptosis and angiogenesis: molecular targets for nutritional preemption of cancer. *Semin Oncol* 37, 243–257.
15. Teng, X. and Xiao, H. (2009) Perspectives of DNA microarray and next-generation DNA sequencing technologies. *Sci China C Life Sci* 52, 7–16.
16. Masotti, A., Da Sacco, L, Bottazzo, G.F., et al. (2010) Microarray technology: a promising tool in nutrigenomics. *Crit Rev Food Sci Nutr* 50, 693–698.
17. Wheatley, K.E., Nogueira, L.M., Perkins, S.N., et. al (2011) Differential effects of calorie restriction and exercise on the adipose transcriptome in diet-induced obese mice. *J Obes* 2011, 265417.
18. Satih, S., Chalabi, N., Rabiau, N., et al. (2010) Gene expression profiling of breast cancer cell lines in response to soy isoflavones using a pangenomic microarray approach. *OMICS* 14, 231–238.
19. Thomas, P. and Fenech, M. (2011) Cytokinesis-block micronucleus cytome assay in lymphocytes. *Methods Mol Biol* 682, 217–234.
20. Bull, C.F., Beetstra-Hill, S., Benassi-Evans, B.J., et al. (2011) Application and adaptation of the in vitro micronucleus assay for the assessment of nutritional requirements of cells for DNA damage prevention. *Mutagenesis* 26, 193–197.
21. Davis, C.D. (2007) Nutrigenomics and the prevention of colon cancer. *Pharmacogenomics* 8, 121–124.
22. Jacob, R.A., Gretz, D.M., Taylor, P.C., et al. (1995) Moderate folate depletion increases plasma homocysteine and decreases lymphocyte DNA methylation in postmenopausal women. *Cancer Res* 55, 1894–901.
23. Pogribny, I.P., Basnakian., A.G., Miller, B.J, et al. (1995) Breaks in genomic DNA and within the p53 gene are associated with hypomethylation in livers of folate/methyl-deficient rats. *Cancer Res* 55, 1894–1901.
24. Wallwork, J.C. and Duerre, J.A. (1985) Effect of zinc deficiency on methionine metabolism, methylation reaction and protein synthesis in isolated perfused rat liver. *J.Nutr* 115, 252–262.
25. Davis, C.D., Uthus, E.O., and Finley, J.W. (2000) Dietary selenium and arsenic affect DNA methylation in vitro in Caco -2 cells and in vivo in rat liver and colon. *J Nutr* 130, 2903–2909.
26. Wolff,G.L., Kodell, R.L., Moore, S.R., et al. (1998) Maternal epigenetics and methyl supplements affect agouti gene expression in Avy/a mice. *FASEB J* 12, 949–957.
27. Cooney, C.A., Dave, A.A., and Wolff, G.L. (2002) Maternal methyl supplements in mice affect epigenetic variation and DNA methylation of offspring. *J Nutr* 132, 2393 S–2400 S.
28. Fraga, M.F., Ballestar, E., and Villar-Garea, A. (2005) Loss of acetylation at Lys16 and trimethylation at Lys20 of histone H4 is a common hallmark of human cancer. *Nat Genet* 37, 391–400.
29. Ho, E, Clarke, J.D., and Dashwood, R.H. (2009) Dietary sulforaphane, a histone deacetylase inhibitor for cancer prevention. *J Nutr* 139, 2393–2396.
30. Nian, H., Delage, B., Ho, E., et al. (2009) Modulation of histone deacetylase activity by dietary isothiocyanates and allyl sulfides: studies with sulforaphane and garlic organosulfur compounds. *Environ Mol Mutagen* 50, 213–221.
31. American Cancer Society. Cancer Facts and Figures 2010. (2010). Atlanta, Georgia, American Cancer Society.
32. http://www.cancer.gov/clinicaltrials/results/summary/2010/prophylactic-surgery0910
33. Ghadirian, P., Narod, S., and Fafard, E. (2009) Breast cancer risk in relation to the joint effect of BRCA mutations and diet diversity. *Breast Cancer Res Treat* 117, 417–422.
34. Vissac-Sabatier, C., Bignon, Y.J., and Bernard–Gallon, D.J. (2003) Effects on the phytoestrogens genistein and daidzein on BRCA2 tumor

suppressor gene expression in breast cell lines. *Nutr Cancer* 45, 247–255.

35. Vissac-Sabatier, C., Coxam, V., Dechelotte, P., et al. (2003) Phytoestrogen-rich diets modulate expression of BRCA-1 and BRCA-2 tumor suppressor genes in mammary gland in female Wistar rats. *Cancer Res* 63, 6607–6612.
36. Cabanes, A., Wang, M., Olivo, S., et al. (2004) Prepubertal estradiol and genistein exposures up-regulate BRCA1 mRNA and reduce mammary tumorigenesis. *Carcinogenesis* 25, 741–748.
37. Fink, B.N., Gaudet, M.M., Britton, J.A., et al. (2006) Fruits, vegetables, and micronutrient intake in relation to breast cancer survival. *Breast Cancer Res Treat* 98, 199–208.
38. Chlebowski, R.T., Blackburn, G.L., Thomson, C.A., et al. (2006) Dietary fat reduction and breast cancer outcome: interim efficacy results from the Women's Intervention Nutrition Study. *J Natl Cancer Inst* 98, 1767–1776.
39. Terry, P., Suzuki, R., and Hu, F.B. (2001) A prospective study of major dietary patterns and the risk of breast cancer. *Cancer Epidemiol Biomarkers Prev* 10, 1281–1285.
40. Bissonauth,V., Shatenstein, B., and Ghadirian, P. (2008) Nutrition and breast cancer among sporadic cases and gene mutation carriers: An overview. *Cancer Detect Prev* 32, 52–64.
41. Pierce, J.P., Natarajan, L., and Caan, B.J. (2007) Influence of a diet very high in vegetables, fruit, and fiber and low in fat on prognosis following treatment for breast cancer: the Women's Healthy Eating and Living (WHEL) randomized trial. *JAMA* 298, 289–298.
42. Egeberg, R., Olsen, A., Autrup, H., et al. (2008) Meat consumption, N-acetyl transferase 1 and 2 polymorphism and risk of breast cancer in Danish postmenopausal women. *Eur J Cancer Prev* 17, 39–47.
43. Ericson, U., Sonestedt, E., and Ivarsson, M.I., (2009) Folate intake, methylenetetrahydrofolate reductase polymorphisms, and breast cancer risk in women from the Malmö Diet and Cancer cohort. Cancer *Epidemiology Biomarkers Prev* 18, 1101–1110.
44. Maruti, S.S., Ulrich, C.M., Jupe, E.R., et al. (2009) MTHFR C677T and postmenopausal breast cancer risk by intakes of one-carbon metabolism nutrients: a nested case–control study. *Breast* 11, R91
45. Sohn, K.J., Jang, H., Campan, M., et al. (2009) The methylenetetrahydrofolate reductase C677T mutation induces cell-specific changes in genomic DNA methylation and uracil misincorporation: a possible molecular basis for the site-specific cancer risk modification. *Int J Cancer* 124, 1999–2005.
46. Li,Y., Yuan, Y.Y., Meeran, S.M., et al. (2010) Synergistic epigenetic reactivation of estrogen receptor-α (ERα) by combined green tea polyphenol and histone deacetylase inhibitor in ERα-negative breast cancer cells. *Mol Cancer.* 14, 274.
47. Berletch JB, Liu C, Love WK, et al. (2008) Epigenetic and genetic mechanisms contribute to telomerase inhibition by EGCG. *J Cell Biochem* 103, 509–519.
48. Wu, A.H., Yu, M.C., and Tseng, C.C. (2003) Green tea and risk of breast cancer in Asian Americans. *Int J Cancer* 106, 574–579.
49. Wu, A.H., Tseng, C.C., Van Den Berg, D., et al. (2003) Tea intake, COMT genotype, and breast cancer in Asian-American women. *Cancer* 63, 7526–7529.
50. Lee, S.A., Fowke, J.H., Lu, W., et al. (2008) Cruciferous vegetables, the GSTP1 Ile105Val genetic polymorphism, and breast cancer risk. *Am J Clin Nutr* 87,753–760.
51. Antosiewicz, J., Ziolkowski,W., Kar,S., et al. (2008) Role of reactive oxygen intermediates in cellular responses to dietary cancer chemopreventive agents. *Planta Med* 74, 1570–1579.
52. Hail, N. Jr., Cortes, M., Drake, E.N., et al. (2008) Cancer chemoprevention: a radical perspective. *Free Radic Biol Med* 45, 97–110.
53. Syed Alwi, S.S., Cavell, B.E., Telang, U., et al. (2010) In vivo modulation of 4E binding protein 1 (4E-BP1) phosphorylation by watercress: a pilot study.*Br J Nutr* 104, 1288–1296.
54. Wang, J., John, E., Ingles, S.E., (2008) 5-Lipoxygenase and 5-Lipoxygenase-Activating Protein Gene Polymorphisms, Dietary Linoleic Acid, and Risk for Breast Cancer. *Cancer Epidemiology Biomarkers Prev.* 17, 2748–2754.
55. Dimri M., Bommi P.V., Sahasrabuddhe A.A., et al. (2010) Dietary omega-3 polyunsaturated fatty acids suppress expression of EZH2 in breast cancer cells. *Carcinogenesis* 31, 489–495.
56. Li, Y., Ambrosone, C.B. and McCullough, M.J. (2009) Oxidative stress-related genotypes, fruit and vegetable consumption and breast cancer risk. *Carcinogenesis* 777–784.
57. Iwasaki, M., Hamada, G.S., Nishimoto, I.N., et al. (2010) Dietary isoflavone intake, polymorphisms in the CYP17, CYP19, 17beta-HSD1, and SHBG genes, and risk of breast cancer in case–control studies in Japanese, Japanese Brazilians, and non-Japanese Brazilians. *Nutr Cancer* 62,466–475.
58. Qin, W., Zhu,W., Shi, H., et al. (2009) Soy isoflavones have an antiestrogenic effect and alter mammary promoter hypermethylation in

healthy premenopausal women. *Nutr Cancer* 61, 238–244.
59. Jawaid, K., Crane, S.R., Nowers, J.L., et al. (2010) Long-term genistein treatment of MCF-7 cells decreases acetylated histone 3 expression and alters growth responses to mitogens and histone deacetylase inhibitors. *J Steroid Biochem Mol Biol* 120, 164–171.
60. Aiyer, H.S. and Gupta, R.C. (2010) Berries and ellagic acid prevent estrogen-induced mammary tumorigenesis by modulating enzymes of estrogen metabolism. *Cancer Prev Res (Phila)* 3, 727–737.
61. Lauber, S.N. and Gooderham, N.J. (2010) The cooked meat-derived mammary carcinogen 2-amino-1-methyl-6-phenylimidazo[4,5-b] pyridine promotes invasive behaviour of breast cancer cells. *Toxicology* 279, 139–145.
62. Taioli, E., Garza, M.A., Ahn, Y.O., et al. (2009) Meta- and pooled analyses of the methylenetetrahydrofolate reductase (MTHFR) C677T polymorphism and colorectal cancer: a HuGE-GSEC review. *Am J Epidemiol* 170, 1207–1221.
63. Liu, J.J. and Ward, R.L. (2010) Folate and one-carbon metabolism and its impact on aberrant DNA methylation in cancer. *Adv Genet* 71, 79–121.
64. Cravo, M.L., Pinto, A.G., Chaves, P., et al. (1998) Effect of folate supplementation on DNA methylation of rectal mucosa in patients with colonic adenomas: correlation with nutrient intake. *Clin Nutr* 17, 45–49.
65. Figueiredo, J.C., Grau, M.V, Wallace, K., et al. (2009) Global DNA hypomethylation (LINE-1) in the normal colon and lifestyle characteristics and dietary and genetic factors. *Cancer Epidemiol Biomarkers Prev* 18, 1041–1049.
66. Economopoulos, K.P. and Sergentanis, T.N. (2010) GSTM1, GSTT1, GSTP1, GSTA1 and colorectal cancer risk: a comprehensive meta-analysis. *Eur J Cancer* 46, 1617–1631.
67. Ross, S.A. (2007) Nutritional genomic approaches to cancer prevention research. *Exp Oncol* 29, 250–256.
68. Novakovic, B., Sibson, M., Ng, H.K., et al. (2009) Placenta-specific methylation of the vitamin D 24-hydroxylase gene: implications for feedback autoregulation of active vitamin D levels at the fetomaternal interface. *J Biol Chem* 284, 14838–14848.
69. Dai, Q., Shrubsole, M.J., Ness, R.M., et al. (2007) The relation of magnesium and calcium intakes and a genetic polymorphism in the magnesium transporter to colorectal neoplasia risk. *Am J Clin Nutr* 86, 743–751.
70. Brevik, A., Joshi, A.D., Corral, R., et al. (2010) Polymorphisms in base excision repair genes as colorectal cancer risk factors and modifiers of the effect of diets high in red meat. *Cancer Epidemiol Biomarkers Prev* 19, 3167–3173.
71. Wong, H.L., Peters, U., Hayes, R.B., et al. (2010) Polymorphisms in the adenomatous polyposis coli (APC) gene and advanced colorectal adenoma risk. *Eur J Cancer* 46, 2457–2466.
72. Biswas, S.K., McClure, D., Jimenez, L.A., et al. (2005) Curcumin induces glutathione biosynthesis and inhibits NF-kappaB activation and interleukin-8 release in alveolar epithelial cells: mechanism of free radical scavenging activity. *Antioxid Redox Signal* 7, 32–41.
73. Li, L., Aggarwal, B.B., Shishodia, S., et al. (2004) Nuclear factor-kappaB and IkappaB kinase are constitutively active in human pancreatic cells, and their down-regulation by curcumin (diferuloylmethane) is associated with the suppression of proliferation and the induction of apoptosis. *Cancer* 101, 2351–2362.
74. Mudduluru, G., George-William, J.N., Muppala, S., et al. (2011) Curcumin regulates miR-21 expression and inhibits invasion and metastasis in colorectal cancer. *Biosci Rep* 31,185–197.
75. Reuter, S., Gupta, S.C., Park, B., et al. (2011) Epigenetic changes induced by curcumin and other natural compounds. *Genes Nutr* 6, 93–108.
76. Ströhle, A., Maike, W., and Hahn, A. (2007) Nutrition and colorectal cancer. *Med Monatsschr Pharm* 30, 25-32.

Chapter 23

Dietary and Lifestyle Factors of DNA Methylation

Unhee Lim and Min-Ae Song

Abstract

Lifestyle factors, such as diet, smoking, physical activity, and body weight management, are known to constitute the majority of cancer causes. Epigenetics has been widely proposed as a main mechanism that mediates the reversible effects of dietary and lifestyle factors on carcinogenesis. This chapter reviews human studies on potential dietary and lifestyle determinants of DNA methylation. Apart from a few prospective investigations and interventions of limited size and duration, evidence mostly comes from cross-sectional observational studies and supports some associations. Studies to date suggest that certain dietary components may alter genomic and gene-specific DNA methylation levels in systemic and target tissues, affecting genomic stability and transcription of tumor suppressors and oncogenes. Most data and supportive evidence exist for folate, a key nutritional factor in one-carbon metabolism that supplies the methyl units for DNA methylation. Other candidate bioactive food components include alcohol and other key nutritional factors of one-carbon metabolism, polyphenols and flavonoids in green tea, phytoestrogen, and lycopene. Some data also support a link of DNA methylation with physical activity and energy balance. Effects of dietary and lifestyle exposures on DNA methylation may be additionally modified by common genetic variants, environmental carcinogens, and infectious agents, an aspect that remains largely unexplored. In addition, growing literature supports that the environmental conditions during critical developmental stages may influence later risk of metabolic disorders in part through persistent programming of DNA methylation. Further research of these modifiable determinants of DNA methylation will improve our understanding of cancer etiology and may present certain DNA methylation markers as attractive surrogate endpoints for prevention research. Considering the plasticity of epigenetic marks and correlated nature of lifestyle factors, more longitudinal studies of healthy individuals of varying age, sex, and ethnic groups are warranted, ideally with comprehensive data collection on various lifestyle factors.

Key words: Diet, Developmental origins, DNA methylation, Folate, Lifestyle, Obesity, Bioactive food components, Gene-nutrient interactions, Metabolic disorders, Nutrition, One-carbon metabolism, Physical activity, Smoking, Supplement

1. Introduction

Dietary and other lifestyle factors explain a large proportion of cancer incidence and mortality (1, 2). DNA methylation, along with other epigenetic marks, is broadly proposed to be the mediator of

Ramona G. Dumitrescu and Mukesh Verma (eds.), *Cancer Epigenetics: Methods and Protocols*, Methods in Molecular Biology, vol. 863, DOI 10.1007/978-1-61779-612-8_23, © Springer Science+Business Media, LLC 2012

the reversible effects of lifestyle factors on chronic diseases (3). However, human data are yet limited to characterize the mediating effects. Even for DNA methylation that has been studied most extensively among epigenetic marks, the majority of research compared the analysis of specific tumor tissue with normal counterparts. Variations in DNA methylation patterns have been less frequently examined in relation to lifestyle practice prior to cancer diagnosis. The lack of data may be also in part due to much smaller variations in DNA methylation found in healthy individuals, as well as the difficulty in accessing specific tissue samples or otherwise relating systemic findings to the patterns in distant target tissues. Also, studies of determinants require more resources: ideally, repeated measures of DNA methylation markers and comprehensive data collection on various lifestyle covariates in a representative sample of the general population. Nevertheless, certain lifestyle factors have emerged from cross-sectional or short-term intervention studies as more likely candidates than others to influence DNA methylation. This chapter summarizes such candidate determinants based on human studies, with more focus on data in a healthy state than postdiagnostic alterations in tumor tissue.

2. Considerations in Interpreting the Literature

As in the critical review of any biomarker determinants, there are some general issues to consider. Most human data regarding the correlates of DNA methylation come from observational studies that only allow concluding associations, not causality. Even the rarely available intervention studies that assessed changes in DNA methylation levels after modification of one or more factors are limited in generalizability in terms of the studied population and efficacy of the type, dose/intensity, and duration of the intervention. More observational data are warranted, preferentially from well-designed epidemiologic studies with comprehensive covariate information, to understand independent associations of the potential lifestyle determinants with DNA methylation markers. Also, more prospective studies are needed to avoid recall bias by patients regarding lifestyle exposures before diagnosis or experiencing clinical symptoms.

Comparing study findings is further complicated by differences in DNA methylation markers, for the types (global or gene-specific), specimen sources (systemic or target-tissue), and analytic methods (4). DNA methylation patterns are characterized for overall genome-wide CpG dinucleotides or for targeted CpG island sites, typically in specific gene promoters. These methylation patterns differ in systemic (blood, urine) vs. target-tissue samples and can show heterogeneity even within each biological sample of mixed cells. *Global or genomic DNA methylation* patterns in relation to lifestyle have been studied either through direct measures of 5-methylcytosine (5mC) in proportion to total cytosine content in genomic DNA or through indirect measures of percent methylation in selected loci of common repetitive sequences, such as long interspersed nuclear element 1 (LINE1) or Alu. Analytic methods for 5mC content are mainly based on PCR of the sample DNA digested with methylation-sensitive restriction-enzyme (RE) or bisulfite-treated to have unmethylated cytosine converted to uracil (4). Depending on the specificity of the RE used, the outcome can be limited to only a fraction of the whole genomic CpG sites. Percent 5mC is most accurately quantified by RE-digestion followed by high performance liquid chromatography (HPLC) (5), which can be further combined with mass spectrometry for higher sensitivity and specificity (6, 7). This method, however, requires relatively large amounts of high-quality genomic DNA. Others have used a luminometric assay on a pyrosequencing platform (8) or an indirect approach of the in vitro radiolabeled methyl ((^{3}H)-methyl) acceptance assay, output of which is in an inverse association with 5mC (9). Genomic DNA methylation can be also estimated from methylation in repeat elements as a proxy—with a caution that although these repetitive DNA sequences are highly common, their genomic distribution is not random (10, 11). Repeat element methylation is often analyzed using comprehensive methods such as pyrosequencing (12) that allows the quantification of partial allelic methylation of 25–30 bp at a time or more targeted approaches such as MethyLight (13) that assumes complete methylation or complete unmethylation. Similarly, assessment of *gene- or locus-specific CpG island DNA methylation* utilizes various techniques, including comprehensive pyrosequencing and targeted approaches of quantitative methylation-specific PCR (QMSP) (14), MethyLight (4, 15), and a mass-spectrometry-based method (16–18). These methods differ in the specific location and number of the CpG sites analyzed and presumably can lead to different outcomes, even assessing the same samples. CpG island methylation can be also examined on a genome-wide scale using high-throughput oligonucleotide arrays—bead arrays, lithographic arrays, or inkjet arrays from different manufacturers (19). High-throughput sequencing called next-generation sequencing is also on the horizon, which will enable powerful global mapping of 5mC at single-base resolution for allele-specific DNA methylation analysis, while avoiding hybridization artifacts (20). In summary, continued rapid improvements in technology make the study of DNA methylation more feasible and comprehensive. However, no one method of DNA methylation analysis will be appropriate for every study, and studies based on different approaches will continue to require caution in the interpretation and comparisons.

3. Heritability vs. Acquired Variations in DNA Methylation

So, how much of the variation in DNA methylation can be explained by acquired modifications due to nongenetic determinants? A monozygotic twin study demonstrated that the acquired non-heritable variation in DNA methylation and histone acetylation is substantial. A cohort study of 80 monozygotic twins of ages 3–74 observed that both global and locus-specific DNA methylation patterns in several cell types (lymphocytes, mouth endothelium, intra-abdominal fat, skeletal muscle) were very similar between young twins, but showed greater divergence between older twins—in both continuous and dichotomized analysis around age 28 (21). Total 5mC content, along with acetylation levels of histones H3 and H4, was very similar in 65% of the twin pairs examined, but significantly different in the remaining 35% of the pairs. Most notably, there was a significant positive association of the epigenetic differences in the pair with the age of the twins and also with the lifetime spent separately. Interestingly, their analysis of DNA methylation fingerprint sites (amplification of intermethylated sites or AIMS) from older divergent twins, as compared to younger twins, revealed 2.5 times as many differences in CpG islands. Also, AIMS were frequently found in differentially methylated repeat elements (43% Alus and 9% LINEs and other repetitive sequences out of 53 selected AIMS), often involving specific genomic areas (most telomeres and a few chromosomal regions) (21). These findings support that DNA methylation and other epigenetic mechanisms may mediate the phenotypic discordance in monozygotic twins who share identical genetic composition yet increasingly develop anthropometric and behavioral differences and different disease susceptibility with age. In contrast, heritability of DNA methylation appears greater in imprinted genomic regions, where varying degrees of loss of epigenetic control by parent-of-origin allele-specific methylation patterns yield more substantial consequences, ranging from long-term metabolic abnormality to developmental disorders. A large study of adolescent and middle-aged twins observed high interindividual variation in DNA methylation of the imprinted *IGF2* and *H19* differentially methylated regions (DMR) and estimated the heritability in each DMR to be about 75–80% and 35%, respectively, without much differences by age (22, 23).

3.1. Intraindividual Variability in DNA Methylation

The best characterization of intraindividual variation in global DNA methylation is available from an Icelandic cohort of older adults, where a subset of participants provided two repeat DNA samples on average 11 years apart (23). About 70% of the 111 subjects examined showed less than 10% changes in global leukocyte DNA methylation over time of about a decade, but in the remaining 30%, global methylation either increased or decreased by 10% or more over time. For a shorter duration of over 12 weeks, five repeated measures of total 5mC content for global lymphocyte DNA methylation in eight monozygotic twin pairs did not vary significantly (21). As for gene-specific DNA methylation, the variability or stability over time appears to depend on the target CpG site. In a pilot study with repeat samples of blood and buccal cells, with time intervals ranging several years to a decade between sampling, 5 of the 8 loci examined showed stable CpG island methylation over time, with a significant correlation between DNA methylation in blood and buccal cells for four loci (24). DNA methylation in imprinted regions of *IGF2/H19* ($n=133$) and *IGF2R* DMRs ($n=75$) did not show notable intraindividual variation over about 20 years of observation, with a paired correlation coefficient of 0.78 (25).

4. Demographic Factors: Age, Sex, and Race/Ethnicity

Certain demographic factors have been associated with DNA methylation levels, part of which may be due to lifestyle or environmental exposure differences in the subgroups. Older age is associated with decreased levels of global DNA methylation and increased levels of gene-specific methylation in animals (26). In humans, the relationship is less consistent (21, 23, 27–29), in part possibly due to marker-specific nonlinear changes with increasing age (28). Men were observed to have higher levels of DNA methylation than women in repeat elements and certain promoters in one study (30), but were observed with lower Alu methylation and higher LINE1 methylation in another (29). Also, certain racial/ethnic heterogeneity has been observed in global leukocyte DNA methylation among African Americans and Hispanics compared with Caucasians (31). In a study of LINE1 methylation in colonic mucosa samples, Hispanics showed higher levels of global DNA methylation than Caucasians or African Americans, but this finding was largely limited to DNA from the right (proximal, ascending) colon (32). Whether the demographic correlations are inherent traits or due to confounding environmental exposures, it would be important to control for the demographic factors when comparing studies or investigating determinants of DNA methylation markers.

5. Dietary Factors

5.1. Folate, Alcohol, and One-Carbon Metabolism

Nutrients that are methyl-unit carriers or coenzymes for one-carbon metabolism (Fig. 1), which supplies the universal methyl donor compound, *S*-adenosylmethionine (SAM), have been studied the

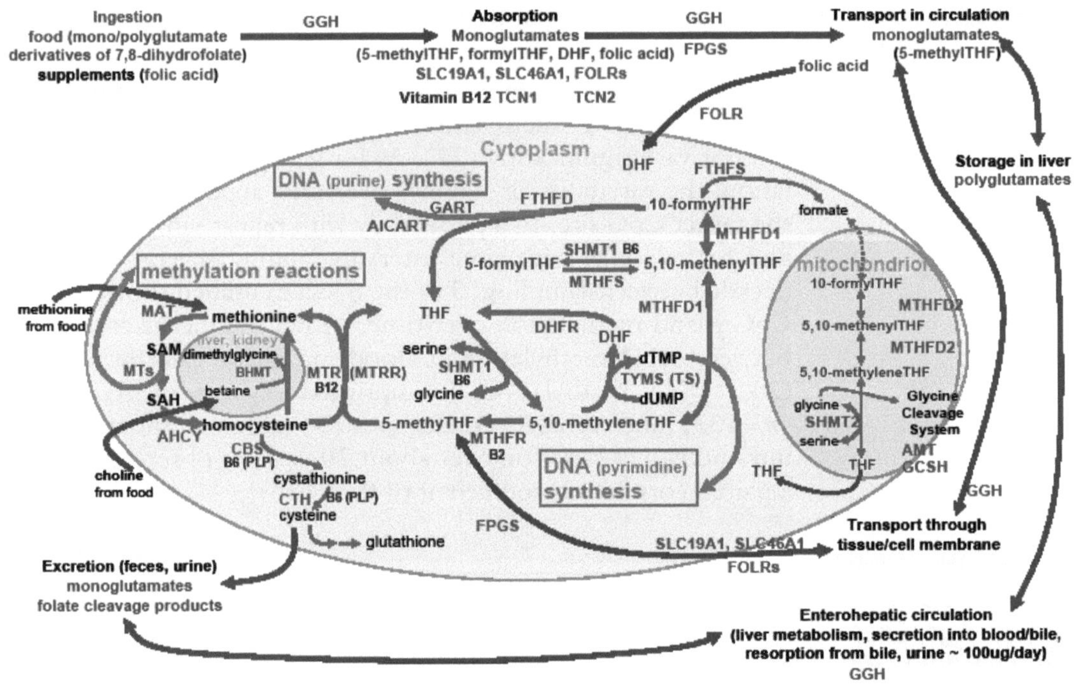

Fig. 1. Nutrients and genes involved in folate and one-carbon metabolism (modified from Lim et al. (75)). This diagram illustrates absorption, transport, and metabolism of folate along with other nutritional and genetic factors of intracellular one-carbon metabolism (76–82) that provides the methyl unit for DNA methylation through synthesis of *S*-adenosylmethionine (SAM). Folates in food, mostly polyglutamates, are hydrolyzed to monoglutamates by *GGH* in the gut and are absorbed across the intestinal mucosa by active transporters (reduced folate carriers, encoded by *SLC19A1*; folate receptors, *FOLR1*, *FOLR2*, and *FOLR3*; and proton-coupled folate transporter, *SLC46A1*) and minimally by passive diffusion at high levels of folate consumption. Once absorbed into the portal circulation, folates are taken up by the liver and retained or released into blood or bile as 5-methylTHF. About two thirds of 5-methylTHF, the predominant form of folate in circulation, is bound to low-affinity proteins, mostly albumin. Blood 5-methylTHF is transported into various organ cells by the active transporters noted above. The predominant cytoplasmic folate, 5-methylTHF, donates its one-carbon moiety to methylate homocysteine and yield methionine and THF. THF is a much preferred substrate to *FPGS* that lengthens the glutamate chain of the monoglutamate folate, so folates can be retained in the cell. This polyglutamylation also enables folates to be utilized by one-carbon metabolizing enzymes better than monoglutamates. The conversion of 5-methylTHF to THF is inhibited in deficiency of vitamin B12, which is a coenzyme for methionine synthase (MTR), or with insufficient transcobalamins (TCN1, TCN2) for vitamin B12 absorption. In such a condition, deficiency of functional folate (THF) occurs despite sufficient folate (5-methylTHF) in circulation—a phenomenon called "methyl-trap." The conversion is also affected when *MTR* loses its activity from the oxidation of its vitamin B12-derived coenzyme, cobalamin: *MTRR* reactivates *MTR* using the methyl supply from SAM. Homocysteine can be remethylated via an alternative mechanism of *BHMT* using betaine, supplied from dietary choline, in the kidney and liver. Methionine, from homocysteine and also directly from diet, is converted to SAM, a universal donor of one-carbon unit for various methylation reactions by methyltransferases (MTs), including DNA methylation by *DNMTs*. Resulting SAH is hydrolyzed to homocysteine, which then gets remethylated or catabolyzed via the transsulfuration pathway initiated by *CBS*. The active folate coenzyme THF obtains one-carbon moiety also from amino acid serine via *SHMT1* catalysis, yielding 5,10-methyleneTHF, which is an important common substrate to methylation pathway described above via *MTHFR* or to nucleic acid synthesis pathways via *TYMS* (uridylate to thymidylate conversion; pyrimidine synthesis) or *MTHFD1/FTHFD* (purine synthesis). DHF, the remaining folate after the *TYMS* reaction on THF, is also supplied from folic acid that is reported to be found in blood in higher proportion than usual when a large dose is consumed from fortified foods or supplements. 5,10-methenylTHF can be interconverted with 5-formylTHF (also known as folinic acid or leucovorin; thought to be the storage form of folate) via *SHMT1/MTHFS*. Although less understood, mitochondrial one-carbon metabolism is proposed to be in equilibrium with cytoplasmic metabolism and contains the glycine cleavage system. *AHCY* *S*-adenosylhomocysteine hydrolase; *AICART* phosphoribosylaminoimidazolecarboxamide formyltransferase;

most in relation to DNA methylation (3). In particular, most human studies have examined folate, and some on alcohol—antagonist to folate and one-carbon metabolism. Only a few human studies examined other nutrients involved in one-carbon metabolism (vitamins B2, B6 and B12, methionine, choline, and betaine) that have shown weaker modulating effects on DNA methylation than in animals (3).

Controlled feeding studies of folate are mostly consistent in demonstrating the effect on global DNA methylation. Global DNA methylation levels in lymphocytes of postmenopausal women decreased on a folate-deficient diet (56 μg/day for 5 weeks and 111 μg/day for 4 weeks) and increased on a folate-replete diet (286–516 μg/day for 3 weeks) (33). In older women of ages 60–85, leukocyte DNA global methylation declined on a moderately deplete folate diet (118 μg/day for 7 weeks), but did not significantly improve even after 7 weeks on a replete diet (415 μg/day) (34). Similarly, a randomized and double-blinded intervention of folic acid supplements (400 μg/day) or placebo for 10 weeks led to increased leukocyte DNA global methylation by 31% in the supplemented group (35). These series of findings suggest that a relatively short-term depletion in total folate intake reduces global DNA methylation and a recovery may be achieved with supplementation at levels of folic acid found in common multivitamin supplement (400 μg/day), but the efficacy may be lower in older ages.

Alcohol is a known antagonist to folate metabolism and methionine synthase (MTR; Fig. 1) activity, and frequent consumption was associated with lower leukocyte DNA global methylation in breast cancer cases and healthy controls (36). This was further supported in a large pooled study of leukocyte DNA methylation of repeat elements, where higher alcohol intake was inversely correlated with lower Alu methylation ($r = -0.214$) (29).

A few intervention studies examined the effect of folic acid supplementation on global DNA methylation in the colon or rectal

Fig. 1. (continued) *AMT* aminomethyltransferase; *B2* vitamin B2; *B6* vitamin B6; *B12* vitamin B12; *BHMT* betaine-homocysteine methyltransferase; *CBS* cystathionine beta-synthase; *CTH* cystathionase; *DHF* dihydrofolate; *DHFR* dihydrofolate reductase; *DNMT* DNA methyltransferase; *FPGS* folylpolyglutamate synthase; *dTMP* deoxythymidine monophosphate; *dUMP* deoxyuridine monophosphate; *FOLRs* folate receptors; *FTHFD* 10-formyltetrahydrofolate dehydrogenase; *FTHFS* 10-formyltetrahydrofolate synthase; *FTHFSDC1* 10-formyltetrahydrofolate synthetase domain containing 1; *GART* glycinamide ribonucleotide formyltransferase; *GCPII* glutamate carboxypeptidase II; *GCSH* glycine cleavage system protein H; *GGH* gamma-glutamylhydrolase; *MAT* methionine *S*-adenosyltransferase; *MTs* a group of methyltransferases; *MTHFD1* cytoplasmic 5,10-methylenetetrahydrofolate dehydrogenase; *MTHFD2* mitochondrial 5,10-methylenetetrahydrofolate dehydrogenase; *MTHFR* 5,10-methylenetetrahydrofolate reductase; *MTHFS* 5,10-methenyltetrahydrofolate synthetase; *MTR* methionine synthase; *MTRR* methionine synthase reductase; *PLP* pyridoxal 5′-phosphate; *SAH* *S*-adenosylhomocysteine; *SAM* *S*-adenosylmethionine; *SHMT1* cytoplasmic serine hydroxymethyltransferase; *SHMT2* mitochondrial serine hydroxymethyltransferase; *SLC19A1* reduced folate carrier; *SLC46A1* proton-coupled folate transporter; *TCN1* transcobalamin 1; *TCN2* transcobalamin 2; *THF* tetrahydrofolate; *TYMS* thymidylate synthetase. (copyright Symbol) The American Society of Hematology.

mucosa of adenoma patients after the resection of the lesions. A high-dose folic acid supplementation (5 mg/day for 3 months) increased global DNA methylation levels of rectal mucosa, which was reversed in a cross-over phase of placebo supplementation (37). These folate-induced responses appeared stronger in single polyp cases compared to multiple polyp cases. The folic acid supplementation trial (400 μg/day for 10 weeks) by Pufulete et al. observed an increase in global DNA methylation in the colonic mucosa of adenoma patients by 25% with borderline significance, which was smaller than the increment seen in leukocyte DNA, about 31% (35). In another study of healthy individuals free of colorectal adenoma or cancer who underwent folic acid supplementation, serum and erythrocyte folate levels showed a borderline significant inverse association with global DNA methylation in colonic mucosa (38). However, data from a long-term randomized, placebo-controlled folic acid supplementation trial (1 mg/day for 3 years) on efficacy of recurrent adenoma prevention are less consistent (32). In a subset of the participants (388 out of 768) whose left and right colon biopsy samples were analyzed after the intervention, the folic acid supplement group showed nonsignificantly higher global DNA methylation in LINE1 repeat elements compared to the placebo group. Global DNA methylation was not associated with the overall risk of adenoma recurrence, but showed a nonsignificant inverse association with advanced adenoma recurrence. Also, there were no significant differences in global DNA methylation by age, sex, body mass index (BMI), genotypes of one-carbon metabolism enzymes (methylenetetrahydrofolate reductase (*MTHFR*), *MTR*, methionine synthase reductase (*MTRR*), cystathionine beta-synthase (*CBS*)), total folate intake, or baseline nonfasting blood levels of relevant B vitamins, except vitamin B6 (32). Some anatomic site-specific associations were noted: colonic DNA global methylation was significantly higher in the left (distant) colon compared to the right (proximal) colon, and plasma vitamin B6 was positively associated with global DNA methylation of the left colon.

A recent prospective study investigated an association of prediagnostic dietary intake of folate and other nutritional factors of one-carbon metabolism with LINE1 global methylation in the tumor DNA of 609 incident colon cancer patients (39). Higher dietary folate intake before diagnosis (≥400 vs. <200 μg/day) was associated with significantly less LINE1 hypomethylation in colon tumor DNA, while higher alcohol consumption (≥15 g/day or 1 drink/day vs. none) was associated with a higher risk of LINE1 hypomethylation. Other nutrients, including vitamins B2, B6, and B12 and methionine, did not show any association. The same study group had reported that the degree of LINE1 hypomethylation in colon tumor had a dose–response association with poor prognosis and higher mortality (40).

Some studies support main effects and gene-nutrient interactions by genetic polymorphisms related to one-carbon metabolism, such as the *MTHFR* 677C>T variant, on global DNA methylation. Friso and Choi et al. compared healthy adults who were homozygous carriers of the *MTHFR* 677TT genotype ($n = 105$) vs. CC carriers ($n = 187$) and observed lower levels of global DNA methylation in peripheral blood mononuclear cells (PBMC) of TT carriers, specifically among TT carriers with low folate status (41). Likewise, the overall positive correlation between plasma or erythrocyte folate and global methylation in PBMC was largely due to a strong association in the subgroup of *MTHFR* 677TT carriers.

In studies of tissue DNA, the relationship of genetic variants and global DNA methylation appears less consistent. Global methylation of colonic DNA was higher among cancer-free carriers of the *MTR* 2756A>G variant, but did not differ by genotypes of the *MTHFR* 677C>T, *MTHFR* 1298A>C or *CBS* 844ins68 variant (38). Similarly, colonic DNA methylation in LINE1 promoters did not differ by genotypes of the *MTHFR* C677T and A1298C, *MTR* A2756G, *MTRR* A66G, and *CBS* C1080T and C699T variants (32). On the other hand, a study of 233 patients with colorectal, breast, or lung tumors showed that carriers of the *MTHFR* 677T allele had significantly lower global methylation in tumor and adjacent normal tissue DNA (42). This study also observed an average 22% loss of global DNA methylation in tumor genome compared to normal tissue (5.5 vs. 4.3%).

Much less data are available on CpG island methylation, which is typically examined in target tissues in relation to specific tumors. In studies of several solid tumors, data appear to support an association between methyl donor nutrient status or related genetic variants and CpG island methylation in the key genes of cancer etiology. In a study that examined colon tumor DNA for the promoter methylation of six genes related to colorectal cancer etiology (*APC*, $p14^{ARF}$, $p16^{INK4A}$, *hMLH1*, O^{8}-*MGMT*, and *RASSF1A*), the prevalence of hypermethylation in each of the gene promoters was higher in cases who consumed low folate and high alcohol ($n = 61$) than those who reported high folate and low alcohol ($n = 61$), although the difference did not reach statistical significance (43). Among cancer patients of the colorectum, breast, or lung, carriers of the *MTR* 2756G allele, compared to noncarriers, had significantly fewer hypermethylated CpG islands on average for each cancer-specific tumor suppressor genes, which included $p16^{INK4\alpha}$, $p14^{ARF}$, *hMLH1*, *MGMT*, *APC*, *LKB1*, *DAPK*, *GSTP1*, *BRCA1*, *RARβ2*, *CDH1*, and *RASSF1* (42). A recent prospective study examined prediagnostic blood DNA for promoter methylation of several genes (*CDKN2A/p16*, *RASSF1A*, *GSTP1*, *MTHFR*, and *MGMT*) that are frequently hypermethylated in various malignancies (44). In addition to an association between *RASSF1A* promoter methylation and cancer incidence, they found a positive association between dietary intake of folate and the promoter methylation levels of *RASSF1A* and *MTHFR*, in particular among never smokers, and also an inverse association between dietary methionine, another methyl donor nutrient, and *RASSF1A* methylation. No significant associations were detected between the intake levels of folate or its antagonist, alcohol, and promoter methylation of selected genes (*CDH1*, *CDKN2A*, *GSTP1*, *MTHFR*, *RASSF1A*) in lung tumor DNA (45).

5.2. Green Tea and Components

In Japanese studies of gastric carcinoma tumor DNA, high consumption of green tea (seven cups or more per day compared to six cups or less) was associated with lower methylation of *CDX2* and *BMP-2* genes, which are frequently hypermethylated in gastric cancers (46, 47). These findings are consistent with cancer cell culture study data, where polyphenols such as catechin, epicatechin, and (−)-epigallocatechin-3-*O*-gallate (EGCG) and flavonoids such as quercetin that are high in green tea, have been observed to inhibit the DNA methyltransferase (*DNMT*) activity, with most potency from EGCG, and to reactivate silenced tumor suppressor genes (48, 49). Catechins appear to inhibit DNMT activity through increasing the intracellular *S*-adenosylhomocysteine (SAH) levels, whereas EGCG may directly inhibit the catalytic site of DNMT.

6. Other Bioactive Food Components

Although human data are sparse, animal studies support that other bioactive food components, including genistein (50) and lycopene (51), may modulate DNA methylation.

7. Physical Activity

There is limited but suggestive evidence that higher or increased physical activity may alter DNA methylation. In an intervention study of high-intensity interval walking exercise conducted in older adults, the promoter methylation of *ASC* gene (apoptosis-association speck-like protein containing a caspase recruitment domain), which facilitates cytokine release (e.g., IL-1β, IL-18), increased after the 6-month intervention, close to the levels found in younger adult controls (52). This finding supports that exercise may reduce the levels of inflammatory cytokines by increasing the promoter methylation of *ASC* and suppressing the transcription. However, it was not clear whether the difference in *ASC* promoter methylation was independent of other correlates, such as changes in weight, body fat, or dietary intake, which were brought on by the intervention.

Another study of gastric carcinoma tumor DNA showed a borderline inverse association between promoter methylation of calcium channel voltage-dependent $\alpha 2/\delta$ subunit 3 (*CACNA2D3*) and self-reported levels of physical activity before the cancer onset (47). On the other hand, physical inactivity from 9-day bed rest, compared to an active state, was associated with a trend of higher promoter methylation of peroxisome proliferator-activated receptor-γ coactivator-1α (*PPARGC1A*) in the skeletal muscle tissue DNA of young men, which may contribute to dyslipidemia (53).

8. Overweight and Obesity

A recent large pooled study of global repeat element methylation in about 1,500 healthy individuals did not find an association with BMI (29). However, there are some reports of an association between adiposity indicators and blood DNA methylation of specific regions. For example, promoter methylation in transcription factor A (*TFAM*) was associated with adolescent obesity and waist-to-hip ratio (54). As for DNA methylation in imprinted regions, higher methylation of the *H19* DMR, but not of *IGF2* DMR, was associated with smaller waist circumference and waist-to-hip ratio in middle-aged twins (22). In an exercise intervention study of older adults, where leukocyte *ASC* promoter methylation increased after the intervention, percent body fat was also borderline inversely associated with *ASC* methylation (52).

9. Smoking

Although not all consistent (29), there is some evidence that smoking may be a correlate of DNA methylation. In individuals without known cancers, global DNA methylation levels in both peripheral blood leukocytes (55) and colonic mucosa (38) were lower among current smokers, which may be in part due to lower folate status in smokers but also possibly through an independent mechanism (56). Methylation in the *MTHFR* promoter of lung tumor DNA was significantly higher in current smokers than in never smokers, although without a dose–response association (45). Interestingly, there was a weak but significant inverse correlation between the *MTHFR* promoter methylation and LINE1 global methylation in the lung tumor DNA ($r = -0.16$), indicating a possible effect of suppressed *MTHFR* on lowering global DNA methylation. In addition, as with folate, cigarette smoking has been associated with specific molecular subtype of colorectal cancers—the microsatellite instability (MSI)-high, CpG island methylator phenotype (CIMP)-positive, and *BRAF* mutation-positive cancer (57).

10. Hormone Replacement Therapy

Estrogen has long been inversely associated with blood levels of homocysteine, a metabolite that in elevation reflects folate insufficiency and that could inhibit methylation reactions. In a small cross-over intervention study of eight healthy postmenopausal women, an 8-week estrogen treatment led to reduced homocysteine and increased global DNA methylation, but no significant changes in promoter methylation of estrogen receptors (*ESR1* and *ESR2*) and p16 (*CDKN2A*) genes (58). In a population-based case–control study of colorectal cancer, current users of hormone replacement therapy, compared to never and former users, had higher promoter methylation of progesterone receptor (*PGR*) in normal colonic tissue and higher promoter methylation of *ESR1* in tumor (59), which may explain the protective effect of the therapy on colorectal cancer. It would be of interest to examine whether phytoestrogens, such as genistein found high in soy, have similar effects on global and gene-specific DNA methylation.

11. Environmental Toxins

Increasing evidence suggests that cumulative exposures to common environmental toxins and carcinogens, such as benzene, arsenic, lead, polycyclic aromatic hydrocarbons (PAH), and ionizing radiation, may lead to DNA methylation alterations from normally high levels of global methylation and normally low levels of CpG island-specific methylation (56, 60). What remains to be explored is whether such detrimental effects of environmental toxins interact with lifestyle factors, leading certain groups to be more susceptible to disturbances in DNA methylation.

12. Early Nutrition and Environmental Conditions

Strong evidence supports developmental origins of health and diseases, also known as the "fetal origins hypothesis" or "Barker's thrifty phenotype hypothesis" (61). Poor in-utero nutrition, most often assessed with birth size, followed by accelerated growth in early childhood due to excess foods leads to increased risk of central adiposity and metabolic diseases in childhood through adult life, most strikingly demonstrated in individuals who were prenatally exposed to the Dutch famine in 1944–1945 (62–67). Some recent studies (68, 69) specifically support the hypothesis of "metabolic imprinting"—that prenatal and early postnatal nutrition and other environmental conditions lead to persistent epigenetic programming for long-term health consequences (70). In a comparison of individuals who were exposed to the Dutch famine during peri-conceptional period to their unexposed, same-sex siblings, the exposure was associated with significantly lower DNA methylation in imprinted genes *IGF2* (18) and *INSIGF* (71) and higher promoter methylation in *IL10*, *LEP*, *ABCA1*, *GNASAS*, and *MEG2*, with further sex-interactions observed for *INSIGF*, *LEP*, and *GNASAS* (71). These findings confirmed the suspected long-term impact mediated by altered methylation of imprinted genes (*IGF2*, *INSR*, *INSIGF*, *GNASAS*), but also demonstrated significant and large relative differences in the methylation levels of nonimprinted genes (*IL10*, *LEP*). However, the evidence is not as strong on the association between intrauterine growth restriction due to less severe conditions and DNA methylation of selected development-related genes (72).

Among a milieu of peri-conceptional nutritional factors that could affect intrauterine programming of the offspring's epigenome, maternal folate status has been studied with special interest as in other research of DNA methylation. Children of mothers who used peri-conceptional folic acid supplements had significantly higher levels of DNA methylation in imprinted *IGF2* DMR at ages around 17 months, compared to children whose mothers did not take supplements (73). In the same study of a generally well-nourished population, where higher than average birth weight as well as low birth weight has been associated with later obesity, *IGF2* DMR methylation was inversely associated with children's birth weight. Maternal BMI has also been associated with the promoter methylation of *PPARGC1A* in umbilical cord samples (74).

13. Conclusions

Studies appear to support some effect of folate status on global DNA methylation in healthy individuals and tumor patients and also on promoter methylation of certain genes. Data are far less available on other dietary components. Increasing evidence suggests that physical activity and obesity may also influence DNA methylation. Nutritional and other conditions during early developmental stages, in particular, may have lasting effects on metabolism through DNA methylation programming. More observational studies in humans, preferentially from well-designed epidemiologic studies with high-quality data on dietary and lifestyle practices, are warranted for a valid assessment of various potential determinants of DNA methylation. Also, more comprehensive and reproducible analytic methods suitable for large-scale human studies are likely to move the field forward to enhance our understanding of the relationship between lifestyle factors and DNA methylation in health and disease.

References

1. Doll, R., and Peto, R. (1981) The causes of cancer: quantitative estimates of avoidable risks of cancer in the United States today, *J.Natl. Cancer Inst. 66*, 1191–1308.
2. Danaei, G., Ding, E. L., Mozaffarian, D., Taylor, B., Rehm, J., Murray, C. J., and Ezzati, M. (2009) The preventable causes of death in the United States: comparative risk assessment of dietary, lifestyle, and metabolic risk factors, *PLoS Med* 6, e1000058.
3. Choi, S. W., Corrocher, R., and Friso, S. (2009) Nutrients and DNA methylation, In *Nutrients and Epigenetics* (Choi, S. W., and Friso, S., Eds.), CRC Press Taylor & Francis Group, Boca Raton, FL.
4. Laird, P. W. (2003) The power and the promise of DNA methylation markers, *Nat Rev Cancer* 3, 253–266.
5. Fraga, M. F., Rodriguez, R., and Canal, M. J. (2000) Rapid quantification of DNA methylation by high performance capillary electrophoresis, *Electrophoresis* 21, 2990–2994.
6. Friso, S., Choi, S. W., Dolnikowski, G. G., and Selhub, J. (2002) A method to assess genomic DNA methylation using high-performance liquid chromatography/electrospray ionization mass spectrometry, *Anal Chem* 74, 4526–4531.
7. Song, L., James, S. R., Kazim, L., and Karpf, A. R. (2005) Specific method for the determination of genomic DNA methylation by liquid chromatography-electrospray ionization tandem mass spectrometry, *Anal Chem* 77, 504–510.
8. Karimi, M., Johansson, S., Stach, D., Corcoran, M., Grander, D., Schalling, M., Bakalkin, G., Lyko, F., Larsson, C., and Ekstrom, T. J. (2006) LUMA (LUminometric Methylation Assay)—a high throughput method to the analysis of genomic DNA methylation, *Exp Cell Res* 312, 1989–1995.
9. Balaghi, M., and Wagner, C. (1993) DNA methylation in folate deficiency: use of CpG methylase, *Biochem Biophys Res Commun* 193, 1184–1190.
10. Lander, E. S., Linton, L. M., Birren, B., Nusbaum, C., Zody, M. C., Baldwin, J., Devon, K., Dewar, K., Doyle, M., FitzHugh, W., Funke, R., Gage, D., Harris, K., Heaford, A., Howland, J., Kann, L., Lehoczky, J., LeVine, R., McEwan, P., McKernan, K., Meldrim, J., Mesirov, J. P., Miranda, C., Morris, W., Naylor, J., Raymond, C., Rosetti, M., Santos, R., Sheridan, A., Sougnez, C., Stange-Thomann, N., Stojanovic, N., Subramanian, A., Wyman, D., Rogers, J., Sulston, J., Ainscough, R., Beck, S., Bentley, D., Burton, J., Clee, C., Carter, N., Coulson, A., Deadman, R., Deloukas, P., Dunham, A., Dunham, I., Durbin, R., French, L., Grafham, D., Gregory, S., Hubbard, T., Humphray, S., Hunt, A., Jones, M., Lloyd, C., McMurray, A., Matthews, L., Mercer, S., Milne, S., Mullikin, J. C., Mungall, A., Plumb, R., Ross, M., Shownkeen, R., Sims, S., Waterston, R. H., Wilson, R. K., Hillier, L. W., McPherson, J. D., Marra, M. A., Mardis, E. R., Fulton, L. A., Chinwalla, A. T., Pepin, K. H., Gish, W. R., Chissoe, S. L., Wendl, M. C., Delehaunty, K. D., Miner, T. L., Delehaunty, A., Kramer, J. B., Cook, L. L., Fulton, R. S., Johnson, D. L., Minx, P. J., Clifton, S. W., Hawkins, T., Branscomb, E., Predki, P., Richardson, P., Wenning, S., Slezak, T., Doggett, N., Cheng, J. F., Olsen, A., Lucas, S., Elkin, C., Uberbacher, E., Frazier, M., Gibbs, R. A., Muzny, D. M., Scherer, S. E., Bouck, J. B., Sodergren, E. J., Worley, K. C., Rives, C. M., Gorrell, J. H., Metzker, M. L., Naylor, S. L., Kucherlapati, R. S., Nelson, D. L., Weinstock, G. M., Sakaki, Y., Fujiyama, A., Hattori, M., Yada, T., Toyoda, A., Itoh, T., Kawagoe, C., Watanabe, H., Totoki, Y., Taylor, T., Weissenbach, J., Heilig, R., Saurin, W., Artiguenave, F., Brottier, P., Bruls, T., Pelletier, E., Robert, C., Wincker, P., Smith, D. R., Doucette-Stamm, L., Rubenfield, M., Weinstock, K., Lee, H. M., Dubois, J., Rosenthal, A., Platzer, M., Nyakatura, G., Taudien, S., Rump, A., Yang, H., Yu, J., Wang, J., Huang, G., Gu, J., Hood, L., Rowen, L., Madan, A., Qin, S., Davis, R. W., Federspiel, N. A., Abola, A. P., Proctor, M. J., Myers, R. M., Schmutz, J., Dickson, M., Grimwood, J., Cox, D. R., Olson, M. V., Kaul, R., Shimizu, N., Kawasaki, K., Minoshima, S., Evans, G. A., Athanasiou, M., Schultz, R., Roe, B. A., Chen, F., Pan, H., Ramser, J., Lehrach, H., Reinhardt, R., McCombie, W. R., de la Bastide, M., Dedhia, N., Blocker, H., Hornischer, K., Nordsiek, G., Agarwala, R., Aravind, L., Bailey, J. A., Bateman, A., Batzoglou, S., Birney, E., Bork, P., Brown, D. G., Burge, C. B., Cerutti, L., Chen, H. C., Church, D., Clamp, M., Copley, R. R., Doerks, T., Eddy, S. R., Eichler, E. E., Furey, T. S., Galagan, J., Gilbert, J. G., Harmon, C., Hayashizaki, Y., Haussler, D., Hermjakob, H., Hokamp, K., Jang, W., Johnson, L. S., Jones, T. A., Kasif, S., Kaspryzk, A., Kennedy, S., Kent, W. J., Kitts, P., Koonin, E. V., Korf, I., Kulp, D., Lancet, D., Lowe, T. M., McLysaght, A., Mikkelsen, T., Moran, J. V., Mulder, N., Pollara, V. J., Ponting, C. P., Schuler, G., Schultz, J., Slater, G., Smit, A. F., Stupka, E., Szustakowski, J., Thierry-Mieg, D., Thierry-Mieg, J., Wagner, L., Wallis, J.,

Wheeler, R., Williams, A., Wolf, Y. I., Wolfe, K. H., Yang, S. P., Yeh, R. F., Collins, F., Guyer, M. S., Peterson, J., Felsenfeld, A., Wetterstrand, K. A., Patrinos, A., Morgan, M. J., de Jong, P., Catanese, J. J., Osoegawa, K., Shizuya, H., Choi, S., and Chen, Y. J. (2001) Initial sequencing and analysis of the human genome, *Nature* 409, 860–921.

11. Rollins, R. A., Haghighi, F., Edwards, J. R., Das, R., Zhang, M. Q., Ju, J., and Bestor, T. H. (2006) Large-scale structure of genomic methylation patterns, *Genome Res* 16, 157–163.
12. Irahara, N., Nosho, K., Baba, Y., Shima, K., Lindeman, N. I., Hazra, A., Schernhammer, E. S., Hunter, D. J., Fuchs, C. S., and Ogino, S. (2010) Precision of pyrosequencing assay to measure LINE-1 methylation in colon cancer, normal colonic mucosa, and peripheral blood cells, *J Mol Diagn* 12, 177–183.
13. Weisenberger, D. J., Campan, M., Long, T. I., Kim, M., Woods, C., Fiala, E., Ehrlich, M., and Laird, P. W. (2005) Analysis of repetitive element DNA methylation by MethyLight, *Nucleic Acids Res.* 33, 6823–6836.
14. Herman, J. G., Graff, J. R., Myohanen, S., Nelkin, B. D., and Baylin, S. B. (1996) Methylation-specific PCR: a novel PCR assay for methylation status of CpG islands, *Proc Natl Acad Sci U S A* 93, 9821–9826.
15. Eads, C. A., Danenberg, K. D., Kawakami, K., Saltz, L. B., Blake, C., Shibata, D., Danenberg, P. V., and Laird, P. W. (2000) MethyLight: a high-throughput assay to measure DNA methylation, *Nucleic Acids Res.* 28, E32.
16. Ehrich, M., Nelson, M. R., Stanssens, P., Zabeau, M., Liloglou, T., Xinarianos, G., Cantor, C. R., Field, J. K., and van den Boom, D. (2005) Quantitative high-throughput analysis of DNA methylation patterns by base-specific cleavage and mass spectrometry, *Proc Natl Acad Sci U S A* 102, 15785–15790.
17. Coolen, M. W., Statham, A. L., Gardiner-Garden, M., and Clark, S. J. (2007) Genomic profiling of CpG methylation and allelic specificity using quantitative high-throughput mass spectrometry: critical evaluation and improvements, *Nucleic Acids Res* 35, e119.
18. Heijmans, B. T., Tobi, E. W., Stein, A. D., Putter, H., Blauw, G. J., Susser, E. S., Slagboom, P. E., and Lumey, L. H. (2008) Persistent epigenetic differences associated with prenatal exposure to famine in humans, *Proc.Natl.Acad. Sci.U.S.A* 105, 17046–17049.
19. Zilberman, D., and Henikoff, S. (2007) Genome-wide analysis of DNA methylation patterns, *Development* 134, 3959–3965.
20. Bibikova, M., Lin, Z., Zhou, L., Chudin, E., Garcia, E. W., Wu, B., Doucet, D., Thomas, N. J., Wang, Y., Vollmer, E., Goldmann, T., Seifart, C., Jiang, W., Barker, D. L., Chee, M. S., Floros, J., and Fan, J. B. (2006) High-throughput DNA methylation profiling using universal bead arrays, *Genome Res* 16, 383–393.
21. Fraga, M. F., Ballestar, E., Paz, M. F., Ropero, S., Setien, F., Ballestar, M. L., Heine-Suner, D., Cigudosa, J. C., Urioste, M., Benitez, J., Boix-Chornet, M., Sanchez-Aguilera, A., Ling, C., Carlsson, E., Poulsen, P., Vaag, A., Stephan, Z., Spector, T. D., Wu, Y. Z., Plass, C., and Esteller, M. (2005) Epigenetic differences arise during the lifetime of monozygotic twins, *Proc. Natl.Acad.Sci.U.S.A* 102, 10604–10609.
22. Heijmans, B. T., Kremer, D., Tobi, E. W., Boomsma, D. I., and Slagboom, P. E. (2007) Heritable rather than age-related environmental and stochastic factors dominate variation in DNA methylation of the human IGF2/H19 locus, *Hum.Mol.Genet.* 16, 547–554.
23. Bjornsson, H. T., Sigurdsson, M. I., Fallin, M. D., Irizarry, R. A., Aspelund, T., Cui, H., Yu, W., Rongione, M. A., Ekstrom, T. J., Harris, T. B., Launer, L. J., Eiriksdottir, G., Leppert, M. F., Sapienza, C., Gudnason, V., and Feinberg, A. P. (2008) Intra-individual change over time in DNA methylation with familial clustering, *JAMA* 299, 2877–2883.
24. Talens, R. P., Boomsma, D. I., Tobi, E. W., Kremer, D., Jukema, J. W., Willemsen, G., Putter, H., Slagboom, P. E., and Heijmans, B. T. (2010) Variation, patterns, and temporal stability of DNA methylation: considerations for epigenetic epidemiology, *FASEB J* 24, 3135–3144.
25. Sandovici, I., Leppert, M., Hawk, P. R., Suarez, A., Linares, Y., and Sapienza, C. (2003) Familial aggregation of abnormal methylation of parental alleles at the IGF2/H19 and IGF2R differentially methylated regions, *Hum Mol Genet* 12, 1569–1578.
26. Keyes, M. K., Jang, H., Mason, J. B., Liu, Z., Crott, J. W., Smith, D. E., Friso, S., and Choi, S. W. (2007) Older age and dietary folate are determinants of genomic and p16-specific DNA methylation in mouse colon, *J Nutr* 137, 1713–1717.
27. Christensen, B. C., Houseman, E. A., Marsit, C. J., Zheng, S., Wrensch, M. R., Wiemels, J. L., Nelson, H. H., Karagas, M. R., Padbury, J. F., Bueno, R., Sugarbaker, D. J., Yeh, R. F., Wiencke, J. K., and Kelsey, K. T. (2009) Aging and environmental exposures alter tissue-specific DNA methylation dependent upon CpG island context, *PLoS Genet* 5, e1000602.
28. Jintaridth, P., and Mutirangura, A. (2010) Distinctive patterns of age-dependent

hypomethylation in interspersed repetitive sequences, *Physiol Genomics.*

29. Zhu, Z. Z., Hou, L., Bollati, V., Tarantini, L., Marinelli, B., Cantone, L., Yang, A. S., Vokonas, P., Lissowska, J., Fustinoni, S., Pesatori, A. C., Bonzini, M., Apostoli, P., Costa, G., Bertazzi, P. A., Chow, W. H., Schwartz, J., and Baccarelli, A. (2010) Predictors of global methylation levels in blood DNA of healthy subjects: a combined analysis, *Int J Epidemiol.*
30. El-Maarri, O., Becker, T., Junen, J., Manzoor, S. S., Diaz-Lacava, A., Schwaab, R., Wienker, T., and Oldenburg, J. (2007) Gender specific differences in levels of DNA methylation at selected loci from human total blood: a tendency toward higher methylation levels in males, *Hum Genet* 122, 505–514.
31. Terry, M. B., Ferris, J. S., Pilsner, R., Flom, J. D., Tehranifar, P., Santella, R. M., Gamble, M. V., and Susser, E. (2008) Genomic DNA methylation among women in a multiethnic New York City birth cohort, *Cancer Epidemiol. Biomarkers Prev.* 17, 2306–2310.
32. Figueiredo, J. C., Grau, M. V., Wallace, K., Levine, A. J., Shen, L., Hamdan, R., Chen, X., Bresalier, R. S., McKeown-Eyssen, G., Haile, R. W., Baron, J. A., and Issa, J. P. (2009) Global DNA hypomethylation (LINE-1) in the normal colon and lifestyle characteristics and dietary and genetic factors, *Cancer Epidemiol Biomarkers Prev* 18, 1041–1049.
33. Jacob, R. A., Gretz, D. M., Taylor, P. C., James, S. J., Pogribny, I. P., Miller, B. J., Henning, S. M., and Swendseid, M. E. (1998) Moderate folate depletion increases plasma homocysteine and decreases lymphocyte DNA methylation in postmenopausal women, *J Nutr* 128, 1204–1212.
34. Rampersaud, G. C., Kauwell, G. P., Hutson, A. D., Cerda, J. J., and Bailey, L. B. (2000) Genomic DNA methylation decreases in response to moderate folate depletion in elderly women, *Am J Clin Nutr* 72, 998–1003.
35. Pufulete, M., Al Ghnaniem, R., Khushal, A., Appleby, P., Harris, N., Gout, S., Emery, P. W., and Sanders, T. A. (2005) Effect of folic acid supplementation on genomic DNA methylation in patients with colorectal adenoma, *Gut* 54, 648–653.
36. Choi, J. Y., James, S. R., Link, P. A., McCann, S. E., Hong, C. C., Davis, W., Nesline, M. K., Ambrosone, C. B., and Karpf, A. R. (2009) Association between global DNA hypomethylation in leukocytes and risk of breast cancer, *Carcinogenesis* 30, 1889–1897.
37. Cravo, M. L., Pinto, A. G., Chaves, P., Cruz, J. A., Lage, P., Nobre Leitao, C., and Costa Mira, F. (1998) Effect of folate supplementation on DNA methylation of rectal mucosa in patients with colonic adenomas: correlation with nutrient intake, *Clin Nutr* 17, 45–49.
38. Pufulete, M., Al Ghnaniem, R., Rennie, J. A., Appleby, P., Harris, N., Gout, S., Emery, P. W., and Sanders, T. A. (2005) Influence of folate status on genomic DNA methylation in colonic mucosa of subjects without colorectal adenoma or cancer, *Br.J.Cancer* 92, 838–842.
39. Schernhammer, E. S., Giovannucci, E., Kawasaki, T., Rosner, B., Fuchs, C. S., and Ogino, S. (2010) Dietary folate, alcohol and B vitamins in relation to LINE-1 hypomethylation in colon cancer, *Gut* 59, 794–799.
40. Ogino, S., Nosho, K., Kirkner, G. J., Kawasaki, T., Chan, A. T., Schernhammer, E. S., Giovannucci, E. L., and Fuchs, C. S. (2008) A cohort study of tumoral LINE-1 hypomethylation and prognosis in colon cancer, *J Natl Cancer Inst* 100, 1734–1738.
41. Friso, S., Choi, S. W., Girelli, D., Mason, J. B., Dolnikowski, G. G., Bagley, P. J., Olivieri, O., Jacques, P. F., Rosenberg, I. H., Corrocher, R., and Selhub, J. (2002) A common mutation in the 5,10-methylenetetrahydrofolate reductase gene affects genomic DNA methylation through an interaction with folate status, *Proc Natl Acad Sci U S A* 99, 5606–5611.
42. Paz, M. F., Avila, S., Fraga, M. F., Pollan, M., Capella, G., Peinado, M. A., Sanchez-Cespedes, M., Herman, J. G., and Esteller, M. (2002) Germ-line variants in methyl-group metabolism genes and susceptibility to DNA methylation in normal tissues and human primary tumors, *Cancer Res* 62, 4519–4524.
43. van Engeland, M., Weijenberg, M. P., Roemen, G. M., Brink, M., de Bruine, A. P., Goldbohm, R. A., van den Brandt, P. A., Baylin, S. B., de Goeij, A. F., and Herman, J. G. (2003) Effects of dietary folate and alcohol intake on promoter methylation in sporadic colorectal cancer: the Netherlands cohort study on diet and cancer, *Cancer Res* 63, 3133–3137.
44. Vineis, P., Chuang, S. C., Vaissiere, T., Cuenin, C., Ricceri, F., Johansson, M., Ueland, P., Brennan, P., and Herceg, Z. (2011) DNA methylation changes associated with cancer risk factors and blood levels of vitamin metabolites in a prospective study, *Epigenetics* 6.
45. Vaissiere, T., Hung, R. J., Zaridze, D., Moukeria, A., Cuenin, C., Fasolo, V., Ferro, G., Paliwal, A., Hainaut, P., Brennan, P., Tost, J., Boffetta, P., and Herceg, Z. (2009) Quantitative analysis of DNA methylation profiles in lung cancer identifies aberrant DNA methylation of specific genes and its association

with gender and cancer risk factors, *Cancer Res* 69, 243–252.

46. Yuasa, Y., Nagasaki, H., Akiyama, Y., Sakai, H., Nakajima, T., Ohkura, Y., Takizawa, T., Koike, M., Tani, M., Iwai, T., Sugihara, K., Imai, K., and Nakachi, K. (2005) Relationship between CDX2 gene methylation and dietary factors in gastric cancer patients, *Carcinogenesis* 26, 193–200.
47. Yuasa, Y., Nagasaki, H., Akiyama, Y., Hashimoto, Y., Takizawa, T., Kojima, K., Kawano, T., Sugihara, K., Imai, K., and Nakachi, K. (2009) DNA methylation status is inversely correlated with green tea intake and physical activity in gastric cancer patients, *Int J Cancer* 124, 2677–2682.
48. Fang, M. Z., Wang, Y., Ai, N., Hou, Z., Sun, Y., Lu, H., Welsh, W., and Yang, C. S. (2003) Tea polyphenol (−)-epigallocatechin-3-gallate inhibits DNA methyltransferase and reactivates methylation-silenced genes in cancer cell lines, *Cancer Res* 63, 7563–7570.
49. Lee, W. J., Shim, J. Y., and Zhu, B. T. (2005) Mechanisms for the inhibition of DNA methyltransferases by tea catechins and bioflavonoids, *Mol Pharmacol* 68, 1018–1030.
50. Dolinoy, D. C., Weidman, J. R., Waterland, R. A., and Jirtle, R. L. (2006) Maternal genistein alters coat color and protects Avy mouse offspring from obesity by modifying the fetal epigenome, *Environ Health Perspect* 114, 567–572.
51. King-Batoon, A., Leszczynska, J. M., and Klein, C. B. (2008) Modulation of gene methylation by genistein or lycopene in breast cancer cells, *Environ Mol Mutagen* 49, 36–45.
52. Nakajima, K., Takeoka, M., Mori, M., Hashimoto, S., Sakurai, A., Nose, H., Higuchi, K., Itano, N., Shiohara, M., Oh, T., and Taniguchi, S. (2010) Exercise effects on methylation of ASC gene, *Int J Sports Med* 31, 671–675.
53. Alibegovic, A. C., Sonne, M. P., Hojbjerre, L., Bork-Jensen, J., Jacobsen, S., Nilsson, E., Faerch, K., Hiscock, N., Mortensen, B., Friedrichsen, M., Stallknecht, B., Dela, F., and Vaag, A. (2010) Insulin resistance induced by physical inactivity is associated with multiple transcriptional changes in skeletal muscle in young men, *Am J Physiol Endocrinol Metab* 299, E752–763.
54. Gemma, C., Sookoian, S., Dieuzeide, G., Garcia, S. I., Gianotti, T. F., Gonzalez, C. D., and Pirola, C. J. (2010) Methylation of TFAM gene promoter in peripheral white blood cells is associated with insulin resistance in adolescents, *Mol Genet Metab* 100, 83–87.
55. Lim, U., Flood, A., Choi, S. W., Albanes, D., Cross, A. J., Schatzkin, A., Sinha, R., Katki, H. A., Cash, B., Schoenfeld, P., and Stolzenberg-Solomon, R. (2008) Genomic methylation of leukocyte DNA in relation to colorectal adenoma among asymptomatic women, *Gastroenterology* 134, 47–55.
56. Mathers, J. C., Strathdee, G., and Relton, C. L. (2010) Induction of epigenetic alterations by dietary and other environmental factors, *Adv Genet* 71, 3–39.
57. Limsui, D., Vierkant, R. A., Tillmans, L. S., Wang, A. H., Weisenberger, D. J., Laird, P. W., Lynch, C. F., Anderson, K. E., French, A. J., Haile, R. W., Harnack, L. J., Potter, J. D., Slager, S. L., Smyrk, T. C., Thibodeau, S. N., Cerhan, J. R., and Limburg, P. J. (2010) Cigarette smoking and colorectal cancer risk by molecularly defined subtypes, *J Natl Cancer Inst* 102, 1012–1022.
58. Friso, S., Lamon-Fava, S., Jang, H., Schaefer, E. J., Corrocher, R., and Choi, S. W. (2007) Oestrogen replacement therapy reduces total plasma homocysteine and enhances genomic DNA methylation in postmenopausal women, *Br J Nutr* 97, 617–621.
59. Wu, A. H., Siegmund, K. D., Long, T. I., Cozen, W., Wan, P., Tseng, C. C., Shibata, D., and Laird, P. W. (2010) Hormone therapy, DNA methylation and colon cancer, *Carcinogenesis* 31, 1060–1067.
60. Pavanello, S., Bollati, V., Pesatori, A. C., Kapka, L., Bolognesi, C., Bertazzi, P. A., and Baccarelli, A. (2009) Global and gene-specific promoter methylation changes are related to anti-B(a)PDE-DNA adduct levels and influence micronuclei levels in polycyclic aromatic hydrocarbon-exposed individuals, *Int J Cancer* 125, 1692–1697.
61. Hales, C. N., and Barker, D. J. (2001) The thrifty phenotype hypothesis, *Br Med Bull* 60, 5–20.
62. Ravelli, G. P., Stein, Z. A., and Susser, M. W. (1976) Obesity in young men after famine exposure in utero and early infancy, *N Engl J Med* 295, 349–353.
63. Ravelli, A. C., van Der Meulen, J. H., Osmond, C., Barker, D. J., and Bleker, O. P. (1999) Obesity at the age of 50 y in men and women exposed to famine prenatally, *Am J Clin Nutr* 70, 811–816.
64. Roseboom, T. J., van der Meulen, J. H., Ravelli, A. C., Osmond, C., Barker, D. J., and Bleker, O. P. (2001) Effects of prenatal exposure to the Dutch famine on adult disease in later life: an overview, *Twin Res* 4, 293–298.
65. Painter, R. C., De Rooij, S. R., Bossuyt, P. M., Osmond, C., Barker, D. J., Bleker, O. P., and Roseboom, T. J. (2006) A possible link between prenatal exposure to famine and

breast cancer: a preliminary study, *Am J Hum Biol* 18, 853–856.

66. Painter, R. C., Osmond, C., Gluckman, P., Hanson, M., Phillips, D. I., and Roseboom, T. J. (2008) Transgenerational effects of prenatal exposure to the Dutch famine on neonatal adiposity and health in later life, *BJOG* 115, 1243–1249.
67. Lussana, F., Painter, R. C., Ocke, M. C., Buller, H. R., Bossuyt, P. M., and Roseboom, T. J. (2008) Prenatal exposure to the Dutch famine is associated with a preference for fatty foods and a more atherogenic lipid profile, *Am J Clin Nutr* 88, 1648–1652.
68. Waterland, R. A., and Michels, K. B. (2007) Epigenetic epidemiology of the developmental origins hypothesis, *Annu.Rev.Nutr.* 27, 363–388.
69. Gluckman, P. D., Hanson, M. A., Cooper, C., and Thornburg, K. L. (2008) Effect of in utero and early-life conditions on adult health and disease, *N Engl J Med* 359, 61–73.
70. Waterland, R. A., and Garza, C. (1999) Potential mechanisms of metabolic imprinting that lead to chronic disease, *Am J Clin Nutr* 69, 179–197.
71. Tobi, E. W., Lumey, L. H., Talens, R. P., Kremer, D., Putter, H., Stein, A. D., Slagboom, P. E., and Heijmans, B. T. (2009) DNA methylation differences after exposure to prenatal famine are common and timing- and sex-specific, *Hum Mol Genet* 18, 4046–4053.
72. Tobi, E. W., Heijmans, B. T., Kremer, D., Putter, H., Delemarre-van de Waal, H. A., Finken, M. J., Wit, J. M., and Slagboom, P. E. (2011) DNA methylation of IGF2, GNASAS, INSIGF and LEP and being born small for gestational age, *Epigenetics* 6.
73. Steegers-Theunissen, R. P., Obermann-Borst, S. A., Kremer, D., Lindemans, J., Siebel, C., Steegers, E. A., Slagboom, P. E., and Heijmans, B. T. (2009) Periconceptional maternal folic acid use of 400 microg per day is related to increased methylation of the IGF2 gene in the very young child, *PLoS One* 4, e7845.
74. Gemma, C., Sookoian, S., Alvarinas, J., Garcia, S. I., Quintana, L., Kanevsky, D., Gonzalez, C. D., and Pirola, C. J. (2009) Maternal Pregestational BMI Is Associated With Methylation of the PPARGC1A Promoter in Newborns, *Obesity.(Silver.Spring)*.
75. Lim, U., Wang, S. S., Hartge, P., Cozen, W., Kelemen, L. E., Chanock, S., Davis, S., Blair, A., Schenk, M., Rothman, N., and Lan, Q. (2007) Gene-nutrient interactions among determinants of folate and one-carbon metabolism on the risk of non-Hodgkin lymphoma: NCI-SEER case-control study, *Blood* 109, 3050–3059.
76. Shane, B. (2000) Folic Acid, Vitamin B12, and Vitamin B6, In *Biochemical and physiological aspects of human nutrition* (Stipanuk, M. H., Ed.), pp 453–518, W.B. Saunders Company, Philadelphia.
77. Choi, S. W., and Mason, J. B. (2000) Folate and carcinogenesis: an integrated scheme, *J Nutr* 130, 129–132.
78. Bailey, L. B. (1995) *Folate in health and disease*, Marcel Dekker, Inc., New York.
79. Institute of Medicine. (1998) Dietary reference intakes for thiamin, riboflavin, niacin, vitamin B6, folate, vitamin B12, pantothenic acid, biotin, and choline, National Academy Press, Washington, DC.
80. Stover, P. J., and Garza, C. (2006) Nutrition and developmental biology--implications for public health, *Nutr Rev* 64, S60-71; discussion S72–91.
81. Kelemen, L. E. (2006) The role of folate receptor alpha in cancer development, progression and treatment: cause, consequence or innocent bystander?, *Int.J.Cancer* 119, 243–250.
82. Zhao, R., Matherly, L. H., and Goldman, I. D. (2009) Membrane transporters and folate homeostasis: intestinal absorption and transport into systemic compartments and tissues, *Expert Rev Mol Med* 11, e4.

Chapter 24

Diet, Epigenetics, and Cancer

L. Joseph Su

Abstract

Cancer encompasses a highly heterogeneous group of diseases. It has been thought that transition from promotion to progression in carcinogenesis may be driven primarily by epigenetic abnormalities. Diet is known to play crucial roles in cancer etiology and has an important role in epigenetics. Current knowledge in the interrelationship among cancer, nutrition and epigenetics is reviewed.

Key words: Nutrition, Epigenetics, Cancer

1. Background: Epigenetics and Nutrition

Cancer is thought as a group of diseases initiated and driven by heritable genetic aberrations in important genes as the result of exposure to endogenous and environmental agents (1, 2). Therefore, the general approach for elucidating key events for cancer development has been focused on identification of genetic lesions associated with carcinogenesis. However, the presence of genetic abnormality by itself is not sufficient for tumor formation. Mainly, the inability of cells to maintain and control accurate expression of genetic information is responsible for tumorigenesis. Additionally, genetic alternations alone cannot explain the extremely diverse phenotypic changes observed in preneoplastic and malignant cells. These findings have led to the hypothesis that the transition from promotion, a stage that may be reversible in carcinogenesis, to progression, a stage on the other hand may be irreversible, may be driven primarily by epigenetic abnormalities (3).

Epigenetics is defined as processes that regulate heritable changes in gene activity that are transmitted through meiosis and mitosis but not accompanied by changes in the coding sequence of DNA (4). Gene expression is controlled by epigenetic signals through remodeling of chromatin, which consists of DNA and

Ramona G. Dumitrescu and Mukesh Verma (eds.), *Cancer Epigenetics: Methods and Protocols*, Methods in Molecular Biology, vol. 863, DOI 10.1007/978-1-61779-612-8_24, © Springer Science+Business Media, LLC 2012

DNA-binding proteins, such as histone. It is critically important for epigenetic control of gene expression in regulating embryonic development, cellular differentiation and organogenesis, and imprinting and silencing of large chromosomal domains, such as the X chromosome in females. Dysregulation of any of these processes has severe consequences for the phenotype and function of the cell, which may be causal for several human diseases, including cancer (5). During the malignant transformation, cancer cells can exhibit global changes in the chromatin structure affecting the whole epigenome, altering the expression of hundreds of genes and perturbing entire metabolic pathways. As a result, epigenetic dysregulation has been hypothesized to be detrimental to the cell as mutation in DNA coding (5).

Diet and lifestyle play crucial roles in cancer etiology. It has been estimated that poor choice of diet could account for more than one-third of cancer death in the USA (6). Several different mechanisms, such as antioxidant, anti-inflammatory, antiestrogenic, etc., have been proposed regarding the protective nature of certain nutrients. However, the exact mechanistic pathways where these effects exert on the cells to avoid, delay, or reverse carcinogenesis were not as clear. Epigenetic marks are influenced by aging and by the environment exposures (7, 8). The observation that epigenetic changes are reversible makes them an attractive target for cancer prevention.

Established epigenetic patterns during the fetal period can be changed in adult life by environmental factors including nutrition. Diet can profoundly alter epigenetic patterns in animals. The Agouti mouse has been used extensively to demonstrate the impact of maternal nutrition on the fetal epigenome and the phenotype of the offspring (9). The coat color is linked to the methylation status of the agouti gene, which is highly dependent on maternal diet. Most importantly, altered epigenetic change is associated with the increased risk of diabetes-like condition, obesity, and tumorigenesis (10–12). There are also some evidences that specific nutrients in the human diet that are strongly associated with the risk of cancer can modulate DNA methylation (13). For example, it is found that identical twins possess the same genotype and no distinguishable epigenetic differences in their early life but showed remarkable differences in genomic methylation and histone acetylation patterns in their later life (14). These epigenetic differences may result in different gene expression and disease susceptibility.

Nutrient intakes play an important role in regulating one-carbon metabolism (15, 16). Excessive or deficient nutrient status may have an effect on DNA methylation. This is based on the observation that the primary methyl donor, *S*-adenosylmethionine (SAM) may be regenerated from *S*-adenosylhomocysteine (SAH) through a series of several chemical reactions that rely on the presence of several nutrients, such as folate, betaine, choline, zinc,

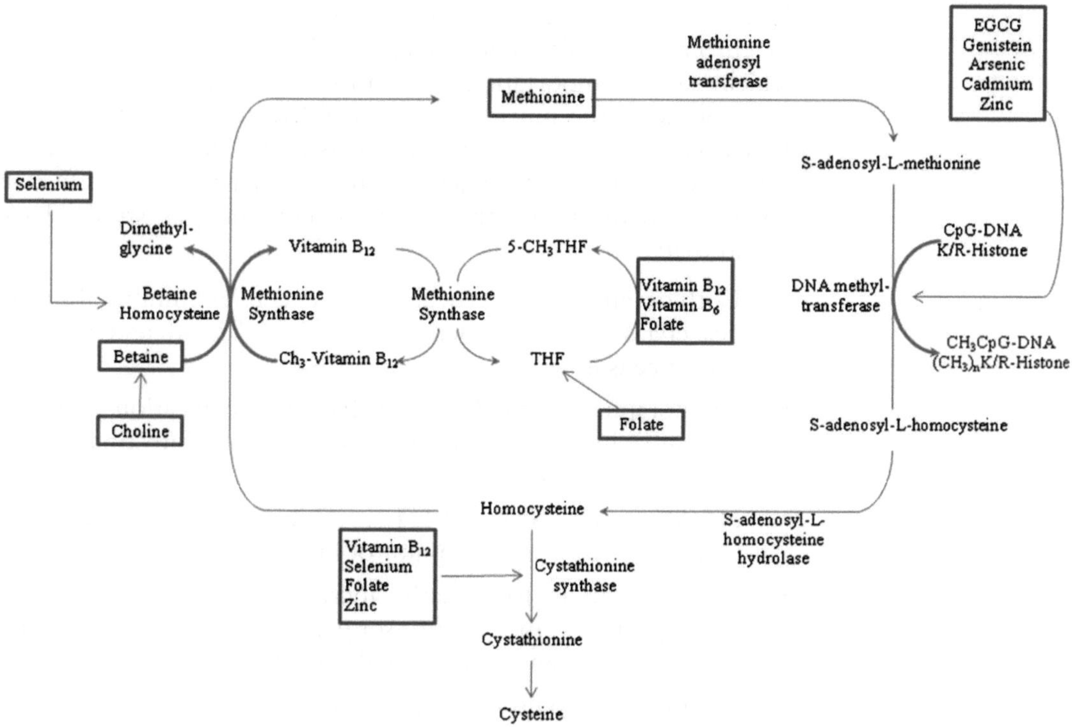

Fig. 1. Overview of the menthionine-homocysteine-folate-B_{12} cycle, which provides methyl donors for methyltransferase. Nutritional regulations of the cycle are identified by rectangle frames (adapted from (17)).

vitamin B_6, and vitamin B_{12}, as cofactors or intermediates (Fig. 1). Deficiency on any of these nutrients can result in a depletion of cellular pools of SAM, which may cause aberrant DNA methylation (18). Folate, vitamin B_6, vitamin B_{12}, methionine, and choline are involved in the one-carbon metabolism and provide the most compelling data for the interaction between nutrients and DNA methylation because they influence the supply of methyl groups and hence the biochemical pathways of methylation process (19). Other dietary factors, such as alcohol, arsenic, cadmium, coumestrol, equol, genistein, nickel, selenium, tea polyphenol, vitamin A, and zinc are also known to influence DNA methylation and cancer susceptibility (15). Certain bioactive food components, such as sulforaphanes in broccoli, diallyl disulfides in garlic, and resveratrol in wine, have been shown to alter epigenetic processes in cell functions, such as control of proliferation, upregulated apoptosis, and reduction in inflammation (20).

It is still unclear what the causal link between diet and epigenetics in the development of cancer is and whether diet is differentially effective at various stages in the lifespan of humans despite observations on abnormal epigenetic control of gene expression increases cancer risk (12). Hypermethylation as the result of excess or deficient of certain nutrients or food components may affect the binding of transcription factors to DNA and change the structure of chromatin resulting in silencing of tumor suppressor genes, which plays an important role in cancer initiation and progression (21). Some of the nutrients, such as folate and other B vitamins have been explored more on their effects on cancer. Other nutrients, on the other hand, have only limited information indicative of epigenetic pathway in carcinogenesis. For example, studies have found that:

- Isothiocyanates in cruciferous vegetables inhibit histone deacetylase (HDAC) activity in colon, breast, and prostate cancer cells in vitro.
- Sulphoraphane, an inducer for phase 2 detoxification enzymes, increases histone acetylation and inhibits intestinal polyp formation in *Apc*-min mice.
- HDAC activity (H3 and H4) is inhibited in blood cells from volunteers fed a small amount of broccoli sprouts.
- Diallyl disulfide from garlic increases H3 and H4 histone deacetylation, tumor suppressor gene *p21* gene expression and inhibits colon cancer cell growth in culture.
- Polyphenol curcumin in spice tumeric and resveratrol in red wine (strong antioxidant, anti-inflammatory, and anticarcinogenic) modify histone acetylation patterns in circulating inflammatory cells and induce HDAC activity (22).

This chapter is by no means to serve as a comprehensive summary of published information, in particular because this is a fast growing research field with new publications quickly becoming available. It intends to offer a review of major evidences regarding diet, epigenetics, and cancer.

2. Nutrients

2.1. Folate

Folate probably is one of the most studied nutrients on DNA methylation because it's position on the one-carbon metabolism pathway. Folate is a group of water-soluble B vitamins that is found in high concentration mostly in green leafy vegetables. Folate deficiency has been implicated in the development of several human epithelial cell malignancies, including cancer of breast, ovary, pancreas, brain, lung, cervix, and colon (23–26).

As a coenzyme in one-carbon metabolism, folate participates in both nucleotide synthesis (genetic pathway) and DNA methylation (epigenetic pathway). Folate and aging interact genetically and epigenetically in a complex manner thus to promote cancer development (27). Inadequate folate intake reduces the synthesis of thymidylate from deoxyuridylate, resulting in excessive uracil misincorporation into DNA thus leading to mutagenesis (28, 29).

It has been demonstrated that increased uracil content in elder rat colonic DNA when compared to young rats; and dietary folate depletion further increased uracil misincorporation (30). Folate can also affect the integrity of mitochondrial DNA, which is thought to play an important role in tumorigenesis (31–33). On the methylation front, folate depletion decreases SAM, the universal methyl donor, and increases SAH, an inhibitor of methyltransferases. Aberrant DNA methylation mediated by folate depletion has also been regarded as one of the candidate mechanisms that explain the association between folate and cancer (34).

It has been suggested that under conditions of limiting folate or methionine, SAM synthesis has metabolic priority over DNA biosynthesis, and one-carbon units are directed preferentially through the methionine cycle to facilitate methylation reactions at the expense of DNA synthesis and repairs (24). The enzyme methyltetrafolate reductase (MTHFR) catalyzes the irreversible conversion of 5,10-methylene THF into 5-methyl THF, which remethylates homocysteine to methionine. This key protein thus controls whether folate is partitioned toward DNA precursor synthesis or DNA methylation. Polymorphisms at *MTHFR* gene modulate the risk of human cancers. Impaired MTHFR activity would be expected to increase cancer risk due to low blood 5-methyl THF, DNA hypomethylation, and proto-oncogene activation.

Genomic DNA hypomethylation is observed in many malignant tissues. Decreased DNA methylation is thought to promote chromosomal instability, eventually leading to carcinogenesis (35, 36). Genome-wide DNA hypomethylation also affects transcription through loss of imprinting, ectopic oncofetal gene expression, and upregulation of silent genes, all of which might induce tumor development (37, 38). It is hypothesized that folate deficiency may induce both gene-specific DNA hypermethylation and global hypomethylation by its DNA-damaging effect. DNA methyltransferase (DNMT), an ancestral DNA repair protein, is sequestered away from the DNA replication folk to regions of folate-deficiency-induced DNA damage, resulting in both genomic hypomethylation and site-specific hypermethylation in gene promoter regions (39). Global and gene-specific DNA hypomethylation and site-specific hypermethylation are common features in tumorigenesis (40).

Inhibition of methyl transfer or reduced folate intake could increase the risk of neural tube defects in humans by reducing level of DNA methylation (13, 41, 42). Folate status is positively associated with DNA methylation status during pregnancy (43). A study using hyperhomocysteinemia rat model demonstrated that folate-supplemented diet increased placenta DNA methylation while folate-depleted diet decreased the methylation in placenta. Placenta DNA methylation was also positively correlated with hepatic folate and hepatic SAM, the unique methyl donor for DNA methylation (44).

Rats fed a protein-restricted diet during pregnancy showed decreased promoter methylation and increased expression of the glucocorticoid receptor gene (*GR*) and peroxisome proliferator-activated receptor gene (*PPARα*) in the liver of adult offspring along with reduced *DNMT1* expression (45, 46). However, folate supplementation could reverse DNA hypomethylation and reduced the expression of these genes (47, 48). Similarly, methyl-deficient diet in female mature sheep during early development also resulted in alterations of promoter DNA methylation and leads to offspring obesity, altered immune responses, insulin resistance and elevated blood pressure, in particular male offspring (49). It has been proposed by Waterland and Michels that these epigenetic effects of maternal nutrients on phenotype of their offspring may be explained by (1) reduced methyl availability alters the establishment of DNA methylation at metastable epialleles by affecting either one-carbon metabolism or the activity of *DNMT1* and (2) repression of critical genes may occur during *de novo* DNA methylation in early fetal development (50). Furthermore, this early nutritional effect can result in a permanent defect of epigenetic regulation through DNA methylation, suggesting a possible mechanism for the development of later life diseases (51).

Epigenetic effect of folate on cancer has been most studied in colorectal cancer since the early study finding suggesting the preventive effect of folate on colorectal cancer (52). DNA methylation is high in human colonocytes expressing the *MTHFR* TT mutation cultured in adequate or high folic acid but is hypomethylated in folate-deficient cells (53). Combined high-dose synthetic folic acids and vitamin B_{12} supplementation increased uracil misincorporation and tumor suppressor gene promoter methylation in rectal biopsies from colorectal adenoma patients (54).

Animal and human studies demonstrated that folate deficiency induces epigenetic changes by attenuating remethylation of SAH to SAM in methionine cycle, which leads to cytosine demethylation, global DNA hypomethylation, proto-oncogene activation, and chromosomal instability (26). The effect of folate status on DNA methylation and potentially on colon carcinogenesis are profoundly dependent not only on the severity and duration of folate depletion but also on the gene, tissue, and stage of malignant transformation. At this time, the available evidence does not strongly support the hypothesis that altered genome-wide DNA methylation, as the result of folate deficiency, increases human colon cancer risk. Similarly, whereas the evidence for folate deficiency decreasing genomic instability by inducing DNA damage, inhibiting DNA repair and increasing malignant transformation are more consistent across in vitro, animal, and human studies (26).

In elder rat liver, folate supplementation increases genomic DNA methylation in a dose-dependent manner (55). It is also found that genomic DNA methylation and promoter methylation of *p16*^{INK4a} increased in parallel with increase of dietary folate level in old mice colon (56). DNA methylation may interact with genetic mechanism because genomic DNA hypomethylation is associated with instability of chromosome and DNA and specific allelic sequence variation such as single nucleotide polymorphism (SNPs) may act in *cis* or *trans* to influence DNA methylation. Genetic variations in genes that regulate epigenetic phenomena such as *DNMT* genes or polymorphisms of gene involves in one-carbon metabolism, such as 5,10-methyltetrahydrofolate reductase gene (*MTHFR*), can affect DNA methylation. 5-methyltetradrofolate remethylates homocysteine to methionine and subsequently metabolized to SAM within the methionine cycle. SAM serves as one carbon donor in the methylation of DNA. Under conditions of low dietary folate, SAM concentrations are depleted causing hypomethylation of newly synthesized DNA and increased proto-oncogene expression. Although abnormal DNA methylation and gene expression is a consistent event in tumorigenesis, aberrant cytosine methylation and proto-oncogene activation may also be a common mechanism linking malignant transformation in cancer.

2.2. Vitamin B_{12}

Vitamin B_{12} is involved as cofactor for the synthesis of methionine from homocysteine. Deficiency in vitamin B_{12} leads to accumulation of serum homocysteine (57, 58). Homocysteine metabolism is strongly linked to its function as a methyl group donor in transmethylation reaction. Two possible consequences of disturbed remethylation caused by vitamin B_{12} deficiency are decreased synthesis of SAM and the reversible synthesis of SAH from homocysteine. SAH is a potent inhibitor of methyl transferase. In case of elevated homocysteine concentration, the process that SAH is hydrolysized to homocysteine is reversed. Because of their role in methylation, the SAM/SAH ratio has been suggestive as marker of cellular methylation capacity (59).

2.3. Vitamin B_1

Vitamin B_1 (thiamine) is metabolized to thiamine pyrophosphate, a cofactor of transketolase, which is involved in ribose synthesis and necessary for cell replication (60). A study of colorectal cancer patients found promoter hypermethylation in *p16*^{INK4a} among those with low vitamin B_1 intake, which may be explained by the relationship between DNA synthesis and DNA methylation through one-carbon metabolism (19).

2.4. Polyphenols

Polyphenols is a group of plant phytochemicals consumed in significant amounts in human diet. Phytochemicals may be responsible for the maintenance of normal DNA methylation and gene expression patterns as well as reversal of methylation-induced inactivation of tumor suppressor genes, which may be an alternative approach for cancer prevention and treatment. Polyphenols in tea, berries, vegetables, apples, and wines have been shown to be potent anticarcinogenic agent in vitro and in animal models that prevent DNA instability at several sites in the carcinogenic pathway (61–63). Polyphenols can directly insert into the binding pocket of *DNMT* and indirectly decrease intracellular SAM concentration thus inhibit *DNMT* activity in vitro, capable of reversing DNA hypermethylation and reactivating tumor suppressor gene activity (64).

Polyphenols, including (–)-epigallocatechin 3-gallate (EGCG), quercetin, myricetin, and fisetin, may decrease DNA methylation by altering the cellular ratio SAM/SAH and indirectly inhibit DNMT activity. Genistein from soybean and EGCG from green tea are the most potent DNMT inhibitors. EGCG and other green tea metabolites dose-dependently inhibit DNMT activity in human esophageal cancer cells (64). The gallate moiety on the D ring of EGCG interacts strongly with the cytosine-active site on the DNMT enzyme and hydrogen bonds formed between hydroxyl groups of the A and B ring and *Sr1229* and *Cys1225* on the protein contribute to the high-affinity binding of EGCG and inhibition of activity (64). Genistein was also found to interact strongly with DNMT and inhibit the enzyme activity.

Tumor suppressor genes that were silenced as a result of hypermethylation of CpG islands in the promoter regions include $p16^{INK4a}$, retinoic acid receptor β (*RARβ*), methylguanine methyltransferase (*MGMT*), *mMLH1* and glutathione *S*-transferase π (*GSTP*) in cancer cells. Reactivation of tumor suppressor genes is associated with a corresponding increase in mRNA and protein expression. EGCG is found to reverse DNA methylation and increases expression of *MGMT*, $p16^{INK4a}$, and *hMLH1* in esophageal cancer cell line. Levels of cytosine methylation and mRNA expression were altered after 48-h exposure to the green tea polyphenol and continued to progress over time. Reversal of DNA hypermethylation was found to be increased with protein expression. EGCG can also reactivate RARβ in prostate and breast cancer cells, $p16^{INK4}$ in colon cancer cells, and GSTP in prostate cancer cells (16, 65). Genistein partially reversed DNA hypermethylation and reactivated $p16^{INK4}$, *RARβ* and *MGMT* gene expression (66). The isoflavones biochanin A and daidzein and the flavonoids, myricetin, quercetin, hesperitin, naringenein, apigenin, and luteolin were active but less effective in altering DNA methylation and reactivating tumor suppressor genes.

Malignant transformation involves phenotypic changes in initiated cells that promote invasion into extracellular tissue matrices. EGCG decreased *RECK*, which encodes an inhibitor of the angiogenesis, invasion and metastasis, DNA methylation, and increased mRNA in cell lines. More importantly, this is associated with a subsequent decrease in *MMP-2* and *MMP-9* expression and in the ability of the cancer cells to invade a 3-D collagen model.

EGCG reduced the cell proliferation, depth of migration, and frequency, and size of invasive loci (67). However, the ability of EGCG to decrease DNA hypermethylation and reactivate tumor suppressor gene expression and activity was inconsistent (68, 69).

In addition, to be an inhibitor for *DNMT* activity in human cancer cells, the major polyphenols in tea, EGCG, is a potent inhibitor of catechol-*O*-methyltransferase (*COMT*) activity (70). Both COMT and DNMT belong to the same family of SAM dependent methyltransferases. Inhibition by certain drugs, such as 5-aza-deoxycytidine, has been shown to inhibit cancer growth, induce apoptosis and reduce tumor volume in mice (71). In an in vivo study, competitive inhibition of *DNMT1* was evident in carcinogenesis prevention (64). Reversal of methylation in $p16^{INK4a}$, *RARβ*, *MGMT*, and *hMLH1* genes was also observed. Therefore, green tea EGCG, even at a dose as low as 20 μmol, may inhibit *DNMT* causing CpG demethylation and reactivation of previously silenced genes by methylation. EGCG provides a good example of a food component with the capacity for reversal of aberrant methylation.

2.5. Phytoestrogens

Phytoestrogens include coumestans, isoflavones and lignans are plant-derived estrogen-like compounds, which occur naturally in many foods, such as fruits, legumes, and grains (40). Phytoestrogens have been suggested to have several biological actions that may attenuate cancer risk, including antiestrogenic, anti-inflammatory, and anticarcinogenic effects (72, 73). The estrogen receptor (*ESR*) gene has shown age-related methylation and is methylated in both sporadic and familial colorectal adenoma (8, 74). It is hypothesized that *ESR* methylation may predispose to colorectal neoplasia. Aberrant *ESR* hypermethylation of the promoter region of the *ESR* gene has been shown to result in transcriptional silencing in breast cell line (75). As a result, no *ESR* was available for binding so that increased circulating estrogen level and breast cancer risk were observed. Phytoestrogens may not have any beneficial effect once *ESR* is hypermethylated. It is suggested that the health benefit of phytoestrogens may only be effective prior to *ESR* gene methylation and is heterogeneous and dependent on target tissues (40).

2.6. Flavonoids

Flavonoids are a group of polyphenolic plant secondary metabolites that may have numerous health benefits, such as antioxidant properties and anti-inflammatory and antitumor activities (18). Various cancer cell lines showed reduced promoter methylation status and increased mRNA expression of numerous tumor suppressor genes when exposed to flavonoids or isoflavones. In animals and humans, flavonoids are extensively metabolized after ingestion through glucoronidation, sulfation, or methylation.

2.7. Sulforaphane/ Isothiocyanates

Sulforaphane is an isothiocyanate found in cruciferous vegetables, such as broccoli and broccoli sprouts. This anticarcinogen was first identified as a potent inducer of phase II detoxification enzymes. However, mounting evidence suggests that sulforaphane acts through other chemopreventive mechanisms (76–78). Sulforaphane have been reported to inhibit HDAC activity in human colon cancer (79), prostate cancer (80), and breast cancer (81) cell lines to increase both global and local histone acetylation status, such as on the promoter region of *p21* and *bax* genes. Sulforaphane altered histone deacetylation status and histone acetylase inhibition thus suppressed the growth of prostate cancer xenographs and inhibited spontaneous intestinal polyps in the Apc^{min} mouse (82, 83). In human subjects, a single ingestion of one cup of broccoli sprouts inhibited histone acetylase activity in circulating peripheral blood mononuclear cells 3–6 h after consumption. A simultaneous induction of histone H3 and H4 acetylation was also noted (82). It is hypothesized that isothiocyanates might inhibit HDAC activity if they are metabolized via the mercapturic acid pathway (84).

2.8. Vitamin A

Vitamin A and their metabolites are thought to be involved in DNA methylation through a different mechanism than the one-carbon metabolism (15). Glycine *N*-methyltransferase (GNMT) is a key enzyme essential in optimizing methyl group supply and subsequent functioning of the methyltransferase enzyme. It was found in rats that vitamin A and its derivates, such as retinoic acids, regulate the *GNMT* which resulted in DNA hypomethylation (85). Similarly, a study in colorectal cancer patients found that vitamin A deficiency was associated with promoter hypermethylation in three loci analyzed, i.e., $p16^{INK4a}$, $p14^{ARF}$, and *hMLH1* (19). These results suggest an important role for vitamin A and *GNMT* in the regulation of DNA methylation.

2.9. Fat

An animal study showed that offspring of rats fed high-fat diet had structural changes to mammary tissue, lowered estrogen receptor-α, insulin receptor, and insulin-like growth factor (IGF-1) receptor expression and increased levels of activated mitogen-activated protein kinase (86). Other study reported that offspring of rats fed a protein-restricted diet during pregnancy and lactation had a two-fold increased sensitivity to mammary gland tumor induction by nitrosomethylurea (87).

It is believed that noncoding microRNAs (miRNAs) control the expression of approximately one-third of the mammalian messenger RNAs (mRNAs) (88). miRNAs act through partial complementation to 3′-untranslated regions of their target mRNAs and regulate mRNA degradation and translation thus inhibit gene expression (88, 89). Altered expressions of a number of noncoding RNAs have been linked to the development and prognosis of colorectal neoplasia (90–94). Additionally, cellular phenotypes, such as apoptosis are regulated by miRNAs and upstream and downstream genes have been linked to the epigenetic silencing of miRNAs (95–97). These findings suggest that miRNA expression profile could contribute to a more precise colonic tumor classification and predict outcomes of chemotherapy (98). A study suggested that common global miRNA expression patterns exist in human azoxymethane (a carcinogen)-induced colon tumor and *n*-3 polyunsaturated fatty acids modulated carcinogen-directed noncoding miRNA signatures (98).

2.10. Trace Elements

Deficiency of trace elements such as zinc and selenium can cause genomic DNA hypomethylation by altering one-carbon metabolism in the elderly (99). Interest in selenium and cancer prevention started up from early ecologic study that found an inverse relation between selenium status and carcinogenesis in geographic area where selenium was low in soil (100). Cell culture and animal studies have demonstrated that selenium deficiency causes global hypomethylation and promoter methylation of *p53* and $p16^{INK4a}$ genes (101). In human colon cancer, selenium has been shown to play a role in chemoprevention by inhibiting *DNMT* and subsequently suppressing aberrant DNA methylation (102).

2.11. Other Compounds

Dietary agents such as butyrate, biotin, lipoic acid, garlic organosulfur compounds, and metabolites of vitamin E have structural features compatible with HDAC inhibition (103). A study found a higher methylation level of $p16^{INK4a}$ among colorectal cancer patients who consumed significant less potassium ($p=0.03$) and iron ($p=0.02$) when compared to controls (19).

3. Concluding Remarks

Cancer encompasses a highly heterogeneous group of diseases. It has been considered that cancer is the result of unrepaired genetic alternations that damage the structure of DNA and subsequently induces mutations which result in abnormal protein functioning. Both epidemiological data and animal experiments support the hypothesis that environmental agents, including diet, may exert their oncogenic effects through epigenetics as well as genetic mechanisms. The ability of dietary compounds to depress epigenetically silenced genes in cancer cells has important implications for cancer prevention and therapy. However, important questions remain to be answered, such as the possible nonselectivity of inhibition toward multiple HDACs and the downstream regulating pathways. There are needs to have a greater understanding of the epigenetic basis of cancer and how nutrients and various compounds influence epigenetic modification (18).

One of the major developments in the field of cancer epigenetics in the past decade has been the rapid advance in genome-wide technologies, initially employing microarrays but increasingly high throughput sequencing. In the foreseeable near future, cancer epigenomic methods will be able to sufficiently address issues of tissue heterogeneity and the often limiting amount of DNA present in clinical and observational study samples. Nevertheless, many challenges are still lying ahead for further understanding the exact roles of diet on epigenetics for designing better strategies for cancer prevention. For example, it is now known that epigenetic mechanisms consist of a combination of interactions among histone tail modifications, DNA methylation, and histone- and DNA-modifying enzymes, which are responsible for the regulation of chromatin structure and function. Despite of significant greater amount of data that are available on effect of diet on DNA methylation, less knowledge is available on the involvement of histone modifications in the regulation of chromatin structure and gene expression and the identification on the nature of metabolic pathways that are controlled by nutrition through epigenetic mechanisms, both in early life and adulthood. Furthermore, the relationship between epigenetic events and latent nature of cancer in humans may need to be explored through prospective cohort study with multiple measurements of diet and biomarkers through the critical time point in life. A new paradigm shift with focus on improving knowledge on the interplay relationship between diet and epigenetics could move the field of diet and cancer into an era of targeted lifestyle modification for cancer prevention.

References

1. Loeb, L.A. and Harris, C.C. (2008) Advances in chemical carcinogenesis: a historical review and prospective. *Cancer Res* 68, 6863–6872.
2. Pogribny, I.P., Shpyleva, S.I., Muskhelishvili, L., Bagnyukova, T.V., James, S.J., and Beland, F.A. (2009) Role of DNA damage and alterations in cytosine DNA methylation in rat liver carcinogenesis induced by a methyl-deficient diet. *Mutat Res* 669, 56–62.
3. Pitot, H.C. (2007) Adventures in hepatocarcinogenesis. *Annu Rev Pathol* 2, 1–29.
4. Duthie, S.J. (2011) Epigenetic modifications and human pathologies: cancer and CVD. *Proc Nutr Soc* 70, 47–56.
5. Jones, P.A. and Baylin, S.B. (2007) The epigenomics of cancer. *Cell* 128, 683–692.
6. Doll, R. and Peto, R. (1981) The causes of cancer: quantitative estimates of avoidable risks of cancer in the United States today. *J Natl Cancer Inst* 66, 1191–308.
7. Issa, J.P. (2003) Age-related epigenetic changes and the immune system. *Clin Immunol*109, 103–108.
8. Issa, J.P., Ottaviano, Y.L., Celano, P., Hamilton, S.R., Davidson, N.E., and Baylin, S.B. (1994) Methylation of the oestrogen receptor CpG island links ageing and neoplasia in human colon. *Nat Genet* 7, 536–540.
9. Wolff, G.L., Kodell, R.L., Moore, S.R., and Cooney, C.A. (1998) Maternal epigenetics and methyl supplements affect agouti gene expression in Avy/a mice. *FASEB J* 12, 949–957.
10. Yen, T.T., Gill, A.M., Frigeri, L.G., Barsh, G.S., and Wolff, G.L. (1994) Obesity, diabetes, and neoplasia in yellow A(vy)/- mice: ectopic expression of the agouti gene. *FASEB J* 8, 479–488.
11. Dolinoy, D.C. (2008) The agouti mouse model: an epigenetic biosensor for nutritional

and environmental alterations on the fetal epigenome. *Nutr Rev*, 66 Suppl 1, S7–11.

12. Duthie, S.J. Epigenetic modifications and human pathologies: cancer and CVD. *Proc Nutr Soc* 70, 47–56.
13. Kim, K.C., Friso, S., and Choi, S.W. (2009) DNA methylation, an epigenetic mechanism connecting folate to healthy embryonic development and aging. *J Nutr Biochem* 20, 917–926.
14. Fraga, M.F., Ballestar, E., Paz, M.F., Ropero, S., Setien, F., Ballestar, M.L., Heine-Suner, D., Cigudosa, J.C., Urioste, M., Benitez, J., Boix-Chornet, M., Sanchez-Aguilera, A., Ling, C., Carlsson, E., Poulsen, P., Vaag, A., Stephan, Z., Spector, T.D., Wu, Y.Z., Plass, C., and Esteller, M. (2005) Epigenetic differences arise during the lifetime of monozygotic twins. *Proc Natl Acad Sci U S A* 102, 10604–10609.
15. Davis, C.D. and Uthus, E.O. (2004) DNA methylation, cancer susceptibility, and nutrient interactions. *Exp Biol Med (Maywood)* 229, 988–995.
16. Lee, W.J., Shim, J.Y., and Zhu, B.T. (2005) Mechanisms for the inhibition of DNA methyltransferases by tea catechins and bioflavonoids. *Mol Pharmacol* 68, 1018–1030.
17. Delage, B. and Dashwood, R.H. (2008) Dietary manipulation of histone structure and function. *Annu Rev Nutr* 28, 347–366.
18. Gilbert, E.R. and Liu, D. (2010) Flavonoids influence epigenetic-modifying enzyme activity: structure—function relationships and the therapeutic potential for cancer. *Curr Med Chem* 17, 1756–1768.
19. Mas, S., Lafuente, M.J., Crescenti, A., Trias, M., Ballesta, A., Molina, R., Zheng, S., Wiencke, J.K., and Lafuente, A. (2007) Lower specific micronutrient intake in colorectal cancer patients with tumors presenting promoter hypermethylation in p16(INK4a), p4(ARF) and hMLH1. *Anticancer Res* 27, 1151–1156.
20. Ross, S.A., Dwyer, J., Umar, A., Kagan, J., Verma, M., Van Bemmel, D.M., and Dunn, B.K. (2008) Introduction: diet, epigenetic events and cancer prevention. *Nutr Rev* 66 Suppl 1, S1–6.
21. Zhang, Y.W., Miao, Y.F., Yi, J., Geng, J., Wang, R., and Chen, L.B. (2010) Transcriptional inactivation of secreted frizzled-related protein 1 by promoter hypermethylation as a potential biomarker for non-small cell lung cancer. *Neoplasma* 57, 228–233.
22. Rahman, I. (2008) Dietary polyphenols mediated regulation of oxidative stress and chromatin remodeling in inflammation. *Nutr Rev*, 66 Suppl 1, S42–45.
23. Glynn, S.A. and Albanes, D. (1994) Folate and cancer: a review of the literature. *Nutr Cancer* 22, 101–119.
24. Kim, Y.I. (2007) Folate and colorectal cancer: an evidence-based critical review. *Mol Nutr Food Res* 51, 267–292.
25. Yang, Q., Bostick, R.M., Friedman, J.M., and Flanders, W.D. (2009) Serum folate and cancer mortality among U.S. adults: findings from the Third National Health and Nutritional Examination Survey linked mortality file. *Cancer Epidemiol Biomarkers Prev* 18, 1439–1447.
26. Duthie, S.J. (2011) Folate and cancer: how DNA damage, repair and methylation impact on colon carcinogenesis. *J Inherit Metab Dis* 34, 101–109.
27. Rampersaud, G.C., Kauwell, G.P., Hutson, A.D., Cerda, J.J., and Bailey, L.B. (2000) Genomic DNA methylation decreases in response to moderate folate depletion in elderly women. *Am J Clin Nutr* 72, 998–1003.
28. Mason, J.B. and Choi, S.W. (2000) Folate and carcinogenesis: developing a unifying hypothesis. *Adv Enzyme Regul* 40, 127–141.
29. Blount, B.C., Mack, M.M., Wehr, C.M., MacGregor, J.T., Hiatt, R.A., Wang, G., Wickramasinghe, S.N., Everson, R.B., and Ames, B.N. (1997) Folate deficiency causes uracil misincorporation into human DNA and chromosome breakage: implications for cancer and neuronal damage. *Proc Natl Acad Sci U S A* 94, 3290–3295.
30. Choi, S.W., Friso, S., Dolnikowski, G.G., Bagley, P.J., Edmondson, A.N., Smith, D.E., and Mason, J.B. (2003) Biochemical and molecular aberrations in the rat colon due to folate depletion are age-specific. *J Nutr* 133, 1206–1212.
31. Shay, J.W. and Werbin, H. (1992) New evidence for the insertion of mitochondrial DNA into the human genome: significance for cancer and aging. *Mutat Res* 275, 227–235.
32. Zhu, W., Qin, W., and Sauter, E.R. (2004) Large-scale mitochondrial DNA deletion mutations and nuclear genome instability in human breast cancer. *Cancer Detect Prev* 28, 119–126.
33. Crott, J.W., Choi, S.W., Branda, R.F., and Mason, J.B. (2005) Accumulation of mitochondrial DNA deletions is age, tissue and

folate-dependent in rats. *Mutat Res* 570, 63–70.

34. Choi, S.W. and Mason, J.B. (2000) Folate and carcinogenesis: an integrated scheme. *J Nutr* 130, 129–132.
35. Eden, A., Gaudet, F., Waghmare, A., and Jaenisch, R. (2003) Chromosomal instability and tumors promoted by DNA hypomethylation. *Science* 300, 455.
36. Gaudet, F., Hodgson, J.G., Eden, A., Jackson-Grusby, L., Dausman, J., Gray, J.W., Leonhardt, H., and Jaenisch, R. (2003) Induction of tumors in mice by genomic hypomethylation. *Science* 300, 489–492.
37. Holm, T.M., Jackson-Grusby, L., Brambrink, T., Yamada, Y., Rideout, W.M., 3 rd and Jaenisch, R. (2005) Global loss of imprinting leads to widespread tumorigenesis in adult mice. *Cancer Cell* 8, 275–285.
38. Walsh, C.P., Chaillet, J.R., and Bestor, T.H. (1998) Transcription of IAP endogenous retroviruses is constrained by cytosine methylation. *Nat Genet* 20, 116–117.
39. James, S.J., Pogribny, I.P., Pogribna, M., Miller, B.J., Jernigan, S., and Melnyk, S. (2003) Mechanisms of DNA damage, DNA hypomethylation, and tumor progression in the folate/methyl-deficient rat model of hepatocarcinogenesis. *J Nutr* 133, 3740 S–3747 S.
40. Arasaradnam, R.P., Commane, D.M., Bradburn, D., and Mathers, J.C. (2008) A review of dietary factors and its influence on DNA methylation in colorectal carcinogenesis. *Epigenetics* 3, 193–198.
41. Weingartner, J., Lotz, K., Fanghanel, J., Gedrange, T., Bienengraber, V., and Proff, P. (2007) Induction and prevention of cleft lip, alveolus and palate and neural tube defects with special consideration of B vitamins and the methylation cycle. *J Orofac Orthop* 68, 266–277.
42. Dunlevy, L.P., Burren, K.A., Mills, K., Chitty, L.S., Copp, A.J., and Greene, N.D. (2006) Integrity of the methylation cycle is essential for mammalian neural tube closure. *Birth Defects Res A Clin Mol Teratol* 76, 544–552.
43. Park, B.H., Kim, Y.J., Park, J.S., Lee, H.Y., Ha, E.H., Min, J.W., and Park, H.S. (2005) (Folate and homocysteine levels during pregnancy affect DNA methylation in human placenta). *J Prev Med Public Health* 38, 437–442.
44. Kim, J.M., Hong, K., Lee, J.H., Lee, S., and Chang, N. (2009) Effect of folate deficiency on placental DNA methylation in hyperhomocysteinemic rats. *J Nutr Biochem* 20, 172–6.
45. Watkins, A.J., Wilkins, A., Cunningham, C., Perry, V.H., Seet, M.J., Osmond, C., Eckert, J.J., Torrens, C., Cagampang, F.R., Cleal, J., Gray, W.P., Hanson, M.A., and Fleming, T.P. (2008) Low protein diet fed exclusively during mouse oocyte maturation leads to behavioural and cardiovascular abnormalities in offspring. *J Physiol* 586, 2231–2244.
46. Lillycrop, K.A., Phillips, E.S., Jackson, A.A., Hanson, M.A., and Burdge, G.C. (2005) Dietary protein restriction of pregnant rats induces and folic acid supplementation prevents epigenetic modification of hepatic gene expression in the offspring. *J Nutr* 135, 1382–1386.
47. Kappen, C. (2005) Folate supplementation in three genetic models: implications for understanding folate-dependent developmental pathways. *Am J Med Genet C Semin Med Genet* 135 C, 24–30.
48. Lillycrop, K.A., Slater-Jefferies, J.L., Hanson, M.A., Godfrey, K.M., Jackson, A.A., and Burdge, G.C. (2007) Induction of altered epigenetic regulation of the hepatic glucocorticoid receptor in the offspring of rats fed a protein-restricted diet during pregnancy suggests that reduced DNA methyltransferase-1 expression is involved in impaired DNA methylation and changes in histone modifications. *Br J Nutr* 97, 1064–1073.
49. Sinclair, K.D., Allegrucci, C., Singh, R., Gardner, D.S., Sebastian, S., Bispham, J., Thurston, A., Huntley, J.F., Rees, W.D., Maloney, C.A., Lea, R.G., Craigon, J., McEvoy, T.G., and Young, L.E. (2007) DNA methylation, insulin resistance, and blood pressure in offspring determined by maternal periconceptional B vitamin and methionine status. *Proc Natl Acad Sci U S A* 104, 19351–19356.
50. Waterland, R.A. and Michels, K.B. (2007) Epigenetic epidemiology of the developmental origins hypothesis. *Annu Rev Nutr* 27, 363–388.
51. McKay, J.A., Williams, E.A., and Mathers, J.C. (2004) Folate and DNA methylation during in utero development and aging. *Biochem Soc Trans* 32, 1006–7.
52. Giovannucci, E., Stampfer, M.J., Colditz, G.A., Rimm, E.B., Trichopoulos, D., Rosner, B.A., Speizer, F.E., and Willett, W.C. (1993) Folate, methionine, and alcohol intake and risk of colorectal adenoma. *J Natl Cancer Inst* 85, 875–884.
53. Sohn, K.J., Jang, H., Campan, M., Weisenberger, D.J., Dickhout, J., Wang, Y.C., Cho, R.C., Yates, Z., Lucock, M., Chiang, E.P., Austin, R.C., Choi, S.W., Laird, P.W.,

and Kim, Y.I. (2009) The methylenetetrahydrofolate reductase C677T mutation induces cell-specific changes in genomic DNA methylation and uracil misincorporation: a possible molecular basis for the site-specific cancer risk modification. *Int J Cancer* 124, 1999–2005.

54. van den Donk, M., Pellis, L., Crott, J.W., van Engeland, M., Friederich, P., Nagengast, F.M., van Bergeijk, J.D., de Boer, S.Y., Mason, J.B., Kok, F.J., Keijer, J., and Kampman, E. (2007) Folic acid and vitamin B-12 supplementation does not favorably influence uracil incorporation and promoter methylation in rectal mucosa DNA of subjects with previous colorectal adenomas. *J Nutr* 137, 2114–2120.
55. Choi, S.W., Friso, S., Keyes, M.K., and Mason, J.B. (2005) Folate supplementation increases genomic DNA methylation in the liver of elder rats. *Br J Nutr* 93, 31–35.
56. Keyes, M.K., Jang, H., Mason, J.B., Liu, Z., Crott, J.W., Smith, D.E., Friso, S., and Choi, S.W. (2007) Older age and dietary folate are determinants of genomic and p16-specific DNA methylation in mouse colon. *J Nutr* 137, 1713–1717.
57. Herrmann, W., Schorr, H., Obeid, R., and Geisel, J. (2003) Vitamin B-12 status, particularly holotranscobalamin II and methylmalonic acid concentrations, and hyperhomocysteinemia in vegetarians. *Am J Clin Nutr* 78, 131–136.
58. Bissoli, L., Di Francesco, V., Ballarin, A., Mandragona, R., Trespidi, R., Brocco, G., Caruso, B., Bosello, O., and Zamboni, M. (2002) Effect of vegetarian diet on homocysteine levels. *Ann Nutr Metab* 46, 73–79.
59. Yi, P., Melnyk, S., Pogribna, M., Pogribny, I.P., Hine, R.J., and James, S.J. (2000) Increase in plasma homocysteine associated with parallel increases in plasma S-adenosylhomocysteine and lymphocyte DNA hypomethylation. *J Biol Chem* 275, 29318–29323.
60. Comin-Anduix, B., Boren, J., Martinez, S., Moro, C., Centelles, J.J., Trebukhina, R., Petushok, N., Lee, W.N., Boros, L.G., and Cascante, M. (2001) The effect of thiamine supplementation on tumour proliferation. A metabolic control analysis study. *Eur J Biochem* 268, 4177–4182.
61. Duthie, G.G., Duthie, S.J., and Kyle, J.A. (2000) Plant polyphenols in cancer and heart disease: implications as nutritional antioxidants. *Nutr Res Rev* 13, 79–106.
62. Ferguson, L.R. (2001) Role of plant polyphenols in genomic stability. *Mutat Res* 475, 89–111.
63. Duthie, S.J. (2007) Berry phytochemicals, genomic stability and cancer: evidence for chemoprotection at several stages in the carcinogenic process. *Mol Nutr Food Res* 51, 665–674.
64. Fang, M., Chen, D., and Yang, C.S. (2007) Dietary polyphenols may affect DNA methylation. *J Nutr* 137, 223 S–228 S.
65. Fang, M.Z., Wang, Y., Ai, N., Hou, Z., Sun, Y., Lu, H., Welsh, W., and Yang, C.S. (2003) Tea polyphenol (−)-epigallocatechin-3-gallate inhibits DNA methyltransferase and reactivates methylation-silenced genes in cancer cell lines. *Cancer Res* 63, 7563–7570.
66. Fang, M.Z., Chen, D., Sun, Y., Jin, Z., Christman, J.K., and Yang, C.S. (2005) Reversal of hypermethylation and reactivation of p16INK4a, RARbeta, and MGMT genes by genistein and other isoflavones from soy. *Clin Cancer Res* 11, 7033–7041.
67. Kato, K., Long, N.K., Makita, H., Toida, M., Yamashita, T., Hatakeyama, D., Hara, A., Mori, H., and Shibata, T. (2008) Effects of green tea polyphenol on methylation status of RECK gene and cancer cell invasion in oral squamous cell carcinoma cells. *Br J Cancer* 99, 647–654.
68. Chuang, J.C., Yoo, C.B., Kwan, J.M., Li, T.W., Liang, G., Yang, A.S., and Jones, P.A. (2005) Comparison of biological effects of non-nucleoside DNA methylation inhibitors versus 5-aza-2′-deoxycytidine. *Mol Cancer Ther* 4, 1515–1520.
69. Stresemann, C., Brueckner, B., Musch, T., Stopper, H., and Lyko, F. (2006) Functional diversity of DNA methyltransferase inhibitors in human cancer cell lines. *Cancer Res* 66, 2794–2800.
70. Lu, H., Meng, X., Li, C., Sang, S., Patten, C., Sheng, S., Hong, J., Bai, N., Winnik, B., Ho, C.T., and Yang, C.S. (2003) Glucuronides of tea catechins: enzymology of biosynthesis and biological activities. *Drug Metab Dispos* 31, 452–461.
71. Christman, J.K. (2002) 5-Azacytidine and 5-aza-2′-deoxycytidine as inhibitors of DNA methylation: mechanistic studies and their implications for cancer therapy. *Oncogene* 21, 5483–5495.
72. Adlercreutz, H., Mousavi, Y., and Hockerstedt, K. (1992) Diet and breast cancer. *Acta Oncol* 31, 175–181.
73. Dijsselbloem, N., Vanden Berghe, W., De Naeyer, A., and Haegeman, G. (2004) Soy isoflavone phyto-pharmaceuticals in interleukin-6 affections. Multi-purpose nutraceuticals at the crossroad of hormone replacement, anti-cancer and anti-inflammatory therapy. *Biochem Pharmacol* 68, 1171–1185.

74. Woodson, K., Weisenberger, D.J., Campan, M., Laird, P.W., Tangrea, J., Johnson, L.L., Schatzkin, A., and Lanza, E. (2005) Gene-specific methylation and subsequent risk of colorectal adenomas among participants of the polyp prevention trial. *Cancer Epidemiol Biomarkers Prev* 14, 1219–1223.
75. Ottaviano, Y.L., Issa, J.P., Parl, F.F., Smith, H.S., Baylin, S.B., and Davidson, N.E. (1994) Methylation of the estrogen receptor gene CpG island marks loss of estrogen receptor expression in human breast cancer cells. *Cancer Res* 54, 2552–2555.
76. Juge, N., Mithen, R.F., and Traka, M. (2007) Molecular basis for chemoprevention by sulforaphane: a comprehensive review. *Cell Mol Life Sci* 64, 1105–1127.
77. Myzak, M.C. and Dashwood, R.H. (2006) Chemoprotection by sulforaphane: keep one eye beyond Keap1. *Cancer Lett* 233, 208–218.
78. Dashwood, R.H., and Ho, E. (2008) Dietary agents as histone deacetylase inhibitors: sulforaphane and structurally related isothiocyanates. *Nutr Rev* 66 Suppl 1, S36–38.
79. Myzak, M.C., Karplus, P.A., Chung, F.L., and Dashwood, R.H. (2004) A novel mechanism of chemoprotection by sulforaphane: inhibition of histone deacetylase. *Cancer Res* 64, 5767–5774.
80. Myzak, M.C., Hardin, K., Wang, R., Dashwood, R.H., and Ho, E. (2006) Sulforaphane inhibits histone deacetylase activity in BPH-1, LnCaP and PC-3 prostate epithelial cells. *Carcinogenesis* 27, 811–819.
81. Pledgie-Tracy, A., Sobolewski, M.D., and Davidson, N.E. (2007) Sulforaphane induces cell type-specific apoptosis in human breast cancer cell lines. *Mol Cancer Ther* 6, 1013–1021.
82. Myzak, M.C., Tong, P., Dashwood, W.M., Dashwood, R.H., and Ho, E. (2007) Sulforaphane retards the growth of human PC-3 xenografts and inhibits HDAC activity in human subjects. *Exp Biol Med (Maywood)* 232, 227–234.
83. Myzak, M.C., Dashwood, W.M., Orner, G.A., Ho, E., and Dashwood, R.H. (2006) Sulforaphane inhibits histone deacetylase in vivo and suppresses tumorigenesis in Apc-minus mice. *FASEB J* 20, 506–508.
84. Ho, E., Clarke, J.D., and Dashwood, R.H. (2009) Dietary sulforaphane, a histone deacetylase inhibitor for cancer prevention. *J Nutr* 139, 2393–2396.
85. Rowling, M.J., McMullen, M.H., and Schalinske, K.L. (2002) Vitamin A and its derivatives induce hepatic glycine N-methyltransferase and hypomethylation of DNA in rats. *J Nutr* 132, 365–369.
86. de Assis, S., Wang, M., Goel, S., Foxworth, A., Helferich, W., and Hilakivi-Clarke, L. (2006) Excessive weight gain during pregnancy increases carcinogen-induced mammary tumorigenesis in Sprague-Dawley and lean and obese Zucker rats. *J Nutr* 136, 998–1004.
87. Fernandez-Twinn, D.S., Ekizoglou, S., Gusterson, B.A., Luan, J., and Ozanne, S.E. (2007) Compensatory mammary growth following protein restriction during pregnancy and lactation increases early-onset mammary tumor incidence in rats. *Carcinogenesis* 28, 545–552.
88. Esquela-Kerscher, A., and Slack, F.J. (2006) Oncomirs—microRNAs with a role in cancer. *Nat Rev Cancer* 6, 259–269.
89. Sood, P., Krek, A., Zavolan, M., Macino, G., and Rajewsky, N. (2006) Cell-type-specific signatures of microRNAs on target mRNA expression. *Proc Natl Acad Sci U S A* 103, 2746–2751.
90. Michael, M.Z., SM, O.C., van Holst Pellekaan, N.G., Young, G.P., and James, R.J. (2003) Reduced accumulation of specific microRNAs in colorectal neoplasia. *Mol Cancer Res* 1, 882–891.
91. Akao, Y., Nakagawa, Y., and Naoe, T. (2006) let-7 microRNA functions as a potential growth suppressor in human colon cancer cells. *Biol Pharm Bull* 29, 903–906.
92. Bandres, E., Cubedo, E., Agirre, X., Malumbres, R., Zarate, R., Ramirez, N., Abajo, A., Navarro, A., Moreno, I., Monzo, M., and Garcia-Foncillas, J. (2006) Identification by Real-time PCR of 13 mature microRNAs differentially expressed in colorectal cancer and non-tumoral tissues. *Mol Cancer* 5, 29.
93. Monzo, M., Navarro, A., Bandres, E., Artells, R., Moreno, I., Gel, B., Ibeas, R., Moreno, J., Martinez, F., Diaz, T., Martinez, A., Balague, O., and Garcia-Foncillas, J. (2008) Overlapping expression of microRNAs in human embryonic colon and colorectal cancer. *Cell Res* 18, 823–833.
94. Schepeler, T., Reinert, J.T., Ostenfeld, M.S., Christensen, L.L., Silahtaroglu, A.N., Dyrskjot, L., Wiuf, C., Sorensen, F.J., Kruhoffer, M., Laurberg, S., Kauppinen, S., Orntoft, T.F., and Andersen, C.L. (2008) Diagnostic and prognostic microRNAs in stage II colon cancer. *Cancer Res* 68, 6416–6424.
95. Cheng, A.M., Byrom, M.W., Shelton, J., and Ford, L.P. (2005) Antisense inhibition of human miRNAs and indications for an

involvement of miRNA in cell growth and apoptosis. *Nucleic Acids Res* 33, 1290–1297.

96. Carthew, R.W. (2006) Gene regulation by microRNAs. *Curr Opin Genet Dev* 16, 203–208.
97. Grady, W.M., Parkin, R.K., Mitchell, P.S., Lee, J.H., Kim, Y.H., Tsuchiya, K.D., Washington, M.K., Paraskeva, C., Willson, J.K., Kaz, A.M., Kroh, E.M., Allen, A., Fritz, B.R., Markowitz, S.D., and Tewari, M. (2008) Epigenetic silencing of the intronic microRNA hsa-miR-342 and its host gene EVL in colorectal cancer. *Oncogene* 27, 3880–3888.
98. Davidson, L.A., Wang, N., Shah, M.S., Lupton, J.R., Ivanov, I., and Chapkin, R.S. (2009) n-3 Polyunsaturated fatty acids modulate carcinogen-directed non-coding microRNA signatures in rat colon. *Carcinogenesis* 30, 2077–2084.
99. Cooney, C.A. (2001) Dietary selenium and arsenic affect DNA methylation. *J Nutr* 131, 1871–1872.
100. Clark, L.C., Cantor, K.P., and Allaway, W.H. (1991) Selenium in forage crops and cancer mortality in U.S. counties. *Arch Environ Health* 46, 37–42.
101. Davis, C.D., Uthus, E.O., and Finley, J.W. (2000) Dietary selenium and arsenic affect DNA methylation in vitro in Caco-2 cells and in vivo in rat liver and colon. *J Nutr*,130, 2903–2909.
102. Fiala, E.S., Staretz, M.E., Pandya, G.A., El-Bayoumy, K., and Hamilton, S.R. (1998) Inhibition of DNA cytosine methyltransferase by chemopreventive selenium compounds, determined by an improved assay for DNA cytosine methyltransferase and DNA cytosine methylation. *Carcinogenesis* 19, 597–604.
103. Dashwood, R.H., Myzak, M.C., and Ho, E. (2006) Dietary HDAC inhibitors: time to rethink weak ligands in cancer chemoprevention? *Carcinogenesis* 27, 344–349.

Chapter 25

Role of Epigenetics in Cancer Health Disparities

Sulma I. Mohammed, Sanya Springfield, and Rina Das

Abstract

Cancer disparities in incidence and death rates exist among various racial and ethnic groups. These disparities are thought to be due to socioeconomic status, culture, diet, stress, the environment, and biology. Biological functions, such as epigenetic processes, are affected by all these causal factors and extend throughout the life course. Epigenetic processes, in particular DNA methylation, may play a role in the induction of phenotypes with increased cancer risk due to exposure to these multiple factors. DNA methylation is known to cause changes in gene expression of key regulatory genes in cancer. There are limited studies in which epigenetic changes have been explored to address cancer disparities in various racial and ethnic populations. These few studies have reported significant epigenetic differences in various racial and ethnic groups that could account for the differences seen in tumor initiation, progression, aggressiveness, and outcome of these cancers. Genes differentially methylated among these racially and ethnically diverse populations were involved in important cellular functions, such as tumor growth, tumor suppression, hormone receptors, and genes involved in tumor metastasis. Epigenetic research with the advancement in technology has helped identify biomarkers, therapeutic targets, and understand cancer causation in the general population. Unfortunately, these advances in technology have not been applied to explore the basis for cancer health disparities. More research in epigenetics is needed that will enhance our understanding of the determinants of cancer across various diverse populations and ultimately reduce cancer health disparities.

Key words: Cancer disparities, Epigenetics, Race, Ethnic, DNA methylation

1. Introduction on Cancer Disparities

Cancer disparities are defined as differences in the incidence, prevalence, mortality, and burden of cancer that exist between diverse racial, ethnic, and underserved populations when compared to the general population. These racial and ethnic populations include African Americans; American Indians and Alaska Natives; Asians; Hispanics; and Native Hawaiians and Other Pacific Islanders; low socioeconomic status (SES), rural persons; and other underserved

Ramona G. Dumitrescu and Mukesh Verma (eds.), *Cancer Epigenetics: Methods and Protocols*, Methods in Molecular Biology, vol. 863, DOI 10.1007/978-1-61779-612-8_25,

populations. Because of the projected large increases in these diverse populations, cancer health disparities represent a major public health concern in the world and in the United States.

1.1. Cancers Disparities in Racial and Ethnic Populations

The cancer incidence and death rates vary significantly among various racial and ethnic groups. Certain populations are prone to certain types of cancer, such as the fact that African American (AA) men have a 14% and 34% higher incidence and death rates, respectively, than White men (1). It is also known that although Asians are less affected with cancer compared to Whites, however, the incidence and death rates for cancers caused by infection, such as stomach, liver, esophagus, and cervix are higher in these populations (2). In addition, the incidence and death rates for liver cancer due to infection with hepatitis B virus (HBV) and stomach cancer due to Helicobacter pylori, are twice as high in Asian American/ Pacific Islanders when compared to White Americans (2, 3).

When one compares survival rates among various populations, similar cancer disparities have been observed. When racial disparities in survival were evaluated in several cancers, it was found that AA patients had worse survival than White patients for early-stage premenopausal and postmenopausal breast cancer, advanced staged ovarian cancer, and advanced stage prostate cancer (4). African Americans are also less likely to survive cancer after a diagnosis compared to Whites. Although access to quality health care is implicated in this disparity, AA experience worst outcomes even after receiving similar cancer treatment and medical care as Whites (5). Furthermore, the lowest SES groups have the highest disparity for colorectal, breast, and prostate cancer (6). The causes for such cancer disparities in incidence, mortality, and survival rates among these racial and ethnic populations are not clear and seem to be a complex phenomenon.

1.2. Possible Causes of Disparities

Cancer disparities are caused by the complex interplay of multiple factors such as socioeconomic status, culture, biology, and access to care. Research in the field of cancer health disparities has shown that there is a disconnect between what is discovered and what is delivered to diverse populations in the form of prevention, screening, detection, diagnosis, and treatment of cancer (7). The decline in mortality rates in the general population can be attributed to cancer prevention, early detection, and effective cancer screening tests such as Pap smears for cervical cancer, mammography for breast cancer, prostate-specific antigen testing for prostate cancer, and smoking prevention for lung cancer (7). These screening tests have not been equally available to all racial and ethnic populations and may account, in part, for the higher mortality rates for various cancers among some racial and ethnic groups. Many investigators are trying to address various sociocultural determinants as the major causes of cancer disparities and designing better community-specific interventions for different populations in the USA and across the world. However, there is growing evidence that cancer disparities could be a more complex problem that may involve the interplay of biological and environmental factors, as well as behavioral, socioeconomic, cultural, health care system, institutional, and community influences.

1.2.1. Biological Factors

To understand the intricacies of cancer disparities, one needs to determine if there are biological differences in these diverse populations, assess the effect of the environment, and explore the interplay of these multiple factors in cancer disparities. There have been very limited research efforts on understanding the role of biological determinants on cancer disparities.

One way to explore the biological determinants of cancer disparities is to examine the molecular factors resulting from genetic and epigenetic changes in various racial and ethnic populations. Evidence is accumulating in the literature on differences in inherited mutations (8), differences in cancer causing somatic mutations that vary with race and ethnicity that could help explain why certain populations disproportionately suffer from cancer compared to others (8). Similarly, genetic variations have also been shown to affect the efficacy of drugs and therapeutic interventions for specific populations which can influence health outcomes (9, 10).

It is well known that cancer is an epigenetic disease characterized by the dysregulation of DNA methylation and histone modification patterns that may turn on or off certain genes (11, 12). Social and environmental determinants, such as diet, stress, infection, and exposure to environmental chemicals throughout all stages of human development, can cause epigenetic changes (13, 14). This provides a strong rationale for examining the role of epigenetics in cancer disparities since global histone modifications and DNA methylation are affected by environmental factors throughout the course of life. Factors that cause such epigenetic changes are known to disproportionately affect various racial and ethnic populations, which may ultimately result in cancer disparities.

Diet, lifestyle, environmental exposures, or infection are known to initiate epigenetic changes. For example, flavonoids from tea and soya are potent inhibitors of DNA methyl transferases (DNMT), capable of reversing hypermethylation (15). Folates, a group of water-soluble B vitamins found in high concentration in green leafy vegetables, regulate DNA methylation through their ability to generate *S*-adenosylmethionine (16). It is therefore important to examine the relationship between diet and cancer in racially diverse populations in order to better understand how these factors might influence epigenetic changes (17, 18). For example, AAs have been found to have statistically significantly lower plasma concentrations of certain antioxidants such as vitamin E, alpha-carotene, beta-carotene, and lutein and zeaxanthin than Whites (19).

Epigenetics provides, within different populations, a link between genetics, environment, and cancer. It is important to identify how these epigenetic patterns may modify cancer pathogenesis in these diverse populations. These epigenetic changes induced by environment, diet, or lifestyle may provide clues to the mystery of cancer disparities.

Recent advances in molecular technologies for measuring DNA methylation across the whole genome have enabled investigators to better understand the role of such epigenetic changes in various diseases including cancer (12, 20, 21). To date, however, these technological advances have not been utilized to address some of the critical questions in cancer health disparities across diverse populations. For a better understanding of biological basis for cancer disparities, highlights from the literature of some of the epigenetic findings in breast, prostate, colon, and liver cancer in various racial and ethnic populations are reported below.

2. Breast Cancer Disparities

Disparities in the incidence and mortality rates of breast cancer among various racial and ethnic populations are well established. For example, the breast cancer incidence rate is lower in Africa American (AA) women, but the mortality rates are higher compared with White women (22). African American women are more often diagnosed with breast cancer at an earlier age and with more aggressive disease, characterized by higher-grade, negative-estrogen, progesterone, and Her2-receptor status (23–25) and poor outcome (26, 27).

Genetic variations have been reported in the literature that could account in part for such breast cancer disparities in various racial and ethnic populations (28–30). Genetic variations in *BRCA1* and *BRCA2* (28, 31), *p53* (32), *CYP1A1* (29), *H-ras*-1 (33), and *Cyclin D1* genes (34) have been associated more strongly with breast cancers in AA than breast cancers in Caucasian (CA) women. The prevalence of *BRCA1* mutation was reported to be different between diverse groups such as 3.5% for Hispanics, 1.3% for AA, 0.5% for Asian Americans, 8.3% for Ashkenazi Jews, and 2.2% for other non-Hispanic Whites (35).

2.1. Epigenetic Changes

The disparities observed among these diverse populations, however, cannot be fully explained by the genetic variations alone. Although, epigenetic modifications of key regulatory genes such as *BRCA1* and *ER* in breast cancer have been reported (36–39), few studies have examined differences in epigenetic alterations among various racial and ethnic groups.

A recent study indicated that differences in gene promoter hypermethylation of tumor suppressor genes, *p16* and *BRAC1*, in healthy breast tissues of CA and AA women were associated with family history of cancer (40). Another study by Mehrotra et al. (41) showed a significantly higher frequency of hypermethylation of DNA in AA than in CA women that resulted in loss of expression of a number of regulatory genes in tumors. The authors compared DNA promoter hypermethylation profiles of AA and CA breast cancers for a panel of five genes known to be frequently hypermethylated in breast cancer in the general population: *HIN-1*, *Twist*, *Cyclin D2*, *RAR-beta*, and *RASSF1A*. They reported that the group with ER/PR negative and less than 50 years of age had the highest differences in methylation of these genes between the two populations (41). African American tumors had higher frequency of methylation in four of these five genes as compared with CA. The significance of these methylated genes can be determined by the cellular function each of these genes control. Ras-association domain family 1A (*RASSF1A*) gene, a tumor suppressor gene, is reported to be methylated in 50–60% of primary breast carcinomas (42). There was also evidence of a significant association of frequent *Cyclin D2* methylation with cancer-related death. Interestingly, the percentage of methylation of *Cyclin D2* gene was significantly more prevalent in AA (64%) than CA women (19%) with breast cancer which may have led to the negative prognostic factors seen in AA. Another recent study reported gene hypermethylation in basal-like breast cancer (predominant in AA women) to be significantly higher than luminal subtype (37). Another study reported that the methylation of the RASSF1A was associated strongly with poor survival in Tunisian breast cancer patients (43).

These studies suggest that epigenetic alteration may account in part for breast cancer disparities observed in AA women. Silencing of these tumor suppressor genes by hypermethylation may be the contributing factor for poor outcome and such disparities. Therefore, a better understanding of these epigenetic changes is needed that may help unravel how these differences may account for breast cancer disparities in various populations.

3. Prostate Cancer Disparities

Differences in prostate cancer in both incidence and mortality exist between different racial groups. It has been shown that the incidence rates, as well as mortality rates, from prostate cancer are higher, almost twofold, in AA compared to CA (44). African American men have the highest prostate cancer morbidity and mortality rates than any other racial or ethnic group in the USA.

This disparity between AA and CA men is thought to be due to interaction between socioeconomic, environmental, and biological factors (45).

The genetic alterations are probably important biological contributors to malignant transformation, progression, and metastasis among these various populations. Admixture mapping studies of prostate cancer in AA men identified region on chromosome 8q24 as a susceptibility region, and three loci in that region are associated with prostate cancer risk in AA (46, 47). Mutations in tumor suppressor gene, *HPC2/ELAC2* at 17p11, 2′-5′-oligoadenylate-dependent *RNASEL* at 1q25, and *MSR1* at 8p22 (48) have been found to increase risk of prostate cancer in AA men. Additionally, mutations in androgen receptor (*AR*) gene (49) and polymorphism in *SRD5A2* enzyme were found to be associated with prostate cancer in AA men. The product of 5-alpha-reductase gene (*SRD5A2*) converts testosterone to more active metabolite, dihydrotestosterone, which interacts with (*AR*). This polymorphism may result in elevation of enzyme activity, leading to increased prostatic level of dihydrotestosterone which is known to contribute to prostatic cancer development (50).

3.1. Epigenetic Changes

Genetic variations, although important, may not account for all the racial differences in outcome for prostate cancer. Epigenetic changes, such as methylation of genes in prostate tissue samples from various racial and ethnic populations, have been reported in the literature (51–54). Recently, a pyrosequencing technique was used to quantitatively measure the methylation status of many genes such as *GSTP1*, *AR*, *RARbeta2*, *SPARC*, *TIMP3*, and *NKX2-5* and examine racial differences that contribute to prostate cancer pathogenesis. The studies showed that many of the genes examined above were found to be methylated, and their methylation frequencies differ among AA men when compared to CA men (51). Hypermethylation of *GSTP1*, an enzyme involved in DNA repair, was confirmed by other studies and found to be significantly higher in prostate cancer samples in AA men compared with CA men (52, 53). Additionally, racial differences in methylation status of *CD44* and *CDH1* genes were reported by Woodson et al. (54) in prostate cancer tissues of AA when compared to those of CA men. In addition, significant higher methylation prevalence for *AR* gene in AA men when compared with CA samples was reported recently (51).

The differences in rates of clinically significant prostate cancer among various populations could be attributed to epigenetic changes caused by diet or the environment. It has been shown that prostate cancer rates are 15-fold higher in men from the United States than in men from Asian countries. The high levels of soy consumed in Asian countries are thought to be a contributing factor that may be responsible for this discrepancy in prostate cancer among these populations. The average intake of soy isoflavone in Asian diets is high which may have an effect on DNA methylation (53). Smoking may also affect DNA methylation. One study demonstrated significant correlation of methylation status of multiple genes with smoking status in prostate cancer (55). All these studies indicate that environmental and dietary factors may influence the risk of prostate cancer via epigenetic pathways, and some of these factors may possess preventive and therapeutic potential in prostate cancer. Thus, high prevalence of promoter hypermethylation of many important genes associated with prostate cancer in AA (Table 1) indicate that more research is needed for a thorough investigation of these differences and how these differences impact prostate cancer disparities.

4. Colorectal Cancer Disparities

Cancers of the colon and rectum are the second leading cause of cancer deaths in the USA (56). African Americans are at high risk of developing colorectal cancer (CRC) (57, 58). Population-based studies reported 30–50% higher rates of colon cancer mortality in AA compared to CA (58). About 10–60% of AA, Chinese, and Mexican are likely to be diagnosed with stages III or IV CRC compared to Caucasian men (58). CRC in AA has been shown to be more advanced and right-sided.

The analysis of the various biological factors that might play a role in the CRC disparity among diverse population is of great clinical importance. Genetic alterations that may provide evidence for racial disparities have been reported in the literature for arachidonate lipoxygenase polymorphisms (59), microsatellite instability (60, 61), folate metabolic gene polymorphisms in methylene tetrahydrofolate reductase (62), and vitamin D receptor haplotypes (63). Furthermore, deletion of *EXOC4, EPHB6, GNAS, MLL3,* and *TBX22* genes and amplification of *HAPLN1, ADAM29, SMAD2* genes were reported in AA (64). Mutation in adenomatous polyposis coli (APC), a tumor suppressor gene, was associated with colon cancer in Korean (65), Chinese (66), and AA patients (62).

4.1. Epigenetic Changes

Genes that are hypermethylated in colon cancer may be considered as a marker of colon carcinogenesis among the general populations. Although various racial and ethnic populations have higher rates of CRC, only a few studies have explored the epigenetic changes as a possible explanation for such disparities. One of the hypotheses for CRC disparities may be due to transcriptional silencing of important genes by hypermethylation of CpG islands.

In few recent studies, racial differences in the methylation status of genes associated with CRC progression were examined

Table 1
Summary of epigenetic changes reported among various racial and ethnic populations

Gene	Gene product	Cancer pathway	Cancer site	Racial variations	References
BRCA	BRCA protein	Regular cellular proliferation and DNA repair	Breast	BRCA-1 hypermethylation occurred in AA women; BRCA1 hypermethylation frequencies for Tunisian breast cancer were 46%	(31, 39)
HIN-1	Tumor suppressor gene	Inhibitor of cell growth invasion	Breast	Higher methylation—79% in AA vs. 19% in CA women	(41)
Twist	Transcription factor	A gene implicated in apoptosis	Breast	Higher methylation—67% in AA vs. 16% in CA	(41)
Cyclin D2	Cyclin D	Involved in cell cycle regulation	Breast	Cyclin D2 methylation—64% in AA vs. 19% in CA	(41)
RASSF1A	Ras-association domain family 1A	Tumor suppressor gene	Breast, liver	RASSF1A methylation—76% in AA vs. 29% in CA; 87% in breast cancer in Tunisian women; also methylated in liver cancer	(41, 43, 80)
GSTP1	Glutathione *S*-transferase P1	DNA repair	Prostate	Highly methylated in AA compared to CA men	(53)
AR	Androgen receptor	Hormone receptor gene, metabolism of androgens and testosterone	Prostate	Higher methylation in AA compared to CA men	(51)
RARβ	Retinoic acid receptor, beta	Gene transcription	Prostate, breast	Higher methylation in AA compared to CA men for prostate cancer; for breast cancer 40% in AA vs. 8% in CA	(41, 51)
SPARC	Secreted protein, acidic and rich cysteine	Involved in cell-matrix interactions, migration, and angiogenesis	Prostate	SPARC is more frequently methylated in AA prostate cancer	(51)
TIMP3	Tissue inhibitors of metalloproteinase inhibitors 3	Involved in degradation of extracellular matrix	Prostate	More methylated in AA men with prostate cancer	(51)

NKX2-5	Homeobox protein	Transcription factor	Prostate	More methylated in AA prostate cancer	(51)
CD44	CD44 antigen	Involve in lymphocyte activation, recirculation and homing, and tumor metastasis	Prostate	More methylated in AA men with prostate cancer	(54)
MGMT	*O*(6)-methylguanine-DNA methyltransferase	Involved in DNA repair	Prostate	Frequently methylated in prostate cancer in AA men	(51)
CDH1	E-cadherin protein	Adhesion molecule and its loss contribute to progression in cancer by increasing proliferation, invasion, and/or metastasis	Prostate	Altered methylation in AA men	(54)
CHD5	Chromodomain-helicase-DNA-binding protein 5	Involved in early tumorigenic processes at the chromatin remodeling level	Colon	Frequently methylated in prostate cancer in AA than CA men	(67)
ICAM5	Intercellular adhesion molecule (ICAM) family	Involved in invasiveness and metastatic potential of the tumors	Colon	Frequently methylated in prostate cancer in AA than CA men	(67)
MLH1	mutL homolog 1	DNA repair	Colon	Frequently methylated in prostate cancer in AA than CA men	(61)
APC2	Adenomatous polyposis coli	Tumor suppressor	Colon	Frequently methylated in prostate cancer in AA than CA men	(61)
GPNMB	Transmembrane glycoprotein	Involved in invasiveness and metastatic potential of the tumors	Colon	Frequently methylated in prostate cancer in AA than CA men	(67)
HOXA9	Homeobox protein	Transcription factor regulates gene expression, morphogenesis, and differentiation	Liver	Frequently methylated in HBV-positive HCC cases in Chinese	(79)
SFRP1	Secreted frizzled-related protein 1	Tumor suppressor	Liver	Frequently methylated in HBV-positive HCC cases in Chinese	(79)
CDKN2A	Cyclin-dependent kinase inhibitors 2A	Tumor suppressor	Liver	Frequently methylated in HBV-positive HCC cases in Chinese	(79)
DNMT3B	DNA methyltransferase 3B	DNA methylation	Liver	More frequently methylated in HCV-positive HCC cases in Chinese	(79)

for AA and compared to White Iranians (67). Genes, found to be significantly methylated in AA when compared to Whites, were *CHD5*, *ICAM5*, and *GPNMB* (67). *GPNMB* and *ICAM5* gene products are involved in growth delay and reduction of metastatic potential. Higher methylation level of *GPNMB* and *ICAM5* in AA silences these important genes, which might partly account for the aggressiveness and invasiveness of colon tumors in AA. *ICAM5* encodes a type I transmembrane glycoprotein that is a member of the intercellular adhesion molecule (ICAM) family. The high methylation level of *ICAM5* decreases the cell-to-cell adhesion in the tumor cells, thus increasing their invasive potential. Thus, methylation of *GPNMB* and *ICAM5* genes in AA patients may lead to an increase in the invasiveness and metastatic potential of the tumors. *CHD-5* (chromodomain-helicase-DNA-binding protein 5) seems to be involved in early tumorigenic processes at the chromatin remodeling level (67).

Another study reported a high level of methylation for *MLH1*, *APC*, and *APC2* genes in AA (61) and aberrant global histone (*H3* and *H4*) acetylation and histone deacetylase 2 (*HDAC2*) expression in AA patient samples (68). The high methylation level of these genes in AA compared to Whites may help explain the increase of incidence of colon cancer in AA (Table 1).

Environmental and dietary factors that affect DNA methylation could result in different genotypes for colon cancer risk in diverse populations. Williams (69) showed an association between antioxidant nutrients, and risk of CRC in CA and AA. The study evaluated the relationships between antioxidant nutrients (such as vitamin C, vitamin E, β-carotene, selenium) and DNA methylation-related nutrients (such as folate, vitamin B6, vitamin B12) and its association with the risk of distal CRC and found differences among CA and AA. These initial reports on differences in dietary factors and methylation patterns of key regulatory genes in different racial and ethnic populations provide key evidence that epigenetics could play a role in colon cancer disparities.

5. Liver Cancer Disparities

Significant disparities in hepatocellular carcinoma (HCC) have been observed in selected racial and ethnic populations in the USA. (70). Chronic HBV and hepatitis C virus (HCV) infections account for the majority of these cases. Chronic hepatitis B infection is the greatest in the Asian and Pacific Islander (API) populations in the USA. Within the Asian community, Laotian/Hmong and the

Cambodian community seem to have the highest incidence of HCC (71). These disparities could be attributed to race, culture, socioeconomic status, and biology.

Genomic studies have provided initial evidence for the disparity in liver cancer among Asian population. Recently, a genome-wide association study identified that the 1p36.22 locus confers susceptibility to HBV-related HCC and suggested that *KIF1B*-, *UBE4B*-, or *PGD*-related pathways might be involved in the pathogenesis of liver cancer in Chinese populations (72). Furthermore, *EGF 61* GG genotype was reported to be associated with liver cancer in Chinese patients (73). Vascular endothelial growth factor (*VEGF*), an important regulator of angiogenesis and vascular permeability, is involved in various steps of many malignancies (74). Recent data suggest that polymorphism rs3025035 in the *VEGF* gene may be a potential genetic marker for HCC recurrence in Chinese populations (75). The *hGSTA1* gene has been reported to be polymorphic in the Chinese population that is different from other racial populations (76) and is linked to differences in tumor incidences in various Asian groups (77).

5.1. Epigenetic Changes

Epigenetic changes associated with HCC due to infection with HBV and HCV have been found to be different in various racial and ethnic populations. HBV and HCV, for example, were associated with over 90% of HCC cases in Asian Americans (78). Among these HCC cases, genes such as *HOXA9*, *RASSF1,* and *SFRP1* were frequently methylated in HBV-positive HCC cases, while *CDKN2A* were significantly more frequently methylated in HCV-positive HCC cases (79). In addition, *RASSF1A* and DNA methyltransferase 3B (*DNMT3B*) hypermethylation were shown to predict a poor outcome in Japanese and Moroccan patients, respectively (80, 81). These genes may play an oncogenic role during tumorigenesis of HCC (Table 1). There are also some interesting findings showing significant differences in the prevalence of allelic imbalance (AI) and CpG island methylation in HCC from Australian and South African patients. Allelic imbalance was examined at 1p, 4p, 4q, 8p, 9p, 13q, 16q, and 17p and was reported to be significantly higher in South African HCC patients. Methylation status of several genes such as *p14*, *p16*, *p15*, *RIZ1*, *E-cadherin*, and *O6-MGMT* was significantly higher in Australian HCC cases compared to South African patients (82).

These few reports indicate that there could be differences in epigenetic modifications in HCCs from different racial and ethnic populations, which could lead to different clinical outcome. More research is needed to fully understand how these epigenetic modifications take place and then subsequently affect the overall outcome of in liver cancer in diverse populations.

6. Conclusion

While some progress has been made, cancer health disparities affecting racial and ethnic populations still persist and need to be addressed. Epigenetic processes, in particular, DNA methylation, may play a role in the induction of certain phenotypes with increased cancer risk due to exposure to environmental factors throughout the life course. With the advances in molecular technologies, epigenetic approaches may prove useful in identifying the environmental and lifestyle factors that contribute to the cancer disparities in certain high-risk populations. Epigenetic alterations in tumor suppressor genes and genes involved in control of cell proliferation, DNA repair and metastasis, and hormone receptor expression, have shown to play a role in tumor causation and progression. The prevalence of these epigenetic alterations may provide a basis for understanding the unequal cancer burden in early onset, aggressiveness, and poor outcomes observed in these various racial and ethnic populations. Identification of these differences in epigenetic processes in various diverse populations may help in developing biomarkers of disease risk and design better therapeutic interventions. Epigenetic research has the potential to enhance our understanding of the determinants of cancer burden among diverse populations and ultimately reduce cancer health disparities.

References

1. Jemal, A., Siegel, R., Xu, J. and Ward, E. (2010) Cancer Statistics, 2010. *CA Cancer J Clin* 60, 277–300.
2. McCracken, M., Olsen, M., Chen, M.S. Jr., Jemal, A., Thun, M., Cokkinides, V., Deapen, D. and Ward, E. (2007) Cancer Incidence, Mortality, and Associated Risk Factors Among Asian Americans of Chinese, Filipino, Vietnamese, Korean, and Japanese Ethnicities. *CA Cancer J Clin* 57, 190–205.
3. Chen, M.S. Jr. (2005) Cancer health disparities among Asian Americans: what we do and what we need to do. *Cancer* 104, 2895–902.
4. Albain, K.S., Unger, J.M., Crowley, J.J., Coltman, C.A. Jr. and Hershman, D.L. (2009) Racial disparities in cancer survival among randomized clinical trials patients of the Southwest Oncology Group. *J Natl Cancer Inst* 101, 984–992.
5. Godley, P.A., Schenck, A.P., Amamoo, M.A., Schoenbach, V.J., Peacock, S., Manning, M., Symons, M. and Talcott, J.A. (2003) Racial differences in mortality among Medicare recipients after treatment for localized prostate cancer. *J Natl Cancer Inst* 95, 1702–1710.
6. Chu, K.C., Miller, B.A., and Springfield, S. A. (2007) Measures of racial/ethnic health disparities in cancer mortality rates and the influence of socioeconomic status. *J Nat Med Assoc* 99, 1092–1100.
7. Freedman, H. and Chu, K. (2005) Determinants of cancer disparities: barriers to cancer screening, diagnosis, and treatment. *Surg Oncol Clin N Am* 14, 655–669.
8. Rotimi, C.N. and Jorde, L.B. (2010) Ancestry and disease in the age of genomic medicine. *N Engl J Med* 363, 1551–1558.
9. Ingelman-Sundberg, M. (2008) Pharmacogenomic biomarkers for prediction of severe adverse drug reactions. *N Engl J Med* 358, 637–639.
10. Phan, V.H., Moore, M.M., McLachlan, A.J., Piquette-Miller, M., Xu, H. and Clarke, S.J. (2009) Ethnic differences in drug metabolism and toxicity from chemotherapy. *Expert Opin. Drug Metab. Toxicol* 5, 243–257.
11. Verma, M. and Srivastava, S. (2002) Epigenetics in cancer: implications for early detection and prevention. *Lancet Oncol* 3, 755–763.

12. Jones, P.A. and Baylin, S.B. (2007) The epigenomics of cancer. *Cell* 128, 683–692.
13. McGowan, P.O., Meaney, M.J. and Szyf, M. (2008) Diet and the epigenetic (re)programming of phenotypic differences in behavior. *Brain Res* 1237, 12–24.
14. Mathers, J.C., Strathdee, G. and Relton, C.L. (2010) Induction of epigenetic alterations by dietary and other environmental factors *Advances in Genetics* 71, 3–39.
15. Fang, M.Z., Chen, D., Sun, Y., Jin, Z., Christman, J.K. and Yang, C.S. (2005) Reversal of hypermethylation and reactivation of p16INK4a, RARbeta, and MGMT genes by genistein and other isoflavones from soy. *Clin Cancer Res* 11, 7033–7041.
16. Duthie, S.J. (2010) Epigenetic modifications and human pathologies: cancer and CVD. *Proc Nutr Soc* 11, 1–10.
17. Williams, C.D., Satia, J.A., Adair, L.S., Stevens, J., Galanko, J., Keku, T.O. and Sandler, R.S. (2009) Dietary patterns, food groups, and rectal cancer risk in Whites and African-Americans. *Cancer Epidemiol Biomarkers Prev* 18, 1552–1561.
18. Krukowski, R.A. and West, D.S. (2010) Consideration of the food environment in cancer risk reduction. *J Am Diet Assoc* 110, 842–844.
19. Watters, J.L., Satia, J.A., Kupper, L.L., Swenberg, J.A., Schroeder, J.C. and Switzer, B.R. (2007) Associations of antioxidant nutrients and oxidative DNA damage in healthy African-American and White adults. *Cancer Epidemiol Biomarkers Prev* 16, 1428–1436.
20. Lechner, M., Boshoff, C. and Beck, S. (2010) Cancer epigenome. *Adv Genet* 70, 247–276.
21. Feinberg, A.P. (2010) Epigenomics reveals a functional genome anatomy and a new approach to common disease. *Nat Biotechnol 28*, 1049–1052.
22. Ray, M. and Polite, B. N. (2010) Triple Negative Breast Cancers- A view from 10,000 feet. *Cancer J* 16, 17–22.
23. Amend, K., Hicks, D. and Ambrosone, C.B. (2006) Breast Cancer in African-American Women: Differences in Tumor Biology from European-American Women. *Cancer Res* 66, 8327–8330.
24. Hayanga, A.J. and Newman, L.A. (2007) Investigating the phenotypes and genotypes of breast cancer in women with African ancestry: the need for more genetic epidemiology. *Surg Clin North Am* 87, 551–568.
25. Agurs-Collins, T., Dunn, B.K., Browne, D., Johnson, K.A. and Lubet, R. (2010) Epidemiology of health disparities in relation to the biology of estrogen receptor-negative breast cancer. *Semin Oncol* 37, 384–401.
26. Rakha, E. and Reis-Filho, J. (2009) Basal like Breast carcinoma. *Arch Pathol Lab Med* 133, 860–868.
27. Patel, T. A., Colon-Otero, G., Bueno Hume, C., Copland, J.A. 3 rd. and Perez, E.A. (2010) Breast cancer in Latinas: Gene Expression, Differential Response to Treatments, and Differential Toxicities in Latinas Compared with Other Population Groups. *The Oncologist* 15, 466–475.
28. Kurian, A.W. (2010) BRCA1 and BRCA2 mutations across race and ethnicity: distribution and clinical implications. *Curr Opin Obstet Gynecol* 22, 72–78.
29. Kato, I., Cichon, M., Yee, C.L., Land, S., and Korczak, J.F. (2009) African American-preponderant single nucleotide polymorphisms (SNPs) and risk of breast cancer. *Cancer Epidemiol* 33, 24–30.
30. Sowers, M. R., Wilson, A.L., Kardia, S.R., Chu, J. and McConnell, D.S. (2006) CYP1A1 and CYP1B1 Polymorphisms and Their Association with Estradiol and Estrogen Metabolites in Women Who Are Premenopausal and Perimenopausal. *The Am J of Med* 119, S44–S51.
31. Olopade, O. I., Fackenthal, J.D., Dunston, G., Tainsky, M.A., Collins, F. and Whitfield-Broome, C. (2003) Breast cancer genetics in African Americans. *Cancer* 97, 236–245.
32. Rose, D.P. and Royak-Schaler, R. (2001) Tumor biology and prognosis in black breast cancer patients: a review. *Cancer Detect Prev* 25, 16–31.
33. Weston, A. and Godbold, J.H. (1997) Polymorphisms of H-ras-1 and p53 in breast cancer and lung cancer: a meta-analysis. *Environ Health Perspect* 105, 919–926.
34. Joe, A.K., Arber, N., Bose, S., Heitjan, D., Zhang, Y., Weinstein, I.B. and Hibshoosh, H. (2001) Cyclin D1 overexpression is more prevalent in non-Caucasian breast cancer. *Anticancer Res* 21, 3535–3539.
35. John, E.M., Miron, A., Gong,G., Phipps, A.I., Felberg, A., Li, F.P., West, D.W. and Whittemore, A.S. (2007) Prevalence of pathogenic BRCA1 mutation carriers in 5 US racial/ethnic groups. *JAMA* 298, 2869–2876.
36. Jing, F., Yuping, W., Yong, C., Jie, L., Jun, L., Xuanbing, T. and Lihua, H. (2010) CpG island methylator phenotype of multigene in serum of sporadic breast carcinoma. *Tumour Biol* 31, 321–331.
37. Guendel, I., Carpio, L., Pedati, C., Schwartz, A., Teal, C., Kashanchi, F. and Kehn-Hall, K.

(2010) Methylation of the tumor suppressor protein, BRCA1, influences its transcriptional cofactor function. *PLoS One* 5, e11379.

38. Lee, J. S., Fackler, M.J., Lee, J.H., Choi, C., Park, M.H., Yoon, J.H., Zhang, Z. and Sukumar, S. (2010) Basal-like breast cancer displays distinct patterns of promoter methylation. *Cancer Biol Ther* 9, 1017–1024.
39. Karray-Chouayekh, S., Trifa, F., Khabir, A., Boujelbane, N., Sellami-Boudawara, T., Daoud, J., Frikha, M., Gargouri, A. and Mokdad-Gargouri, R. (2009) Clinical Significance of Epigenetic Inactivation of hMLH1 and BRCA1 in Tunisian Patients with Invasive Breast Carcinoma. *J of Biomed and Biotech* 2009, 369129.
40. Dumitrescu, R.G., Marian, C., Krishnan, S.S., Spear, S.L., Kallakury, B.V., Perry, D.J., Convit, J.R., Seillier-Moiseiwitsch, F., Yang, Y., Freudenheim, J.L. and Shields, P.G. (2010) Familial and racial determinants of tumour suppressor genes promoter hypermethylation in breast tissues from healthy women. *J Cell Mol Med* 14, 1468–1475.
41. Mehrotra, J., Ganpat, M.M., Kanaan, Y., Fackler, M.J., McVeigh, M., Lahti-Domenici, J., Polyak, K., Argani, P., Naab, T., Garrett, E., Parmigiani, G., Broome, C. and Sukumar, S. (2004) Estrogen Receptor/Progesterone Receptor-Negative Breast Cancers of Young African-American Women Have a Higher Frequency of Methylation of Multiple Genes than Those of Caucasian Women. *Clin Cancer Res* 10, 2052–2057.
42. Fackler, M. J., McVeigh, M., Evron, E., Garrett, E., Mehrotra, J., Polyak, K., Sukumar, S. and Argani, P. (2003) DNA methylation of RASSF1A, HIN-1, RAR-b, Cyclin D2 and Twist in in situ invasive and lobular carcinoma. *Int J Cancer* 107, 970–975.
43. Karray-Chouayekh, S., Trifa, F., Khabir, A., Boujelbane, N., Sellami-Boudawara, T., Daoud, J., Frikha, M., Jlidi, R., Gargouri, A. and Mokdad-Gargouri, R. (2010) Aberrant methylation of RASSF1A is associated with poor survival in Tunisian breast cancer patients. *J Cancer Res Clin Oncol* 136, 203–210.
44. Hsing, A.W., Tsao L., and Devesa S.S. (2000) International trends and patterns of prostate cancer incidence and mortality. *Int J Cancer* 85, 60–67.
45. Odedina, F.T., Akinremi, T.O., Chinegwundoh, F., Roberts, R., Yu, D., Reams, R.R., Freedman, M.L., Rivers, B., Green, B.L., Kumar, N. (2009) Prostate cancer disparities in Black men of African descent: a comparative literature review of prostate cancer burden among Black men in the United States, Caribbean, United Kingdom, and West Africa. *Infect Agent Cancer* 4, Suppl 1:S2
46. Robbins, C., Torres, J.B., Hooker, S., Bonilla, C., Hernandez, W., Candreva, A., Ahaghotu, C., Kittles, R. and Carpten, J. (2007) Confirmation study of prostate cancer risk variants at 8q24 in African Americans identifies a novel risk locus. *Genome Res* 17, 1717–1722.
47. Xu, J., Kibel, A.S., Hu, J.J., Turner, A.R., Pruett, K., Zheng, S.L., Sun, J., Isaacs, S.D., Wiley, K.E., Kim, S.T., Hsu, F.C., Wu, W., Torti, F.M., Walsh, P.C., Chang, B.L. and Isaacs, W.B. (2007) Prostate cancer risk associated loci in African Americans. *Cancer Epidemiol Biomarkers Prev* 18, 2145–2149.
48. Rokman, A., Ikonen, T., Seppälä, E.H., Nupponen, N., Autio, V., Mononen, N., Bailey-Wilson, J., Trent, J., Carpten, J., Matikainen, M.P., Koivisto, P.A., Tammela, T.L., Kallioniemi, O.P. and Schleutker, J. (2004) Germline alterations of the RNASEL gene, a candidate HPC1 gene at 1q25, in patients and families with prostate cancer. *Am J Hum Genet* 70, 1299–1304.
49. Kittles, R., Young, D., Weinrich, S., Hudson, J., Argyropoulos, G., Ukoli, F., Adams-Campbell, L. and Dunston, G.M. (2001) Extent of linkage disequilibrium between the androgen receptor gene CAG and GGC repeats in human populations: implications for prostate cancer risk. *Hum Genet* 109, 253–261.
50. Rose, R.K., Bernstein, L., Lobo, R.A., Shimizu, H., Stanczyk, F.Z., Pike, M.C. and Henderson, B.E. (1992) 5-alpha-reducing activity and risk of prostate cancer among Japanese and US white and black males. *Lancet* 339, 887–889.
51. Kwabi-Addo, B., Wang, S., Chung, W., Jelinek, J., Patierno, S.R., Wang, B.D., Andrawis, R., Lee, N.H., Apprey, V., Issa, J.P. and Ittmann, M. (2010) Identification of differentially methylated genes in normal prostate tissues from African American and Caucasian men. *Clin Cancer Res* 16, 3539–3547.
52. Enokida, H., Shiina, H., Urakami, S., Igawa, M., Ogishima, T., Pookot, D., Li, L.C., Tabatabai, Z.L., Kawahara, M., Nakagawa, M., Kane, C.J., Carroll, P.R. and Dahiya, R. (2005) Ethnic group-related differences in CpG hypermethylation of the GSTP1 gene promoter among African-American, Caucasian and Asian patients with prostate cancer. *Int J Cancer* 116, 174–181.
53. Li, L.C. and Dahiya, R. (2007) Epigenetics of prostate cancer. *Frontiers in Bioscience* 12, 3377–3397.
54. Woodson, K., Hayes, R., Wideroff, L., Villaruz, L. and Tangrea, J. (2003) Hypermethylation of GSTP1, CD44, and E-cadherin genes in prostate

cancer among US Blacks and Whites. *Prostate* 55, 199–205.

55. Enokida, H., Shiina, H., Urakami, S., Terashima, M., Ogishima, T., Li, L.C., Kawahara, M., Nakagawa, M., Kane, C.J., Carroll, P.R., Igawa, M. and Dahiya, R. (2006) Smoking influences aberrant CpG hypermethylation of multiple genes in human prostate carcinoma. *Cancer* 106, 79–86.
56. SEER Cancer Statistics Review 1975-2007 http://seer.cancer.gov/csr/1975_2007/index.html
57. Sharma, S.O. and Keefe, S. J. (2007) Environmental influences on the high mortality from colorectal cancer in African Americans. *Postgrad Med J* 83, 583–589.
58. Chien, C., Morimoto, L.M., Tom, J. and Li, C.I. (2005) Differences in colorectal carcinoma stage and survival by race and ethnicity. *Cancer* 104, 629–639.
59. Goodman, J.E., Bowman, E.D., Chanock, S.J., Alberg, A.J. and Harris, C.C. (2004) Arachidonate lipoxygenase (ALOX) and cyclooxygenase (COX) polymorphisms and colon cancer risk. *Carcinogenesis* 25: 2467–2472.
60. Brim, H., Mokarram, P., Naghibalhossaini, F., Saberi-Firoozi, M., Al-Mandhari, M., et al. (2008) Impact of BRAF, MLH1 on the incidence of microsatellite instability high colorectal cancer in populations based study. *Mol Cancer* 7, 68.
61. Kumar, K., Brim, H., Giardiello, F., Smoot, D.T., Nouraie, M., Lee, E.L. and Ashktorab, H. (2009) Distinct BRAF (V600E) and KRAS mutations in high microsatellite instability sporadic colorectal cancer in African Americans. *Clin Cancer Res* 15, 1155–1161.
62. Ashktorab, H., Begum, R., Akhgar, A., Smoot, D.T., Elbedawi, M., Daremipouran, M., Zhao, A., Momen, B. and Giardiello, F.M. (2007) Folate status and risk of colorectal polyps in African Americans. *Dig Dis Sci* 52, 1462–1470.
63. Sweeney, C., Curtin, K., Murtaugh, M.A., Caan, B.J., Potter, J.D. and Slattery, M.L. (2006) Haplotype analysis of common vitamin D receptor variants and colon and rectal cancers. *Cancer Epidemiol Biomarkers Prev* 15, 744–749.
64. Ashktorab, H., Schäffer, A.A., Daremipouran, M., Smoot, D.T., Lee, E. and Brim, H. (2010) Distinct genetic alterations in colorectal cancer. *PLoS One* 5, e8879.
65. Jang, Y.H., Lim, S.B., Kim, M.J., Chung, H.J., Yoo, H.W., Byeon, J.S., Myung, S.J., Lee, W., Chun, S. and Min, W.K. (2010) Three novel mutations of the APC gene in Korean patients with familial adenomatous polyposis. *Cancer Genet Cytogenet* 200, 34–39.
66. Sheng, J.Q., Cui, W.J., Fu, L., Jin, P., Han, Y., Li, S.J., Fan, R.Y., Li, A.Q., Zhang, M.Z. and Li, S.R. (2010) APC gene mutations in Chinese familial adenomatous polyposis patients. *World J Gastroenterol* 16, 1522–1526.
67. Mokarram, P., Kumar, K., Brim, H., Naghibalhossaini, F., Saberi-firoozi, M., Nouraie, M., Green, R., Lee, E., Smoot, D.T. and Ashktorab, H. (2009)Distinct high-profile methylated genes in colorectal cancer. *PLoS One* 4, e7012.
68. Ashktorab, H., Belgrave, K., Hosseinkhah, F., Brim, H., Nouraie, M., Takkikto, M., Hewitt, S., Lee, E.L., Dashwood, R.H. and Smoot, D. (2009) Global Histone H4 acetylation and HDAC2 expression in colon adenoma and carcinoma. *Dig Dis Sci* 54, 2109–2117.
69. Williams, C.D. (2010) Antioxidant and DNA methylation-related nutrients and risk of distal colorectal cancer. *Cancer Causes Control* 21, 1171–1181.
70. Ma, G.X., Shive, S.E., Fang, C.Y., Feng, Z., Parameswaran, L., Pham, A. and Khanh, C. (2007) Knowledge, attitudes, and behaviors of hepatitis B screening and vaccination and liver cancer risks among Vietnamese Americans. *J Health Care Poor Underserved*18, 62–73.
71. Kwong, S.L., Stewart, S.L., Aoki, C.A. and Chen, M.S. Jr. (2010) Disparities in Hepatocellular Carcinoma Survival among Californians of Asian Ancestry, 1988 to 2007. *Cancer Epidemiol Biomarkers Prev* 19, 2747–2757.
72. Zhang, H., Zhai, Y., Hu, Z., Wu, C., Qian, J., Jia, W., Ma, F., Huang, W., Yu, L., Yue, W., Wang, Z., Li, P., Zhang, Y., Liang, R., Wei, Z., Cui, Y., Xie, W., Cai, M., Yu, X., Yuan, Y., Xia, X., Zhang, X., Yang, H., Qiu, W., Yang, J., Gong, F., Chen, M., Shen, H., Lin, D., Zeng, Y.X., He, F. and Zhou, G. (2010) Genome-wide association study identifies 1p36.22 as a new susceptibility locus for hepatocellular carcinoma in chronic hepatitis B virus carriers. *Nat Genet* 42, 755–758.
73. Li, Y., Xie, Q., Lu, F., Zhao, J., Mao, P., Li, Z., Liu, S. and Zhuang, H. (2010) Association between epidermal growth factor 61A/G polymorphism and hepatocellular carcinoma susceptibility in Chinese patients. *Liver Int* 30, 112–118.
74. Podar, K., and Anderson, K.C. (2005) The pathophysiologic role of VEGF in hematologic malignancies: therapeutic implications. *Blood* 105, 1383–1395.
75. Wu, L.M., Xie, H.Y., Zhou, L., Yang, Z., Zhang, F. and Zheng, S.S. (2009) A single nucleotide polymorphism in the vascular endothelial growth factor gene is associated with

recurrence of hepatocellular carcinoma after transplantation. *Arch Med Res* 40, 565–570.

76. Ping, J., Wang, H., Huang, M. and Liu, Z.S. (2006) Genetic analysis of glutathione S-transferase A1 polymorphism in the Chinese population and the influence of genotype on enzymatic properties. *Toxicol Sci* 89, 438–443.
77. Fang, W., Piao, Z., Buyse, I.M., Simon, D., Sheu, J.C., Perucho, M. and Huang, S. (2001) Preferential loss of a polymorphic RIZ allele in human hepatocellular carcinoma. *Br J Cancer* 84, 743–747.
78. Tong, M. J., Chavalitdhamrong, D., Lu, D.S., Raman, S.S., Gomes, A., Duffy, J.P., Hong, J.C. and Busuttil, R.W. (2010) Survival in Asian Americans after treatments for hepatocellular carcinoma: a seven-year experience at UCLA. *J Clin Gastroenterol* 44, e63.
79. Feng, Q., Stern, J.E., Hawes, S.E., Lu, H., Jiang, M. and Kiviat, N.B. (2010) DNA methylation changes in normal liver tissues and hepatocellular carcinoma with different viral infection. *Exp Mol Pathol* 88, 287–292.
80. Sugawara, W., Haruta, M., Sasaki, F., Watanabe, N., Tsunematsu, Y., Kikuta, A. and Kaneko, Y. (2007) Promoter hypermethylation of the RASSF1A gene predicts the poor outcome of patients with hepatoblastoma. *Pediatr Blood Cancer* 49, 240249.
81. Ezzikouri, S., El Feydi, A.E., Benazzouz, M., Afifi, R., El Kihal, L., Hassar, M., Akil, A., Pineau, P. and Benjelloun, S. (2009) Single nucleotide polymorphism in DNMT3B promoter and its association with hepatocellular carcinoma in a Moroccan population. *Infect Genet Evol* 9, 877–881.
82. Herath, N.I., Purdie, D.M., Kew, M.C., Smith, J.L., Young, J., Leggett, B.A. and MacDonald, G.A. (2009) Varying etiologies lead to different molecular changes in Australian and South African hepatocellular carcinomas. *Int J Oncol* 35, 1081–1089.

Chapter 26

Multifactorial Etiology of Gastric Cancer

Jovanny Zabaleta

Abstract

The prevalence of gastric cancer is associated with several factors including geographical location, diet, and genetic background of the host. However, it is evident that infection with *Helicobacter pylori* (*H. pylori*) is crucial for the development of the disease. Virulence of the bacteria is also important in modulating the risk of the disease. After infection, *H. pylori* gains access to the gastric mucosa and triggers the production of cytokines that promote recruitment of inflammatory cells, probably involved in tissue damage. Once the infection is established, a cascade of inflammatory steps associated with changes in the gastric epithelia that may lead to cancer is triggered. *H. pylori*-induced gastritis and *H. pylori*-associated gastric cancer have been the focus of extensive research aiming to discover the underlying mechanisms of gastric tissue damage. This research has led to the association of host genetic components with the risk of the disease. Among these is the presence of single nucleotide polymorphisms (SNPs) in several genes, including cytokine genes, which are able to differentially modulate the production of inflammatory cytokines and then modulate the risk of gastric cancer. Interestingly, the frequency of some of these SNPs is different among populations and may serve as a predictive factor for gastric cancer risk within that specific population. However, the role played by other genetic modifications should not be minimized. Methylation of gene promoters has been recognized as a major mechanism of gene expression regulation without changing the primary structure of the DNA. Most DNA methylation occurs in cytosine residues in CpG dinucleotide, but it can also be found in other DNA bases. DNA methyltransferases add methyl groups to the CpG dinucleotide, and when this methylation level is too high, the gene expression is turned off. In *H. pylori* infection as well as in gastric cancer, hypermethylation of promoters of genes involved in cell cycle control, metabolism of essential nutrients, and production of inflammatory mediators, among others, has been described. Interestingly, DNA changes like SNPs or mutations can create CpG sites in sequences where transcription factors normally sit, affecting transcription.

In this chapter, we review the literature about the role of SNPs and methylation on *H. pylori* infection and gastric cancer, with big emphasis to the *H. pylori* role in the development of the disease due to the strong association between both.

Key words: *Helicobacter pylori*, Gastric cancer, Single nucleotide polymorphisms, Methylation

Ramona G. Dumitrescu and Mukesh Verma (eds.), *Cancer Epigenetics: Methods and Protocols*, Methods in Molecular Biology, vol. 863, DOI 10.1007/978-1-61779-612-8_26, © Springer Science+Business Media, LLC 2012

1. Introduction

In 2008, close to one million new cases of gastric cancer (7.8% of the total cases) were estimated, with 736,000 deaths (9.7% of the total) due to the disease in the same period, making gastric cancer the second leading cause of cancer-related deaths worldwide (1). However, the incidence and mortality of gastric cancer around the world varies significantly according to the geographical location. The incidence in Asia and Eastern Europe is more than 20 cases per 100,000 individuals, contrasting with incidence rates lower than 10 cases per 100,000 individuals in North America, New Zealand, and Oceania (2, 3). The contrast in the survival rate of stomach cancer is significant as well. Japan, North America, and Western Europe have the highest survival rates (52, 21, and 27%, respectively) compared with only 6% survival in the sub-Saharan regions (2). Parkin et al. suggested that the incidence of stomach cancer is higher in men than in women in most of these regions (2). In the United States, it is estimated that approximately 13,000 men and 8,000 women were diagnosed with gastric cancer in 2010 (4); more than 10,000 of them are expected to have died as a direct result of the neoplasia.

Several classifications of gastric cancer have been proposed over the years, based on different aspects including histopathology, clinical aspects, and endoscopic characteristics (5–9). However, the most widely followed classification is the one by Laurén (8), which, after few later updates, classifies cancer into intestinal and diffuse types, according to structural characteristics of the tumors. In general, the diffuse type seems to be diagnosed at earlier stages, more frequent in women than in men, and to be associated with specific blood types and associated to pangastritis without atrophy (10, 11). In contrast, the intestinal type of gastric cancer is more associated with gastritis in the corpus that leads to atrophy and intestinal metaplasia, dysplasia, and finally cancer (see below) (10). In addition, the intestinal type seems to be more common in men and diagnosed at later ages (11, 12). The observed decline in gastric cancer globally seems to be associated to a reduction in the incidence of the intestinal type, while there is an increase of the diffuse-type gastric cancer (13, 14).

2. Risk Factors: *Helicobacter pylori* Is Fundamental for Gastric Cancer Development

Infection with *Helicobacter pylori* (*H. pylori*) is considered essential for the development of gastric cancer, such that *H. pylori* has been classified as a type I carcinogen by the International Agency for

Research in Cancer (IARC) (15). It is estimated that nearly half of the world's population is infected with this bacterium; however, most people are asymptomatic, and approximately 1–3% develop cancer (16–18). This infection induces an inflammatory response that increases the infiltration of lymphocytes, macrophages, and plasma cells into the gastric mucosa. Neutrophils can also be found when acute inflammation is present. When the inflammatory response is not accompanied by loss of gastric glands (atrophy), it is referred to as non-atrophic gastritis (NAG), according to the updated Sydney classification (19). NAG lesions are associated with the development of duodenal ulcer, especially if it is localized to the gastric antrum (20). A small percentage of patients with NAG progress to multifocal atrophic gastritis (MAG). MAG is characterized by the loss of gastric glands and the appearance of fibrotic tissue (21). This disease can later progress to MAG with intestinal metaplasia (MAG-IM), in which cells of the gastric epithelium are replaced by intestinal absorptive and goblet cells (for a graphical view of the lesions, please see refs. (21, 22)). MAG-IM is considered to be a true preneoplastic lesion leading to the development of dysplasia, with abnormal nuclear morphology and abnormal tissue architecture. It is estimated that up to 85% of patients with dysplasia and a high degree of atypical features progress to invasive carcinomas (23). Even though some of these lesions may regress to the previous, less malignant states, the rate of progression is higher than the rate of regression (24).

It is widely accepted that gastric cancer is the result of the above-described cascade of histological events leading from normal epithelia to cancer. However, the molecular and cellular events controlling the transition from one step to the next are not yet fully understood. Inflammation is a common finding in cancer (25). The inflammatory process is mediated by pro- and anti-inflammatory cytokines, the levels of which are controlled, among other things, by changes in the primary sequence of the DNA sequence. Several single nucleotide polymorphisms (SNPs) in genes encoding cytokines involved in the inflammatory process have been associated with risk of gastric cancer among several populations (26–29). Our work with premalignant inflammatory stages in African-American and Caucasian individuals from the southern region of the United States has suggested that many of these SNPs associations observed in gastric cancer are also present in the premalignant stages and that there is a significant difference in the frequency of these SNPs between the two ethnic groups (22, 30). These findings are important because it would help to identify people at increased risk of developing cancer at an earlier stage, allowing for better intervention strategies and remediation of the possible mucosal damage already inflicted by the inflammatory reaction.

3. Biology of *H. pylori* Infection

H. pylori is a gram-negative bacterium that infects humans early in life (31). Infection occurs at earlier ages in developing countries than in more advanced areas (31, 32) and is related to socioeconomic status (33, 34). Upon infection, *H. pylori* gains access to the mucosa overlying the gastric epithelia, delivering several pathogenic factors. Vacuolating cytotoxin (VacA) can be secreted as a soluble protein (35) but can also be found attached to the membrane of the bacteria (36). VacA is responsible for the formation of large intracellular vacuoles in mammalian cells (37) and for opening channels on the membrane of the gastric epithelial cells (38), allowing molecules like urea to enter the gastric lumen (39). Once in the gastric lumen, the urea is broken down into ammonia and carbon dioxide by the *H. pylori* urease, a metalloenzyme that uses nickel as a cofactor (40). The importance of *H. pylori* urease is evidenced by the fact that *urease* (−) *H. pylori* strains are unable to colonize the stomachs of several animal models (41, 42). In addition, *H. pylori* urease accounts for up to 10% of the total protein produced by the bacteria (43). The ammonia generated by the breakdown of urea can, by itself, neutralize the gastric acid (44), thus helping the bacteria survive and causing damage to the gastric epithelia (45).

The cytotoxin-associated antigen (CagA) is injected into the membranes of the gastric cells by a type IV secretion system (46, 47). Once inserted into the host's cell membrane, CagA is activated by phosphorylation at the carboxy-terminal end of the protein by c-Src/Lyn kinases (48). This phosphorylation occurs at the tyrosine residues of the EPIYA motifs (protein domains formed by glutamic acid, proline, isoleucine, tyrosine, and alanine residues) (48, 49). Phosphorylation-activated CagA recruits the cytoplasmic SRC homology 2 domain-containing tyrosine phosphatase (SHP-2 tyrosine phosphatase) to the membrane and deregulates the phosphatase domain (49). Tyrosine phosphorylation of the CagA protein and its subsequent binding to the SHP-2 phosphatase are essential for the induction of the cellular changes associated with CagA since *H. pylori* harboring *cagA* genes without the EPIYA motifs are able to translocate the protein into the cell membranes, but once there, it is not phosphorylated nor able to induce any cellular changes (48, 49). Activated and SHP-2 associated CagA triggers a cascade of phosphorylation events (50) that lead to changes in the cell shape (46, 48). Interestingly, the promoter activity of the *H. pylori cagA* gene was found to be increased in the presence of NaCl in a dose-dependent manner (48, 51). Furthermore, the levels of the CagA protein were higher in *H. pylori* grown in higher salt concentrations and resulted in increased interaction with gastric epithelial cells and increased phenotypic changes associated with CagA (51, 52). CagA is also responsible for the induction of inflammatory responses, including interleukin (IL) 8 released by gastric epithelia, which serves as a chemotactic factor for inflammatory cells (53–56). Once recruited to the gastric mucosa, the inflammatory cells mount a response essentially mediated by lymphocyte-derived cytokines which, if not controlled, can promote tissue damage.

Another important factor produced by *H. pylori* is the arginase enzyme which is encoded by the *rocF* gene (57–59). This enzyme is found in many other organisms (60) and is involved in the generation of urea and ornithine, the latter being the primary source for the production of polyamines (61). In Leishmania, the generation of polyamines is essential for the survival of the parasite, such that arginase gene knockout parasites are unable to survive in culture media unless supplemented with polyamines (62). In *H. pylori*, the enzyme seems to be critical for survival of the *H. pylori* in acidic environments, but the lack of the gene does not affect colonization of mouse stomach (57). Mendz and Hazell (63) have shown that *H. pylori* lacks some of the enzymes required for the synthesis of L-arginine (L-Arg) and depends on L-Arg generated by the host. We and others have shown that *H. pylori* arginase can inhibit functions of both macrophages and T cells, making the bacterium able to control both acquired and innate immune responses to the infection (64, 65).

4. Immune Dysfunction Caused by *H. pylori* Products in T Cells

H. pylori antigens, including urease and *H. pylori* DNA, can impair T-cell function (66, 67). It has been shown that lysates of *H. pylori* reduce the proliferation of both peripheral blood lymphocytes (PBL) and Jurkat cells (68). This effect is not limited to T cells but also includes human monocytic cell lines and even human gastric cell lines (67, 69). Several studies have been designed to identify the factors involved in the modulation of the immune response to *H. pylori*. VacA and CagA antigens have been associated with virulence in *H. pylori* and are believed to be the mediators of T-cell dysfunction. Paziak-Domanska et al. (70) have shown that crude extracts of CagA+VacA– *H. pylori* G27 leads to downregulation of PHA-induced proliferation of T cells. This effect was not observed when crude extracts of the isogenic CagA–VacA+ was used. On the other hand, *H. pylori* CagA and VacA are responsible for the downregulation of the proliferation of gastric cell lines (71, 72), an effect not mediated by apoptosis (73). Interestingly, the dysfunction of T cells observed in *H. pylori* infection is also seen in gastric cancer (74, 75).

We have shown that *H. pylori* arginase contributes to the depletion of L-Arg in culture media, leading to the downregulation of the CD3ξ molecule, essential for activation of T cells (64). Some studies have shown that in gastric cancer there is a reduced expression of CD3ξ in T cells in local lymph nodes (76). Whether this happens in response to the infection with *H. pylori*, or if the virulence of the bacteria is differentially associated with this event, is still to be determined.

5. Cytokine Production in Response to *H. pylori* Infection

It has been shown that mice deficient in B and T cells ($RAG\text{-}1^{-/-}$), or mice deficient in T cells alone ($TCR\beta\delta^{-/-}$), do not develop gastritis when infected with *Helicobacter felis* (77). This supports the idea that the immune response is essential for the development of gastritis after infection with *Helicobacter*. In addition, interferon response factor element 1-deficient mice ($IRF\text{-}1^{-/-}$), which do not produce IFNγ, also fail to develop gastritis after infection with *H. pylori*. Mohammadi et al. (78) and Nedrud et al. (79) clearly demonstrated that C57Bl/6 mice infected with *H. felis* develop aggressive gastritis due to a strong Th1 response. In contrast, Balb/c mice that have a preferential Th2 response developed a protective immune response. Therefore, the type of cytokine response is closely associated with the pathological outcome of the infection.

In humans, most reports agree that a Th1 response is elicited both *in vitro* and *in vivo* after *H. pylori* exposure, while a Th2 response is absent or negligible. Increased levels of IFNγ in the mucosa of patients infected with *H. pylori* were observed both in situ and after purifying the epithelia-infiltrating lymphocytes. No production of IL4 or IL5 could be detected (80, 81). Cytokines like IL8 and IL6 have also been reported to be increased; however, the increase of IL8 appears to be independent of the presence of *H. pylori* and may be more of a response to the inflammatory process initiated by the infection (82). In contrast, increased expression of IL6 within the gastric mucosa is largely associated with the presence of the bacteria, such that its levels significantly decrease after clearance of the infection (82).

6. *H. pylori* Infection, Arginine, Arginase, and Immunity

In humans, the metabolism of the amino acid L-Arg has been associated with regulation of the immune responses (83). In patients with trauma, liver transplantation, and some tumors, an increase production of arginase I has been linked to significantly decreased responses of T cells (84, 85). The lack of L-Arg induces a low expression of CD3ζ, which has been associated with reduction in T-cell proliferation and decreased production of cytokines (85–87). However, it is possible to suggest that in addition to the CD3ζ molecule, other mechanisms might be important in the induction of this altered state of the T lymphocytes. Recent data has shown that one of the mechanisms associated with L-Arg reduction includes an increased expression of the cationic amino acid transporter (CAT-2B) in murine myeloid-derived suppressor cells (MDSC, characterized as macrophages in mice), which increase the uptaking of L-Arg by CAT-2B (86). This mechanism is not present in human MDSC, which are characterized as polymorphonuclear neutrophils (PMN). In contrast, human MDSC release arginase I into the microenvironment, where it depletes L-Arg and induces T-cell dysfunction by impairing all the described functions of T cells (88, 89). Interestingly, the same phenomenon has been described in the placenta of pregnant women, suggesting some role of L-Arg metabolism in the tolerance of the fetus (90).

The enzyme arginase (EC 3.5.3.1) is one of the enzymes involved in the metabolism of L-Arg, producing L-ornithine and urea, the first needed for the synthesis of polyamines required for cell proliferation (91, 92). Additionally, nitric oxide synthase (EC 1.14.13.39) metabolizes L-Arg into citrulline and nitric oxide, an innate mechanism involved in cytotoxic cellular responses mediated by macrophages (93, 94).

L-Arg metabolism by arginase is emerging as an important regulator of T-cell responses in human diseases, including infectious diseases and cancer (95–101). Our work with *H. pylori* has shown that the presence of an arginase enzyme, previously characterized in the bacteria (102), is responsible for reducing the expression of the CD3ξ molecule in Jurkat T cells and primary T lymphocytes cultured in the presence of *H. pylori* (64). In addition, *H. pylori* arginase plays an important role in reducing the levels of nitric oxide production by macrophages, an event that may be associated to increased survival of the bacteria (65). On the other hand, *H. pylori* infection also induces the expression of macrophage arginase II, which reduces intracellular availability of arginine with subsequent reduction of nitric oxide responses (103, 104). In fact, the critical role of arginase II in *H. pylori* infection has been shown in arginase knockout mice ($arg2^{-/-}$) (105). This study suggested that arginase II affects the degree of cellular immunity against *H. pylori*, by reducing the levels of Th1/Th17 cytokines, including IFNγ, IL17a, and IL12p40 (105). The latter has been shown also in macrophages in the intestinal muscularis (jejunum and ileum) of mice infected with *Helicobacter hepaticus* (106). Even though these macrophages did not show any signs of infection by the *Helicobacter*, those obtained from infected mice had significantly reduced induction of inflammatory cytokines than those obtained from uninfected, after being stimulated *in vitro* with LPS and IFNγ (106). These results indicate that even if the *Helicobacter* never encounters cells of the immune system, soluble factors released by the bacteria, or by the inflamed gastric epithelia, may influence the immune response associated with gastric damage. The possibility about *H. pylori* being able to invade the gastric mucosa and interact directly with cells of the immune system is still controversial, but there are some research showing actual *in vivo* phagocytosis of *H. pylori* at the gastric level (107–109). This controversy is far from being solved, but some *in vitro* assays suggest that, even if ingested, *H. pylori* is able to delay the intracellular killing, at least by macrophages (110–113). If this is a phenomenon that actually happens *in vivo*, it may lead to intracellular *H. pylori* replication, as shown *in vitro* (114), and explain the persistence of the infection, which in turns may lead to antibiotic resistance, selecting more aggressive strains able to induce stronger inflammatory responses associated to mucosal damage.

7. Single Nucleotide Polymorphisms and the Regulation of Cytokine Genes

Under normal circumstances, modulation of the immune response is achieved at several levels, including gene expression. SNPs are, in general, biallelic variations of one nucleotide occurring throughout the genome. SNPs can cause alteration of the primary structure of a protein. If, on the other hand, the allelic variation does not involve changes in the amino acid sequence, it is referred to as synonymous or conservative. SNPs in noncoding regions may be involved in splicing or in the formation of transcription factor-binding regions. Several SNPs in cytokine genes have been associated with the regulation of cytokine levels. For example, one haplotype on the *IL10* gene (*IL10−1082A/IL10−819T/IL10−592A*) has been associated with reduced levels of IL10 production (115). On the other hand, *IL1B−511T/T* and the presence of allele 2 of the IL1 receptor antagonist gene (*IL1RN*2*) is associated with increased levels of IL1β production in the mucosa (116). This has been associated with gastric inflammation and intestinal metaplasia (116, 117). Pociot et al. (118) have also shown that a C to T change at *IL1B+3954* position is associated with increased secretion of IL1β from monocytes after stimulation with LPS. Other studies (119, 120) using transiently transfected cells have shown that allele A at position −308 of the *TNFA* gene (*TNF*2*) is associated with increased levels of TNF-α, suggesting a role for this SNP in inflammatory and infectious processes. The proinflammatory IL6 is responsible for inducing fever after injection of IL1 in animals (121). The levels of IL6 are also controlled by genetic mechanisms. An SNP at position −174 (G>C change) has been associated with differential production of IL6 with increased activity of promoters containing G (121). After stimulation with LPS, PBMCs obtained from healthy individuals with *IL6-174GG* or *IL1-174GC* genotypes produced significantly higher amounts of IL6 in response to LPS than individuals with the *IL6-174CC* (121). Furthermore, haplotype analysis of the *IL6* promoter has suggested that the IL6 expression is controlled by the interaction of at least four polymorphisms in the *IL6* promoter (122). The clinical importance of genetically controlled levels of cytokines has been demonstrated in transplantation (123, 124), autoimmune diseases (125), and infectious diseases (126, 127).

8. Cancer Health Disparities, Ethnicity, and SNPs

The incidence of most cancers is higher in African-Americans than in Caucasians (128). Many factors may be playing a significant role in these disparities. According to the National Institutes of Health, cancer health disparities are defined as "all adverse differences in cancer incidence, cancer prevalence, cancer death, cancer survivorship, and burden of cancer or related health conditions that exist among specific population groups in the United States" (129). Even though the socioeconomic status is highlighted as one of the major factors leading to lack of appropriate health care, it is possible to suggest that ethnic differences are also playing some role in defining such disparities. Recent reports have shown that the composition of genetic blocks between African-Americans and Caucasians is different, with more heterogeneity observed in the African-American group (130, 131). This could be associated to a differential genetic background that makes one individual more susceptible to suffer specific diseases, including cancer (132). These differences may include differential transcription of regulatory genes, increased transcription of genes that promote inflammation and reduced transcription of those that are anti-inflamatory. Because gene transcription may be affected by the presence of SNPs at the promoter level, these may potentially be used as determinants of risk of disease in specific ethnic groups. An example of differential SNPs distribution between ethnic groups and its possible association with disease is given by the gene of the multidrug transporter (*MDR1*), which mediates the transport of many types of drugs including anticancer drugs (133, 134). The frequency of one SNP in exon 26 of the *MDR1* gene (a C>T change at position 3435) has been found to be differentially associated with African-Americans, Caucasians, and Asian populations (135), as well as with differential expression of the MDR1 protein and with plasma levels of several drugs (136–142). Additional work has shown that such SNP is in linkage disequilibrium with two other nearby SNPs forming haplotype blocks differentially associated with three ethnic groups in Asia (143). Regarding to inflammatory mediators, several cytokine SNPs have been associated with the development of gastric cancer. A seminal work by El-Omar et al. (26) associated a transition from C to T at position −511 of the *IL1B* gene (*ILB−511C>T*) with gastric cancer in European populations. This finding has been later confirmed by other groups (28, 29, 144, 145), even though racial and ethnicity factors have been associated with differential gastric cancer risk in various populations worldwide. However, most studies agree that the presence of allele *IL1B−511T* increases the risk of intestinal-type and noncardia gastric cancer in Caucasian but not in Asian populations, a fact that has been validated by several meta-analyses (146–149). Interestingly, this SNP has also been linked to increased secretion of IL1β (116, 117); this, in turn, is associated with reduction of gastric acid secretion (150), promoting the colonization by *H. pylori*. *IL1B−511* is in near complete linkage disequilibrium with another SNP at position −31 (*IL1B−31*) (26), and its capacity to modulate *IL1B* gene transcription is modified depending on the presence of other nearby SNPs (151). This strongly suggests that SNP's association with disease needs to be studied not only individually but also as haplotypes.

The biological activity of the IL1β is regulated by the presence of a natural antagonist, the interleukin 1 receptor antagonist (IL1ra), which is encoded by the *IL1RN* gene (152). Allele 2 of a variable number of tandem repeats (VNTR) on intron 2 of the *IL1RN* gene (*IL2RN*2*) has been associated with reduced levels of IL1ra (153, 154) and with the increased risk of several types of cancer, including gastric cancer (26–28).

Another cytokine important in the initiation and maintenance of immune responses is tumor necrosis factor alpha (TNF-α), in which SNPs have been associated with gastric cancer as well as other types of cancer. The presence of allele A at position −308 of the *TNFA* gene (*TNF−308A*) has been associated with an increased risk of gastric cancer and non-small cell lung carcinoma (28, 29, 155). In addition to the effect of the *TNF−308* SNP, *TNF−857T* has been linked to the development of gastric intestinal metaplasia (156) and gastric B-cell lymphoma (157).

Interleukin 8 (IL8) is a member of the CXC chemokine family and functions as a chemoattractant for neutrophils (53–56). Its role in gastric cancer is suggested by the high levels of mRNA and IL8 protein in gastric cancer cell lines (82, 158, 159). Gastric cancer patients carrying the *IL8−251A* allele or the haplotype of *IL8 AGT/AGC* (*−251/+396/+781*) had a two- and fourfold increased risk of developing adenocarcinoma of gastric cardia, respectively (160). Interestingly, the *IL8−251AA* genotype increases the risk of gastric cancer only in individuals infected with *H. pylori* CagA+ strains (161).

IL10 is an anti-inflammatory cytokine (162). The level of IL10, as mentioned before, is associated with the presence of specific SNPs and haplotypes in its promoter region, and these, in turn, have been associated with differential risk of gastric cancer and other malignancies (29, 115, 163–165).

Recent genome-wide association studies (GWAS) using Japanese and Korean populations found that two SNPs in the prostate stem cell antigen gene (*PSCA*) were significantly associated with diffuse-type gastric cancer (166). A later study showed that one of those SNPs, rs2976392, is associated with a significant increase risk of both gastric cancer types, intestinal and diffuse, in a Chinese population (167). These results were further confirmed by a more recent GWAS in a Chinese population, which, in addition to finding that the same two SNPs in the *PSCA* gene were associated with noncardia gastric cancer, also found that risk of gastric cardia cancer was associated with two SNPs, rs22742223 and rs3765524, that create missense mutations in the region 10q23 encoding the phospholipase Cε1 (*PLCE1*) (168).

Our work with African-American and Caucasian individuals from Louisiana has identified SNPs, alone or arranged in haplotypes, in several cytokine genes differentially associated with more severe forms of gastritis (22, 30). Interestingly, African-Americans have higher frequency of proinflammatory SNPs and haplotypes in both *IL1B* and *IL10* genes (22, 30), present higher incidence of more aggressive forms of the disease (22, 30), and are infected more frequently with aggressive *H. pylori* strains (30). Taken together, and considering that these inflammatory stages may lead to gastric malignancy, our results may help explain in part why African-Americans have increased risk of developing gastric cancer than Caucasian individuals.

In summary, the balance of the pro- and anti-inflammatory responses to an offending agent (*H. pylori*) appears to play a central role in gastric mucosal damage and repair. Defects on the type of the response elicited, or in their balance, result in an abnormal environment that can be detrimental for the host and favor the development of malignancy. However, the interplay between the virulence of the bacteria and the genetic background of the host is crucial in determining the fate of the inflammation initiated by the *H. pylori* infection.

9. DNA Methylation, *H. pylori* Infection, and Gastric Cancer

DNA methylation has been described as one important way of gene regulation that occurs normally in imprinted genes, X-chromosome inactivation, and silencing of tumor suppressor genes, among other situations (169). Most DNA methylation events occur in CpG dinucleotides and very especially in those located in gene promoters (170). Even though the mechanisms of this regulation are no totally understood, many clues point to either a direct interference (by the methyl groups) of the binding of transcription factors or by the formation of protein complexes by the recruitment of methyl-binding proteins, which ultimately inhibit transcription (171–176).

DNA methylation is carried out by several DNA methyltransferase (DNMT) enzymes, DNMT1, DNMT22, and DNMT3 (comprising 3A, 3B and 3L) involved in *de novo* and maintenance methylation of hemi- and unmethylated DNA sequences (177, 178). Interestingly, there is an increased expression of DNMT proteins in gastric cancer tissues, as compared to tissues with normal histology. A recent study has found an SNP at position −448 of the *DNMT3A* gene (*DNMT3A*−*448A*) highly associated with risk of gastric cancer in a Chinese population (179). The presence of *DNMT3A*−*448A* increases more than twofold the activity of the promoter, and homozygous carriers of this SNP (*DNMT3A*−*448AA*) have more than sixfold increased risk of gastric cancer when compared with *GG* carriers (179).

Hypermethylation of gene promoters has been described in gastric tissues, and this process seems to be directly associated with the inactivation of specific genes in gastric cancer samples (180, 181). However, as different population may have differences in their genetic contents, differences in the methylation patterns may also vary. In a sample from Colombia, South America, when comparing two populations with different risks of gastric cancer, hypermethylation of the *RPRM* gene was associated with the disease and with infection with virulent *H. pylori* strains (*cagA+/vacA s1m1+*) in the high-risk population (182), as compared with an area of low risk for gastric cancer. *H. pylori* virulence seem to be also associated with differential methylation on enzymes involved in the pathway that generates *S*-adenosylmethionine, the universal donor of methyl groups in humans (183). In a study from Brazil, it was found that infection with virulent strains of *H. pylori* is associated with a polymorphism in the methylenetetrahydrofolate reductase gene (*MTHFR*) enzyme (*MTHFR C677T*) in patients 60 years old or older (184). In addition, hypermethylation of cell cycle controlling genes (E-cadherin and *CDKN2A*) have been reported in patients infected with *H. pylori* (184–188). Regarding to E-cadherin (encoded by the gene *CDH1*), the hypermethylation of this gene seems to be directly related to the infection with *H. pylori* since its eradication by antibiotic treatment lead to a significant reduction of the methylation level (188). This type of inactivation of this gene adds to the importance of CDH1 in the process of the progression of malignancy associated with gastric cancer. One study using New Zealand families have found that a G to T mutation in the sequence of exon 7 leads to an aberrant product and is associated with familial gastric cancer (189).

Many factors may influence the degree of methylation on one specific genomic region. One of those factors is the presence of SNPs that either create CpG sites at the promoter levels, maybe modifying the binding of proteins involved in the transcription machinery, or increase the binding of transcription factor that promotes the increased transcription of the gene. One example of the latter is the effect that C to T change at position −511 in the *IL1B* gene (*IL1B−511T*) has on the methylation of CpG islands of several genes, including *TWIST1* and *CYPB1* (190). It was noted that gastric cancer patients with the allele *IL1B−511T* had significantly increased methylation on genes like *TWIST1*, *CAGNA1G*, *GRIN2B*, *CYPB1*, and *CRABP1*, when compared to individuals with the allele *IL1B−511C* (190). One possible explanation of these results may be the association between the levels of IL1β at the gastric mucosa and the *IL1B* gene polymorphisms. It has been shown that individuals with the *IL1BTT* genotype have significantly higher IL1β at the gastric level than those with the genotype *IL1BCC* genotype (117). This cytokine has a plethora of effects, and among them are both the increased expression of *DNMT1* and the increased activity of the enzyme, which, as discussed before, is involved in the transfer of *S*-adenosylmethionine to cytosine residues in CpG sites (183).

10. Other Risk Factors Associated with Gastric Cancer

It is very clear that environmental factors are involved in the development of gastric cancer. Studies have shown that the risk of gastric cancer changes if people move to geographical areas with different gastric cancer risk, either increasing or decreasing, according to the risk of the new area of settlement (191, 192). Several factors have been associated with the development of gastric cancer, including environmental, microbial, and genetic factors (33, 193). It has been shown that fruits and vegetables reduce the risk of gastric cancer, without regard to the anatomical position or histological type of cancer (194). A large study involving more than 10,000 individuals reported that those with the very low to none intake of fruits and vegetables had a relative risk (RR) of developing gastric cancer of 5.5 (95% CI 1.7–18.3), compared to those with a high intake of these foods (195). In addition, a study with more than 12,000 individuals from seven countries reported a reduced risk for gastric cancer in individuals with high consumption of fruits, even though no effect was associated with vegetable consumption (196). Such studies have helped identify the specific micronutrients that are involved in preventing this malignancy. Despite conflicting results (197–199), it is commonly found that beta-carotene intake is inversely associated with the risk of gastric cancer (200–203), while the consumption of salted meats seem to increase the risk of the disease (204, 205).

11. Models of *H. pylori*-Induced Gastric Inflammation

The role of the immune system in response to infection with *Helicobacter* strains has been extensively studied using animal models. These models have helped to clarify the process of the infection, the preneoplastic steps, and the severity and different outcomes of the neoplasia. Mongolian gerbils have been used as *H. pylori* infection models because they develop a disease very similar to human gastritis (206). However, phenotypic studies in gerbils are limited because of the lack of many gerbil cell-specific reagents. Mice infected with *H. felis* have also been used to study the human gastritis. Furthermore, *H. pylori* strains have been adapted to infect mice and are preferred because the *Helicobacter* infection seems to be highly host specific (77, 207, 208).

In humans, it has been shown that T cells isolated from the antral mucosa of patients with active gastritis or duodenal ulcer disease, associated with *H. pylori* infection, are preferentially producing Th1 cytokine (77, 80, 209–211). Other studies have shown that $CD4^+$ T-cell clones isolated from the gastric mucosa of these patients proliferate in response to specific *H. pylori* antigens, including CagA, VacA, and urease, thus showing antigen specificity (209, 210). This enhanced proliferation is related to the cytokine response which appears to be associated with the presence of CagA and VacA (73). Patients infected with *H. pylori* strains expressing these two proteins show an activation of nuclear transcription factors AP-1 and NFkB and several tyrosine kinases including MAP kinases. All of these factors participate in the transactivation of proinflammatory cytokine genes (212–214).

Even though most of the research on *H. pylori*-induced gastritis has focused on T cells, other cells involved in the inflammatory reaction including the gastric epithelium, polymorphonuclear cells, and macrophage/dendritic cells play an important role in the response to *H. pylori* infection. Gastric epithelial cells can produce IL6 and IL10 upon contact with *H. pylori* (215). Furthermore, they express B7.1 and B7.2 costimulatory molecules, suggesting they could play an important role as antigen-presenting cells (216). Initial reports about the role of macrophage/dendritic cells suggested that *H. pylori* severely impairs phagocytosis and antigen processing in these cells, a mechanism that may be dependent on the presence of the CagA protein (217). Furthermore, urease from *H. pylori* can degrade urea which is needed to produce CO_2 and NH_3, effectively blocking the bactericidal function of peroxynitrite, a metabolite derived from nitric oxide (218). Thus, it is possible that the detrimental effects of *H. pylori* on macrophages could lead to the T-cell dysfunction observed in chronic infections.

12. Concluding Remarks

Even though many advances in the understanding of gastric cancer have been made, the disease is still one of the malignancies with the highest incidence and mortality rates worldwide. The identification of *H. pylori* as a crucial player in the pathology of gastric cancer was a pivotal step in the understanding and control of the disease. However, it is important to fully understand the inflammatory response initiated by the infection in order to fully block the cascade of events that lead to gastric cancer. This pathogen–host interaction is one of the highest hierarchies since *H. pylori* has evolved mechanisms to hijack the immune responses of the host and make its survival easier. Even though the environment, the host's genetic background, diet, and gender, among other factors, add to the *H. pylori*-associated risk of gastric cancer, making the disease very complex and difficult to understand and devise strategies to prevent, cure, and/or better treat patients diagnose with the disease, our efforts should converge in finding the commonalities of the disease: what is common among individuals who become infected with *H. pylori* and also among the different strains of the bacteria able to colonize and induce inflammation in humans. Genetic and epigenetic markers of the infection and of the damage induced by it are necessary tools to devise strategies aiming at limiting the degree of inflammation and to restore the homeostasis of the gastric environment. These markers will probably show differences among populations and related to *H. pylori* virulence, but our actual capacity to fully sequence the human genome will, for sure, identify those common DNA sequences and transcripts able to modify the risk not only of being infected with the bacteria but also of developing gastric cancer.

Acknowledgment

This work was supported by a NCRR-NIH grant number 149740220B to J. Zabaleta

References

1. GLOBOCAN. Stomach Cancer Incidence and Mortality Worldwide in 2008. http://globocan.iarc.fr/. 2008.
2. Parkin, D.M., Bray, F., Ferlay, J., and Pisani, P. (2005) Global cancer statistics, 2002. *CA Cancer J. Clin.*, 55, 74–108.
3. Parkin, D.M. (2004) International variation. *Oncogene*, 23, 6329–6340.
4. Jemal, A., Siegel, R., Xu, J., and Ward, E. (2010) Cancer statistics, 2010. *CA Cancer J Clin.*, 60, 277–300.
5. Jass, J.R., Sobin, L.H., and Watanabe, H. (1990) The World Health Organization's histologic classification of gastrointestinal tumors. A commentary on the second edition. *Cancer*, 66, 2162–2167.

6. Mulligan, R.M. (1972) Histogenesis and biologic behavior of gastric carcinoma. *Pathol. Annu.*, 7, 349–415.
7. Ming, S.C. (1977) Gastric carcinoma. A pathobiological classification. *Cancer*, 39, 2475–2485.
8. LAURÉN, P. (1965) The two histological main types of gastric carcinoma: diffuse and so-called intestinal-type carcinoma. An attempt at histo-clinical classification. *Acta Pathol. Microbiol. Scand.*, 64, 31–49.
9. Goseki, N., Takizawa, T., and Koike, M. (1992) Differences in the mode of the extension of gastric cancer classified by histological type: new histological classification of gastric carcinoma. *Gut*, 33, 606–612.
10. Crew, K.D. and Neugut, A.I. (2006) Epidemiology of gastric cancer. *World J Gastroenterol.*, 12, 354–362.
11. Correa, P., Sasano, N., Stemmermann, G.N., and Haenszel, W. (1973) Pathology of gastric carcinoma in Japanese populations: comparisons between Miyagi prefecture, Japan, and Hawaii. *J Natl. Cancer Inst.*, 51, 1449–1459.
12. Mohar, A., Suchil-Bernal, L., Hernandez-Guerrero, A., Podolsky-Rapoport, I., Herrera-Goepfert, R., Mora-Tiscareno, A. et al. (1997) Intestinal type: diffuse type ratio of gastric carcinoma in a Mexican population. *J Exp. Clin. Cancer Res.*, 16, 189–194.
13. Kaneko, S. and Yoshimura, T. (2001) Time trend analysis of gastric cancer incidence in Japan by histological types, 1975-1989. *Br. J Cancer*, 84, 400–405.
14. Henson, D.E., Dittus, C., Younes, M., Nguyen, H., and Bores-Saavedra, J. (2004) Differential trends in the intestinal and diffuse types of gastric carcinoma in the United States, 1973-2000: increase in the signet ring cell type. *Arch. Pathol. Lab Med.*, 128, 765–770.
15. IARC. IARC monograph on the evaluation of carcinogenic risks to humans:Schistosomes, liver flukes and *Helicobacter pylori*. IARC 61, 177–240. 1994.
16. Suerbaum, S. and Michetti, P. (2002) Helicobacter pylori infection. *N. Engl. J Med.*, 347, 1175–1186.
17. Uemura, N., Okamoto, S., Yamamoto, S., Matsumura, N., Yamaguchi, S., Yamakido, M. et al. (2001) Helicobacter pylori infection and the development of gastric cancer. *N. Engl. J Med.*, 345, 784–789.
18. Wroblewski, L.E., Peek, R.M., Jr., and Wilson, K.T. (2010) Helicobacter pylori and gastric cancer: factors that modulate disease risk. *Clin. Microbiol. Rev.*, 23, 713–739.
19. Dixon, M.F., Genta, R.M., Yardley, J.H., and Correa, P. (1996) Classification and grading of gastritis. The updated Sydney System. International Workshop on the Histopathology of Gastritis, Houston 1994. *Am. J. Surg. Pathol.*, 20, 1161–1181.
20. Hansson, L.E., Nyren, O., Hsing, A.W., Bergstrom, R., Josefsson, S., Chow, W.H. et al. (1996) The risk of stomach cancer in patients with gastric or duodenal ulcer disease. *N. Engl. J Med.*, 335, 242–249.
21. Correa, P. and Houghton, J. (2007) Carcinogenesis of Helicobacter pylori. *Gastroenterology*, 133, 659–672.
22. Zabaleta, J., Camargo, M.C., Piazuelo, M.B., Fontham, E., Schneider, B.G., Sicinschi, L.A. et al. (2006) Association of interleukin-1beta gene polymorphisms with precancerous gastric lesions in African Americans and Caucasians. *Am. J. Gastroenterol.*, 101, 163–171.
23. Rugge, M., Correa, P., Dixon, M.F., Hattori, T., Leandro, G., Lewin, K. et al. (2000) Gastric dysplasia: the Padova international classification. *Am. J Surg. Pathol.*, 24, 167–176.
24. Correa, P., Haenszel, W., Cuello, C., Zavala, D., Fontham, E., Zarama, G. et al. (1990) Gastric precancerous process in a high risk population: cohort follow-up. *Cancer Res.*, 50, 4737–4740.
25. Coussens, L.M. and Werb, Z. (2002) Inflammation and cancer. *Nature*, 420, 860–867.
26. El-Omar, E.M., Carrington, M., Chow, W.H., McColl, K.E., Bream, J.H., Young, H.A. et al. (2000) Interleukin-1 polymorphisms associated with increased risk of gastric cancer. *Nature*, 404, 398–402.
27. Alpizar-Alpizar,W., Perez-Perez, G.I., Une, C., Cuenca, P., and Sierra, R. (2005) Association of interleukin-1B and interleukin-1RN polymorphisms with gastric cancer in a high-risk population of Costa Rica. *Clin. Exp. Med.*, 5, 169–176.
28. Machado, J.C., Figueiredo, C., Canedo, P., Pharoah, P., Carvalho, R., Nabais, S. et al. (2003) A proinflammatory genetic profile increases the risk for chronic atrophic gastritis and gastric carcinoma. *Gastroenterology*, 125, 364–371.
29. El-Omar, E.M., Rabkin, C.S., Gammon, M.D., Vaughan, T.L., Risch, H.A., Schoenberg, J.B. et al. (2003) Increased risk of noncardia gastric cancer associated with proinflammatory cytokine gene polymorphisms. *Gastroenterology*, 124, 1193–1201.
30. Zabaleta, J., Camargo, M.C., Ritchie, M.D., Piazuelo, M.B., Sierra, R.A., Turner, S.D.

et al. (2011) Association of haplotypes of inflammation-related genes with gastric pre-neoplastic lesions in African Americans and Caucasians. *Int. J Cancer*, 128, 668–675.

31. Banatvala, N., Mayo, K., Megraud, F., Jennings, R., Deeks, J.J., and Feldman, R.A. (1993) The cohort effect and Helicobacter pylori. *J Infect. Dis.*, 168, 219–221.
32. Lindkvist, P., Asrat, D., Nilsson, I., Tsega, E., Olsson, G.L., Wretlind, B. et al. (1996) Age at acquisition of Helicobacter pylori infection: comparison of a high and a low prevalence country. *Scand. J Infect. Dis.*, 28, 181–184.
33. Fiedorek, S.C., Malaty, H.M., Evans, D.L., Pumphrey, C.L., Casteel, H.B., Evans, D.J., Jr. et al. (1991) Factors influencing the epidemiology of Helicobacter pylori infection in children. *Pediatrics*, 88, 578–582.
34. Sitas, F., Yarnell, J., and Forman, D. (1992) Helicobacter pylori infection rates in relation to age and social class in a population of Welsh men. *Gut*, 33, 1582.
35. Cover, T.L. and Blaser, M.J. (1992) Purification and characterization of the vacuolating toxin from Helicobacter pylori. *J Biol. Chem.*, 267, 10570–10575.
36. Ilver, D., Barone, S., Mercati, D., Lupetti, P., and Telford, J.L. (2004) Helicobacter pylori toxin VacA is transferred to host cells via a novel contact-dependent mechanism. *Cell Microbiol.*, 6, 167–174.
37. Leunk, R.D., Johnson, P.T., David, B.C., Kraft, W.G., and Morgan, D.R. (1988) Cytotoxic activity in broth-culture filtrates of Campylobacter pylori. *J Med. Microbiol.*, 26, 93–99.
38. Szabo, I., Brutsche, S., Tombola, F., Moschioni, M., Satin, B., Telford, J.L. et al. (1999) Formation of anion-selective channels in the cell plasma membrane by the toxin VacA of Helicobacter pylori is required for its biological activity. *EMBO J*, 18, 5517–5527.
39. Tombola, F., Morbiato, L., Del, G.G., Rappuoli, R., Zoratti, M., and Papini, E. (2001) The Helicobacter pylori VacA toxin is a urea permease that promotes urea diffusion across epithelia. *J Clin. Invest*, 108, 929–937.
40. Mobley, H.L., Island, M.D., and Hausinger, R.P. (1995) Molecular biology of microbial ureases. *Microbiol. Rev.*, 59, 451–480.
41. Eaton, K.A., Brooks, C.L., Morgan, D.R., and Krakowka, S. (1991) Essential role of urease in pathogenesis of gastritis induced by Helicobacter pylori in gnotobiotic piglets. *Infect. Immun.*, 59, 2470–2475.
42. Eaton, K.A. and Krakowka, S. (1994) Effect of gastric pH on urease-dependent colonization of gnotobiotic piglets by Helicobacter pylori. *Infect. Immun.*, 62, 3604–3607.
43. Bauerfeind, P., Garner, R., Dunn, B.E., and Mobley, H.L. (1997) Synthesis and activity of Helicobacter pylori urease and catalase at low pH. *Gut*, 40, 25–30.
44. Goodwin, C.S., Armstrong, J.A., and Marshall, B.J. (1986) Campylobacter pyloridis, gastritis, and peptic ulceration. *J Clin. Pathol.*, 39, 353–365.
45. Smoot, D.T., Mobley, H.L., Chippendale, G.R., Lewison, J.F., and Resau, J.H. (1990) Helicobacter pylori urease activity is toxic to human gastric epithelial cells. *Infect. Immun.*, 58, 1992–1994.
46. Odenbreit, S., Puls, J., Sedlmaier, B., Gerland, E., Fischer, W., and Haas, R. (2000) Translocation of Helicobacter pylori CagA into gastric epithelial cells by type IV secretion. *Science*, 287, 1497–1500.
47. Backert, S., Ziska, E., Brinkmann, V., Zimny-Arndt, U., Fauconnier, A., Jungblut, P.R. et al. (2000) Translocation of the Helicobacter pylori CagA protein in gastric epithelial cells by a type IV secretion apparatus. *Cell Microbiol.*, 2, 155–164.
48. Stein, M., Bagnoli, F., Halenbeck, R., Rappuoli, R., Fantl, W.J., and Covacci, A. (2002) c-Src/Lyn kinases activate Helicobacter pylori CagA through tyrosine phosphorylation of the EPIYA motifs. *Mol. Microbiol.*, 43, 971–980.
49. Higashi, H., Tsutsumi, R., Muto, S., Sugiyama, T., Azuma, T., Asaka, M. et al. (2002) SHP-2 tyrosine phosphatase as an intracellular target of Helicobacter pylori CagA protein. *Science*, 295, 683–686.
50. Puls, J., Fischer, W., and Haas, R. (2002) Activation of Helicobacter pylori CagA by tyrosine phosphorylation is essential for dephosphorylation of host cell proteins in gastric epithelial cells. *Mol. Microbiol.*, 43, 961–969.
51. Loh, J.T., Torres, V.J., and Cover, T.L. (2007) Regulation of Helicobacter pylori cagA expression in response to salt. *Cancer Res.*, 67, 4709–4715.
52. Segal, E.D., Cha, J., Lo, J., Falkow, S., and Tompkins, L.S. (1999) Altered states: involvement of phosphorylated CagA in the induction of host cellular growth changes by Helicobacter pylori. *Proc. Natl. Acad. Sci. U. S. A*, 96, 14559–14564.
53. Kunkel, S.L., Standiford, T., Kasahara, K., and Strieter, R.M. (1991) Interleukin-8 (IL-8): the major neutrophil chemotactic factor in the lung. *Exp. Lung Res.*, 17, 17–23.

54. Papoff, P., Fiorucci, P., Ottaviano, C., and Bucci, G. (1995) Interleukin-8: a potent neutrophil chemotactic factor. *Arch. Dis. Child Fetal Neonatal Ed*, 73, F54.
55. Matsushima, K., Baldwin, E.T., and Mukaida, N. (1992) Interleukin-8 and MCAF: novel leukocyte recruitment and activating cytokines. *Chem. Immunol.*, 51, 236–265.
56. Roebuck, K.A. (1999) Regulation of interleukin-8 gene expression. *J. Interferon Cytokine Res.*, 19, 429–438.
57. McGee, D.J., Radcliff, F.J., Mendz, G.L., Ferrero, R.L., and Mobley, H.L. (1999) Helicobacter pylori rocF is required for arginase activity and acid protection in vitro but is not essential for colonization of mice or for urease activity. *J. Bacteriol.*, 181, 7314–7322.
58. Tomb, J.F., White, O., Kerlavage, A.R., Clayton, R.A., Sutton, G.G., Fleischmann, R.D. et al. (1997) The complete genome sequence of the gastric pathogen Helicobacter pylori. *Nature*, 388, 539–547.
59. Alm, R.A., Ling, L.S., Moir, D.T., King, B.L., Brown, E.D., Doig, P.C. et al. (1999) Genomic-sequence comparison of two unrelated isolates of the human gastric pathogen Helicobacter pylori. *Nature*, 397, 176–180.
60. Sekowska, A., Danchin, A., and Risler, J.L. (2000) Phylogeny of related functions: the case of polyamine biosynthetic enzymes. *Microbiology*, 146 (Pt 8), 1815–1828.
61. Tabor, C.W. and Tabor, H. (1984) Polyamines. *Annu. Rev. Biochem.*, 53, 749–790.
62. Roberts, S.C., Tancer, M.J., Polinsky, M.R., Gibson, K.M., Heby, O., and Ullman, B. (2004) Arginase plays a pivotal role in polyamine precursor metabolism in Leishmania. Characterization of gene deletion mutants. *J. Biol. Chem.*, 279, 23668–23678.
63. Mendz, G.L. and Hazell, S.L. (1995) Aminoacid utilization by Helicobacter pylori. *Int. J. Biochem. Cell Biol.*, 27, 1085–1093.
64. Zabaleta, J., McGee, D.J., Zea, A.H., Hernandez, C.P., Rodriguez, P.C., Sierra, R.A. et al. (2004) Helicobacter pylori arginase inhibits T cell proliferation and reduces the expression of the TCR zeta-chain (CD3zeta). *J. Immunol.*, 173, 586–593.
65. Gobert, A.P., McGee, D.J., Akhtar, M., Mendz, G.L., Newton, J.C., Cheng, Y. et al. (2001) Helicobacter pylori arginase inhibits nitric oxide production by eukaryotic cells: a strategy for bacterial survival. *Proc. Natl. Acad. Sci. U. S. A*, 98, 13844–13849.
66. Chmiela, M., Lelwala-Guruge, J.A., Wadstrom, T., and Rudnicka, W. (1996) The stimulation and inhibition of T cell proliferation by Helicobacter pylori components. *J. Physiol Pharmacol.*, 47, 195–202.
67. Rudnicka, W., Covacci, A., Wadstrom, T., and Chmiela, M. (1998) A recombinant fragment of Helicobacter pylori CagA affects proliferation of human cells. *J. Physiol Pharmacol.*, 49, 111–119.
68. Meyer, F., Wilson, K.T., and James, S.P. (2000) Modulation of innate cytokine responses by products of Helicobacter pylori. *Infect. Immun.*, 68, 6265–6272.
69. Knipp, U., Birkholz, S., Kaup, W., and Opferkuch, W. (1996) Partial characterization of a cell proliferation-inhibiting protein produced by Helicobacter pylori. *Infect. Immun.*, 64, 3491–3496.
70. Paziak-Domanska, B., Chmiela, M., Jarosinska, A., and Rudnicka, W. (2000) Potential role of CagA in the inhibition of T cell reactivity in Helicobacter pylori infections. *Cell Immunol.*, 202, 136–139.
71. Ricci, V., Ciacci, C., Zarrilli, R., Sommi, P., Tummuru, M.K., Del Vecchio, B.C. et al. (1996) Effect of Helicobacter pylori on gastric epithelial cell migration and proliferation in vitro: role of VacA and CagA. *Infect. Immun.*, 64, 2829–2833.
72. Smoot, D.T., Wynn, Z., Elliott, T.B., Allen, C.R., Mekasha, G., Naab, T. et al. (1999) Effects of Helicobacter pylori on proliferation of gastric epithelial cells in vitro. *Am. J. Gastroenterol.*, 94, 1508–1511.
73. Rokkas, T., Ladas, S., Liatsos, C., Petridou, E., Papatheodorou, G., Theocharis, S. et al. (1999) Relationship of Helicobacter pylori CagA status to gastric cell proliferation and apoptosis. *Dig. Dis. Sci.*, 44, 487–493.
74. Kim, C.W., Choi, S.H., Chung, E.J., Lee, M.J., Byun, E.K., Ryu, M.H. et al. (1999) Alteration of signal-transducing molecules and phenotypical characteristics in peripheral blood lymphocytes from gastric carcinoma patients. *Pathobiology*, 67, 123–128.
75. Takahashi, A., Kono, K., Amemiya, H., Iizuka, H., Fujii, H., and Matsumoto, Y. (2001) Elevated caspase-3 activity in peripheral blood T cells coexists with increased degree of T-cell apoptosis and down-regulation of TCR zeta molecules in patients with gastric cancer. *Clin. Cancer Res.*, 7, 74–80.
76. Ishigami, S., Natsugoe, S., Miyazono, F., Tokuda, K., Nakajo, A., Matsumoto, M. et al. (2004) CD3 zeta expression of regional lymph node and peripheral blood lymphocytes in gastric cancer. *Anticancer Res.*, 24, 2123–2126.

77. Roth, K.A., Kapadia, S.B., Martin, S.M., and Lorenz, R.G. (1999) Cellular immune responses are essential for the development of Helicobacter felis-associated gastric pathology. *J. Immunol.*, 163, 1490–1497.
78. Mohammadi, M., Nedrud, J., Redline, R., Lycke, N., and Czinn, S.J. (1997) Murine CD4 T-cell response to Helicobacter infection: TH1 cells enhance gastritis and TH2 cells reduce bacterial load. *Gastroenterology*, 113, 1848–1857.
79. Nedrud, J.G., Mohammadi, M., Blanchard, T., Redline, R., and Czinn, S.J. (1998) TH1/TH2 lymphocyte responses in Helicobacter infections. In Hunt,R. and Tycgat,S. (eds.) *Helicobacter pylori. Mechanisms to clinical cure.* Kluwer Academics Publishers, Boston, pp 101–9.
80. Bamford, K.B., Fan, X., Crowe, S.E., Leary, J.F., Gourley, W.K., Luthra, G.K. et al. (1998) Lymphocytes in the human gastric mucosa during Helicobacter pylori have a T helper cell 1 phenotype. *Gastroenterology*, 114, 482–492.
81. Lindholm, C., Quiding-Jarbrink, M., Lonroth, H., Hamlet, A., and Svennerholm, A.M. (1998) Local cytokine response in Helicobacter pylori-infected subjects. *Infect. Immun.*, 66, 5964–5971.
82. Yamaoka, Y., Kodama, T., Kita, M., Imanishi, J., Kashima, K., and Graham, D.Y. (2001) Relation between cytokines and Helicobacter pylori in gastric cancer. *Helicobacter.*, 6, 116–124.
83. Morris, S.M., Jr. (2004) Recent advances in arginine metabolism. *Curr. Opin. Clin. Nutr. Metab Care*, 7, 45–51.
84. Roth, E., Steininger, R., Winkler, S., Langle, F., Grunberger, T., Fugger, R. et al. (1994) L-Arginine deficiency after liver transplantation as an effect of arginase efflux from the graft. Influence on nitric oxide metabolism. *Transplantation*, 57, 665–669.
85. Zea, A.H., Rodriguez, P.C., Atkins, M.B., Hernandez, C., Signoretti, S., Zabaleta, J. et al. (2005) Arginase-producing myeloid suppressor cells in renal cell carcinoma patients: a mechanism of tumor evasion. *Cancer Res.*, 65, 3044–3048.
86. Rodriguez, P.C., Quiceno, D.G., Zabaleta, J., Ortiz, B., Zea, A.H., Piazuelo, M.B. et al. (2004) Arginase I production in the tumor microenvironment by mature myeloid cells inhibits T-cell receptor expression and antigen-specific T-cell responses. *Cancer Res.*, 64, 5839–5849.
87. Rodriguez, P.C., Zea, A.H., Culotta, K.S., Zabaleta, J., Ochoa, J.B., and Ochoa, A.C. (2002) Regulation of T cell receptor CD3zeta chain expression by L-arginine. *J. Biol. Chem.*, 277, 21123–21129.
88. Munder, M., Mollinedo, F., Calafat, J., Canchado, J., Gil-Lamaignere, C., Fuentes, J.M. et al. (2005) Arginase I is constitutively expressed in human granulocytes and participates in fungicidal activity. *Blood*, 105, 2549–2556.
89. Munder, M., Schneider, H., Luckner, C., Giese, T., Langhans, C.D., Fuentes, J.M. et al. (2006) Suppression of T-cell functions by human granulocyte arginase. *Blood*, 108, 1627–1634.
90. Kropf, P., Baud, D., Marshall, S.E., Munder, M., Mosley, A., Fuentes, J.M. et al. (2007) Arginase activity mediates reversible T cell hyporesponsiveness in human pregnancy. *Eur. J. Immunol.*, 37, 935–945.
91. Chang, C.I., Liao, J.C., and Kuo, L. (2001) Macrophage arginase promotes tumor cell growth and suppresses nitric oxide-mediated tumor cytotoxicity. *Cancer Res.*, 61, 1100–1106.
92. Mendez, J.D. and Arreola, M.A. (1992) Effect of L-arginine on pancreatic arginase activity and polyamines in alloxan treated rats. *Biochem. Int.*, 28, 569–575.
93. Mori, M. and Gotoh, T. (2000) Regulation of nitric oxide production by arginine metabolic enzymes. *Biochem. Biophys. Res. Commun.*, 275, 715–719.
94. Murray, H.W. and Teitelbaum, R.F. (1992) L-arginine-dependent reactive nitrogen intermediates and the antimicrobial effect of activated human mononuclear phagocytes. *J Infect. Dis.*, 165, 513–517.
95. Das, P., Lahiri, A., Lahiri, A., and Chakravortty, D. (2010) Modulation of the arginase pathway in the context of microbial pathogenesis: a metabolic enzyme moonlighting as an immune modulator. *PLoS. Pathog.*, 6, e1000899.
96. Hung, C.Y., Xue, J., and Cole, G.T. (2007) Virulence mechanisms of coccidioides. *Ann. N. Y. Acad. Sci.*, 1111, 225–235.
97. Luiking, Y.C., Poeze, M., Dejong, C.H., Ramsay, G., and Deutz, N.E. (2004) Sepsis: an arginine deficiency state? *Crit Care Med.*, 32, 2135–2145.
98. Luiking, Y.C., Poeze, M., Ramsay, G., and Deutz, N.E. (2005) The role of arginine in infection and sepsis. *JPEN J Parenter. Enteral Nutr.*, 29, S70–S74.
99. Molnar, B., Galamb, O., Sipos, F., Leiszter, K., and Tulassay, Z. (2010) Molecular pathogenesis of Helicobacter pylori infection: the role of bacterial virulence factors. *Dig. Dis.*, 28, 604–608.

100. Mori, M. and Gotoh, T. (2004) Arginine metabolic enzymes, nitric oxide and infection. *J Nutr.*, 134, 2820S–2825S.
101. Wanasen, N. and Soong, L. (2008) L-arginine metabolism and its impact on host immunity against Leishmania infection. *Immunol. Res.*, 41, 15–25.
102. Mendz, G.L., Holmes, E.M., and Ferrero, R.L. (1998) In situ characterization of Helicobacter pylori arginase. *Biochim. Biophys. Acta*, 1388, 465–477.
103. Lewis, N.D., Asim, M., Barry, D.P., Singh, K., de, S.T., Boucher, J.L. et al. (2010) Arginase II restricts host defense to Helicobacter pylori by attenuating inducible nitric oxide synthase translation in macrophages. *J Immunol.*, 184, 2572–2582.
104. Gobert, A.P., Cheng, Y., Wang, J.Y., Boucher, J.L., Iyer, R.K., Cederbaum, S.D. et al. (2002) Helicobacter pylori induces macrophage apoptosis by activation of arginase II. *J Immunol.*, 168, 4692–4700.
105. Lewis, N.D., Asim, M., Barry, D.P., de, S.T., Singh, K., Piazuelo, M.B. et al. (2011) Immune Evasion by Helicobacter pylori Is Mediated by Induction of Macrophage Arginase II. *J Immunol.*, 186, 3632–3641.
106. Hoffman, S.M. and Fleming, S.D. (2010) Natural Helicobacter infection modulates mouse intestinal muscularis macrophage responses. *Cell Biochem. Funct.*, 28, 686–694.
107. el-Zimaity, H.M. and Graham, D.Y. (2001) Ultrastructural evidence of in vivo phagocytosis of Helicobacter pylori. *Ultrastruct. Pathol.*, 25, 159.
108. Zu, Y., Cassai, N.D., and Sidhu, G.S. (2000) Light microscopic and ultrastructural evidence of in vivo phagocytosis of Helicobacter pylori by neutrophils. *Ultrastruct. Pathol.*, 24, 319–323.
109. Ozbek, A., Ozbek, E., Dursun, H., Kalkan, Y., and Demirci, T. (2010) Can Helicobacter pylori invade human gastric mucosa?: an in vivo study using electron microscopy, immunohistochemical methods, and real-time polymerase chain reaction. *J Clin. Gastroenterol.*, 44, 416–422.
110. Ramarao, N., Gray-Owen, S.D., Backert, S., and Meyer, T.F. (2000) Helicobacter pylori inhibits phagocytosis by professional phagocytes involving type IV secretion components. *Mol. Microbiol.*, 37, 1389–1404.
111. Allen, L.A., Schlesinger, L.S., and Kang, B. (2000) Virulent strains of Helicobacter pylori demonstrate delayed phagocytosis and stimulate homotypic phagosome fusion in macrophages. *J Exp. Med.*, 191, 115–128.
112. Zheng, P.Y. and Jones, N.L. (2003) Helicobacter pylori strains expressing the vacuolating cytotoxin interrupt phagosome maturation in macrophages by recruiting and retaining TACO (coronin 1) protein. *Cell Microbiol.*, 5, 25–40.
113. Ramarao, N. and Meyer, T.F. (2001) Helicobacter pylori resists phagocytosis by macrophages: quantitative assessment by confocal microscopy and fluorescence-activated cell sorting. *Infect. Immun.*, 69, 2604–2611.
114. Wang, Y.H., Wu, J.J., and Lei, H.Y. (2009) When Helicobacter pylori invades and replicates in the cells. *Autophagy.*, 5, 540–542.
115. Turner, D.M., Williams, D.M., Sankaran, D., Lazarus, M., Sinnott, P.J., and Hutchinson, I.V. (1997) An investigation of polymorphism in the interleukin-10 gene promoter. *Eur. J. Immunogenet.*, 24, 1–8.
116. Rad,R., Dossumbekova, A., Neu, B., Lang, R., Bauer, S., Saur, D. et al. (2004) Cytokine gene polymorphisms influence mucosal cytokine expression, gastric inflammation, and host specific colonisation during Helicobacter pylori infection. *Gut*, 53, 1082–1089.
117. Hwang, I.R., Kodama, T., Kikuchi, S., Sakai, K., Peterson, L.E., Graham, D.Y. et al. (2002) Effect of interleukin 1 polymorphisms on gastric mucosal interleukin 1beta production in Helicobacter pylori infection. *Gastroenterology*, 123, 1793–1803.
118. Pociot, F., Molvig, J., Wogensen, L., Worsaae, H., and Nerup, J. (1992) A TaqI polymorphism in the human interleukin-1 beta (IL-1 beta) gene correlates with IL-1 beta secretion in vitro. *Eur. J. Clin. Invest*, 22, 396–402.
119. Kroeger, K.M., Carville, K.S., and Abraham, L.J. (1997) The -308 tumor necrosis factor-alpha promoter polymorphism effects transcription. *Mol. Immunol.*, 34, 391–399.
120. Wilson, A.G., Symons, J.A., McDowell, T.L., McDevitt, H.O., and Duff, G.W. (1997) Effects of a polymorphism in the human tumor necrosis factor alpha promoter on transcriptional activation. *Proc. Natl. Acad. Sci. U. S. A*, 94, 3195–3199.
121. Fishman, D., Faulds, G., Jeffery, R., Mohamed-Ali, V., Yudkin, J.S., Humphries, S. et al. (1998) The effect of novel polymorphisms in the interleukin-6 (IL-6) gene on IL-6 transcription and plasma IL-6 levels, and an association with systemic-onset juvenile chronic arthritis. *J. Clin. Invest*, 102, 1369–1376.
122. Terry, C.F., Loukaci, V., and Green, F.R. (2000) Cooperative influence of genetic polymorphisms on interleukin 6 transcriptional

regulation. *J. Biol. Chem.*, 275, 18138–18144.

123. Abdallah, A.N., Cucchi-Mouillot, P., Biteau, N., Cassaigne, A., Haras, D., and Iron, A. (1999) Analysis of the polymorphism of the tumour necrosis factor (TNF) gene and promoter and of circulating TNF-alpha levels in heart-transplant patients suffering or not suffering from severe rejection. *Eur. J. Immunogenet.*, 26, 249–255.
124. Bunnapradist, S. and Jordan, S.C. (2000) The role of cytokines and cytokine gene polymorphism in T-cell activation and allograft rejection. *Ann. Acad. Med. Singapore*, 29, 412–416.
125. Hajeer, A.H., Lazarus, M., Turner, D., Mageed, R.A., Vencovsky, J., Sinnott, P. et al. (1998) IL-10 gene promoter polymorphisms in rheumatoid arthritis. *Scand. J. Rheumatol.*, 27, 142–145.
126. Cabrera, M., Shaw, M.A., Sharples, C., Williams, H., Castes, M., Convit, J. et al. (1995) Polymorphism in tumor necrosis factor genes associated with mucocutaneous leishmaniasis. *J. Exp. Med.*, 182, 1259–1264.
127. Wilkinson, R.J., Patel, P., Llewelyn, M., Hirsch, C.S., Pasvol, G., Snounou, G. et al. (1999) Influence of polymorphism in the genes for the interleukin (IL)-1 receptor antagonist and IL-1beta on tuberculosis. *J. Exp. Med.*, 189, 1863–1874.
128. SEER. SEER Cancer Statistics Review 1975-2004.http://seer.cancer.gov/csr/1975_2004/results_merged/topic_inc_trends.pdf. 2004.
129. Cancer Health Disparities. http://www.cancer.gov/cancertopics/types/disparities. 2008.
130. Gabriel, S.B., Schaffner, S.F., Nguyen, H., Moore, J.M., Roy, J., Blumenstiel, B. et al. (2002) The structure of haplotype blocks in the human genome. *Science*, 296, 2225–2229.
131. Huang, W., He, Y., Wang, H., Wang, Y., Liu, Y., Wang, Y. et al. (2006) Linkage disequilibrium sharing and haplotype-tagged SNP portability between populations. *Proc Natl. Acad. Sci. U. S. A*, 103, 1418–1421.
132. Epplein, M., Signorello, L.B., Zheng, W., Peek, R.M., Jr., Michel, A., Williams, S.M. et al. (2011) Race, African ancestry, and Helicobacter pylori infection in a low-income United States population. *Cancer Epidemiol. Biomarkers Prev.*.
133. Lee, C.G., Gottesman, M.M., Cardarelli, C.O., Ramachandra, M., Jeang, K.T., Ambudkar, S.V. et al. (1998) HIV-1 protease inhibitors are substrates for the MDRl multidrug transporter. *Biochemistry*, 37, 3594–3601.
134. Lee, C.G. and Gottesman, M.M. (1998) HIV-1 protease inhibitors and the MDRl multidrug transporter. *J. Clin. Invest*, 101, 287–288.
135. Balram, C., Sharma, A., Sivathasan, C., and Lee, E.J. (2003) Frequency of C3435T single nucleotide MDRl genetic polymorphism in an Asian population: phenotypic-genotypic correlates. *Br. J. Clin. Pharmacol.*, 56, 78–83.
136. Hitzl, M., Drescher, S., van der, K.H., Schaffeler, E., Fischer, J., Schwab, M. et al. (2001) The C3435T mutation in the human MDRl gene is associated with altered efflux of the P-glycoprotein substrate rhodamine 123 from CD56+ natural killer cells. *Pharmacogenetics*, 11, 293–298.
137. Hoffmeyer, S., Burk, O., von, R.O., Arnold, H.P., Brockmoller, J., Johne, A. et al. (2000) Functional polymorphisms of the human multidrug-resistance gene: multiple sequence variations and correlation of one allele with P-glycoprotein expression and activity in vivo. *Proc. Natl. Acad. Sci. U. S. A*, 97, 3473–3478.
138. Tanabe, M., Ieiri, I., Nagata, N., Inoue, K., Ito, S., Kanamori, Y. et al. (2001) Expression of P-glycoprotein in human placenta: relation to genetic polymorphism of the multidrug resistance (MDR)-1 gene. *J. Pharmacol. Exp. Ther.*, 297, 1137–1143.
139. Kim, R.B., Leake, B.F., Choo, E.F., Dresser, G.K., Kubba, S.V., Schwarz, U.I. et al. (2001) Identification of functionally variant MDRl alleles among European Americans and African Americans. *Clin. Pharmacol. Ther.*, 70, 189–199.
140. Sakaeda, T., Nakamura, T., Horinouchi, M., Kakumoto, M., Ohmoto, N., Sakai, T. et al. (2001) MDRl genotype-related pharmacokinetics of digoxin after single oral administration in healthy Japanese subjects. *Pharm. Res.*, 18, 1400–1404.
141. Fellay, J., Marzolini, C., Meaden, E.R., Back, D.J., Buclin, T., Chave, J.P. et al. (2002) Response to antiretroviral treatment in HIV-1-infected individuals with allelic variants of the multidrug resistance transporter 1: a pharmacogenetics study. *Lancet*, 359, 30–36.
142. von, A.N., Richter, M., Grupp, C., Ringe, B., Oellerich, M., and Armstrong, V.W. (2001) No influence of the MDR-1 C3435T polymorphism or a CYP3A4 promoter polymorphism (CYP3A4-V allele) on dose-adjusted cyclosporin A trough concentrations or rejection incidence in stable renal transplant recipients. *Clin. Chem.*, 47, 1048–1052.
143. Tang, K., Ngoi, S.M., Gwee, P.C., Chua, J.M., Lee, E.J., Chong, S.S. et al. (2002)

Distinct haplotype profiles and strong linkage disequilibrium at the MDR1 multidrug transporter gene locus in three ethnic Asian populations. *Pharmacogenetics*, 12, 437–450.

144. Machado, J.C., Pharoah, P., Sousa, S., Carvalho, R., Oliveira, C., Figueiredo, C. et al. (2001) Interleukin 1B and interleukin 1RN polymorphisms are associated with increased risk of gastric carcinoma. *Gastroenterology*, 121, 823–829.
145. Sicinschi, L.A., Lopez-Carrillo, L., Camargo, M.C., Correa, P., Sierra, R.A., Henry, R.R. et al. (2006) Gastric cancer risk in a Mexican population: role of Helicobacter pylori CagA positive infection and polymorphisms in interleukin-1 and -10 genes. *Int. J. Cancer*, 118, 649–657.
146. Xue, H., Lin, B., Ni, P., Xu, H., and Huang, G. (2010) Interleukin-1B and interleukin-1 RN polymorphisms and gastric carcinoma risk: a meta-analysis. *J Gastroenterol. Hepatol.*, 25, 1604–1617.
147. Wang, P., Xia, H.H., Zhang, J.Y., Dai, L.P., Xu, X.Q., and Wang, K.J. (2007) Association of interleukin-1 gene polymorphisms with gastric cancer: a meta-analysis. *Int. J Cancer*, 120, 552–562.
148. Camargo, M.C., Mera, R., Correa, P., Peek, R.M., Jr., Fontham, E.T., Goodman, K.J. et al. (2006) Interleukin-1beta and interleukin-1 receptor antagonist gene polymorphisms and gastric cancer: a meta-analysis. *Cancer Epidemiol. Biomarkers Prev.*, 15, 1674–1687.
149. Persson, C., Canedo, P., Machado, J.C., El-Omar, E.M., and Forman, D. (2011) Polymorphisms in inflammatory response genes and their association with gastric cancer: A HuGE systematic review and meta-analyses. *Am. J Epidemiol.*, 173, 259–270.
150. Beales, I.L. and Calam, J. (1998) Interleukin 1 beta and tumour necrosis factor alpha inhibit acid secretion in cultured rabbit parietal cells by multiple pathways. *Gut*, 42, 227–234.
151. Chen, H., Wilkins, L.M., Aziz, N., Cannings, C., Wyllie, D.H., Bingle, C. et al. (2006) Single nucleotide polymorphisms in the human interleukin-1B gene affect transcription according to haplotype context. *Hum. Mol. Genet.*, 15, 519–529.
152. Arend, W.P., Malyak, M., Guthridge, C.J., and Gabay, C. (1998) Interleukin-1 receptor antagonist: role in biology. *Annu. Rev. Immunol.*, 16, 27–55.
153. Andus, T., Daig, R., Vogl, D., Aschenbrenner, E., Lock, G., Hollerbach, S. et al. (1997) Imbalance of the interleukin 1 system in colonic mucosa--association with intestinal inflammation and interleukin 1 receptor antagonist (corrected) genotype 2. *Gut*, 41, 651–657.
154. Tountas, N.A., Casini-Raggi, V., Yang, H., Di Giovine, F.S., Vecchi, M., Kam, L. et al. (1999) Functional and ethnic association of allele 2 of the interleukin-1 receptor antagonist gene in ulcerative colitis. *Gastroenterology*, 117, 806–813.
155. Shih, C.M., Lee, Y.L., Chiou, H.L., Chen, W., Chang, G.C., Chou, M.C. et al. (2006) Association of TNF-alpha polymorphism with susceptibility to and severity of non-small cell lung cancer. *Lung Cancer*, 52, 15–20.
156. Zambon, C.F., Basso, D., Navaglia, F., Belluco, C., Falda, A., Fogar, P. et al. (2005) Pro- and anti-inflammatory cytokines gene polymorphisms and Helicobacter pylori infection: interactions influence outcome. *Cytokine*, 29, 141–152.
157. Hellmig, S., Fischbach, W., Goebeler-Kolve, M.E., Folsch, U.R., Hampe, J., and Schreiber, S. (2005) A functional promotor polymorphism of TNF-alpha is associated with primary gastric B-Cell lymphoma. *Am. J. Gastroenterol.*, 100, 2644–2649.
158. Kido, S., Kitadai, Y., Hattori, N., Haruma, K., Kido, T., Ohta, M. et al. (2001) Interleukin 8 and vascular endothelial growth factor—prognostic factors in human gastric carcinomas? *Eur. J. Cancer*, 37, 1482–1487.
159. Kitadai, Y., Haruma, K., Mukaida, N., Ohmoto, Y., Matsutani, N., Yasui, W. et al. (2000) Regulation of disease-progression genes in human gastric carcinoma cells by interleukin 8. *Clin. Cancer Res.*, 6, 2735–2740.
160. Savage, S.A., Abnet, C.C., Mark, S.D., Qiao, Y.L., Dong, Z.W., Dawsey, S.M. et al. (2004) Variants of the IL8 and IL8RB genes and risk for gastric cardia adenocarcinoma and esophageal squamous cell carcinoma. *Cancer Epidemiol. Biomarkers Prev.*, 13, 2251–2257.
161. Kato, I., Van Doorn, L.J., Canzian, F., Plummer, M., Franceschi, S., Vivas, J. et al. (2006) Host-bacterial interaction in the development of gastric precancerous lesions in a high risk population for gastric cancer in Venezuela. *Int. J. Cancer*, 119, 1666–1671.
162. Mege, J.L., Meghari, S., Honstettre, A., Capo, C., and Raoult, D. (2006) The two faces of interleukin 10 in human infectious diseases. *Lancet Infect. Dis.*, 6, 557–569.
163. Havranek, E., Howell, W.M., Fussell, H.M., Whelan, J.A., Whelan, M.A., and Pandha, H.S. (2005) An interleukin-10 promoter polymorphism may influence tumor development

in renal cell carcinoma. *J. Urol.*, 173, 709–712.

164. Nikolova, P.N., Pawelec, G.P., Mihailova, S.M., Ivanova, M.I., Myhailova, A.P., Baltadjieva, D.N. et al. (2007) Association of cytokine gene polymorphisms with malignant melanoma in Caucasian population. *Cancer Immunol. Immunother.*, 56, 371–379.
165. Seifart, C., Plagens, A., Dempfle, A., Clostermann, U., Vogelmeier, C., von, W.P. et al. (2005) TNF-alpha, TNF-beta, IL-6, and IL-10 polymorphisms in patients with lung cancer. *Dis. Markers*, 21, 157–165.
166. Sakamoto, H., Yoshimura, K., Saeki, N., Katai, H., Shimoda, T., Matsuno, Y. et al. (2008) Genetic variation in PSCA is associated with susceptibility to diffuse-type gastric cancer. *Nat. Genet.*, 40, 730–740.
167. Lu, Y., Chen, J., Ding, Y., Jin, G., Wu, J., Huang, H. et al. (2010) Genetic variation of PSCA gene is associated with the risk of both diffuse- and intestinal-type gastric cancer in a Chinese population. *Int. J Cancer*, 127, 2183–2189.
168. Abnet, C.C., Freedman, N.D., Hu, N., Wang, Z., Yu, K., Shu, X.O. et al. (2010) A shared susceptibility locus in PLCE1 at 10q23 for gastric adenocarcinoma and esophageal squamous cell carcinoma. *Nat. Genet.*, 42, 764–767.
169. Bird, A. (2002) DNA methylation patterns and epigenetic memory. *Genes Dev.*, 16, 6-21.
170. Wang, Y. and Leung, F.C. (2004) An evaluation of new criteria for CpG islands in the human genome as gene markers. *Bioinformatics.*, 20, 1170–1177.
171. Tate, P.H. and Bird, A.P. (1993) Effects of DNA methylation on DNA-binding proteins and gene expression. *Curr. Opin. Genet. Dev.*, 3, 226–231.
172. Nan, X., Meehan, R.R., and Bird, A. (1993) Dissection of the methyl-CpG binding domain from the chromosomal protein MeCP2. *Nucleic Acids Res.*, 21, 4886–4892.
173. Prendergast, G.C. and Ziff, E.B. (1991) Methylation-sensitive sequence-specific DNA binding by the c-Myc basic region. *Science*, 251, 186–189.
174. Watt, F. and Molloy, P.L. (1988) Cytosine methylation prevents binding to DNA of a HeLa cell transcription factor required for optimal expression of the adenovirus major late promoter. *Genes Dev.*, 2, 1136–1143.
175. Jones, P.L., Veenstra, G.J., Wade, P.A., Vermaak, D., Kass, S.U., Landsberger, N. et al. (1998) Methylated DNA and MeCP2 recruit histone deacetylase to repress transcription. *Nat. Genet.*, 19, 187–191.
176. Nan, X., Ng, H.H., Johnson, C.A., Laherty, C.D., Turner, B.M., Eisenman, R.N. et al. (1998) Transcriptional repression by the methyl-CpG-binding protein MeCP2 involves a histone deacetylase complex. *Nature*, 393, 386–389.
177. Kim, G.D., Ni, J., Kelesoglu, N., Roberts, R.J., and Pradhan, S. (2002) Co-operation and communication between the human maintenance and de novo DNA (cytosine-5) methyltransferases. *EMBO J*, 21, 4183–4195.
178. Okano, M., Bell, D.W., Haber, D.A., and Li, E. (1999) DNA methyltransferases Dnmt3a and Dnmt3b are essential for de novo methylation and mammalian development. *Cell*, 99, 247–257.
179. Fan, H., Liu, D., Qiu, X., Qiao, F., Wu, Q., Su, X. et al. (2010) A functional polymorphism in the DNA methyltransferase-3A promoter modifies the susceptibility in gastric cancer but not in esophageal carcinoma. *BMC. Med.*, 8, 12.
180. Esteller, M. (2002) CpG island hypermethylation and tumor suppressor genes: a booming present, a brighter future. *Oncogene*, 21, 5427–5440.
181. Yamashita, S., Tsujino, Y., Moriguchi, K., Tatematsu, M., and Ushijima, T. (2006) Chemical genomic screening for methylation-silenced genes in gastric cancer cell lines using 5-aza-2′-deoxycytidine treatment and oligonucleotide microarray. *Cancer Sci.*, 97, 64–71.
182. Schneider, B.G., Peng, D.F., Camargo, M.C., Piazuelo, M.B., Sicinschi, L.A., Mera, R. et al. (2010) Promoter DNA hypermethylation in gastric biopsies from subjects at high and low risk for gastric cancer. *Int. J Cancer*, 127, 2588–2597.
183. Shen, H., Xu, Y., Zheng, Y., Qian, Y., Yu, R., Qin, Y. et al. (2001) Polymorphisms of 5,10-methylenetetrahydrofolate reductase and risk of gastric cancer in a Chinese population: a case-control study. *Int. J Cancer*, 95, 332–336.
184. Neves Filho, E.H., Alves, M.K., Lima, V.P., and Rabenhorst, S.H. (2010) MTHFR C677T polymorphism and differential methylation status in gastric cancer: an association with Helicobacter pylori infection. *Virchows Arch.*, 457, 627–633.
185. Dong, C.X., Deng, D.J., Pan, K.F., Zhang, L., Zhang, Y., Zhou, J. et al. (2009) Promoter methylation of p16 associated with Helicobacter pylori infection in precancerous gastric lesions: a population-based study. *Int. J Cancer*, 124, 434–439.

186. Kague, E., Thomazini, C.M., Pardini, M.I., de, C.F., Leite, C.V., and Pinheiro, N.A. (2010) Methylation status of CDH1 gene in samples of gastric mucous from Brazilian patients with chronic gastritis infected by Helicobacter pylori. *Arq Gastroenterol.*, 47, 7–12.
187. Alves, M.K., Lima, V.P., Ferrasi, A.C., Rodrigues, M.A., De Moura Campos Pardini MI, and Rabenhorst, S.H. (2010) CDKN2A promoter methylation is related to the tumor location and histological subtype and associated with Helicobacter pylori flaA(+) strains in gastric adenocarcinomas. *APMIS*, 118, 297–307.
188. Chan, A.O., Peng, J.Z., Lam, S.K., Lai, K.C., Yuen, M.F., Cheung, H.K. et al. (2006) Eradication of Helicobacter pylori infection reverses E-cadherin promoter hypermethylation. *Gut*, 55, 463–468.
189. Guilford, P., Hopkins, J., Harraway, J., McLeod, M., McLeod, N., Harawira, P. et al. (1998) E-cadherin germline mutations in familial gastric cancer. *Nature*, 392, 402–405.
190. Yoo, E.J., Park, S.Y., Cho, N.Y., Kim, N., Lee, H.S., Kim, D. et al. (2010) Influence of IL1B polymorphism on CpG island hypermethylation in Helicobacter pylori-infected gastric cancer. *Virchows Arch.*, 456, 647–652.
191. McMichael, A.J., McCall, M.G., Hartshorne, J.M., and Woodings, T.L. (1980) Patterns of gastro-intestinal cancer in European migrants to Australia: the role of dietary change. *Int. J Cancer*, 25, 431–437.
192. Haenszel, W. and Kurihara, M. (1968) Studies of Japanese migrants. I. Mortality from cancer and other diseases among Japanese in the United States. *J Natl. Cancer Inst.*, 40, 43–68.
193. Plummer, M., Franceschi, S., and Munoz, N. (2004) Epidemiology of gastric cancer. *IARC Sci. Publ.*,311–326.
194. Lunet, N., Valbuena, C., Vieira, A.L., Lopes, C., Lopes, C., David, L. et al. (2007) Fruit and vegetable consumption and gastric cancer by location and histological type: case-control and meta-analysis. *Eur. J Cancer Prev.*, 16, 312–327.
195. Terry, P., Nyren, O., and Yuen, J. (1998) Protective effect of fruits and vegetables on stomach cancer in a cohort of Swedish twins. *Int. J Cancer*, 76, 35–37.
196. Jansen, M.C., Bueno-de-Mesquita, H.B., Rasanen, L., Fidanza, F., Menotti, A., Nissinen, A. et al. (1999) Consumption of plant foods and stomach cancer mortality in the seven countries study. Is grain consumption a risk factor? Seven Countries Study Research Group. *Nutr. Cancer*, 34, 49–55.
197. Risch, H.A., Jain, M., Choi, N.W., Fodor, J.G., Pfeiffer, C.J., Howe, G.R. et al. (1985) Dietary factors and the incidence of cancer of the stomach. *Am. J Epidemiol.*, 122, 947–959.
198. Nomura, A.M., Hankin, J.H., Kolonel, L.N., Wilkens, L.R., Goodman, M.T., and Stemmermann, G.N. (2003) Case-control study of diet and other risk factors for gastric cancer in Hawaii (United States). *Cancer Causes Control*, 14, 547–558.
199. Lagiou, P., Samoli, E., Lagiou, A., Peterson, J., Tzonou, A., Dwyer, J. et al. (2004) Flavonoids, vitamin C and adenocarcinoma of the stomach. *Cancer Causes Control*, 15, 67–72.
200. Ramon, J.M., Serra-Majem, L., Cerdo, C., and Oromi, J. (1993) Nutrient intake and gastric cancer risk: a case-control study in Spain. *Int. J Epidemiol.*, 22, 983–988.
201. Kaaks, R., Tuyns, A.J., Haelterman, M., and Riboli, E. (1998) Nutrient intake patterns and gastric cancer risk: a case-control study in Belgium. *Int. J Cancer*, 78, 415–420.
202. Palli, D., Russo, A., and Decarli, A. (2001) Dietary patterns, nutrient intake and gastric cancer in a high-risk area of Italy. *Cancer Causes Control*, 12, 163–172.
203. Mayne, S.T., Risch, H.A., Dubrow, R., Chow, W.H., Gammon, M.D., Vaughan, T.L. et al. (2001) Nutrient intake and risk of subtypes of esophageal and gastric cancer. *Cancer Epidemiol. Biomarkers Prev.*, 10, 1055–1062.
204. De, S.E., Correa, P., Boffetta, P., eo-Pellegrini, H., Ronco, A.L., and Mendilaharsu, M. (2004) Dietary patterns and risk of gastric cancer: a case-control study in Uruguay. *Gastric. Cancer*, 7, 211–220.
205. Campos, F., Carrasquilla, G., Koriyama, C., Serra, M., Carrascal, E., Itoh, T. et al. (2006) Risk factors of gastric cancer specific for tumor location and histology in Cali, Colombia. *World J Gastroenterol.*, 12, 5772–5779.
206. Wirth, H.P., Beins, M.H., Yang, M., Tham, K.T., and Blaser, M.J. (1998) Experimental infection of Mongolian gerbils with wild-type and mutant Helicobacter pylori strains. *Infect. Immun.*, 66, 4856–4866.
207. Dey, A., Yokota, K., Kobayashi, K., Oguma, K., Hirai, Y., and Akagi, T. (1998) Antibody and cytokine responses in Helicobacter pylori-infected various mouse strains. *Acta Med. Okayama*, 52, 41–48.
208. Marchetti, M., Arico, B., Burroni, D., Figura, N., Rappuoli, R., and Ghiara, P. (1995) Development of a mouse model of Helicobacter pylori infection that mimics human disease. *Science*, 267, 1655–1658.

209. D'Elios, M.M., Manghetti, M., Almerigogna, F., Amedei, A., Costa, F., Burroni, D. et al. (1997) Different cytokine profile and antigen-specificity repertoire in Helicobacter pylori-specific T cell clones from the antrum of chronic gastritis patients with or without peptic ulcer. *Eur. J. Immunol.*, 27, 1751–1755.

210. D'Elios, M.M., Manghetti, M., De, C.M., Costa, F., Baldari, C.T., Burroni, D. et al. (1997) T helper 1 effector cells specific for Helicobacter pylori in the gastric antrum of patients with peptic ulcer disease. *J. Immunol.*, 158, 962–967.

211. Sommer, F., Faller, G., Konturek, P., Kirchner, T., Hahn, E.G., Zeus, J. et al. (1998) Antrum- and corpus mucosa-infiltrating CD4(+) lymphocytes in Helicobacter pylori gastritis display a Th1 phenotype. *Infect. Immun.*, 66, 5543–5546.

212. Maeda, S., Yoshida, H., Ogura, K., Mitsuno, Y., Hirata, Y., Yamaji, Y. et al. (2000) H. pylori activates NF-kappaB through a signaling pathway involving IkappaB kinases, NF-kappaB-inducing kinase, TRAF2, and TRAF6 in gastric cancer cells. *Gastroenterology*, 119, 97–108.

213. Yasumoto, K., Okamoto, S., Mukaida, N., Murakami, S., Mai, M., and Matsushima, K. (1992) Tumor necrosis factor alpha and interferon gamma synergistically induce interleukin 8 production in a human gastric cancer cell line through acting concurrently on AP-1 and NF-kB-like binding sites of the interleukin 8 gene. *J. Biol. Chem.*, 267, 22506–22511.

214. Mitsuno, Y., Yoshida, H., Maeda, S., Ogura, K., Hirata, Y., Kawabe, T. et al. (2001) Helicobacter pylori induced transactivation of SRE and AP-1 through the ERK signalling pathway in gastric cancer cells. *Gut*, 49, 18–22.

215. Karttunen, R.A., Karttunen, T.J., Yousfi, M.M., el-Zimaity, H.M., Graham, D.Y., and el-Zaatari, F.A. (1997) Expression of mRNA for interferon-gamma, interleukin-10, and interleukin-12 (p40) in normal gastric mucosa and in mucosa infected with Helicobacter pylori. *Scand. J. Gastroenterol.*, 32, 22–27.

216. Ye, G., Barrera, C., Fan, X., Gourley, W.K., Crowe, S.E., Ernst, P.B. et al. (1997) Expression of B7-1 and B7-2 costimulatory molecules by human gastric epithelial cells: potential role in CD4+ T cell activation during Helicobacter pylori infection. *J. Clin. Invest*, 99, 1628–1636.

217. Allen, L.A., Schlesinger, L.S., and Kang, B. (2000) Virulent strains of Helicobacter pylori demonstrate delayed phagocytosis and stimulate homotypic phagosome fusion in macrophages. *J. Exp. Med.*, 191, 115–128.

218. Kuwahara, H., Miyamoto, Y., Akaike, T., Kubota, T., Sawa, T., Okamoto, S. et al. (2000) Helicobacter pylori urease suppresses bactericidal activity of peroxynitrite via carbon dioxide production. *Infect. Immun.*, 68, 4378–4383.

Part V

Epigenetic Epidemiology

Chapter 27

Epigenetic Epidemiology for Cancer Risk: Harnessing Germline Epigenetic Variation

Kevin Brennan and James M. Flanagan

Abstract

Genetic epidemiology aims to use the natural variation in the genome, namely single nucleotide polymorphisms and copy number variants to look for associations between particular genotypes and disease risk or prognosis. Recent work is now aiming to look further into the genome at the natural variation present in the epigenome, in DNA methylation as well as histone modifications, which both regulate gene expression. Epigenetic epidemiology aims to address the same questions about disease risk and prognosis using the normal epigenetic variability. Some examples of rare "epimutations" that can be detected in peripheral blood DNA have been reported in the genes *MLH1*, *MSH2* and *IGF2*. Other studies have reported increased cancer risk with skewed distributions of the normal pattern in cancer cases compared to controls, showing the promise of harnessing the normal variation in the epigenome. However, some confounding factors need to be considered including the relationship between the epigenome and increasing age and tissue heterogeneity. Future studies using genome-wide approaches will likely find many more novel epigenetic biomarkers for cancer risk and prognosis.

Key words: Epigenetic, Methylation, Cancer risk, Breast cancer, Peripheral blood

1. Introduction

1.1. Epigenetics

Epigenetics is the stable, yet reversible chemical alterations to the genome that affects gene expression and genome function. These encompass mechanisms such as DNA methylation, histone modifications, non-coding RNA and other non-genetic methods of gene regulation. Mammalian DNA is packaged into chromosomes by wrapping the DNA around nucleosomes made up of an octamer of histone proteins. Each of the different histone types have N-terminal protein tails that extend outside of the nucleosome and can be modified by several large families of enzymes. Different histone modifications (e.g. acetylation, methylation, phosphorylation) mark either active or inactive chromatin and define the chromosomal structure and gene expression state for the genes within that chromosomal

Ramona G. Dumitrescu and Mukesh Verma (eds.), *Cancer Epigenetics: Methods and Protocols*, Methods in Molecular Biology, vol. 863, DOI 10.1007/978-1-61779-612-8_27, © Springer Science+Business Media, LLC 2012

domain. DNA methylation refers to a chemical modification to the cytosine base in DNA (also called 5-methylcytosine, 5-mC), predominantly in the context of a cytosine-guanine (CpG) dinucleotide. Other forms have recently been identified, such as 5′ hydroxymethylcytosine, although the biological significance of this mark is yet to be determined. While the majority of studies described in this chapter refer to DNA methylation, reflecting most of the studies to date, many of the same concepts could be applied to histone modification profiles to achieve the same objectives of identifying risk biomarkers and this remains an area for future research.

DNA methylation is heritable through mitosis and is copied to the new strand during DNA replication and represents a mechanism of cellular memory of gene expression states in previous parental cells. This cellular memory is particularly important in the development of tissue-specific and cell-lineage-specific expression patterns. Approximately 60% of human genes contain a high density of CpG dinucleotides at the promoters, known as CpG islands (CGIs). The current dogma describes DNA methylation at the promoter of a gene as a sign of silenced gene expression. It has become apparent over the last 20 years that promoter DNA hypermethylation is one of the most common somatic aberrations in cancer development. However, only over the last few years have studies emerged that show that aberrant epigenetic traits in the normal, non-cancerous, cells of an individual may also be involved in carcinogenesis. These "epimutations" or variation in the normal epigenetic patterns may provide novel biomarkers for cancer risk and prognosis.

1.2. Cancer Risk and Prognosis

The purpose of defining cancer risk is to identify individuals who would benefit from increased surveillance or cancer preventive measures. Using breast cancer as an example, current knowledge draws risk from genetic studies that have identified *BRCA1* and *BRCA2* germline mutations that contribute the most to an individual's chance of developing cancer. Epidemiological studies have shown that various factors, including age, hormonal exposures, family history and to a lesser extent various dietary and environmental factors, all contribute to an individual's risk of developing cancer. Many of these factors can be incorporated into statistical models such as the Gail Model (1) or the Cuzic-Tyrer model (2) among others. More recently, genetic genome-wide association studies (GWAS) in breast cancer have identified ~18 genetic loci tagged by particular single nucleotide polymorphisms (SNPs) that reach genome-wide significance and have been validated (3). The contribution to risk of each of these variants is quite small; however, the utility of combining SNPs with other risk factors is under consideration (3). As a simplified example, a typical 50-year-old woman with no family history of breast cancer has a lifetime risk of breast cancer of 9.9%. If she also is heterozygous for the risk allele

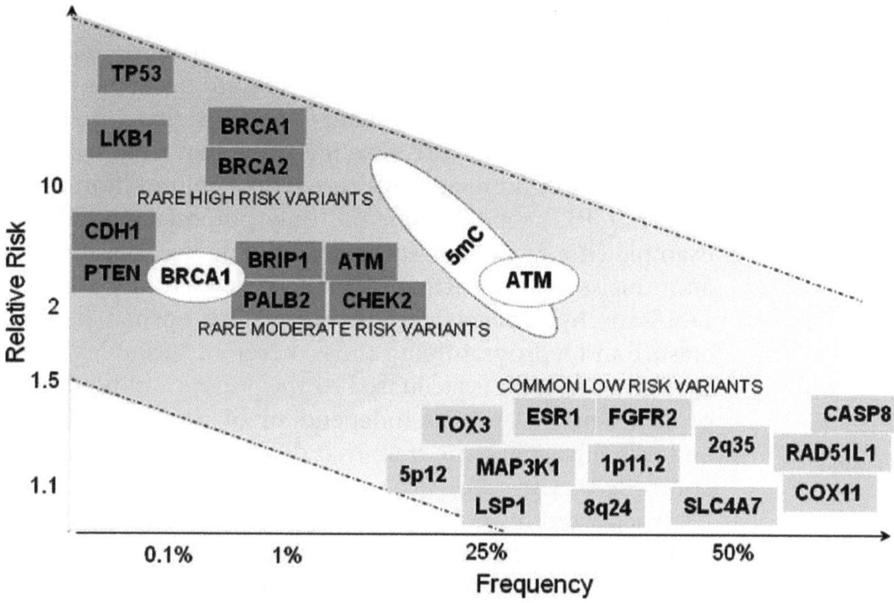

Fig. 1. Relative risk of breast cancer for known genetic risk variants and incorporating candidate epigenetic risk variants. Known genetic mutations that confer high and moderate risk of breast cancer are marked in *dark grey boxes*. Common genetic polymorphisms that confer low increased risk are marked in *light grey boxes*. Epigenetic biomarkers of breast cancer risk are marked in *white ovals* including BRCA1, ATM, and genome-wide methylation levels (5-methylcytosine, 5-mC). Modified from Varghese and Easton (3).

in the *FGFR2* gene polymorphism which confers an average relative risk of 1.26-fold, this particular individual's relative risk would rise to 12.5%. If we include the reported epigenetic biomarker in the *ATM* gene (described later) which confers a relative risk of 1.7-fold, this individual's relative risk would again increase up to 21.2%, which is above the level considered as high risk for screening purposes (15–20%). This simplified example assumes that each biomarker is independent of all other risk factors that are included in the primary relative risk estimate, which is not necessarily a correct assumption. Incorporation of all known genetic and epigenetic risk biomarkers into current models is an area of intense research focus (Fig. 1). Prognostic studies aim to identify biomarkers that define which cancer patients would most benefit from specific therapies, or who will be at risk of certain toxicities. Currently, there have been few studies that have identified useful epigenetic biomarkers of prognosis.

2. Reported Epimutations

2.1. Epimutation Nomenclature

Epimutations may be categorised according to a nomenclature system proposed in 2006, in which "obligatory", "facilitated" and "pure" represent start, mid and end points on a continuous scale of independence from the genetic background (4). Obligatory epimutations, in which an epigenetic state occurs as a result of an underlying genetic lesion, have been described in humans, for example *MSH2* (5). Currently, it is unknown whether pure epimutations exist in humans, with the *MLH1* epimutation in colorectal cancer (CRC) representing the only potential candidate (6). An example of a facilitated epimutation is differential methylation of an intracisternal A particle (IAP), a type of transposons, at which DNA methylation appears to escape the normal developmental erasure and reprogramming and is therefore heritable (4). Although DNA methylation is facilitated by the presence of the IAP, the level of DNA methylation is independent of the genetic background and it is this epigenetic state that determines the expression of the controlled gene (4). Although these types of epimutation have been reported in mouse models such as the Agouti yellow mouse and the kinked tail mouse, no such examples have been identified in humans (7, 8). Genomic imprinting refers to the epigenetic silencing of one allele of a gene on either the maternal or paternal chromosome, resulting in gene dosage regulation (9, 10). There are currently approximately 70 genes verified as imprinted in the human genome (http://www.geneimprint.com/). Loss of imprinting, due to aberration of epigenetic silencing and resulting in biallelic expression, is a phenomenon associated with developmental diseases and cancers (11–13). The best reported example of LOI as an epimutation is *IGF2* LOI in familial CRC patients. Lastly, the use of subtle shifts in the normal distribution of epigenetic variation cannot be called an "epimutation", but rather should be referred to as differentially methylated regions (DMRs).

2.2. IGF2 LOI in Colorectal Cancer

The insulin-like growth factor 2 (*IGF2*) gene is expressed from the paternal allele and is located within a cluster of imprinted genes on chromosome 11p15. Hypomethylation at a DMR of *IGF2*, named differentially methylated region 0 (DMR0), is associated with *IGF2* LOI in Wilm's tumour in which the maternal allele is also unmethylated, resulting in biallelic expression (14). Hypomethylation at this DMR0 region was also found in colorectal neoplasia (15). Interestingly, DMR0 hypomethylation was found not only in colorectal tumour tissue, but also in adenoma, normal colonic mucosa and peripheral blood lymphocytes (PBLs) of cancer patients (16). This was the first account of an epigenetic gene alteration found in the normal tissue and associated with cancer predisposition. The odds ratios of LOI in PBLs of patients with a personal history or family history of colorectal neoplasia were 21.7 and 5.15 times greater, respectively, than patients without personal or family history of neoplasia (16). Similar findings were reported by Woodson et al., who found a 24% greater incidence of LOI in the normal colonic mucosa of women with adenoma compared with women without any neoplasia, and a third study that reported an increase in LOI occurrence in both CRC and normal tissue and an association with poorly differentiated, mucinous cancer (17).

Whether *IGF2* LOI can be detected in PBLs remains disputed (16, 18). In a prospective study, Kaaks et al. failed to find any link between *IGF2* methylation and CRC in PBLs (19). Evidence for the implication of *IGF2* LOI in cancer was supported by the association of LOI with the congenital growth disorder Beckwith-Weidemann syndrome (BWS), in which developmental overgrowth is linked with increased risk of paediatric cancers, especially Wilm's tumour. However, Murrell et al. showed that BWS occurred by hypermethylation at both the *IGF2* and the nearby H19 DMR, with both DMRs on the paternal allele (20). This was in contrast with Wilm's tumour, in which increased methylation at the H19 locus was associated with decreased methylation at the *IGF2* locus, indicating that different methylation states occur at *IGF2* in BWS and cancer. Based on these findings, a new model for DNA methylation changes at *IGF2* was proposed, in which hypermethylation at H19 resulted in the de-methylation of the *IGF2* DMR0 in tumour tissue, but this change was absent in normal tissue and was not associated with *IGF2* LOI. *IGF2* hypomethylation was shown to be more prevalent than LOI per se and the two were not shown to be invariably associated in either colorectal or breast cancer (21). Hypomethylation was age-dependent and was not seen in the colonic mucosa suggesting that *IGF2* LOI is an acquired epigenetic event. Though no association between CRC risk and *IGF2* LOI was found in this study, hypomethylation was found in CRC, and to a lesser extent, breast tumour tissue compared with adjacent normal tissue patients, suggesting a possible role of *IGF2* hypomethylation (but not LOI) as a diagnostic marker. Cheng et al. recently reported a similar picture of *IGF2* hypomethylation in CRC tumour but not adjacent normal tissue (18). Consistent with this, global aberration of DNA methylation patterns in normal colonic tissue may represent an early tissue-specific event leading to colon cancer progression (22).

An important question in relation to any epigenetic biomarker is whether the lesion in question was inherited from the germline or acquired due to environmental exposure later in life. The findings of Cui et al. that *IGF2* LOI was associated with a family history of CRC and was found in normal tissue and PBLs strongly suggested a germline origin and a genetic basis for LOI (16). Using a twin study, Heijmans et al. showed that methylation at the *IGF2* DMR0 was 85% heritable (23). This large contribution of heritability and relatively low contribution of environmental and stochastic factors was similar in 196 adolescent and 176 middle-aged twins, indicating that methylation was not variable at different age groups. *IGF2* methylation has been shown to decrease with increasing age (21, 24). Environmental factors including smoking and BMI have been implicated in *IGF2* hypomethylation, though this association has been disputed (11, 13, 25). *IGF2* hypomethylation may result from exposure to adverse prenatal environmental conditions during epigenetic reprogramming as exposure to prenatal famine around the time of conception is associated with *IGF2* hypomethylation in later life (24). The absolute methylation variation at this locus was small, but extremely stable, being detectable 60 years later (24).

However, other evidence suggested that *IGF2* LOI and hypomethylation is an acquired event and may be environmentally affected. Four studies have failed to find any strong association between *IGF2* hypomethylation in normal tissue or PBLs of patients with Wilm's tumour (20), breast cancer (21) and CRC (19, 21, 25). Two studies failed to find any association with family history or in a prospective study (13, 21). Hunt et al. reported that an association between *IGF2* LOI in serum and CRC development was mainly found in patients whose samples were taken a maximum of 2 years before diagnosis (25).

In summary, *IGF2* DMR0 hypomethylation occurs in CRCs and methylation at this locus is variable in normal tissues, such as PBLs, and can be influenced by environmental exposures and age. While this has not been confirmed as an epimutation, these studies have provided a clear paradigm for identifying and validating novel epimutations and highlight some of the pitfalls and difficulties in confirming a germline origin for such epimutations.

2.3. *MLH1* and *MSH2* in Lynch Syndrome

Lynch syndrome is a familial mismatch repair deficiency (MMR) syndrome associated with microsatellite instability (MSI) and up to 75% lifetime risk of CRC and endometrial cancer (20, 26). Lynch syndrome includes features of early-onset, specific cancer types, MSI and family history (27). MSI is a direct result of insufficient MMR, due to biallelic inactivation of the MMR genes *MLH1*, *MSH2* and rarely *MSH6* or *PMS2* (26). In one third of clinical Lynch syndrome cases, however, no sequence mutations are identified, indicating that unidentified pathogenic lesions may exist (6). Epigenetic inactivation of MMR genes is also associated with MSI in CRCs as biallelic *MLH1* hypermethylation occurs in roughly 70% of MSI+sporadic CRCs (28, 29). *MLH1* methylation in normal colonic mucosa of sporadic colon cancer patients has been recently described, though this methylation is thought to be somatically acquired in the normal colonic mucosa, similarly to *IGF2* hypomethylation, with methylation typically absent in blood cells (21). *MSH2* methylation is less frequently associated with MSI+CRCs, but usually constitutes a "second hit" in patients with pre-existing germline *MSH2* mutations (29). Rare epimutations in both *MLH1* and *MSH2*, in which promoter methylation in normal tissue is associated with predisposition to Lynch syndrome, have been reported (30–33). The nature of these epimutations, regarding their germline origin and potential heritability, has been the subject of extensive investigation and debate, due to their potential implications for the current understanding of germline epigenetics and transgenerational inheritance of biological information (34–36).

Selecting CRC patients from families suspected of Lynch syndrome, Chan et al. identified a family with *MSH2* promoter methylation in normal colonic mucosa and PBLs, in the absence of identifiable *MSH2* (or other MMR gene) germline mutations (33). *MSH2* methylation was found in ten family members over three generations, showing autosomal-dominant heritability and was associated with disease risk, as three family members were affected by Lynch syndrome spectrum cancers. Extensive genetic screening had failed to identify any genetic determinant of *MSH2* methylation, therefore the possibility that this represented a heritable germline pure epimutation was proposed (33). However, autosomal dominance of the epimutation, coupled with tissue mosaicism of methylation, suggested linkage to an underlying genetic determinant in *cis* (36). *MSH2* methylation was later found to be linked to a deletion in the *TACSTD1* gene directly upstream of *MSH2*, in which deletion of the polyadenylation signal resulted in transcriptional read-through to *MSH2*, resulting in methylation of the *MSH2* promoter (37). In this instance, therefore, *MSH2* methylation represents an obligatory epimutation, as the epigenetic state is determined by an underlying, heritable genetic lesion (38).

In 1999, Deng et al. identified the region of the *MLH1* promoter that had previously been associated with tumour-specific hypermethylation and loss of expression in sporadic CRC (39). Complete methylation at this site (from −248 to −178 bp relative to ATG translation start site) was associated with loss of *MLH1* expression in CRC cell lines. Tumour-specific *MLH1* methylation is found in the majority of MMR-deficient CRCs without mutations in MMR genes and was strongly associated with female gender, late cancer onset and right-sided tumours (40). The first identification of a patient with *MLH1* in normal tissue PBLs was reported by Gazolli et al. (30). Using a heterozygous −93 bp G>A polymorphism, it was shown that CGI promoter methylation occurred exclusively on the G allele (30). Monoallelic methylation was shown to predispose to cancer as the "first hit", with the unmethylated allele being lost in the tumour due to loss of heterozygosity (LOH). As *MLH1* methylation occurred in normal tissue, it was speculated that it may have arisen in the germline. Since this initial report, 29 cases of *MLH1* methylation in normal tissue have been found (27–29, 31, 32, 41–46). In addition to PBLs, methylation was found in other normal tissue samples, such as buccal cells, normal colonic mucosa and saliva DNA. In five studies, methylation was detected in tissues (PBLs, buccal cells and hair follicles) derived from all three embryonic germ layers, suggesting that the epimutation was soma-wide and potentially of germline origin (29, 32, 41, 43, 44). Methylation in sperm cells was proposed as further evidence of a germline origin; however, this was subsequently acknowledged as an artefact due to contamination with somatic cells (29, 32, 41, 43, 44).

Mosaic methylation describes varying levels of methylation in the same tissue or cell type, due to somatic variation, and has been shown for *MLH1* (5, 46). Mosaic methylation may occur due to variation in the susceptibility of different alleles to methylation in the germline, clonal expansion of cells with full *MLH1* methylation or somatic loss of methylation (26, 46). The existence of mosaic methylation may cast doubt over the theory of germline origin of the epimutation, as a germline changes may be expected to occur in most or all cells in the body, as with germline mutations (26). However, it could equally be argued that the epimutation occurred soma-wide, but with mosaic de-methylation in a tissue- and cell-specific manner due to incomplete fidelity of maintenance methylation or by other mechanisms. The level of mosaicism in the *MLH1* epimutation contrasts with the tissue specificity seen in *MSH2* methylation, as mosaicism in the *MLH1* epimutation carriers refers to a state in which *MLH1* is unmethylated only in a small minority of alleles (36).

The most controversial issue relating to the *MLH1* epimutation relates to the question of its heritability (32, 35, 36). Only two studies, to date, have provided evidence for heritability (32, 46). Hitchins et al. showed inheritance of the epimutation from a constitutional epimutation carrier to her son. The mother (patient A) in this instance was a classic epimutation carrier with monoallelic *MLH1* methylation in normal tissue from all germ layers and early-onset, microsatellite unstable tumours of the endometrium and colon (32). *MLH1* methylation was detected in half of the chromosomes of one of patient A's three sons (patient II6-A) which was associated with loss of *MLH1* expression for the maternal allele. No methylation was seen in the spermatozoa of patient II6-A, consistent with erasure of the epimutation in his germline. Non-mendelian inheritance of the *MLH1* methylation was shown, as the epimutation was found in only one of patient A's three sons, though all shared the same *MLH1* haplotype. This non-mendelian transmission was in contrast with the autosomal-dominant inheritance of the *MSH2* epimutation reported by Chan et al. (33) and argued strongly against the presence of an underlying *cis* genetic lesion.

Further evidence for germline inheritance of the epimutation was provided by Morak et al. when they found 8% mosaic methylation in the blood of the mother of an epimutation carrier with colon cancer and 10% methylation in blood (46). No sign of disease, however, was seen in the mother at age 64. Absence of the epimutation in male gametes in this and another case, and the fact that both reports of epimutation inheritance occurred through the female germline, suggested that the *MLH1* epimutation occurs on the maternal allele only and may arise during oogenesis (32, 41, 46). Another potential mechanism could be maternal inheritance of miRNA or non-coding RNA species that influence the germline methylation patterns (47). *MLH1* methylation had not been tested in the female germline, however, due to the difficulty in isolating ova samples. As an alternative to heritability of *MLH1* methylation, "de novo" establishment of the epimutation has been demonstrated in a number of cases as parents and siblings of epimutation carriers were *MLH1* methylation-negative, even when SNP analysis revealed shared inheritance of the same *MLH1* allele (27, 29, 32, 44, 46). This would argue that the *MLH1* epimutation is a facilitated epimutation rather than a pure epimutation.

A basic profile of the pathogenicity and incidence of the *MLH1* epimutation can be drawn from the 12 studies to date (27–32, 41–46). It occurs in early-onset cancers with the average age at first cancer incidence being 37; however, this may be due to selection bias in the current studies, therefore the true population incidence and age range are currently unknown (28, 29). Of 94 highly selected candidates, Morak et al. found 12 (13%) were epimutation carriers (46). However, as few as 0.6% of patients selected for screening were found to be epimutation-positive when less stringent criteria (suspicion of HNPCC due to family history and lack of germline *MLH1* sequence mutations) were used (27, 44). Regardless of selection criteria, the *MLH1* germline epimutation appears to be rare (27, 44). The pathogenicity of the *MLH1* epimutation appears to be equivalent to *MLH1* sequence mutations, with most cases displaying multiple tumours of different histology within the Lynch syndrome spectrum (31, 41–43). Patients with mosaic *MLH1* methylation, associated with partial loss of *MLH1* expression, displayed an equally severe phenotype to those with full methylation, indicating the pathogenic properties of even lower (10–30%) levels of *MLH1* methylation are clinically significant (46).

A major potential confounding factor in all *MLH1* epimutations studies is the possibility that *MLH1* methylation is caused by an underlying genetic lesion in the germline (35). Methylation in the *MSH2*, *HBA2* and *DAPK1* genes results from underlying genetic lesions in *cis* (5, 37, 48). In Fragile X syndrome, methylation at the *FMR1* gene is caused by a CGG repeat expansion, which is heritable through the germline (48). The discovery of an underlying genetic factor causing promoter methylation in the *MSH2* gene which was previously thought to represent a germline epimutation suggests that the interpretation of the *MLH1* epimutation as being a *bona fida* germline epigenetic event is still questionable (35, 37). However, no consistent sequence alteration has been found to explain the *MLH1* epimutation, and until one is found, the possibility that *MLH1* represents a germline epimutation cannot be excluded.

As *MSH2* methylation is dependent on the formation of a *TACSTD1-MSH2* fusion transcript, methylation is expression-dependent and occurs at much greater levels in colonic mucosa, where *TACSTD1* is highly expressed, compared to blood (6, 37). Although *MLH1* methylation does not display the tissue-specific, mosaic patterns of methylation in *MSH2*, linkage of *MLH1* methylation with expression of an underlying genetic factor might explain the variegated pattern of *MLH1* methylation (36, 46). One study did find an example of constitutional *MLH1* methylation associated with a large genomic deletion of *MLH1* exon 1 and 2 associated with strong family history of CRC similar to genetic mutations (45). However, more examples are needed before any conclusions can be drawn.

As an alternative causative factor to genetic lesions in cis, germline mutations in trans-acting epigenetic modifiers, such as DNA methyltransferase enzymes, may result in aberrant DNA methylation of *MLH1* (5, 48). As *trans*-acting epigenetic mediators are not gene-specific, mutations in these genes would be likely to affect changes in methylation of multiple genes (5). In order to determine if the *MLH1* epimutation is caused by underlying genetic events, a genome-wide mutation screen of the *MLH1* epimutation cases would be required (5). Even in the case of such a screen, genetic heterogeneity between individuals would make it almost impossible to rule out the possibility of an underlying genetic event in the establishment of the *MLH1* epimutation (35, 36). Further work to establish the origin and incidence of this *MLH1* epimutation is required.

3. Peripheral Blood DNA Methylation Variation and Cancer Risk

There is a growing desire to identify peripheral blood-based biomarkers for disease risk and prognosis. Foremost is the desire to utilise the many resources of peripheral blood collections from around the world with sample sizes that are appropriate for these types of investigations. A number of studies have now found evidence for epigenetic traits in blood as potential cancer risk markers. To further this goal, it is imperative to first understand the normal pattern of DNA methylation. The most comprehensive map, to date, has been performed on a single Asian individual, at single base-pair resolution using the latest high-throughput sequencing-based approaches (49). Similarly to the first human genome sequence, this can serve as a first reference, but many more individuals will be needed to provide a comprehensive map of normal epigenetic variation with which to compare cancer-specific epigenetic traits.

3.1. BRCA1

BRCA1 is a breast cancer susceptibility gene frequently mutated in familial breast cancer and associated with distinct pathological features including high grade, immunohistochemical triple-negativity for ER, PR and HER-2 and TP53 positivity (50). Sporadic loss of *BRCA1*, due to promoter hypermethylation, occurs in 10–30% of breast tumours and can lead to a *BRCA1*-phenotype (51). Early studies of *BRCA1* promoter methylation failed to detect any methylation in blood or normal breast tissue (50, 52). However, three subsequent studies (51, 53, 54) have reported a modest association between *BRCA1* promoter methylation in blood and breast cancer risk and more significantly when restricted to just individuals with tumours that also contain *BRCA1* promoter hypermethylation. This suggested that methylation of *BRCA1* in blood corresponded to methylation of *BRCA1* in the tumour.

Among seven familial non-*BRCA1/2* breast cancer patients displaying BRCA1-pathology, Snell et al. reported three individuals with mosaic methylation in blood, one of which showed 12% methylation in blood and 6% methylation in buccal mucosa, inferring soma-wide methylation (53). Using a sensitive methylation detection technique (digital methylation-sensitive high-resolution melting), they detected ~1% methylation in the blood of two other patients. Somatic methylation in all three methylation carriers was associated with extensive, biallelic methylation of *BRCA1* in their tumour tissue. Two subsequent reports have validated the occurrence of mosaic methylation ranging between 1 and 17% methylation of *BRCA1* in blood, associated with highly methylated *BRCA1* in tumour DNA (51, 54). Two CpG sites within the *BRCA1* promoter region investigated by these studies have been reported as frequently methylated in both cancer cases and healthy controls; therefore, caution must be taken when assessing blood *BRCA1* methylation as “abnormal” (52).

It is the relative frequency, or a shift in the normal distribution, of *BRCA1* methylation in breast cancer cases compared with controls, rather than the presence of the mark, that is associated with breast cancer risk. Using an unbiased screening approach, Iwamoto et al. detected *BRCA1* methylation in 21.5% of breast cancer cases compared to 13.5% of controls, indicating a significantly higher incidence in breast cancer cases (51). Wong et al. found *BRCA1* methylation in 11% of early-onset breast cancers compared with 3.6% of controls, suggesting a lower overall incidence of hypermethylation, but confirming the significant difference between cases and controls (54). For both studies, blood *BRCA1* methylation was strongly associated with *BRCA1* methylation in tumours and with histological features of *BRCA1* inactivation, suggesting a pathogenic role (51, 54). According to these reports, *BRCA1* methylation in blood confers an 18-fold higher risk of developing tumours that display *BRCA1* methylation (51). Whether *BRCA1* promoter methylation is associated with overall breast cancer risk is unclear. Kontorovich et al. reported detectable *BRCA1* promoter methylation in 6% of a cohort of 230 Jewish individuals, but found no significant difference in the prevalence of methylation among cancer-affected *BRCA1/2* mutation carriers, unaffected *BRCA1/2* mutation carriers, sporadic breast cancers and healthy controls (55). Finding a similar incidence of *BRCA1* methylation in sporadic cancers cases and controls argues against its role as a breast cancer risk factor (55). Furthermore, methylation of *BRCA1* in blood or tumours does not appear to be associated with family history (51). Therefore, similarly to the variable disease penetrance of germline *BRCA1* mutations, it is possible that PBL methylation of *BRCA1* also may have variable influence on disease risk in different populations.

The emergence of *BRCA1* methylation in blood as a mechanism for breast cancer predisposition is a very recent advance, and therefore, further research is required to determine if mosaic methylation confers an inactivating lesion similar to the *BRCA1* mutation and if such a lesion can provide an explanation for any breast cancer cases with *BRCA1* deficiency features with no identified mutations.

3.2. ATM

We have previously shown that it was possible to identify DNA methylation differences in peripheral blood between breast cancer patients and controls within the *ATM* gene (56). We used a tiled microarray covering 17 candidate breast cancer genes to show two things. Firstly, in peripheral blood DNA, these genes were unmethylated and not variable between individuals at the promoter CGIs. This has important implications for the use of commercially available microarray platforms that only target gene promoters and suggested that the most appropriate method for this type of study is to use custom-designed arrays. Secondly, we established a general pattern in which methylation is low at gene promoters but increases and is more variable over the gene body, as has been recently validated (57). Furthermore, methylation variability between individuals (inter-individual methylation) was highest at intragenic repetitive elements. Interestingly, methylation variability at two intragenic repetitive elements within the *ATM* gene in blood was associated with breast cancer risk as methylation at these DMRs was significantly higher among 190 bilateral breast cancer patients than 190 age-matched healthy controls. Patients who displayed methylation within the highest quartile were at a threefold greater risk of breast cancer, and methylation was independent of known demographic risk factors such as BMI or menopausal status (56). Most significantly, this study identified intragenic repetitive element methylation in normal tissue as a risk factor for breast cancer and validated its potential for risk-biomarker development (58, 59).

An important consideration for the investigation of intragenic DNA methylation in cancer risk studies is the mechanistic role of methylation at these loci for transcription both in normal tissue and in cancer (58, 60). Whereas *ATM* hypermethylation appeared to be consistent with the long established role of methylation as a transcriptional repression mechanism, several investigators have reported a widespread association of intragenic methylation with regions of active transcription in the mammalian genome (56, 57, 60–62). The identification of intragenic methylation at both active and inactive loci seems inconsistent with a direct role in transcriptional regulation as is the genome-wide association of highest intragenic methylation with moderate transcription in human brain and plants (57, 60, 62, 63). Maunakea et al. have reported a role for intragenic methylation, in association with H3K4 trimethylation, in positively regulating transcription from cryptic alternative promoters within the gene body (57). Intragenic methylation in this instance was required for specific activation of alternative transcripts in a tissue- and context-specific manner (57). Important for effective communication regarding future study of intragenic DNA methylation will be the concise definition of intragenic DNA methylation, in order to differentiate between non-promoter methylation and methylation at discrete promoters within the transcribed sequence of a neighbouring gene or alternative start site. For this purpose, we propose excluding regions containing alternative start sites from the overall picture of intragenic methylation for a particular gene.

3.3. Genome-Wide Hypomethylation

Genome-wide hypomethylation is a common feature of cancer cells which may or may not have an active role in early carcinogenesis (64). We have previously shown using an in vitro model that genome-wide hypomethylation occurs at a late stage as a consequence of numerous genetic hits (65). Whether there is a predisposition to hypomethylation and, therefore, a predisposition to carcinogenesis is currently not known. Recent studies have found that hypomethylation in peripheral blood DNA may be useful as a risk marker.

Genome-wide DNA hypomethylation has been proposed to confer greater risk of breast, colorectal, bladder and head and neck cancers (66–70). Choi et al. showed that lower 5-mC levels were significantly associated with higher risk of developing breast cancer, in a dose-dependent and family history-associated manner (66). Recently, it has also been shown that *BRCA1*-linked breast tumours have very different genome-wide methylation patterns and present less promoter hypermethylation compared to *BRCA1* wild-type tumours (71). Such a scenario may represent an example of interactions between aberrant epigenetic events in cancer, such that reduced expression of *BRCA1* due to its hypermethylation in blood leads to global DNA hypomethylation, with downstream effects on global gene expression and other epigenetic mechanisms.

Other studies have shown similarly subtle differences between peripheral blood DNA methylation and risk of cancer. Using a global methyl cytosine assay, Moore et al. showed that hypomethylation of leukocyte DNA was associated with increased risk of bladder cancer with an adjusted odds-ratio of 2.5 (95% CI: 1.61–3.88) for the lowest quartile of methylation (68). Using LINE1 methylation as a surrogate marker for genome-wide DNA methylation, Wilhelm et. al. showed a less convincing picture for bladder cancer risk with the lowest decile, showing an odds-ratio of 1.8 (95% CI: 1.12–2.90), with no other decile showing any significant increase in cancer risk (72). A recent study by Teschendorff et al. used a genome-wide approach to identify a large number of CpG sites that were associated with ovarian cancer with an overall picture of lower methylation with higher risk (73). Importantly, this study also showed that the number of CpG sites associated with cancer were typically not within CGIs, supporting our own finding that the promoter CGIs were less likely to show DNA methylation variation between individuals. From these studies, it appears that using a quantitative method that measures the actual level of genomic methylation, such as high performance liquid chromatography (HPLC) or the luminometric methylation assay (LUMA, similar to an ELISA using the methylcytosine antibody), is far superior to using a surrogate assay such as using the LINE1 repetitive element with pyrosequencing. More work is required to determine the usefulness of genomic hypomethylation in blood as a cancer risk marker.

4. Factors That Influence Methylation Variation in Peripheral Blood DNA

4.1. Age

When considering peripheral blood leukocyte (PBL) DNA methylation variation as a risk marker, a number of potentially confounding factors need to be considered, the first of which is age (59, 74, 75). Age is associated with methylation increase at promoter CGIs and overall global decrease in methylation and may also be tissue-specific and dependent on environmental factors such as smoking and alcohol intake (74, 76). Therefore, determining associations between methylation variation and disease risk will need to be controlled for other confounding factors, for instance, age-matching of cases with controls and normalisation for various different environmental factors (59). In the first genome-wide study investigating the association of PBL DNA methylation with age, Rakyan et al. identified 213 loci at which a significant positive correlation was seen between DNA methylation and increasing age and 147 regions at which DNA methylation was inversely correlated with age (75). Ageing-associated differentially methylated regions (aDMR) displaying hypermethylation were enriched at promoter

CGIs with bivalent chromatin states, chromatin at which both active and repressive epigenetic marks are found simultaneously. Hypermethylation at such bivalent state promoters is frequently found in cancer, indicating a potential link between age-associated hypermethylation and disease (75, 77). Teschendorff et al. showed a similar age-related association with genes known to be polycomb group targets, possessing the H3K27me3 histone marks associated with inactive gene promoters (77). This study also showed an effect independent of tissue type, having observed the association in peripheral blood DNA, bone marrow mesenchymal stem cells as well as ovarian, lung and cervical cancer tissues. The effect size in these studies were quite small with an example of methylation values presented for peripheral blood in healthy controls ranging from a median of 19–21% (age range: 51–55 up to >75). This further shows that the effects detectable in peripheral blood will be subtle, but that significant associations can be identified. Age-associated methylation variation are also found at the imprinted genes *H19*, *LIT1*, *NESP55* and *SNRPN* in normal brain cortex and blood tissue, with tissue-dependent differences (78). Further evidence for the effects of age on DNA methylation is provided by the observation that discordance between the levels of DNA methylation in the blood of monozygotic twins is greater in older twin pairs than younger pairs and may also be affected by the degree of shared environment (79). As well as sporadic hypermethylation of tumour suppressor genes, age-associated changes in DNA methylation also include global hypomethylation, which is thought to contribute to genomic instability, increased mutation rate and to human cancer development (80–82). If age-associated methylation variation is a risk factor for cancer, this is an important consideration for experimental design, and studies of inter-individual epigenetic variation should ensure that all research subjects are age-matched where possible.

4.2. Tissue Heterogeneity

In studying inter-individual methylation variation, it is also important to account for the fact that a considerable proportion of DNA methylation is tissue-specific (83–85). Inter-individual epigenetic variation in normal individuals may be largely tissue-specific, as Kaminsky et al. have shown that most epigenetic variation between monozygotic and dizygotic twin pairs was greater in buccal epithelium than in blood of the same individuals (84). By developing a novel algorithm for the prediction of unmethylated regions of the human genome, Straussman et al. identified 750 loci, including 500 CGIs that showed tissue-specific methylation in only one of several different cell types (86). Methylation mapping of coding, non-coding and evolutionarily conserved sequences over chromosomes 6, 20 and 22 revealed that 22% amplicons analysed represented tissue-specific differentially methylated regions (tDMRs). Consistent with this figure, a more recent, genome-wide study has identified 18% of all CGIs included (representing the majority of annotated CGIs in the human genome) were identified as tDMRs, with significant methylation differences over 16 different tissues including between B- and T-lymphocytes (85). tDMRs appear to be enriched at genes of importance during development, especially transcription factors (83, 87), with unmethylated regions in foetal tissue often becoming methylated after differentiation (85). Tissue-specific methylation variation appears to show greater variability at intragenic regions than in promoters both on a locus-specific level and genome-wide (56, 83, 84). Within individual tissues, cell type-specific epigenetic variation may occur and is an important consideration when investigating inter-individual epigenetic variation, as methylation variation between different individual's tissue samples may reflect differences in the proportions of different cell fractions within their tissue samples rather than differences in methylation overall (56, 84). It is important, therefore, to test each blood cell subtype at the loci of interest to determine if each subtype has similar methylation patterns to that in whole blood. An alternative method would be to include blood cell counts, if available, as a factor in the analysis. Lastly, tissue-specific epigenetic variation provides strong evidence of independence of epigenetic variation from the genetic background as different tissue types are genetically identical but phenotypically and epigenetically diverse (84). It is important to determine whether an epimutation occurs in a single, multiple or all tissues, as soma-wide occurrence of an epimutation may suggest an early developmental or germline origin and predisposition to disease in multiple tissues (41), whereas tissue specificity is consistent with somatic acquisition of the abnormality (32, 33, 36).

5. Mechanisms: Cause and Effect of DNA Methylation Variability

5.1. Developmental and Environmental Causes of DNA Methylation Variation in Blood

There is considerable evidence that the human epigenome is sensitive to environmental influence during prenatal development and that environmental stress during critical periods of epigenetic reprogramming may introduce stable epigenetic variations that may contribute to adult phenotype and disease susceptibility (24, 76, 88). The long-term adverse affects of prenatal nutritional stress on the epigenome were demonstrated by investigating the effect of prenatal famine on *IGF2* and six other loci (89). Periconceptual exposure to famine is associated with methylation variation at *IGF2*, *IL10*, *GNASAS*, *INSIGF*, *LEP*, *ABCA1* and *MEG3* (89). Methylation variation at these loci was low, but detectable 60 years later, indicating long-term stability (89). Interestingly, hypermethylation and hypomethylation events were found, which was not consistent with the model in which hypomethylation results simply from the unavailability of methyl donors in the diet (89). Though prenatal famine effects on the epigenome did not show any phenotypic associations, nutrition during early development can affect the postnatal phenotype (90). Furthermore, the effects of maternal diet may have implications for health in later life, as birth weight is a candidate risk factor for some complex disease, including cancer (91–93). Animal studies have further supported an important role of maternal diet, as diets deficient in methyl groups led to extreme phenotypic abnormalities and greater disease predisposition in their exposed young (94, 95). Apart from developmental nutrition, the contribution to disease by potentially harmful lifestyle factors such as smoking and alcohol consumption is potentially epigenetically mediated (96, 97). Developmental exposure to carcinogenic toxins in the prenatal or early developmental environment may introduce stable epigenetic changes that confer cancer risk (98, 99). Prenatal exposure to the synthetic oestrogen diethylstilbestrol (DES), regrettably prescribed to expecting mothers between 1947 and 1971 under the false impression that it prevented miscarriage, is associated with development of reproductive and urethrogenital abnormalities, infertility in both males and females and risk of clear cell adenocarcinoma of the vagina and cervix in women (99–101). Neonatal DES exposure in animal models has revealed aberrant DNA hypomethylation at the oestrogen response element of the Lactoferrin gene and exon 4 hypomethylation of c-fos, associated with over-expression of both genes (99, 101). Emerging evidence for transgenerational effects of DES exposure may indicate a germline affect of DES exposure, though it is not clear if this is via an epigenetic mechanism (101). The association between epigenetic changes at Lactoferrin and oestrogen regulation is consistent with a model in which the developing epigenome is sensitive to changes in the prenatal and developmental endocrine environment, especially with respect to estrogens (92, 99, 100, 102).

5.2. Non-coding RNA-Mediated Epigenetic Silencing as a Cause of Variation

Antisense-mediated silencing of *p15* and the α-globin gene *HBA2* has been demonstrated both in vitro and in vivo, in embryonic stem cells (ESCs) (103, 104). Silencing of *p15* was shown to be initiated in ESCs through heterochromatin formation and histone modifications, followed by DNA methylation of the *p15* during early differentiation (103). Differentiation-dependent acquisition of methylation, via antisense-mediated silencing of the α-globin gene *HBA2*, in an ESC model indicated that methylation occurred as a secondary event (104). Transcriptional read-through from the upstream *LUC7L* gene, caused by a deletion of part of α-globin gene cluster and the polyadenylation signal *LUC7L*, led to generation of antisense transcript and silencing of *HBA2* in ESCs, followed by *HBA2* methylation (104). Epigenetic silencing in this instance was not dependent on the generation of *LUC7L* antisense, as *HBA2* silencing was reproduced when *LUC7L* was replaced with ubiquitin, indicating that antisense RNA may have a general role in developmental epigenetic silencing (104). This RNA-mediated mechanism appears to also be involved in the *MSH2* epimutation described earlier. Antisense RNA is a strong candidate mechanism for epigenetic silencing during early development, as it is well established that genomic imprinting and X-chromosome inactivation, two examples of epigenetic silencing phenomena established during early development, are dependent on antisense RNA for their specification (105). Furthermore, bioinformatic and experimental manipulation of overlapping RNA pairs suggests that most transcribed sequences in the mammalian transcriptome are matched by one or more antisense partners that are involved in their transcriptional regulation (105). The functions of most of these antisense transcripts remain unknown (106), though mitotic heritability of histone modifications is thought to be dependent on non-coding RNA machinery (58).

Taken together, these studies indicate that establishment of DNA methylation likely represents a consequence, rather than a cause, of heterochromatin formation and that association of antisense RNA to DNA may be the initial trigger for epigenetic silencing (103). If DNA methylation is a downstream event in gene silencing, it would seem unlikely that transgenerational inheritance of methylation alone could confer soma-wide silencing of *MLH1*, but rather transgenerational or maternal inheritance of non-coding RNAs. It is more likely that constitutional methylation of *MLH1* and other loci are established during ESC differentiation, as a result of heterochromatin formation in undifferentiated ESCs and this represents an important paradigm for constitutional epimutations. Therefore, it is worth considering that any epigenetic variability identified as candidate cancer risk markers may be caused by an underlying RNA-mediated mechanism.

5.3. Copy Number Variations as Potential Determinants of Epigenetic Specification

Copy number variation (CNV), leading to transcriptional read-through and generation of abnormal transcripts, has been shown to cause abnormal epigenetic silencing of *HBA2*, *MSH2* and *PTRJ7* (37, 38, 104). Abrogation of transcriptional termination from neighbouring genes, due to deletion of duplication of polyadenylation signals, leads to epigenetic silencing of these genes, in the absence of any mutation within the coding sequence of the silenced genes themselves (38). Whereas the extent to which CNV-associated epigenetic silencing contributes to cancer risk is yet to be established (38), constitutional CNVs are thought to represent potential risk markers for cancer predisposition (107). It is, therefore, important to consider copy number analysis in parallel to discovery of epimutations.

5.4. Intragenic DNA Methylation as a Candidate for Risk Biomarkers

Most research focusing on DNA methylation variation in cancer has focused on the promoter CGIs of genes. Reasons for this include the historical identification of methylation at the promoters of tumour suppressor genes in a wide variety of cancers and the mechanistic association of methylation with transcriptional repression at these loci (61, 108). Investigation of constitutional methylation in normal tissue in familial cancers, indicative of germline or constitutional epigenetic abnormality, has only identified four examples of hypermethylation events in tumour suppressor gene promoters, including *MLH1* (30), *MSH2* (33), *BRCA1* (53) and very recently *PTPRJ* (38). Several studies suggest that these epimutations are very rare events (27, 38, 50, 52). This rarity may reflect the overall scarcity of DNA methylation at promoter CGIs, with as little as 2% of CpG sites within promoter CGIs in the human genome being methylated, compared with 34% CpG sites within intragenic regions of "gene-bodies" (57). Given the higher levels of methylation within gene bodies, and specifically intronic repetitive elements, there is a greater potential for methylation variability between individuals which may reflect variability in susceptibility to diseases like cancer in which epigenomic dysregulation is so pronounced (Fig. 2) (58). Therefore, gene bodies may represent better candidate loci for constitutional epimutation discovery and biomarker development (56, 58, 109).

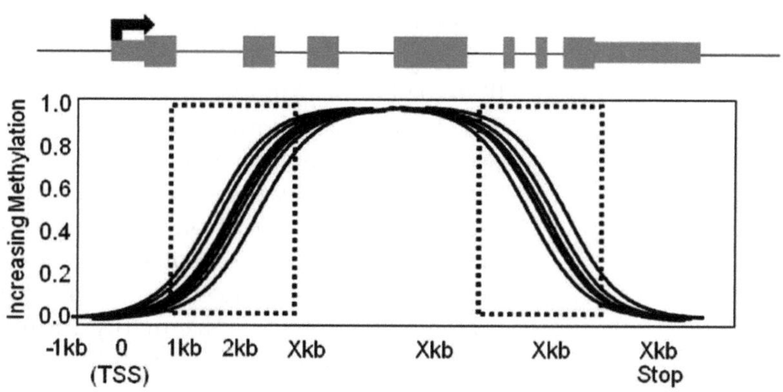

Fig. 2. Intragenic methylation has a greater potential for inter-individual variation for most actively expressed genes. The majority of active genes are unmethylated at the transcription start site (TSS) and highly methylated through the middle of the gene. The genomic regions of transition from unmethylated to methylated represent the areas of most variability.

6. Protocols for Discovery and Validation of Epigenetic Biomarkers

Since the sequencing of the human genome, there have been a large amount of GWAS for many common diseases including cancer. However, it is becoming increasingly clear that these will not identify many common variants for common diseases that will be useful for personalised disease risk prediction. A recent analysis of ten common genetic variants associated with breast cancer risk has shown that the addition of the genetic markers into the pre-existing risk assessment models only provided a very modest increase in performance (110). Therefore, there is hope that epigenetic epidemiology studies, including Epigenome-Wide Association Studies (EWAS), may identify risk biomarkers that can be used for personalised disease risk prediction (59). However, while GWAS studies all have very similar experimental approaches and clear statistical analysis plans, EWAS studies are not so well developed. There are many genome-wide DNA methylation-based approaches, many epigenetic marks that might be investigated and many different regions of the genome that might be interrogated (111). The methods can be broadly classified as based on enrichment of methylated DNA from genomic DNA or based on bisulphite modification of genomic DNA. The DNA can be interrogated via microarray hybridization or via high-throughput sequencing methods such as the Roche-454 or Illumina-Solexa methods. The choice of which method to use depends on cost, numbers of samples to be analysed, desired coverage and validation success rate. The most widely used approach in the last few years for DNA methylation profiling using bisulphite modification has been the use of the Illumina HumanMethylation27 BeadChip. The main disadvantage to this approach is the very low coverage, with generally only two CpG sites interrogated per gene; however, this array has now been superseded by the 450K Beadchip. Given the cost per sample and the requirement of only 500 ng of bisulphite-treated DNA, this array is likely to become the most appropriate and widely used method for genome-wide discovery projects. It is vital that any identified DNA methylation mark is validated using independent quantitative methods such as Pyrosequencing or Epityper. Both of these methods rely on bisulphite conversion of the genomic DNA, followed by PCR amplification of regions of interest and quantitative sequencing. The optimal approach to statistical analysis, as well as the understanding of the level of epigenetic variability that may be biologically significant and associated with risk, remain to be established, and are important considerations for future research.

7. Conclusions

We anticipate that current technology will allow rapid identification and validation of many epigenetic cancer risk biomarkers. The studies conducted thus far have highlighted the difficulty in proving the existence of germline epimutations, the rarity of which suggests that they will not be useful for population-based risk prediction. It is, therefore, more prudent to identify common epigenetic marks or shifts in the normal distribution of epigenetic variation as potential risk markers. Incorporating new information such as this, if independent from other risk factors, can only improve personalised cancer risk modelling.

Acknowledgements

This work was supported by Breast Cancer Campaign UK. JF is a Breast Cancer Campaign Fellow.

References

1. Gail, M.H., Brinton, L.A., Byar, D.P., Corle, D.K., Green, S.B., Schairer, C., and Mulvihill, J.J. (1989) Projecting individualized probabilities of developing breast cancer for white females who are being examined annually. *J Natl Cancer Inst* 81, 1879–1886.
2. Amir, E., Evans, D.G., Shenton, A., Lalloo, F., Moran, A., Boggis, C., Wilson, M., and Howell, A. (2003) Evaluation of breast cancer risk assessment packages in the family history evaluation and screening programme. *J Med Genet* 40, 807–814.
3. Varghese, J.S., and Easton, D.F. (2010) Genome-wide association studies in common cancers—what have we learnt? *Curr Opin Genet Dev* 20, 201–209.
4. Richards, E.J. (2006) Inherited epigenetic variation—revisiting soft inheritance. *Nat Rev Genet* 7, 395–401.
5. Hitchins, M.P. and Ward, R.L. (2009) Constitutional (germline) MLH1 epimutation as an aetiological mechanism for hereditary non-polyposis colorectal cancer. *Journal of Medical Genetics* 46, 793–802.
6. Hesson, L.B., Hitchins, M.P., and Ward, R.L. (2010) Epimutations and cancer predisposition: importance and mechanisms. *Curr Opin Genet Dev* 20, 290–298.
7. Morgan, H.D., Sutherland, H.G., Martin, D.I., and Whitelaw, E. (1999) Epigenetic inheritance at the agouti locus in the mouse. *Nat Genet* 23, 314–318.
8. Rakyan, V.K., Chong, S., Champ, M.E., Cuthbert, P.C., Morgan, H.D., Luu, K.V., and Whitelaw, E. (2003) Transgenerational inheritance of epigenetic states at the murine Axin(Fu) allele occurs after maternal and paternal transmission. *Proc Natl Acad Sci U S A* 100, 2538–2543.
9. Reik, W., Constancia, M., Dean, W., Davies, K., Bowden, L., Murrell, A., Feil, R., Walter, J., and Kelsey, G. (2000) Igf2 imprinting in development and disease. *Int J Dev Biol* 44, 145–150.
10. Feinberg, A.P., Kalikin, L.M., Johnson, L.A., and Thompson, J.S. (1994) Loss of imprinting in human cancer. *Cold Spring Harb. Sym.* 59, 357–364.
11. Cruz-Correa, M., Cui, H., Giardiello, F.M., Powe, N.R., Hylind, L., Robinson, A., Hutcheon, D.F., Kafonek, D.R., Brandenburg, S., Wu, Y., He, X., and Feinberg, A.P. (2004) Loss of imprinting of insulin growth factor II gene: a potential heritable biomarker for colon neoplasia predisposition. *Gastroenterology* 126, 964–970.

12. Reik, W. (2007) Stability and flexibility of epigenetic gene regulation in mammalian development. *Nature* 447, 425–432.
13. Liou, J.M., Wu, M.S., Lin, J.T., Wang, H.P., Huang, S.P., Chiu, H.M., Lee, Y.C., Lin, Y.B., Shun, C.T., and Liang, J.T. (2007) Loss of imprinting of insulin-like growth factor II is associated with increased risk of proximal colon cancer. *Eur J Cancer* 43, 1276–1282.
14. Sullivan, M.J., Taniguchi, T., Jhee, A., Kerr, N., and Reeve, A.E. (1999) Relaxation of IGF2 imprinting in Wilms tumours associated with specific changes in IGF2 methylation. *Oncogene* 18,7527–7534.
15. Cui, H., Onyango, P., Brandenburg, S., Wu, Y., Hsieh, C.L., and Feinberg, A.P. (2002) Loss of imprinting in colorectal cancer linked to hypomethylation of H19 and IGF2. *Cancer Res* 62, 6442–6446.
16. Cui, H., Cruz-Correa, M., Giardiello, F.M., Hutcheon, D.F., Kafonek, D.R., Brandenburg, S., Wu, Y., He, X., Powe, N.R., and Feinberg, A.P. (2003) Loss of IGF2 Imprinting: A Potential Marker of Colorectal Cancer Risk. *Science* 299, 1753–1755.
17. Woodson, K., Flood, A., Green, L., Tangrea, J.A., Hanson, J., Cash, B., Schatzkin, A., and Schoenfeld, P. (2004) Loss of Insulin-Like Growth Factor-II Imprinting and the Presence of Screen-Detected Colorectal Adenomas in Women. *Journal of the National Cancer Institute* 96, 407–410.
18. Cheng, Y.W., Idrees, K., Shattock, R., Khan, S.A., Zeng, Z., Brennan, C.W., Paty, P., and Barany, F. (2010) Loss of imprinting and marked gene elevation are 2 forms of aberrant IGF2 expression in colorectal cancer. *Int J Cancer* 127, 568–577.
19. Kaaks, R., Stattin, P., Villar, S., Poetsch, A.R., Dossus, L., Nieters, A., Riboli, E., Palmqvist, R., Hallmans, G., Plass, C., and Friesen, M.D. (2009) Insulin-like Growth Factor-II Methylation Status in Lymphocyte DNA and Colon Cancer Risk in the Northern Sweden Health and Disease Cohort. *Cancer Research* 69, 5400–5405.
20. Murrell, A., Ito, Y., Verde, G., Huddleston, J., Woodfine, K., Silengo, M.C., Spreafico, F., Perotti, D., De Crescenzo, A., Sparago, A., Cerrato, F., and Riccio, A. (2008) Distinct methylation changes at the IGF2-H19 locus in congenital growth disorders and cancer. *PLoS One* 3, e1849.
21. Ito, Y., Koessler, T., Ibrahim, A.E., Rai, S., Vowler, S.L., Abu-Amero, S., Silva, A.L., Maia, A.T., Huddleston, J.E., Uribe-Lewis, S., Woodfine, K., Jagodic, M., Nativio, R., Dunning, A., Moore, G., Klenova, E., Bingham, S., Pharoah, P.D., Brenton, J.D., Beck, S., Sandhu, M.S., and Murrell, A. (2008) Somatically acquired hypomethylation of IGF2 in breast and colorectal cancer. *Hum Mol Genet* 17, 2633–2643.
22. Belshaw, N.J., Pal, N., Tapp, H.S., Dainty, J.R., Lewis, M.P., Williams, M.R., Lund, E.K., and Johnson, I.T. (2010) Patterns of DNA methylation in individual colonic crypts reveal aging and cancer-related field defects in the morphologically normal mucosa. *Carcinogenesis* 31, 1158–1163.
23. Heijmans, B.T., Kremer, D., Tobi, E.W., Boomsma, D.I., and Slagboom, P.E. (2007) Heritable rather than age-related environmental and stochastic factors dominate variation in DNA methylation of the human IGF2/H19 locus. *Human Molecular Genetics* 16, 547–554.
24. Heijmans, B.T., Tobi, E.W., Stein, A.D., Putter, H., Blauw, G.J., Susser, E.S., Slagboom, P.E., and Lumey, L.H. (2008) Persistent epigenetic differences associated with prenatal exposure to famine in humans. *Proceedings of the National Academy of Sciences* 105, 17046–17049.
25. Hunt, K.J., Toniolo, P., Akhmedkhanov, A., Lukanova, A., Dechaud, H., Rinaldi, S., Zeleniuch-Jacquotte, A., Shore, R.E., Riboli, E., and Kaaks, R. (2002) Insulin-like Growth Factor II and Colorectal Cancer Risk in Women. *Cancer Epidemiology Biomarkers & Prevention* 11, 901–905.
26. Cropley, J.E., Martin, D.I., and Suter, C.M. (2008) Germline epimutation in humans. *Pharmacogenomics* 9, 1861–1868.
27. Niessen, R.C., R.M. Hofstra, Westers, H., Ligtenberg, M.J., Kooi, K., Jager, P.O., de Groote, M.L., Dijkhuizen, T., Olderode-Berends, M.J., Hollema, H., Kleibeuker, J.H., and Sijmons, R.H. (2009) Germline hypermethylation of MLH1 and EPCAM deletions are a frequent cause of Lynch syndrome. *Genes Chromosomes Cancer* 48, 737–744.
28. van Roon, E.H., van Puijenbroek, M., Middeldorp, A., van Eijk, R., de Meijer, E.J., Erasmus, D., Wouters, K.A., van Engeland, M., Oosting, J., Hes, F.J., Tops, C.M., van Wezel, T., Boer, J.M., and Morreau, H. (2010) Early onset MSI-H colon cancer with MLH1 promoter methylation, is there a genetic predisposition? *BMC Cancer* 10, 180.
29. Goel, A., Nguyen, T.P., Leung, H.C., Nagasaka, T., Rhees, J., Hotchkiss, E., Arnold, M., Banerji, P., Koi, M., Kwok, C.T., Packham, D., Lipton, L., Boland, C.R., Ward, R.L., and Hitchins, M.P. (2010) De novo constitutional

MLH1 epimutations confer early-onset colorectal cancer in two new sporadic Lynch syndrome cases, with derivation of the epimutation on the paternal allele in one. *Int J Cancer*

30. Gazzoli, I., Loda, M., Garber, J., Syngal, S., and Kolodner, R.D. (2002) A hereditary nonpolyposis colorectal carcinoma case associated with hypermethylation of the MLH1 gene in normal tissue and loss of heterozygosity of the unmethylated allele in the resulting microsatellite instability-high tumor. *Cancer Res* 62, 3925–3928.
31. Valle, L., Carbonell, P., Fernandez, V., Dotor, A.M., Sanz, M., Benitez, J., and Urioste, M. (2007) MLH1 germline epimutations in selected patients with early-onset non-polyposis colorectal cancer. *Clin Genet* 71, 232–237.
32. Hitchins, M.P., Wong, J.J., Suthers, G., Suter, C.M., Martin, D.I., Hawkins, N.J., and Ward, R.L. (2007) Inheritance of a cancer-associated MLH1 germ-line epimutation. *N Engl J Med* 356, 697–705.
33. Chan, T.L., Yuen, S.T., Kong, C.K., Chan, Y.W., Chan, A.S., Ng, W.F., Tsui, W.Y., Lo, M.W., Tam, W.Y., Li, V.S., and Leung, S.Y. (2006) Heritable germline epimutation of MSH2 in a family with hereditary nonpolyposis colorectal cancer. *Nat Genet* 38, 1178–1183.
34. Horsthemke, B. (2007) Heritable germline epimutations in humans. *Nat Genet* 39, 573–574; author reply 575–576.
35. Chong, S., Youngson, N.A., and Whitelaw, E. (2007) Heritable germline epimutation is not the same as transgenerational epigenetic inheritance. *Nat Genet* 39, 574–575.
36. Suter, C.M. and Martin, D.I. (2007) Inherited epimutation or a haplotypic basis for the propensity to silence? *Nat Genet* 39, 573; author reply 576.
37. Ligtenberg, M.J., Kuiper, R.P., Chan, T.L., Goossens, M., Hebeda, K.M., Voorendt, M., Lee, T.Y., Bodmer, D., Hoenselaar, E., Hendriks-Cornelissen, S.J., Tsui, W.Y., Kong, C.K., Brunner, H.G., van Kessel, A.G., Yuen, S.T., van Krieken, J.H., Leung, S.Y., and Hoogerbrugge, N. (2009) Heritable somatic methylation and inactivation of MSH2 in families with Lynch syndrome due to deletion of the 3′ exons of TACSTD1. *Nat Genet* 41, 112–117.
38. Venkatachalam, R., Ligtenberg, M.J., Hoogerbrugge, N., Schackert, H.K., Gorgens, H., Hahn, M.M., Kamping, E.J., Vreede, L., Hoenselaar, E., van der Looij, E., Goossens, M., Churchman, M., Carvajal-Carmona, L., Tomlinson, I.P., de Bruijn, D.R., Van Kessel, A.G., and Kuiper, R.P. (2010) Germline Epigenetic Silencing of the Tumor Suppressor Gene PTPRJ in Early-Onset Familial Colorectal Cancer. *Gastroenterology*
39. Deng, G., Chen, A., Hong, J., Chae, H.S., and Kim, Y.S. (1999) Methylation of CpG in a small region of the hMLH1 promoter invariably correlates with the absence of gene expression. *Cancer Res* 59, 2029–2033.
40. Poynter, J.N., Siegmund, K.D., Weisenberger, D.J., Long, T.I., Thibodeau, S.N., Lindor, N., Young, J., Jenkins, M.A., Hopper, J.L., Baron, J.A., Buchanan, D., Casey, G., Levine, A.J., Le Marchand, L., Gallinger, S., Bapat, B., Potter, J.D., Newcomb, P.A., Haile, R.W., and Laird, P.W. (2008) Molecular characterization of MSI-H colorectal cancer by MLHI promoter methylation, immunohistochemistry, and mismatch repair germline mutation screening. *Cancer Epidemiol Biomarkers Prev* 17, 3208–3215.
41. Suter, C.M., Martin, D.I., and Ward, R.L. (2004) Germline epimutation of MLH1 in individuals with multiple cancers. *Nat Genet* 36, 497–501.
42. Miyakura, Y., Sugano, K., Akasu, T., Yoshida, T., Maekawa, M., Saitoh, S., Sasaki, H., Nomizu, T., Konishi, F., Fujita, S., Moriya, Y., and Nagai, H. (2004) Extensive but hemiallelic methylation of the hMLH1 promoter region in early-onset sporadic colon cancers with microsatellite instability. *Clin Gastroenterol Hepatol* 2, 147–156.
43. Martin, D.I., Ward, R., and Suter, C.M. (2005) Germline epimutation: A basis for epigenetic disease in humans. *Ann N Y Acad Sci* 1054, 68–77.
44. Hitchins, M., Williams, R., Cheong, K., Halani, N., Lin, V., Packham, D., Ku, S., Buckle, A., Hawkins, N., Burn, J., Gallinger, S., Goldblatt, J., Kirk, J., Tomlinson, I., Scott, R., Spigelman, A., Suter, C., Martin, D., Suthers, G., and Ward, R. (2005) MLH1 germline epimutations as a factor in hereditary nonpolyposis colorectal cancer. *Gastroenterology* 129, 1392–1399.
45. Gylling, A., Ridanpaa, M., Vierimaa, O., Aittomaki, K., Avela, K., Kaariainen, H., Laivuori, H., Poyhonen, M., Sallinen, S.L., Wallgren-Pettersson, C., Jarvinen, H.J., Mecklin, J.P., and Peltomaki, P. (2009) Large genomic rearrangements and germline epimutations in Lynch syndrome. *Int J Cancer* 124, 2333–2340.
46. Morak, M., Schackert, H.K., Rahner, N., Betz, B., Ebert, M., Walldorf, C., Royer-Pokora, B., Schulmann, K., von Knebel-Doeberitz, M., Dietmaier, W., Keller, G., Kerker, B., Leitner, G., and Holinski-Feder,

E. (2008) Further evidence for heritability of an epimutation in one of 12 cases with MLH1 promoter methylation in blood cells clinically displaying HNPCC. *Eur J Hum Genet* 16, 804–811.

47. Teixeira, F.K., Heredia, F., Sarazin, A., Roudier, F., Boccara, M., Ciaudo, C., Cruaud, C., Poulain, J., Berdasco, M., Fraga, M.F., Voinnet, O., Wincker, P., Esteller, M., and Colot, V. (2009) A role for RNAi in the selective correction of DNA methylation defects. *Science* 323, 1600–1604.
48. Dobrovic, A. and Kristensen, L.S. (2009) DNA methylation, epimutations and cancer predisposition. *Int J Biochem Cell Biol* 41, 34–39.
49. Li, Y., Zhu, J., Tian, G., Li, N., Li, Q., Ye, M., Zheng, H., Yu, J., Wu, H., Sun, J., Zhang, H., Chen, Q., Luo, R., Chen, M., He, Y., Jin, X., Zhang, Q., Yu, C., Zhou, G., Sun, J., Huang, Y., Zheng, H., Cao, H., Zhou, X., Guo, S. *et al.*, (2010) The DNA methylome of human peripheral blood mononuclear cells. *PLoS Biol* 8, e1000533.
50. Alvarez, S., Diaz-Uriarte, R., Osorio, A., Barroso, A., Melchor, L., Paz, M.F., Honrado, E., Rodriguez, R., Urioste, M., Valle, L., Diez, O., Cigudosa, J.C., Dopazo, J., Esteller, M., and Benitez, J. (2005) A predictor based on the somatic genomic changes of the BRCA1/BRCA2 breast cancer tumors identifies the non-BRCA1/BRCA2 tumors with BRCA1 promoter hypermethylation. *Clin Cancer Res* 11, 1146–1153.
51. Iwamoto, T., Yamamoto, N., Taguchi, T., Tamaki, Y., and Noguchi, S. (2010) BRCA1 promoter methylation in peripheral blood cells is associated with increased risk of breast cancer with BRCA1 promoter methylation. *Breast Cancer Research and Treatment* 1–9.
52. Chen, Y., Toland, A., McLennan, J., Fridlyand, J., Crawford, B., Costello, J., and Ziegler, J. (2006) Lack of germ-line promoter methylation in BRCA1-negative families with familial breast cancer. *Genet Test* 10, 281–284.
53. Snell, C., Krypuy, M., Wong, E.M., Loughrey, M.B., and Dobrovic, A. (2008) BRCA1 promoter methylation in peripheral blood DNA of mutation negative familial breast cancer patients with a BRCA1 tumour phenotype. *Breast Cancer Res* 10, R12.
54. Wong, E.M., Southey, M.C., Fox, S.B., Brown, M.A., Dowty, J.G., Jenkins, M.A., Giles, G.G., Hopper, J., and Dobrovic, A. (2011) Constitutional Methylation of the BRCA1 promoter is specifically associated with BRCA1 mutation-associated pathology in early-onset breast cancer. *Cancer Prev Res (Phila)* 4, 23–33.
55. Kontorovich, T., Cohen, Y., Nir, U., and Friedman, E. (2009) Promoter methylation patterns of ATM, ATR, BRCA1, BRCA2 and p53 as putative cancer risk modifiers in Jewish BRCA1/BRCA2 mutation carriers. *Breast Cancer Res Treat* 116, 195–200.
56. Flanagan, J.M., Munoz-Alegre, M., Henderson, S., Tang, T., Sun, P., Johnson, N., Fletcher, O., dos Santos Silva, I., Peto, J., Boshoff, C., Narod, S., and Petronis, A. (2009) Gene-body hypermethylation of ATM in peripheral blood DNA of bilateral breast cancer patients. *Human Molecular Genetics* 18, 1332–1342.
57. Maunakea, A.K., Nagarajan, R.P., Bilenky, M., Ballinger, T.J., D'Souza, C., Fouse, S.D., Johnson, B.E., Hong, C., Nielsen, C., Zhao, Y., Turecki, G., Delaney, A., Varhol, R., Thiessen, N., Shchors, K., Heine, V.M., Rowitch, D.H., Xing, X., Fiore, C., Schillebeeckx, M., Jones, S.J., Haussler, D., Marra, M.A., Hirst, M., Wang, T. *et al.*, (2010) Conserved role of intragenic DNA methylation in regulating alternative promoters. *Nature* 466, 253–257.
58. Flanagan, J.M. and Wild, L. (2007) An epigenetic role for noncoding RNAs and intragenic DNA methylation. *Genome Biol* 8, 307.
59. Flanagan, J.M. (2010) Human Methylome Variation and the Rise of Epigenetic Epidemiology. *Current Pharmacogenomics and Personalized Medicine* 8, 89–91.
60. Aran, D., Toperoff, G., Rosenberg, M., and Hellman, A. (2011) Replication timing-related and gene body-specific methylation of active human genes. *Hum Mol Genet* 20, 670–680.
61. Appanah, R., Dickerson, D.R., Goyal, P., Groudine, M., and Lorincz, M.C. (2007) An unmethylated 3′ promoter-proximal region is required for efficient transcription initiation. *PLoS Genet* 3, e27.
62. Wu, X., Rauch, T.A., Zhong, X., Bennett, W.P., Latif, F., Krex, D., and Pfeifer, G.P. (2010) CpG island hypermethylation in human astrocytomas. *Cancer Res* 70, 2718–2727.
63. Zilberman, D., Gehring, M., Tran, R.K., Ballinger, T., and Henikoff, S. (2007) Genome-wide analysis of Arabidopsis thaliana DNA methylation uncovers an interdependence between methylation and transcription. *Nat Genet* 39, 61–69.
64. Wild, L. and Flanagan, J.M. (2010) Genome-wide hypomethylation in cancer may be a passive consequence of transformation. *Biochim Biophys Acta* 1806, 50–57.
65. Wild, L., Funes, J.M., Boshoff, C., and Flanagan, J.M. (2010) In vitro transformation

of mesenchymal stem cells induces gradual genomic hypomethylation. *Carcinogenesis* 31, 1854–1862.

66. Choi, J.Y., James, S.R., Link, P.A., McCann, S.E., Hong, C.C., Davis, W., Nesline, M.K., Ambrosone, C.B., and Karpf, A.R. (2009) Association between global DNA hypomethylation in leukocytes and risk of breast cancer. *Carcinogenesis* 30, 1889–1897.
67. Lim, U., Flood, A., Choi, S.W., Albanes, D., Cross, A.J., Schatzkin, A., Sinha, R., Katki, H.A., Cash, B., Schoenfeld, P., and Stolzenberg-Solomon, R. (2008) Genomic methylation of leukocyte DNA in relation to colorectal adenoma among asymptomatic women. *Gastroenterology* 134, 47–55.
68. Moore, L.E., Pfeiffer, R.M., Poscablo, C., Real, F.X., Kogevinas, M., Silverman, D., Garcia-Closas, R., Chanock, S., Tardon, A., Serra, C., Carrato, A., Dosemeci, M., Garcia-Closas, M., Esteller, M., Fraga, M., Rothman, N., and Malats, N. (2008) Genomic DNA hypomethylation as a biomarker for bladder cancer susceptibility in the Spanish Bladder Cancer Study: a case-control study. *Lancet Oncol* 9, 359–366.
69. Pufulete, M., Al-Ghnaniem, R., Leather, A.J., Appleby, P., Gout, S., Terry, C., Emery, P.W., and Sanders, T.A. (2003) Folate status, genomic DNA hypomethylation, and risk of colorectal adenoma and cancer: a case control study. *Gastroenterology* 124, 1240–1248.
70. Ting Hsiung, D., Marsit, C.J., Houseman, E.A., Eddy, K., Furniss, C.S., McClean, M.D., and Kelsey, K.T. (2007) Global DNA Methylation Level in Whole Blood as a Biomarker in Head and Neck Squamous Cell Carcinoma. *Cancer Epidemiology Biomarkers & Prevention* 16, 108–114.
71. Flanagan, J.M., Cocciardi, S., Waddell, N., Johnstone, C.N., Marsh, A., Henderson, S., Simpson, P., da Silva, L., Khanna, K., Lakhani, S., Boshoff, C., and Chenevix-Trench, G. (2010) DNA methylome of familial breast cancer identifies distinct profiles defined by mutation status. *Am J Hum Genet.* 86, 420–433.
72. Wilhelm, C.S., Kelsey, K.T., Butler, R., Plaza, S., Gagne, L., Zens, M.S., Andrew, A.S., Morris, S., Nelson, H.H., Schned, A.R., Karagas, M.R., and Marsit, C.J. (2010) Implications of LINE1 methylation for bladder cancer risk in women. *Clin Cancer Res* 16, 1682–1689.
73. Teschendorff, A.E., Menon, U., Gentry-Maharaj, A., Ramus, S.J., Gayther, S.A., Apostolidou, S., Jones, A., Lechner, M., Beck, S., Jacobs, I.J., and Widschwendter, M. (2009) An epigenetic signature in peripheral blood predicts active ovarian cancer. *PLoS One* 4, e8274.
74. Christensen, B.C., Houseman, E.A., Marsit, C.J., Zheng, S., Wrensch, M.R., Wiemels, J.L., Nelson, H.H., Karagas, M.R., Padbury, J.F., Bueno, R., Sugarbaker, D.J., Yeh, R.F., Wiencke, J.K., and Kelsey, K.T. (2009) Aging and environmental exposures alter tissue-specific DNA methylation dependent upon CpG island context. *PLoS Genet* 5, e1000602.
75. Rakyan, V.K., Down, T.A., Maslau, S., Andrew, T., Yang, T.P., Beyan, H., Whittaker, P., McCann, O.T., Finer, S., Valdes, A.M., Leslie, R.D., Deloukas, P., and Spector, T.D. (2010) Human aging-associated DNA hypermethylation occurs preferentially at bivalent chromatin domains. *Genome Res* 20, 434–439.
76. Foley, D.L., Craig, J.M., Morley, R., Olsson, C.A., Dwyer, T., Smith, K., and Saffery, R. (2009). Prospects for epigenetic epidemiology. *Am J Epidemiol* 169, 389–400.
77. Teschendorff, A.E., Menon, U., Gentry-Maharaj, A., Ramus, S.J., Weisenberger, D.J., Shen, H., Campan, M., Noushmehr, H., Bell, C.G., Maxwell, A.P., Savage, D.A., Mueller-Holzner, E., Marth, C., Kocjan, G., Gayther, S.A., Jones, A., Beck, S., Wagner, W., Laird, P.W., Jacobs, I.J., and Widschwendter, M. (2010) Age-dependent DNA methylation of genes that are suppressed in stem cells is a hallmark of cancer. *Genome Res* 20, 440–446.
78. Schneider, E., Pliushch, G., El Hajj, N., Galetzka, D., Puhl, A., Schorsch, M., Frauenknecht, K., Riepert, T., Tresch, A., Muller, A.M., Coerdt, W., Zechner, U., and Haaf, T. (2010) Spatial, temporal and interindividual epigenetic variation of functionally important DNA methylation patterns. *Nucleic Acids Res* 38, 3880–3890.
79. Fraga, M.F., Ballestar, E., Paz, M.F., Ropero, S., Setien, F., Ballestar, M.L., Heine-Suner, D., Cigudosa, J.C., Urioste, M., Benitez, J., Boix-Chornet, M., Sanchez-Aguilera, A., Ling, C., Carlsson, E., Poulsen, P., Vaag, A., Stephan, Z., Spector, T.D., Wu, Y.Z., Plass, C., and Esteller, M. (2005) Epigenetic differences arise during the lifetime of monozygotic twins. *Proc Natl Acad Sci U S A* 102, 10604–10609.
80. Gonzalo, S. (2010) Epigenetic alterations in aging. *J Appl Physiol* 109, 586–597.
81. Chen, R.Z., Pettersson, U., Beard, C., Jackson-Grusby, L., and Jaenisch, R. (1998) DNA hypomethylation leads to elevated mutation rates. *Nature* 395, 89–93.
82. Calvanese, V., Lara, E., Kahn, A., and Fraga, M.F. (2009) The role of epigenetics in aging

and age-related diseases. *Ageing Res Rev* 8, 268–276.

83. Eckhardt, F., Lewin, J., Cortese, R., Rakyan, V.K., Attwood, J., Burger, M., Burton, J., Cox, T.V., Davies, R., Down, T.A., Haefliger, C., Horton, R., Howe, K., Jackson, D.K., Kunde, J., Koenig, C., Liddle, J., Niblett, D., Otto, T., Pettett, R., Seemann, S., Thompson, C., West, T., Rogers, J., Olek, A. *et al.*, (2006) DNA methylation profiling of human chromosomes 6, 20 and 22. *Nat Genet* 38, 1378–1385.
84. Kaminsky, Z.A., Tang, T., Wang, S.C., Ptak, C., Oh, G.H., Wong, A.H., Feldcamp, L.A., Virtanen, C., Halfvarson, J., Tysk, C., McRae, A.F., Visscher, P.M., Montgomery, G.W., Gottesman, II, Martin, N.G., and Petronis, A. (2009) DNA methylation profiles in monozygotic and dizygotic twins. *Nat Genet* 41, 240–245.
85. Rakyan, V.K., Down, T.A., Thorne, N.P., Flicek, P., Kulesha, E., Graf, S., Tomazou, E.M., Backdahl, L., Johnson, N., Herberth, M., Howe, K.L., Jackson, D.K., Miretti, M.M., Fiegler, H., Marioni, J.C., Birney, E., Hubbard, T.J., Carter, N.P., Tavare, S., and Beck, S. (2008) An integrated resource for genome-wide identification and analysis of human tissue-specific differentially methylated regions (tDMRs). *Genome Res* 18, 1518–1529.
86. Straussman, R., Nejman, D., Roberts, D., Steinfeld, I., Blum, B., Benvenisty, N., Simon, I., Yakhini, Z., and Cedar, H. (2009) Developmental programming of CpG island methylation profiles in the human genome. *Nat Struct Mol Biol* 16, 564–571.
87. Illingworth, R., Kerr, A., Desousa, D., Jorgensen, H., Ellis, P., Stalker, J., Jackson, D., Clee, C., Plumb, R., Rogers, J., Humphray, S., Cox, T., Langford, C., and Bird, A. (2008) A novel CpG island set identifies tissue-specific methylation at developmental gene loci. *PLoS Biol* 6, e22.
88. Feinberg, A.P. (2007) Phenotypic plasticity and the epigenetics of human disease. *Nature* 447, 433–440.
89. Tobi, E.W., Lumey, L.H., Talens, R.P., Kremer, D., Putter, H., Stein, A.D., Slagboom, P.E., and Heijmans, B.T. (2009) DNA methylation differences after exposure to prenatal famine are common and timing- and sex-specific. *Hum Mol Genet* 18, 4046–4053.
90. Steegers-Theunissen, R.P., Obermann-Borst, S.A., Kremer, D., Lindemans, J., Siebel, C., Steegers, E.A., Slagboom, P.E., and Heijmans, B.T. (2009) Periconceptional maternal folic acid use of 400 microg per day is related to increased methylation of the IGF2 gene in the very young child. *PLoS One* 4, e7845.
91. Xu, X.F. and Du, L.Z. (2010) Epigenetics in neonatal diseases. *Chin Med J (Engl)* 123, 2948–2954.
92. Hilakivi-Clarke, L. and de Assis, S. (2006) Fetal origins of breast cancer. *Trends Endocrinol Metab* 17, 340–348.
93. Burdge, G.C., Lillycrop, K.A., and Jackson, A.A. (2009) Nutrition in early life, and risk of cancer and metabolic disease: alternative endings in an epigenetic tale? *Br J Nutr* 101, 619–630.
94. Waterland, R.A., Lin, J.R., Smith, C.A., and Jirtle, R.L. (2006). Post-weaning diet affects genomic imprinting at the insulin-like growth factor 2 (Igf2) locus. *Hum Mol Genet* 15, 705–716.
95. Dolinoy, D.C., Weidman, J.R., Waterland, R.A., and Jirtle, R.L. (2006) Maternal genistein alters coat color and protects Avy mouse offspring from obesity by modifying the fetal epigenome. *Environ Health Perspect* 114, 567–572.
96. Schwartz, Y.B., Kahn, T.G., Stenberg, P., Ohno, K., Bourgon, R., and Pirrotta, V. (2010) Alternative epigenetic chromatin states of polycomb target genes. *PLoS Genet* 6, e1000805.
97. Christensen, B.C., Kelsey, K.T., Zheng, S., Houseman, E.A., Marsit, C.J., Wrensch, M.R., Wiemels, J.L., Nelson, H.H., Karagas, M.R., Kushi, L.H., Kwan, M.L., and Wiencke, J.K. (2010) Breast cancer DNA methylation profiles are associated with tumor size and alcohol and folate intake. *PLoS Genet* 6, e1001043.
98. Gluckman, P.D. and Hanson, M.A. (2004) Living with the past: evolution, development, and patterns of disease. *Science.* 305, 1733–1736.
99. Li, S., Hursting, S.D., Davis, B.J., McLachlan, J.A., and Barrett, J.C. (2003) Environmental exposure, DNA methylation, and gene regulation: lessons from diethylstilbesterol-induced cancers. *Ann N Y Acad Sci* 983, 161–169.
100. Newbold, R.R. (2008) Prenatal exposure to diethylstilbestrol (DES). *Fertil Steril* 89, e55–56.
101. Sato, K., Fukata, H., Kogo, Y., Ohgane, J., Shiota, K., and Mori, C. (2006) Neonatal exposure to diethylstilbestrol alters the expression of DNA methyltransferases and methylation of genomic DNA in the epididymis of mice. *Endocr J* 53, 331–337.

102. Lagiou, P. (2007) Intrauterine factors and breast cancer risk. *Lancet Oncol* 8, 1047–1048.
103. Yu, W., Gius, D., Onyango, P., Muldoon-Jacobs, K., Karp, J., Feinberg, A.P., and Cui, H. (2008) Epigenetic silencing of tumour suppressor gene p15 by its antisense RNA. *Nature* 451, 202–206.
104. Tufarelli, C., Stanley, J.A., Garrick, D., Sharpe, J.A., Ayyub, H., Wood, W.G., and Higgs, D.R. (2003) Transcription of antisense RNA leading to gene silencing and methylation as a novel cause of human genetic disease. *Nat Genet* 34, 157–165.
105. Katayama, S., Tomaru, Y., Kasukawa, T., Waki, K., Nakanishi, M., Nakamura, M., Nishida, H., Yap, C.C., Suzuki, M., Kawai, J., Suzuki, H., Carninci, P., Hayashizaki, Y., Wells, C., Frith, M., Ravasi, T., Pang, K.C., Hallinan, J., Mattick, J., Hume, D.A., Lipovich, L., Batalov, S., Engstrom, P.G., Mizuno, Y., Faghihi, M.A. *et al.*, (2005) Antisense transcription in the mammalian transcriptome. *Science* 309, 1564–1566.
106. Peters, J. and Williamson, C.M. (2007) Control of imprinting at the Gnas cluster. *Epigenetics* 2, 207–213.
107. Shlien, A. and Malkin, D. (2009) Copy number variations and cancer. *Genome Med* 1, 62.
108. Feinberg, A.P. and Tycko, B. (2004) The history of cancer epigenetics. *Nat Rev Cancer* 4, 143–153.
109. Ordway, J.M., Budiman, M.A., Korshunova, Y., Maloney, R.K., Bedell, J.A., Citek, R.W., Bacher, B., Peterson, S., Rohlfing, T., Hall, J., Brown, R., Lakey, N., Doerge, R.W., Martienssen, R.A., Leon, J., McPherson, J.D., and Jeddeloh, J.A. (2007) Identification of novel high-frequency DNA methylation changes in breast cancer. *PLoS One* 2, e1314.
110. Wacholder, S., Hartge, P., Prentice, R., Garcia-Closas, M., Feigelson, H.S., Diver, W.R., Thun, M.J., Cox, D.G., Hankinson, S.E., Kraft, P., Rosner, B., Berg, C.D., Brinton, L.A., Lissowska, J., Sherman, M.E., Chlebowski, R., Kooperberg, C., Jackson, R.D., Buckman, D.W., Hui, P., Pfeiffer, R., Jacobs, K.B., Thomas, G.D., Hoover, R.N., Gail, M.H. *et al.*, (2010) Performance of common genetic variants in breast-cancer risk models. *N Engl J Med* 362, 986–993.
111. Beck, S. (2010) Taking the measure of the methylome. *Nat Biotechnol* 28, 1026–1028.

Chapter 28

Epigenetic Biomarkers in Cancer Epidemiology

Mukesh Verma

Abstract

Biochemical, epigenetic, genetic, and imaging biomarkers are used to identify people at high risk for developing cancer. In cancer epidemiology, epigenetic biomarkers offer advantages over other types of biomarkers because they are expressed against a person's genetic background and environmental exposure, and because epigenetic events occur early in cancer development. This chapter describes epigenetic biomarkers that are being used to study the epidemiology of different types of cancer. Because epigenetic alterations can be reversed by chemicals and activate gene expression, epigenetic biomarkers potentially have numerous clinical applications in cancer intervention and treatment and significant implications in public health. This review discusses cancer biomarkers, the characteristics of an ideal biomarker for cancer, and technologies for biomarker detection.

Key words: Chromatin, Epidemiology, Epigenetics, Epigenome wide association studies, Histone deacetylase, Histone inhibitors, Infectious agents, Methylation, Methyltransferase, MicroRNAs

1. Introduction: Significance of Biomarkers in Cancer Epidemiology

Cancer epidemiology examines populations exposed to different environmental factors (toxins, chemicals, insecticides, pesticides, radiation, nutrition, infectious agents) to identify causative agents that contribute to the development of cancer (1–3). A perturbed environment during early life has a profound effect on the physiological and cellular adaptations that contribute to disease development (4–7). Adaptive changes may result in permanent changes and contribute to disease development. For example, adaptive responses may be retained by cells and organs and may direct normal development toward pathological states. To detect the initiation and development of diseases, biospecimens and a history of exposure are collected and used to identify biomarkers (1, 4, 8, 9). These biomarkers can be used to follow disease progression, response to treatment, survival, or cancer recurrence.

Ramona G. Dumitrescu and Mukesh Verma (eds.), *Cancer Epigenetics: Methods and Protocols*, Methods in Molecular Biology, vol. 863, DOI 10.1007/978-1-61779-612-8_28, © Springer Science+Business Media, LLC 2012

Biochemical and genetic markers generally are used in cancer epidemiology, but this chapter discusses the use of epigenetic biomarkers in cancer epidemiology.

2. Epigenetics and Cancer

Traditionally, cancer has been considered a genetic disease, although recent evidence supports the idea of it being both a genetic and epigenetic disease, because epigenetics plays a critical role in cell development and differentiation (10–13). Different cancers carry specific "epigenetic signatures" that are associated with risk factors and can be used for cancer detection, diagnosis, and prognosis (14). The epigenetic regulation of gene expression indicates that environmental changes during early life have an impact on epigenetic profiling and gene expression that creates a "memory" of early fetal experience and remains during development and aging (2).

3. Epigenetics and Gene Regulation

Human diseases result from an altered program of gene expression. The genome provides information about what can be done, whereas the epigenome programs the genome and directs it when something should be done (15). The epigenome consists of chromatin modifications and covalent modifications of cytosine residues in GC-rich regions present prominently in the promoter of genes. Gene silencing by epigenetic mechanisms is now well established in cancer and other diseases (16). Multiple genes that are involved in cell cycle regulation, differentiation, tumor suppression, DNA repair, and apoptosis are regulated epigenetically (17). Unlike mutations and other genetic changes, epigenetic alterations do not cause structural changes in the target gene. We know now that dysregulated epigenetic modifications, especially in early neoplastic development, may be as significant as genetic mutations in driving cancer development and growth.

Chromatin is a highly ordered structure. The basic unit of chromatin is the nucleosome (10). Chromatin is composed of histone, nonhistone proteins, and DNA and exists as a condensed nucleoprotein complex. Two conformation states of chromatin, euchromatin and heterochromatin, have been identified; they represent transcriptionally active and inactive states, respectively. The N-terminal regions of histones protrude from the nucleosomes and are modified by posttranslational processes. These posttranslational histone changes govern transcription regulation via chromatin conformational changes. Promoter methylation also contributes to gene regulation. These two processes (promoter methylation and histone modifications) are complex, not necessarily mutually exclusive, and likely to be dynamic processes in which other proteins and enzymes also participate (2). Furthermore, noncoding RNAs also contribute to epigenetic gene regulation by altering the stability of proteins involved in transcriptional regulation. Epigenetic mechanisms allow changes in gene expression in response to environmental factors (10, 16).

4. Epigenetic Biomarkers in Different Cancer Types

Some biomarkers are specific to certain cancer types; others are general cancer biomarkers. Histone demethylase is an example of a general biomarker (12, 13). This enzyme may be overexpressed, mutated, or amplified in different cancers. Examples of histone demethylases include H3K4, H3K9, and H3K27 demethylases, which have been shown to be altered in a variety of cancers. The following sections and Table 1 describe epigenetic biomarkers that have been reported in different cancers.

4.1. Bladder Cancer

Methylated cystein was measured in age- and sex-matched bladder cancer cases and controls to evaluate whether hypomethylation is associated with the progression of bladder cancer. Results indicated that hypomethylation plays a significant role in bladder cancer, and smoking and alcohol are risk factors (18, 19).

4.2. Brain Cancer

Gliomas occur due to genetic and epigenetic changes. Gliomas of astrocytic, oligodendroglial, and ependymal origin account for more than 70% of all brain tumors. The most frequent and most malignant histological type is the glioblastoma. A few genes, such as *MGMT* and *TIMP3*, become inactivated in glioblastoma due to hypermethylation (20, 21). Although epigenetic changes occur independent of genetic changes, the changes are interactive. Methylation profiling and LOH at chromosome 1 are crucial in anaplastic glioma diagnosis (20).

4.3. Breast Cancer

BRCA1 has been studied for the presence of mutation and hypermethylation (22–24). Methylated *RASSF1A* and *PITX2* in PB-P appear to have promising potential as prognostic markers in clinical use. Alcohol consumption, parity, and high estrogen levels are some of the risk factors for this cancer. Methylation of *PTEN* regulates tamoxifen-resistance in breast cancer cells.

4.4. Cervical Cancer

CALCA, *hTERT*, *MYOD1*, *PGR* (progesterone receptor), and *T1MP3* were found to be hypermethylated in cervical cancer cases (25).

Table 1
Epigenetic biomarkers in different cancers

Cancer type	Marker	References
Bladder cancer	Hypermethylation of several genes	(18, 19)
Brain cancer	MGMT, TIMP-3	(20, 21)
Breast cancer	BRCA1, PTEN, RASSF1A	(22–24)
Cervical cancer	CALCA, hTERT, MYOD1, PGR, TIMP-3	(25)
Colon cancer	APC, p14, p16	(26–28)
Endometrial cancer	MLH1	(29)
Esophageal cancer	HPP1, RUNX3, RIZ1, CRBP1, 3-OST-2, APC, TIMP3, p16, MGMT, p14	(32)
Gastric cancer	CDX2	(35)
Head and neck cancer	CYP1A1, CYP2A13, GSTM1	(36)
Leukemia and lymphoma (blood cancer)	miR-29, miR-223	(45–48)
Liver cancer	APC, FHIT, p15, p16, E-cadherin	(36–39)
Lung cancer	P16, CDH13, DAPK, RASSF1A, RARbeta, APC	(41–44)
Oral cancer	P16, CDH1	(50)
Ovarian cancer	ARH1, BRCA1, DR4, GATA4, hMLH1, hMLH2, HOAX10, ICAM1, PACE4, RUNX3, TMS1	(51)
Pancreatic cancer	P14, p16	(52)
Prostate cancer	NKX2-5, CLSTN1, SPOCK2, SLC16A12, DPYS, GSTP1, NSE1	(53, 54)
Rectal cancer	MINT1, MINT3	(55)
Skin cancer (melanoma)	P73, CDH1, DAPK, IGFBP-3, MTAP, SHP-1, SOCS2, T-cadherin	(56)
Thyroid cancer	E-cadherin, DAPK	(57, 58)

MYOD1 methylation has been proposed as a prognostic marker for identifying cervical cancer patients at high risk for lymph node metastasis or relapse.

4.5. Colon Cancer

Epigenetic regulation in colorectal cancer has been observed in several genes, including *APC*, *p14*, and *p16* (26). In a group of more than 100 cancer patients, the distinct phenotype CpG Island Methylator Phenotype (CIMP) was identified and could distinguish people with cancer from the normal, healthy population (27, 28).

4.6. Endometrial Cancer

Endometrial cancer is the most common gynecologic malignancy in the United States, with more than 40,100 new cases every year. Both genetic and epigenetic markers have been studied in endometrial cancer. In one epidemiologic study, the risk of cancer was observed in microsatellite instability (MSI)-positive cells that were negative for *MLH1* methylation (29).

4.7. Esophageal Cancer

Esophageal adenocarcinoma (EAC) incidence is increasing in the United States. Its premalignant stage, Barrett's esophagus (BE), a sequela of chronic gastroesophageal reflux disease (GERD), has attracted the attention of oncologists because methylation markers can distinguish between EAC and BE (30). An individual with BE has a 30–125-fold greater chance of developing EAC (31). Genes that are inactivated by hypermethylation include *HPP1*, *RUNX3*, *RIZ1*, *CRBP1*, *3-OST-2*, *APC*, *TIMP3*, *p16*, *MGMT*, and *p14* (32).

4.8. Gallbladder Cancer

The incidence of gall bladder cancer is higher in Chile and India than in other countries. Risk factors include mutation in *K-ras*, gall bladder stones, air pollutants, and infection. A few genes (*CDH13*, *FHIT*, *SEMA3B*, and *MGMT*) are inactivated due to hypermethylation (33).

4.9. Gastric Cancer

Gastric cancer has been associated with *Helicobacter pylori* infection. The gastric mucosa is affected by *H. pylori* infection, and an abnormal methylation profile has been observed in selected genes (34). Although it is not clear that *H. pylori* is the causative agent for gastric cancer, its role as a risk factor has been well established. The *CDX2* gene is regulated epigenetically in gastric cancer (35).

4.10. Head and Neck Cancer

Hypermethylation of carcinogen metabolism genes *CYP1A1*, *CYP2A13*, and *GSTM1* has been observed (36), although no correlation has been observed between alcohol consumption and polymorphism in *CYP1A1* and *CYP2A13*. This suggests that the regulation of head and neck cancer may be epigenetic.

4.11. Hepatocellular Carcinoma (Liver Cancer)

Hepatocellular carcinoma (HCC) is common in Asian countries, and incidence rates are increasing in Western countries. A few genes have been studied for hypermethylation (*APC*, *FHIT*, *p15*, *p16*, and *E-cadherin* [ECAD)), although the results are not promising (37). A few genes become hypomethylated during liver carcinogenesis, such as estrogen receptor-alpha (38). Global methylation is another biomarker that can be used in determining diagnosis and prognosis in liver cancer (39).

4.12. Lung Cancer

Candidate genes and a genome-wide methylation profile have been used to detect lung cancer-associated genes and their function (40). The common genes regulated by methylation in lung cancer are *p16*, *CDH13*, *DAPK*, *RASSF1A*, *RARbeta*, and *APC* (41).

Views differ regarding the causes of lung cancer in nonsmokers; a majority of scientists think that a combination of genetic and epigenetic regulation contributes to lung cancer in nonsmokers (42–44).

4.13. Leukemia and Lymphoma

The overexpression of miRNAs has been observed in chronic lymphocytic leukemia (CLL). CLL is a frequent $CD5^+$ B cell neoplasia that affects peripheral blood, bone marrow, lymph nodes, and other lymphoid tissues. Two miRNA families, miR-29 and miR-223, are involved with the aggressiveness of this disease (45–48). Levels of these miRNAs decreased with poor prognosis.

4.14. Oral Cancer

Methylation of *CHFR*, a cell cycle regulatory gene, was found to be associated with oral squamous cell carcinoma (OSCC) (49). OSCC progression is correlated with p16 and CDH1 hypermethylation (50). *P16* hypermethylation also was associated with the invasion of lymph nodes in young adults.

4.15. Ovarian Cancer

The most common epigenetic markers of ovarian cancer are: *ARH1*, *BRCA1*, *DR4*, *GATA4*, *hMLH1*, *hMLH2*, *HOAX10*, *ICAM1*, *PACE4*, *RUNX3*, and *TMS1* (51). CIMP also has been reported in a subgroup of ovarian cancer.

4.16. Pancreatic Cancer

The mortality and incidence rates of pancreatic cancer did not change over time. Although this cancer is the fourth leading cause of death in Western countries, early detection markers have yet to be identified. Risk factors for this cancer include long-standing diabetes, alcoholism, and *K-ras* mutation. *P14* and *p16* are hypermethylated when tested in pancreatic fluid (52).

4.17. Prostate Cancer

Numerous reports indicate *GSTP1* hypermethylation as the diagnostic marker for prostate cancer; however, *NKX2-5*, *CLSTN1*, *SPOCK2*, *SLC16A12*, *DPYS*, and *NSE1* also have been reported to be regulated by methylation mechanisms in prostate cancer (53, 54).

4.18. Rectal Cancer

Compared to other cancers, rectal cancer has not been well studied. Methylation at *MINT* loci has been reported, and *MINT1*, *MINT3*, and *MINT31* sometimes are used as rectal cancer epigenetic markers (55).

4.19. Skin Cancer

Several genes become hypermethylated in skin cancer. Genes with hypermethylation in melanoma patient samples include: *p73*, *CDH1*, *DAPK*, *IGFBP-3*, *MTAP*, *PTEN*, *RARbeta*, *SHP-1*, *SOCS2*, and *T-cadherin* (56).

4.20. Thyroid Cancer

Hypermethylation of thyrotropin receptor (TSHR), *ECAD*, *sodium iodide symporter* (*NIS-L*), *ataxia telangiectasia mutated* (*ATM*), and death-associated protein kinase (DAPK) proteins are involved in the development of thyroid cancer (57). Sodium butyrate and acetabine (epigenetics inhibitors) have been found to be effective in treating this cancer (58).

5. Epigenetic Biomarkers in Infectious Agent-Associated Cancers

Approximately 15% of cancers (about 1.5 million cases per year worldwide) are attributed to viral, bacterial, and other pathogens. The number of infectious agents associated with cancer is increasing. Common agents include the human papilloma virus (HPV, cervical cancer); hepatitis B and C (liver cancer); Epstein Barr virus (EBV, nasopharyngeal carcinoma); herpes simplex virus (Kaposi's sarcoma); schistomes (bladder cancer); Markel cell, BK, and JC polyoma virus (kidney cancer); and *H. pylori* (gastric cancer). These agents are known to cause genomic instability, suppress DNA repair genes, and enhance the expression of genes involved in apoptosis. In cervical cancer, *CCNA1*, *PAX1*, *HS3ST2*, *DAPK1*, and *TFPI2* are methylated (13). Lu et al. (59) demonstrated improved HPV vaccine potency when demethylating inhibitors are included. In gastric cancer, methylation of the *CDH1* gene has been reported by Kague et al. (60). Other genes that are involved in epigenetic-mediated gastric cancer in *H. pylori*-infected cells include *CDKN2A* and *RUNX3* (61, 62).

6. Candidate Biomarkers vs. Epigenome Profiling in Cancer Epidemiology

Most of the biomarkers described above were identified by the candidate gene approach. However, profiling of epigenomic components also has been useful in determining cancer-specific signatures (63). The advantage of epigenetic biomarkers over other markers is the availability of technologies for detecting biomarkers in tissue samples and biofluids (16, 64). Epigenome Wide Association Studies (EWAS) should be conducted by determining profiles of methylation, histone modifications, and miRNA in samples from healthy and cancer patients to identify cancer-associated epigenetic marks.

7. Epigenetic Inhibitors in Clinical Trials and FDA-Approved Inhibitors

Methyltransferase inhibitors and histone deacetylase inhibitors (HDACs) have attracted the attention of researchers and clinicians recently because they offer an alternative therapeutic regime for a few diseases, including cancer (65). These inhibitors act on enzymes involved in the epigenetic regulation of genes that does not involve DNA sequence alterations (16). Epigenetic inhibitors work alone or in combination with other therapeutic agents. To date, four epigenetic inhibitors have been approved for cancer treatment. Their mechanisms of action and future prospects are discussed below.

A number of epigenetic inhibitors have been purified from natural resources or developed synthetically. The methyltransferase inhibitors azacitidine and decitabine have been licensed for clinical therapy for patients with myelodysplastic syndrome (66, 67) (Table 2). Zebularine and isothiocynate are among other potential methyltransferase inhibitors. 5-Azacytidine forms a covalent complex with cytosin (C-5)-specific DNA methyltransferases and inhibits their activity. This compound also is activated by uridine-cytidine kinase and thus can be incorporated into both RNA and DNA.

Decitabine (2-deoxy azacitidine) is a hypomethylating agent. It hypomethylates DNA by inhibiting DNA methyltransferases. It functions in a manner similar to azacitidine, although decitabine can be incorporated only into DNA strands, whereas azacitidine can be incorporated into both DNA and RNA chains. Infants, young adults, and pregnant women and their offspring (if treated) may be at risk of developing cardiovascular, musculoskeletal,

Table 2
Epigenetic inhibitors

Inhibitors	Other names	Comments
DNA methyltransferase inhibitors		
5-Azacytidine	Vidaza	FDA-approved (Vidaza by Celgene was approved for treatment of myeloplastic syndrome)
Isothiocynate		Preclinical
Zebularine		Preclinical
Decitabine (5-aza-2′-deoxycytidine)		FDA approved
Arabinosyl-5-azacytidine	Fazarabine	In Phase I/II trial
5-6-Dihydro-5-azacytidine	DHAC	In Phase I/II trial
Hydrazine		In Phase I trial
Histone deacetylase inhibitors		
Vorinostat	Zolinza, suberoylanilide hydroxamic acid (SAHA)	FDA approved for treatment of cutaneous T-cell lymphoma (SAHA is sold by Merck pharmaceutical company)
Butyrates (phenylbutyrate)		For urea cycle disorder
Valproic acid		FDA approved
FK228	Depsipeptide	In Phase I/II trial
Panobinostat	LBH589	In Phase I/II trial
Belinostat	PXD101	In Phase I/II trial

Sources: Refs. (65–68)

neurological, and cognitive problems when treated with azacytidine or decitabine. Clinicians should be cautious.

HDACs present a promising class of compounds for cancer therapy. Histone acetylation is a reversible process in which histone acetyltransferase (HAT) transfers the acetyl moiety from acetyl coenzyme A to an amino acid. Histone deacetylase, as the name suggests, removes the acetyl group. Evidence exists that these compounds are well tolerated and effective. At least 18 forms of HDACs have been reported; these forms differ in their structure and have histones and nonhistones as their substrate (68). Normal cells are relatively resistant to HDAC inhibitors. Epigenetic inhibitors that have been identified so far belong to one of the following classes of agents: short-chain fatty acids, hydroxamic acids, benzamides, cyclic tetrapeptides containing S-2-amino-9, 10-epoxy-8-xodecanoic acid (AOE) moiety, epoxides, and psammaplins (69).

7.1. Advantages of Using Epigenetic Inhibitors

Epigenetic inhibitors, either alone or in combination, are effective in treating cancer (70, 71). EBV infection has been observed in Burkitt's lymphoma and nasopharyngeal carcinoma, and it has been determined that hypermethylation of latency genes allows EBV to stay integrated in the main genome and contribute to these cancers. In myelodisplastic syndrome, with an incidence rate of 20,000, the standard treatment (considered aggressive) is a weekly blood transfusion. Treating these patients with Vidaza was successful, and most did not need transfusion (http://pubs.acs.org/cen/science/87/8714sci1a.html). The survival time and quality of life of these patients also increased substantially.

7.2. Work in Combination Therapy

This section provides examples that indicate the therapeutic potential of epigenetic inhibitors. Vorinostat, an HDAC inhibitor (also called Zolinza), was effective when combined with pelvic palliative radiotherapy for gastrointestinal carcinoma (72). Vorinostat originally was approved by the U.S. Food and Drug Administration (FDA) for the treatment of T-cell lymphoma (73). In more than 400 patients with solid and hematologic malignancies, this agent was well tolerated and produced a therapeutic response. Studies are planned to combine Vorinostat with radiation therapy to treat nonsmall-cell lung cancer, glioblastoma multiforme, multiple myeloma, and myelodysplastic syndrome (a set of bone marrow conditions that often results in terminal blood cancer).

HDAC inhibitors also have been used in combination therapy (74–76). These inhibitors, with tumor necrosis factor-related apoptosis-inducing ligand (TRAIL), were capable of inducing apoptosis in breast, prostate, lung, and other cancer cells (69, 74–76). Reports of epigenetic inhibitors functioning as radiosensitizers in breast, prostate, and glioma cells further suggest the importance of these inhibitors (77–79). Interaction of these inhibitors with DNA repair pathways also has been proposed (80).

According to Shanker and Srivastava (69), combining drugs that target different signaling pathways may cause adverse side effects while increasing treatment efficacy and patient survival. Doxorubicin and decitabine have shown synergistic effects with HDAC inhibitors in cancer treatment (81).

8. Concluding Remarks: Future Directions

Newer and more efficient technologies should be incorporated into population studies that use epigenetic biomarkers. One issue to be resolved is who will support and maintain the large volume of data that is being generated by epigenetics and epidemiology research. The integration of genetic and epigenetic data also is needed in the near future. In risk assessment studies, the question of how long longitudinal measurements should be taken in individuals at high risk before the disease develops needs to be addressed. Resources such as family registries have been underutilized by epigenetic researchers, and they may be useful in identifying cancers that tend to cluster in families. Although few biomarkers have been validated systematically, more markers need to be validated clinically. Early detection of disease onset is possible if biomarkers are assayed in samples collected longitudinally. If disease can be detected at a treatable stage, contributions can be made to improving health.

Thus far, histopathology has been used for EAC and its stages for diagnosis, but the time has come when disease stratification and diagnosis should be based on molecular markers such as epigenetic markers. Incorporating information about a patient's exposure and family history also may improve diagnosis.

The problem of gene-specific targeting remains, and further research is needed to make epigenetic inhibitors gene-specific. The wrong kind of epigenetic intervention may result in the silencing of genes that should not be silenced. Nevertheless, the biological response can be distinguished from responses that occur as a result of deleterious mutational and other genetic changes. Another issue is how to overcome problems that arose during discovery of the first generation of epigenetic inhibitors. Most of the newly identified inhibitors have cytotoxicity problems. A few compounds are not very soluble in aqueous solutions.

Finally, a major challenge in developing cancer biomarkers is the integration of epigenetics with genomics and metabolomics data and their functional interpretation in conjunction with clinical data and epidemiology.

Acknowledgments

We wish to thank Christie Kaefer and Britt Reid of the Epidemiology and Genetics Research Program; and Joanne Brodsky of SCG for reading the manuscript and offering suggestions.

References

1. Kumar, D. and Verma, M. (2009). Methods in cancer epigenetics and epidemiology. *Methods Mol Biol* 471, 273–288.
2. Nise, M. S., Falaturi, P., and Erren, T. C. (2010). Epigenetics: Origins and implications for cancer epidemiology. *Med Hypotheses* 74, 377–382.
3. Verma, M., Seminara, D., Arena, F. J., John, C., Iwamoto, K., and Hartmuller, V. (2006). Genetic and epigenetic biomarkers in cancer: improving diagnosis, risk assessment, and disease stratification. *Mol Diagn Ther* 10, 1–15.
4. Wagner, P. D., Verma, M., and Srivastava, S. (2004). Challenges for biomarkers in cancer detection. *Ann N Y Acad Sci* 1022, 9–16.
5. Arab, L. (2010). Epidemiologic evidence on coffee and cancer. *Nutr Cancer* 62, 271–283.
6. De Silva, M., Senarath, U., Gunatilake, M., and Lokuhetty, D. (2010). Prolonged breastfeeding reduces risk of breast cancer in Sri Lankan women: a case–control study. *Cancer Epidemiol* 34, 267–273.
7. Verma, M. (2010). Pancreatic cancer biomarkers and their implication in cancer diagnosis and epidemiology. *Cancers* 2, 1830–1837.
8. Mishra, A., and Verma, M. (2010). Cancer biomarkers: are we ready for the prime time? *Cancers* 2, 190–208.
9. Verma, M. and Manne, U. (2006). Genetic and epigenetic biomarkers in cancer diagnosis and identifying high risk populations. *Crit Rev Oncol Hematol* 60, 9–18.
10. Feinberg, A. P. (2010). Genome-scale approaches to the epigenetics of common human disease. *Virchows Arch* 456, 13–21.
11. Issa, J.P. (2010). Epigenetic changes in the myelodysplastic syndrome. *Hematol Oncol Clin North Am* 24, 317–330.
12. Lim, S., Metzger, E., Schüle, R., Kirfel, J., and Buettner, R. (2010). Epigenetic regulation of cancer growth by histone demethylases. *Int J Cancer* 127, 1991–1998.
13. Lim, E. H., Ng, S. L., Li, J. L., Chang, A. R., Ng, J., Ilancheran, A., Low, J., Quek, S. C., and Tay, E. H. (2010). Cervical dysplasia: assessing methylation status (Methylight) of CCNA1, DAPK1, HS3ST2, PAX1 and TFPI2 to improve diagnostic accuracy. *Gynecol Oncol* 119, 225–231.
14. Laird, P. W. (2010). Principles and challenges of genome-wide DNA methylation analysis. *Nat Rev Genet* 11, 191–203.
15. Sharma, R., Panda, N. K., and Khullar, M. (2010). Hypermethylation of carcinogen metabolism genes, CYP1A1, CYP2A13 and GSTM1 genes in head and neck cancer. *Oral Dis* 16, 668–673.
16. Banerjee, H. N. and Verma, M. (2009). Epigenetic mechanisms in cancer. *Biomark Med* 3, 397–410.
17. Diamandis, E. P., Sidransky, D., Laird, P. W., Cairns, P., and Bapat, B. (2010). Epigenomics-based diagnostics. *Clin Chem.* 56, 1216–1219.
18. McNeil, B. K. and Getzenberg, R. H. (2008). Urine-based markers in bladder cancer: future prospects. *BJU Int* 101, 668–669.
19. Moore, L. E., Pfeiffer, R. M., Poscablo, C., Real, F. X., Kogevinas, M., Silverman, D., García-Closas, R., Chanock, S., Tardón, A., Serra, C., Carrato, A., Dosemeci, M., García-Closas, M., Esteller, M., Fraga, M., Rothman, N., Malats, N. (2008). Genomic DNA hypomethylation as a biomarker for bladder cancer susceptibility in the Spanish Bladder Cancer Study: a case–control study. *Lancet Oncol* 9, 359–366.
20. DeAngelis, L. M. (2009). Anaplastic glioma: How to prognosticate outcome and choose a treatment strategy. *J Clin Oncol* 27, 5861–5867.
21. Rodriguez, F. J., Thibodeau, S. N., Jenkins, R. B., Schowalter, K. V., Caron, B. L., O'Neill, B. P., James, C. D., Passe, S., Slezak, J., and Giannini, C. (2008). MGMT immunohistochemical expression and promoter methylation in human glioblastoma. *Appl Immunohistochem Mol Morphol* 16, 59–65.
22. Bean, G. R., Ibarra Drendall, C., Goldenberg, V. K., Baker, J. C. Jr., Troch, M. M., Paisie, C., Wilke, L. G., Yee, L., Marcom, P. K., Kimler, B.

F., Fabian, C. J., Zalles, C. M., Broadwater, G., Scott, V., and Seewaldt, V. L. (2007). Hypermethylation of the breast cancer–associated gene 1 promoter does not predict cytologic atypia or correlate with surrogate end points of breast cancer risk. *Cancer Epidemiol Biomarkers Prev* 16, 50–56.

23. Chen, Y., Toland, A. E., McLennan, J., Fridlyand, J., Crawford, B., Costello, J. F., and Ziegler, J.L. (2006). Lack of germ-line promoter methylation in BRCA1-negative families with familial breast cancer. *Genet Test* 10, 281–284.
24. Flanagan, J. M., Popendikyte, V., Pozdniakovaite, N., Sobolev, M., Assadzadeh, A., Schumacher, A., Zangeneh, M., Lau, L., Virtanen, C., Wang, S. C., and Petronis, A. (2006). Intra- and interindividual epigenetic variation in human germ cells. *Am J Hum Genet* 79, 67–84.
25. Widschwendter, A., Müller, H. M., Fiegl, H., Ivarsson, L., Wiedemair, A., Müller-Holzner, E., Goebel, G., Marth, C., and Widschwendter, M. (2004). DNA methylation in serum and tumors of cervical cancer patients. *Clin Cancer Res* 10, 565–571.
26. Moriyama, T., Matsumoto, T., Nakamura, S., Jo, Y., Mibu, R., Yao, T., and Iida, M. (2007). Hypermethylation of p14(ARF) may be predictive of colitic cancer in patients with ulcerative colitis. *Dis Colon Rectum* 50, 1384–1392.
27. Weisenberger, D. J., Siegmund, K. D., Campan, M., Young, J., Long, T. I., Faasse, M. A., Kang, G. H., Widschwendter, M., Weener, D., Buchanan, D., Koh, H., Simms, L., Barker, M., Leggett, B., Levine, J., Kim, M., French, A. J., Thibodeau, S. N., Jass, J., Haile, R., and Laird, P. W. (2006). CpG island methylator phenotype underlies sporadic microsatellite instability and is tightly associated with BRAF mutation in colorectal cancer. *Nat Genet* 38, 787–793.
28. Ogino, S., Nosho, K., Kirkner, G. J., Kawasaki, T., Meyerhardt, J. A., Loda, M., Giovannucci, E. L., and Fuchs, C. S. (2009). CpG island methylator phenotype, microsatellite instability, BRAF mutation and clinical outcome in colon cancer. *Gut* 58, 90–96.
29. Buttin, B. M., Powell, M. A., Mutch, D. G., Rader, J. S., Herzog, T. J., Gibb, R. K., Huettner, P., Edmonston, T. B., and Goodfellow, P. J. (2004). Increased risk for hereditary nonpolyposis colorectal cancer-associated synchronous and metachronous malignancies in patients with microsatellite instability-positive endometrial carcinoma lacking MLH1 promoter methylation. *Clin Cancer Res* 10, 481–490.
30. Wang, S., Zhan, M., Yin, J., Abraham, J. M., Mori, Y., Sato, F., Xu, Y., Olaru, A., Berki, A. T., Li, H., Schulmann, K., Kan, T., Hamilton, J. P., Paun, B., Yu, M. M., Jin, Z., Cheng, Y., Ito, T., Mantzur, C., Greenwald, B. D., Meltzer, S.J. (2006). Transcriptional profiling suggests that Barrett's metaplasia is an early intermediate stage in esophageal adenocarcinogenesis. *Oncogene* 25, 3346–3356.
31. Jin, Z., Cheng, Y., Gu, W., Zheng, Y., Sato, F., Mori, Y., Olaru, A. V., Paun, B. C., Yang, J., Kan, T., Ito, T., Hamilton, J. P., Selaru, F. M., Agarwal, R., David, S., Abraham, J. M., Wolfsen, H. C., Wallace, M. B., Shaheen, N. J., Washington, K., Wang, J., Canto, M. I., Bhattacharyya, A., Nelson, M. A., Wagner, P. D., Romero, Y., Wang, K. K., Feng, Z., Sampliner, R. E., and Meltzer, S. J. (2009). A multicenter, double-blinded validation study of methylation biomarkers for progression prediction in Barrett's esophagus. *Cancer Res* 69, 4112–4115.
32. Schulmann, K., Sterian, A., Berki, A., Yin, J., Sato, F., Xu, Y., Olaru, A., Wang, S., Mori, Y., Deacu, E., Hamilton, J., Kan, T., Krasna, M. J., Beer, D. G., Pepe, M. S., Abraham, J. M., Feng, Z., Schmiegel, W., Greenwald, B. D., and Meltzer, S.J. (2005). Inactivation of p16, RUNX3, and HPP1 occurs early in Barrett's-associated neoplastic progression and predicts progression risk. *Oncogene*. 24, 4138–4148.
33. Goldin, R. D. and Roa, J. C. (2009). Gallbladder cancer: a morphological and molecular update. *Histopathology* 55, 218–229.
34. Nakajima, T., Enomoto, S., Yamashita, S., Ando, T., Nakanishi, Y., Nakazawa, K., Oda, I., Gotoda, T., and Ushijima, T. (2010). Persistence of a component of DNA methylation in gastric mucosae after *Helicobacter pylori* eradication. *J Gastroenterol* 45, 37–44.
35. Yuasa, Y., Nagasaki, H., Akiyama, Y., Sakai, H., Nakajima, T., Ohkura, Y., Takizawa, T., Koike, M., Tani, M., Iwai, T., Sugihara, K., Imai, K., and Nakachi, K. (2005). Relationship between CDX2 gene methylation and dietary factors in gastric cancer patients. *Carcinogenesis* 26, 193–200.
36. Sharma, S., Kelly, T. K., and Jones, P. A. (2010). Epigenetics in cancer. *Carcinogenesis* 31, 27–36.
37. Iyer, P., Zekri, A. R., Hung, C.W., Schiefelbein, E., Ismail, K., Hablas, A., Seifeldin, I.A., and Soliman, A. S. (2010). Concordance of DNA methylation pattern in plasma and tumor DNA of Egyptian hepatocellular carcinoma patients. *Exp Mol Pathol* 88, 107–111.
38. Liu, J. and Waalkes, M. P. (2008). Liver is a target of arsenic carcinogenesis. *Toxicol Sci* 105, 24–32.
39. Guerrero-Preston, R., Santella, R. M., Blanco, A., Desai, M., Berdasco, M., and Fraga, M. (2007). Global DNA hypomethylation in liver cancer cases and controls: a phase I preclinical biomarker development study. *Epigenetics* 2, 223–226.

40. Goto, Y., Shinjo, K., Kondo, Y., Shen, L., Toyota, M., Suzuki, H., Gao, W., An, B., Fujii, M., Murakami, H., Osada, H., Taniguchi, T., Usami, N., Kondo, M., Hasegawa, Y., Shimokata, K., Matsuo, K., Hida, T., Fujimoto, N., Kishimoto, T., Issa, J. P., and Sekido, Y. (2009). Epigenetic profiles distinguish malignant pleural mesothelioma from lung adenocarcinoma. *Cancer Res* 69, 9072–9082.
41. Dubey, S. and Powell, C. A. (2009). Update in lung cancer 2008. *Am J Respir Crit Care Med* 179, 860–868.
42. Georgiou, E., Valeri, R., Tzimagiorgis, G., Anzel, J., Krikelis, D., Tsilikas, C., Sarikos, G., Destouni, C., Dimitriadou, A., and Kouidou, S. (2007). Aberrant p16 promoter methylation among Greek lung cancer patients and smokers: correlation with smoking. *Eur J Cancer Prev* 16, 396–402.
43. Reid, M. E., Santella, R., and Ambrosone, C. B. (2008). Molecular epidemiology to better predict lung cancer risk. *Clin Lung Cancer* 9, 149–153.
44. Subramanian, J. and Govindan, R. (2007). Lung cancer in never smokers: a review. *J Clin Oncol* 25, 561–570.
45. Calin, G. A., Cimmino, A., Fabbri, M., Ferracin, M., Wojcik, S.E., Shimizu, M., Taccioli, C., Zanesi, N., Garzon, R., Aqeilan, R.I., Alder, H., Volinia, S., Rassenti, L., Liu, X., Liu, C.G., Kipps, T.J., Negrini, M., and Croce, C.M. (2008). miR-15a and miR-16-1 cluster functions in human leukemia. *Proc Natl Acad Sci U S A* 105, 5166–5171.
46. Mertens, D., Philippen, A., Ruppel, M., Allegra, D., Bhattacharya, N., Tschuch, C., Wolf, S., Idler, I., Zenz, T., and Stilgenbauer, S. (2009). Chronic lymphocytic leukemia and 13q14: miRs and more. *Leuk Lymphoma* 50, 502–505.
47. Sampath, D. and Calin, G. A. (2009). miRs: fine-tuning prognosis in CLL. *Blood* 113, 5035–5036.
48. Stamatopoulos, B., Meuleman, N., Haibe-Kains, B., Saussoy P., Van Den Neste E., Michaux L., Heimann P., Martiat P., Bron D., and Lagneaux L. (2009). microRNA-29c and microRNA-223 down-regulation has *in vivo* significance in chronic lymphocytic leukemia and improves disease risk stratification. *Blood* 113, 5237–5245.
49. Baba, S., Hara, A., Kato, K., Long, N. K., Hatano, Y., Kimura, M., Okano, Y., Yamada, Y., and Shibata, T. (2009). Aberrant promoter hypermethylation of the CHFR gene in oral squamous cell carcinomas. *Oncol Rep* 22, 1173–1179.
50. Su, P. F., Huang, W. L., Wu, H. T., Wu, C. H., Liu, T. Y., and Kao, S. Y. (2010). p16(INK4A) promoter hypermethylation is associated with invasiveness and prognosis of oral squamous cell carcinoma in an age-dependent manner. *Oral Oncol* 46, 734–739.
51. Asadollahi, R., Hyde, C.A., and Zhong, X. Y. (2010). Epigenetics of ovarian cancer: from the lab to the clinic. *Gynecol Oncol* 118, 81–87.
52. Corn, P. (2008). Genome-wide profiling of methylated promoters in pancreatic adenocarcinoma: defining the pancreatic cancer epigenome. *Cancer Biol Ther.* 7, 1157–1159.
53. Chung, W., Kwabi-Addo, B., Ittmann, M., Jelinek, J., Shen, L., Yu, Y., and Issa, J. P. (2008). Identification of novel tumor markers in prostate, colon and breast cancer by unbiased methylation profiling. *PLoS ONE* 3, e2079.
54. Rogers, C. G., Yan, G., Zha, S., Gonzalgo, M. L., Isaacs, W. B., Luo, J., De Marzo, A. M., Nelson, W. G., and Pavlovich, C. P. (2004). Prostate cancer detection on urinalysis for α methylacyl coenzyme a racemase protein. *J Urol* 172, 1501–1503.
55. Xu, L., Czito, B. G., and Willett, C. G. (2010). Epigenetic markers in rectal cancer. *Clin Cancer Res* 16, 2699–2701.
56. Li, Y., Sawalha, A. H., and Lu, Q. (2009). Aberrant DNA methylation in skin diseases. *J Dermatol Sci* 54, 143–149.
57. Smith, J.A., Fan, C.Y., Zou, C., Bodenner, D., and Kokoska, M. S. (2007). Methylation status of genes in papillary thyroid carcinoma. *Arch Otolaryngol Head Neck Surg* 133, 1006–1011.
58. Provenzano, M. J, Fitzgerald, M. P., Krager, K., and Domann, F. E. (2007). Increased iodine uptake in thyroid carcinoma after treatment with sodium butyrate and decitabine (5-Aza-dC). *Otolaryngol Head Neck Surg* 137, 722–728.
59. Lu, D., Hoory, T., Monie, A., Wu, A., Wang, M. C., and Hung, C. F. (2009). Treatment with demethylating agent, 5-aza-2′-deoxycytidine enhances therapeutic HPV DNA vaccine potency. *Vaccine* 27, 4363–4369.
60. Kague, E., Thomazini, C. M., Pardini, M. I., de Carvalho, F., Leite, C. V., and Pinheiro, N. A. (2010). Methylation status of CDH1 gene in samples of gastric mucous from Brazilian patients with chronic gastritis infected by *Helicobacter pylori*. *Arq Gastroenterol* 47, 7–12.
61. Alves, M. K., Lima, V. P., Ferrasi, A. C., Rodrigues, M. A., De Moura Campos Pardini, M.I., and Rabenhorst, S. H. (2010). CDKN2A promoter methylation is related to the tumor location and histological subtype and associated with *Helicobacter pylori* flaA(+) strains in gastric adenocarcinomas. *APMIS* 118, 297–307.
62. Katayama, Y., Takahashi, M., and Kuwayama, H. (2009). *Helicobacter pylori* causes runx3 gene methylation and its loss of expression in

gastric epithelial cells, which is mediated by nitric oxide produced by macrophages. *Biochem Biophys Res Commun* 388, 496–500.

63. Byun, H. M, Siegmund, K. D., Pan, F., Weisenberger, D. J., Kanel, G., Laird, P. W., and Yang, A. S. (2009). Epigenetic profiling of somatic tissues from human autopsy specimens identifies tissue- and individual-specific DNA methylation patterns. *Hum Mol Genet* 18, 4808–4817.
64. Hoque, M. O., Begum, S., Topaloglu, O., Jeronimo, C., Mambo, E., Westra, W. H., Califano, J. A., and Sidransky, D. (2004). Quantitative detection of promoter hypermethylation of multiple genes in the tumor, urine, and serum DNA of patients with renal cancer. *Cancer Res* 64, 5511–5517.
65. Marks, P. A. (2010). The clinical development of histone deacetylase inhibitors as targeted anticancer drugs. *Expert Opin Investig Drugs* 19, 1049–1066.
66. Cang, S., Lu, Q., Ma, Y., and Liu, D. (2010). Clinical advances in hypomethylating agents targeting epigenetic pathways. *Curr Cancer Drug Targets* 10, 539–545.
67. Ganesan, A., Nolan, L., Crabb, S. J., and Packham, G. (2009). Epigenetic therapy: histone acetylation, DNA methylation and anti-cancer drug discovery. *Curr Cancer Drug Targets* 9, 963–981.
68. Marks, P. A. and Xu, W. S. (2009). Histone deacetylase inhibitors: potential in cancer therapy. *J Cell Biochem* 107, 600–608.
69. Shanker, S. and Srivastava, R.K. (2008). Histone deacetylase inhibitors: mechanisms and clinical significance in cancer: HDAC inhibitor-induced apoptosis. *Adv Exp Med Biol* 615, 261–298.
70. Aparicio, A., North, B., Barske, L., Wang, X., Bollati, V., Weisenberger, D., Yoo, C., Tannir, N., Horne, E., Groshen, S., Jones, P., Yang, A., and Issa, J. P. (2009). LINE-1 methylation in plasma DNA as a biomarker of activity of DNA methylation inhibitors in patients with solid tumors. *Epigenetics* 4, 176–184.
71. Issa, J. P. and Kantarjian, H. M. (2009). Targeting DNA methylation. *Clin Cancer Res* 15, 3938–3946.
72. Ree, A. H., Dueland, S., Folkvord, S., Hole, K. H., Seierstad, T., Johansen, M., Abrahamsen, T. W., and Flatmark, K. (2010). Vorinostat, a histone deacetylase inhibitor, combined with pelvic palliative radiotherapy for gastrointestinal carcinoma: the Pelvic Radiation and Vorinostat (PRAVO) phase 1 study. *Lancet Oncol* 11,459–464.
73. Siegel, D., Hussein, M., Belani, C., Robert, F., Galanis, E., Richon, V. M., Garcia-Vargas, J., Sanz-Rodriguez, C., and Rizvi, S. (2009). Vorinostat in solid and hematologic malignancies. *J Hematol Oncol* 2, 31.
74. Facchetti, F., Previdi, S., Ballarini, M., Minucci, S., Perego, P., and La Porta, C. A. (2004). Modulation of pro- and anti-apoptotic factors in human melanoma cells exposed to histone deacetylase inhibitors. *Apoptosis* 9, 573–582.
75. Fandy, T. E. and Srivastava, R. K. (2006). Trichostatin A sensitizes TRAIL-resistant myeloma cells by downregulation of the anti-apoptotic Bcl-2 proteins. *Cancer Chemother Pharmacol* 58, 471–477.
76. Goldsmith, K. C. and Hogarty, M. D. (2005). Targeting programmed cell death pathways with experimental therapeutics: opportunities in high-risk neuroblastoma. *Cancer Lett* 228, 133–141.
77. Camphausen, K., Burgan, W., Cerra, M., Oswald, K. A., Trepel, J. B., Lee, M. J., and Tofilon, P. J. (2004). Enhanced radiation-induced cell killing and prolongation of gammaH2AX foci expression by the histone deacetylase inhibitor MS-275. *Cancer Res* 64, 316–321.
78. Nome, R. V., Bratland, A., Harman, G., Fodstad, O., Andersson, Y., and Ree, A. H. (2005). Cell cycle checkpoint signaling involved in histone deacetylase inhibition and radiation-induced cell death. *Mol Cancer Ther* 4, 1231–1238.
79. Kim, S. H., Ahn, S., Han, J. W., Lee, H. W., Lee, H. Y., Lee, Y. W., Kim, M. R., Kim, K. W., Kim, W. B., and Hong, S. (2004). Apicidin is a histone deacetylase inhibitor with anti-invasive and anti-angiogenic potentials. *Biochem Biophys Res Commun* 315, 964–970.
80. Paroni, G., Mizzau, M., Henderson, C., Del Sal, G., Schneider, C., and Brancolini, C. (2004). Caspase-dependent regulation of histone deacetylase 4 nuclear-cytoplasmic shuttling promotes apoptosis. *Mol Biol Cell* 15, 2804–2818.
81. Luszczek, W., Cheriyath, V., Mekhail, T. M., and Borden, E. C. (2010). Combinations of DNA methyltransferase and histone deacetylase inhibitors induce DNA damage in small cell lung cancer cells: correlation of resistance with IFN-stimulated gene expression. *Mol Cancer Ther* 9, 2309–2321.

ERRATUM

Screening for miRNA Expression Changes Using Quantitative PCR (Q-PCR)

Richard N. Armstrong, Hilary A.A. Colyer, and Ken I. Mills

Ramona G. Dumitrescu and Mukesh Verma (eds.), *Cancer Epigenetics: Methods and Protocols*, Methods in Molecular Biology, vol. 863, DOI 10.1007/978-1-61779-612-8, © Springer Science+Business Media, LLC 2012

DOI 10.1007/978-1-61779-612-8_29

The publisher regrets that Item 4 on page 298 does not include the 16C step in the cycling conditions but as a stage before the cycling. The text should read as follows: ...40 cycles of: 16C for 2 mins, 42C for 1 min, 50C for 1 sec.

The online version of the original chapter can be found at
http://dx.doi.org/10.1007/978-1-61779-612-8_18

Index

A

B

Ramona G. Dumitrescu and Mukesh Verma (eds.), *Cancer Epigenetics: Methods and Protocols*, Methods in Molecular Biology, vol. 863, DOI 10.1007/978-1-61779-612-8, © Springer Science+Business Media, LLC 2012

C

D

E

F

I

N

O

P

Q

R

U

V

W

X

Z

MIX
Papier aus verantwortungsvollen Quellen
Paper from responsible sources
FSC® C105338

If you have any concerns about our products,
you can contact us on
ProductSafety@springernature.com

In case Publisher is established outside the EU,
the EU authorized representative is:
Springer Nature Customer Service Center GmbH
Europaplatz 3, 69115 Heidelberg, Germany

Printed by Libri Plureos GmbH
in Hamburg, Germany